DATE DUE

The Sinuses

The Sinuses

Paul J. Donald, M.D., F.R.C.S.(C)
Professor
Department of Otolaryngology–Head and Neck
Surgery
University of California, Davis Medical Center
Director, Center for Skull Base Surgery
University of California, Davis
Sacramento, California

Jack L. Gluckman, Ch.B., F.C.S. (S.A.), F.A.C.S.
Professor and Chairman
Department of Otolaryngology–Head and Neck
Surgery
University of Cincinnati Medical Center
Cincinnati, Ohio

Dale H. Rice, M.D.
Tiber/Alpert Professor and Chair
Department of Otolaryngology–Head and Neck
Surgery
University of Southern California Medical School
Los Angeles, California

Raven Press New York

Raven Press, Ltd., 1185 Avenue of the Americas, New York, New York 10036

Made in the United States of America

Library of Congress Cataloging-in-Publication Data

The Sinuses / editors, Paul J. Donald, Jack L. Gluckman, Dale H. Rice.
    p. cm.
    Includes bibliographical references and index.
    ISBN 0-7817-0041-8
    1. Paranasal sinuses—Diseases. I. Donald, Paul J.
II. Gluckman, J. L. (Jack L.) III. Rice, Dale H.
    [DNLM: 1. Paranasal Sinus Diseases. 2. Nose—physiopathology.
WV 340 S6179 1994]
RF421.S56 1994
617.2'23—dc20
DNLM/DLC
for Library of Congress   94-13768
                                 CIP

9 8 7 6 5 4 3 2 1

Dedication

I would like to thank my beloved and loving wife, Roz, the most important person in my life who was closely involved in the process of producing this book. She lovingly sustained and gently encouraged me throughout the entire writing, sacrificing time together during the many hours when I was required to write in isolation. She was completely supportive and unfailingly patient during the entire time this book was being produced.

P.J.D.

To Pam, Kate, Nick, Simon, and Jonathan. Thank you for your understanding and tolerance. To all the residents and fellows for constantly pushing me for answers.

J.L.G.

This effort is dedicated to the members of the Department of Otolaryngology–Head and Neck Surgery at the University of Southern California who have been highly supportive and helpful over the years.

D.H.R.

Contents

vii

III. Trauma

IV. Neoplastic Disease

V. Related Conditions and Procedures

Contributing Authors

John Beumer, D.D.S., M.S. *Department of Removable Prosthodontics, University of California Los Angeles School of Dentistry, 10833 Le Conte Avenue, Los Angeles, California 90024*

Wellington G. Borges, M.D. *Division of Immunology, Harbor-University of California Los Angeles Medical Center, 1000 West Carson Street, Torrance, California 90509; and Clinica Materno-Infantil de Brasilia, 70.000 Brazil*

Paul J. Donald, M.D., F.R.C.S.(C) *Department of Otolaryngology–Head and Neck Surgery, University of California, Davis Medical Center for Skull Base Surgery, University of California, Davis, 2500 Stockton Boulevard, Sacramento, California 95817*

Egbert J. de Vries, M.D. *Department of Otolaryngology–Head and Neck Surgery, University of Cincinnati Medical Center, 231 Bethesda Avenue, Cincinnati, Ohio 45267*

James E. Freije, M.D. *Department of Otolaryngology–Head and Neck Surgery, University of Cincinnati Medical Center, 231 Bethesda Avenue, Cincinnati, Ohio 45267*

Jack L. Gluckman, Ch.B., F.C.S. (S.A.), F.A.C.S. *Department of Otolaryngology–Head and Neck Surgery, University of Cincinnati Medical Center, 231 Bethesda Avenue, Cincinnati, Ohio 45267*

Regina Gandour-Edwards, M.D. *Department of Pathology, University of California, Davis, 2315 Stockton Boulevard, Sacramento, California 95817*

Douglas C. Heiner, M.D., Ph.D. *Department of Pediatrics, Division of Immunology and Allergy, Harbor-University of California Los Angeles Medical Center, 1000 West Carson Street, Torrance, California 90959*

Robert C. Kersten, M.D., F.A.C.S. *University of Cincinnati Medical Center, Barrett Center, 231 Bethesda Avenue, Cincinnati, Ohio 45267*

Dwight R. Kulwin, M.D., F.A.C.S. *Department of Ophthalmology, University of Cincinnati Medical Center, Barrett Center, 231 Bethesda Avenue, Cincinnati, Ohio 45267*

Michael J. Murphy, M.D. *Department of Otolaryngology, University of Washington, 209 South 12th Avenue, Seattle, Washington 98905*

Russell Nishimura, D.D.S. *Department of Removable Prosthodontics, University of California Los Angeles School of Dentistry, 10833 Le Conte Avenue, Los Angeles, California 90024*

Bruce W. Pearson, M.D. *Department of Otolaryngology–Head and Neck Surgery, Mayo Clinic, 4500 San Pablo Road, Jacksonville, Florida 32225*

Dale H. Rice, M.D. *Department of Otolaryngology–Head and Neck Surgery, University of Southern California School of Medicine, 1200 North State Street, Box 795, Los Angeles, California 90033*

Paul D. Righi, M.D. *Department of Otolaryngology–Head and Neck Surgery, University of Cincinnati Medical Center, 231 Bethesda Avenue, Cincinnati, Ohio 45267*

Eleni Roumanas, D.D.S. *Department of Removable Prosthodontics, University of California Los Angeles School of Dentistry, 10833 Le Conte Avenue, Los Angeles, California 90024*

Richard J. Trevino, M.D. *Department of Ears, Nose, and Throat, Louisiana State University-Shreveport, Louisiana State University Medical Center, 1541 Kings Highway, Shreveport, Louisiana 71103*

Jeremy Woodham, M.B., Ch.B., F.R.C.S.(C) *Department of Otolaryngology, University of British Columbia, St. Paul's Hospital, 1081 Burrard Street, Vancouver, British Columbia V6Z 1Y6, Canada*

Preface

For decades following the advent of antibiotics in the early 1940s, the management of sinus inflammation and its sequelae, once one of the keystones of otolaryngologic practice, drifted into relative obscurity. With the exception of cursory chapters on sinus disease, the book of Van Alyea remained as a single definitive source of information on the anatomy, pathology, and surgery of the paranasal sinuses. Interest in the sinuses has been rekindled recently by a number of advances in the understanding of pathophysiology, diagnosis, and therapy of paranasal sinus disease. The development of endoscopic sinus surgery has been one of the most significant stimuli to the rebirth of focus on sinus disease. This modality, developed in the light of the discoveries of Messerklinger and others, radically revised our understanding of the pathophysiology of inflammatory disease of the nose and sinuses. The revolution in radiology with the development of computed tomography and magnetic resonance imaging has remarkably expanded our ability to diagnose sinus disease. The innovation of skull base surgery has produced the ability to resect neoplasms successfully that were previously considered to be inoperable and incurable. Improved diagnostic and therapeutic techniques have greatly enhanced the diagnosis and therapy of allergic disease.

This book reviews the past and current ideas on the management of all disease processes afflicting the paranasal sinuses. The goal is to provide a solid body of knowledge in anatomy, physiology, microbiology, immunology, and pathology on which to base reasonable and logical principles of therapy.

Over the years, numerous ideas and procedures have evolved, unfortunately not altogether based on hard, scientifically derived data. At present, controversy still exists in the arenas of management of inhalant and especially food allergy, the role of septal deviation in the genesis of sinus infection, the significance of septal turbinate abutment as a cause of facial pain, and the most efficacious management of inflammatory disease of the frontal sinuses, to name a few. Some resolution of these issues may be elucidated in the pages to follow—or at least some sound basis for future solution of these conflicts will be provided. We have attempted to make this volume the definitive source of solid information on sinus disease for our fellow practitioners of otolaryngology/head and neck surgery.

Paul J. Donald

xiii

Acknowledgments

As senior editor, I would like to thank those individuals who by their hard work, dedication, and persistence made this work possible. Nelva Richardson was the medical artist responsible for the superlative illustrations in this text. Her rapid grasp of the ideas we wished to portray and her willingness to make changes, especially when the authors made a rather obvious and time-consuming mistake, is greatly appreciated by everyone. My secretary, Amy Petrotta, who regularly produced beautifully edited and accurately typed manuscripts in an unbelievably prompt fashion deserves the highest praise. Kathey Alexander, our editor at Raven Press, did an outstanding job of coordinating all our efforts, patiently nurturing us through the process but firmly keeping us on track, and maintaining her ''cool'' through the passage of numerous production deadlines until we finally completed the work. I hope my fellow authors and contributors are as pleased as I am with the final product.

Paul J. Donald

I would like to acknowledge my co-authors, Paul Donald and Dale Rice for their energy and enthusiasm for the project; Amy Teall, for routinely producing my multiple revisions as if by magic; Nelva Richardson, for the wonderful art work; and finally, Kathey Alexander, who single-handedly kept the project moving when all appeared lost.

Jack L. Gluckman

A project like this does not happen by accident nor in isolation. Much of the credit for this book goes to the Herculean efforts of Paul Donald without whom this book would have been stillborn. Credit must also be given to my mentors at the University of Michigan—Walter P. Work, Roger Boles, Frank Ritter, and Nels Olson,—who taught me much. Since, I have learned an equal amount from my patients.

Dale H. Rice

PART I

Basic Science

CHAPTER 1

History of the Development of Surgery for Sinusitis

Jeremy Woodham

The history of the development in the 20th century of surgery for acute and chronic sinusitis is of great interest at a time that is witnessing the advent of conservative endoscopic sinus surgery (CESS). Many rhinologists during the past 100 years understood the benefits of conservative surgery based on their understanding of the reversibility of sinus mucosal disease. Their efforts in individualizing surgery to the affected sinus cells were hampered by inadequate illumination and also by the ongoing debate between the radical and conservative schools. Rhinologic surgery parallels the development of surgery in the disciplines of otology and laryngology. The common thread was the initial development of radical surgery to excise all "disease" and treat the complications of infection. This often saved lives but at the expense of conservation of function. Over the last 100 years progress toward conservative sinus surgery has been slow and in most centers in the world today such surgery is not yet established practice. Developments occurred simultaneously in Europe, Asia, and North America and the descriptions of earlier surgical procedures are ascribed to many individuals in a variety of languages. This chapter does not attempt to provide the reader with either a chronology of the development of sinus surgery or a listing of the contributions of all rhinologists worldwide over the past 100 years. I apologize in advance for any omissions in this regard. I have attempted to provide the interested endoscopic sinus surgeon with some historical perspectives that will allow him/her to understand better the developing concepts of CESS in 1993.

UNDERSTANDING THE APPLIED ANATOMY OF THE LATERAL NASAL WALL AND PARANASAL SINUSES

It appears that the maxillary sinus was described in the early 17th century by Casserius and later by High-more, who in 1651 described a case of suppurative disease of the maxillary sinus (1). Between 1912 and 1923 great anatomical research was undertaken by Parsons Schaeffer to produce a superbly detailed atlas entitled *The Nose, Paranasal Sinuses, Naso-lachrymal Passageways, and the Olfactory Organ in Man* (2). While Schaeffer remained a pure anatomist, Harris Mosher was more interested in the application of anatomical findings to the development of radical surgery. Mosher, between 1912 and 1929, presented several classical papers on the surgical anatomy of the ethmoid sinuses. He was a descriptive surgical anatomist and was a teacher in the old style. Postgraduate students would attend his lectures and seminars with some trepidation. They were required to dissect and draw the half-head preparations, and then to undergo a full examination of their knowledge, prior to embarking on an ethmoidectomy. At the Annual Meeting of the American Laryngological Association in 1912, Dr. Otto Freer congratulated Dr. Mosher on his original research, which, he said, would mark a great anatomical and surgical advance. He was referring to Dr. Mosher's technique for the intranasal entry into the frontal sinus. The important discovery was the position of the agger nasi cells lying under the anterior attachment of the first part of the middle turbinate where it bridges across the unciform groove (3,4). This discovery completely changed Dr. Mosher's operative approach to the frontal sinus via the intranasal route and marked a reawakening of the applied anatomy of the region.

In 1929, Mosher presented a paper, "The Surgical Anatomy of the Ethmoid Labyrinth," to a symposium dedicated to the ethmoid sinuses, presented at the American Academy of Ophthalmology and Otolaryngology (5). This essay concisely described the surgical anatomy of the ethmoid labyrinth and was based on

Mosher's own work. It described the applied anatomy and gave clear advice for the safe performance of intranasal ethmoidectomy, which remains valid today. This operation still represents one of the most dangerous in modern surgery for the following reasons: the field is variable and usually narrow; instrumentation is through one porthole; the mucosa is frequently infected and bleeds; it is not possible to place a tourniquet around the feeding arteries (cf. arthroscopy); dehiscences may be present in the walls of the labyrinth; the anatomy is frequently altered by scarring from previous resections; and the eye, optic nerve, internal carotid artery, and brain are intimately related to the surgical field. In referring to the ethmoid labyrinth in 1929 Mosher stated: "If it were placed in any other part of the body it would be an insignificant and harmless collection of bony cells. In the place where nature has put it, it has major relationships so that diseases and surgery of the labyrinth often lead to tragedy. Any surgery in this region should be simple but it has proven to be one of the easiest ways to kill a patient!"

The anatomy of the region has been forgotten or perhaps was never adequately learned by many of today's otolaryngologists. With the advent of endoscopic surgery and its advantages including better visualization and therefore a more accurate dissection, the need for a better understanding of the anatomy of the ethmoid labyrinth is obvious.

Since the introduction of CESS in North America in the mid-1980s, there has been a new emphasis on relearning the complicated anatomy of the ethmoid labyrinth. Fresh cadavers are ideal for microdissection but are not always available. Embalmed cadavers have stiff tissues that make it difficult to "get the true feel" of microdissection using heavier traditional ethmoidectomy instruments. However, cadaveric dissection does offer the opportunity for elective exploration of the anatomy beyond the labyrinth into the optic nerve, internal carotid artery, and brain via the skull base. The preparation of skull dissections using the microdrill helps one to understand the detailed osteology without the presence of soft tissue to interfere with essential landmarks (6). There are many fine monographs and books written on the anatomy of the sinuses in the English language; a few of the notable authors are Parsons Schaeffer (1915–1925), Harris Mosher (1912–1930), Van Alyea (1938–1950), Frank Ritter (1978), and Johannes Lang (1990) (2,4–9).

REPLACEMENT OF RADICAL SINUS SURGERY BY CONSERVATIVE SINUS SURGERY

Radical Antrectomy (Caldwell–Luc)

The early approaches into the maxillary sinus were through a large oral antral fistula created in the anterior face of the antrum. Kuster (1889), quoted by Williams in 1935, outlined the prerequisites for maxillary sinus surgery, namely, good visualization of the interior of the sinus, the total removal of disease, and the establishment of adequate drainage (10). The large patent fistula into the oral cavity led to sinus contamination with oral flora and persistant postsurgical drainage. Christopher Heath (1889) of London later produced a small trephination through the canine fossa and William Robertson (1892) of Newcastle upon Tyne, England, removed disease from the maxillary sinus through a similar approach. Nobody made an opening into the nose. In 1893 George Caldwell, an instructor in the Department of Ophthalmology at the New York Polytechnic, described an operation on the maxillary sinus through the canine fossa with the removal of diseased mucosa and sparing of healthy mucosa, and the construction of a drainage window into the inferior meatus. This opening was used for postoperative sinus irrigation. The original description of Caldwell's operation, however, contains other significant statements. He refers to the semilunar hiatus and the relative positions of the ostia of the frontal, ethmoid, and maxillary sinuses. He was aware from cadaveric dissections that the hiatus acted as an imperfect valve, guiding fluid from the higher cells into the lower antrum. For this reason, he states that "the diagnosis of empyema of the antrum is not sufficient until the frontal and anterior ethmoid cells have been excluded. The antrum may be the receptacle not the origin of pus or become involved secondarily." Also, "the frontal sinus may be freely opened by enlarging the infundibulum through the nose with a curette and the sinus irrigated and medicated by means of a soft silver catheter. When the ethmoid cells are affected as well, I prefer to open and resect with a clipper and curette as a preliminary operation." He accurately described the role of the ethmoid sinuses as the central focus of chronic sinusitis (11). In 1893, Henri Luc of Paris reported an operation identical to both Caldwell's and Spicer's (1894) of London, but he advocated the total removal of the maxillary sinus mucosa (12).

Lothrop, an assistant in anatomy in Boston, discussed a new operation for empyema of the antrum in 1897. He studied the anatomy of the maxillary sinus and considered the position of the natural ostium and the difference in heights between the nasal floor and the floor of the antrum. He recognized that antral empyema was often rhinogenic or dental in origin, resulting from the gravitational drainage of fluids from the frontal and ethmoid sinuses (13). None of the earlier recommendations for the complete removal of the ethmoid sinuses in such cases were followed. The common causes of antral empyema at this time were syphilis, foreign bodies, malignant disease, tuberculosis, polypi, dental caries, and cysts (11,13).

Goodyear in 1934 reported on the presence of fibrosis and cystic change within the maxillary sinus following the removal of its lining during the Caldwell–Luc operation (14). Sewall in 1926 and Tilley in 1943 commented on the difficulty experienced during revisional surgery when the radical removal of sinus lining had previously taken place (15,16). Articles again discussed the complications following the Caldwell–Luc procedure. Bell and Stone (1976), Murray (1983), and Sogg (1982) emphasize conservatism with respect to lining excision and discuss the complications of superior alveolar nerve damage with resultant lip and gum anesthesia (17–19). This complication varies in different series and one wonders if it is a result of excessive upper lip reaction causing damage to the infraorbital nerve. Other complications of the Caldwell–Luc procedure were cited by Legler in 1980. These were the development of scar tissue and webs in an incompletely denuded cavity, leading to small contracted ill-draining cavities containing microcysts and pyoceles. These were the same complications reported by Goodyear nearly 50 years earlier.

On the other hand, there were those who claimed that the operation was not always performed properly. The proponents of "modern radical surgery" supported their views with well-documented success. Macbeth (1968) stated that one of the biggest fallacies in rhinology was the intranasal antrostomy. He stated that "the window is made at the level of the floor of the sinus and all that is achieved is the production of a window through which repeated washouts can be made. This impairs ciliary mobility and allows entry of secondary infection." He claimed that the most important reason for failure of the Caldwell–Luc procedure was that irreversibly diseased mucosa had been left behind. He stated that adequate conservative measures prior to surgery were necessary. These included antibiotic and antihistamine treatments, nasal soaks, suction displacement, and repeated direct lavage in an attempt to reverse the sinus lining. If the lining continued to show thickening on radiographs then the correct operation was the Caldwell–Luc procedure. Local anesthesia using Mosher's mud was used. This is a paste containing 25% crystalline cocaine hydrochloride and desiccated suprarenal gland. An oblong hole was made in the anterior wall of the sinus with a dental cutting burr and enlarged in all directions, care being taken not to bruise the infraorbital nerve. Extended too far laterally there may be damage to the anterolateral terminal branch of the sphenopalatine artery. The sinus lining was removed with particular attention to the floor, the inferolateral angle, and the roof. A nasoantral window was constructed to promote outflow of blood into the nose in the postoperative period. Sulfathiazole and penicillin powder were placed in the cavity. The incision was not sewn up as this led to facial swelling.

If the ethmoids were involved, a transantral ethmoidectomy was performed. Postoperatively the patient received sulfur medications and vasoconstricting nasal drops and steam. Mouthwashes after meals were instituted and the patient was told not to blow his/her nose. The antrum was not washed out postoperatively and there were few complications. Macbeth reported on 1259 Caldwell–Luc operations performed in Oxford between 1952 and 1966. He himself performed 700 operations and noticed a decrease in the incidence of sinusitis. This was related to improved nutritional standards in the population. He analyzed the results of 360 procedures in a 5-year period and found a satisfactory success rate of 88% based on objective appraisals by the patients, but the follow-up period was short. The results of the Caldwell–Luc operations were not as good when complicated by ethmopolyposis. Bronchiectasis and persistent ethmoid disease were the commonest causes of failure. Macbeth could find no physiological reason for the intranasal antrostomy or nasal antral window procedure (20).

Intranasal Antrostomy

The earliest recorded intranasal procedures were on the antrum and appeared to focus on the need for a window into the sinus either through the middle or inferior meatus. Each approach had its followers with Zuckerkandl (1882), Schaeffer, Claoue (1886), Siebenmann, and Killian (1900) leading the middle meatal approach. This approach lost favor following orbital complications mainly due to poor illumination, poor visualization, and the radical concepts of the day. Mikulicz (1886), Lothrop (1897), Dahmer (1909), Onodi (1902), and McBride (1900) favored the safer inferior approach. Partial turbinectomies were added for the creation of larger windows to allow better drainage of pus and for easier sinus irrigation by either surgeon or patient. Lothrop recognized the tendency for early closure of the inferior meatal window as early as 1897. Freer (1905) found that the two procedures for the treatment of chronic maxillary sinusitis, namely, alveolar drainage into the mouth and the Caldwell–Luc operation, were too radical. He described an intranasal operation that involved a resection of the anterior two-thirds of the inferior turbinate and the anterior two-thirds of the inner wall of the maxillary sinus. This was one of the earliest antrostomy procedures in North America and the size of Freer's opening from the maxillary sinus into the nose would be acceptable to the proponents of large antrostomy today (21)! Freer believed in conservatism and understood the need for sinus ventilation. Hempstead in 1939 reported 1634 cases of nasal antrostomy and noted the return to normal of the maxillary sinus mucosa following this procedure. He correctly believed that the window had to be made sufficiently large in order to remain patent. He subluxed the anterior border of the inferior turbinate superiorly (22). Hilding (1931) demonstrated that carbon particles would bypass an inferior meatal window and be actively transported to the natural ostium of the maxillary sinus (23). This process of active mucociliary transport was later photographed by Messerklinger and Stammberger (1967) (24). Double antrostomies were described by McKenzie (1927), and Sluder (1927) performed a subtotal medial maxillectomy. King (1935) showed evidence of reversal of hyperplastic antral mucosa after an antrostomy.

Buiter (1988), after the introduction of endoscopic sinus surgery in Europe, reviewed the results of a modified inferior meatal antrostomy in 378 sinuses and found a 92% success rate. These results were similar to Hempstead's 50 years earlier. Buiter created a window 2.5 cm by 1.25 cm and removed the mucosa. The base of the window was level with the floor of the nose and the sinus mucosa was preserved. This procedure was restricted to maxillary sinuses where they were singularly involved and no surgery on the osteomeatal complex was performed (25). Any minor inflammation in this region is regarded as secondary to the action of mucopurulent secretions from the involved maxillary sinus. The choice of maxillary sinus to be operated on was taken following endoscopy of the middle meatus and computed tomography (CT) scanning. The purpose of this approach is to preserve the normal functioning anterior ethmoid anatomy but at the same time to provide aeration to the maxillary sinus. In the presence of ethmoid disease endoscopic clearance is performed. Melen (1986) stated that nasal and sinus ventilation, whether achieved pharmacologically or by surgical intervention, is necessary for the successful treatment of chronic maxillary sinusitis (26). Lund (1987) performed a retrospective study of 108 patients who had undergone inferior meatal antrostomy (IMA) and performed a prospective study on the pre- and postsurgical size of the antrostomy in 65 patients. The effect of patency on the goblet cell population was examined in a prospective manner in another 19 patients. She states that after antral lavage, IMA is the commonest procedure performed on the maxillary sinus in Great Britain. The retrospective analysis of IMA patency showed that the greatest change occurred during the first postoperative year. She indicated that the minimum critical size for an IMA was 1 cm × 1 cm. This was difficult to achieve in children with preservation of the attachment of the inferior turbinate. The position of the inferior meatal artery was also a consideration. The IMA was of no value for the treatment of those patients who demonstrated hypertrophy and hyperplasia of the goblet cell and who consequently had persistent postnasal rhinorrhea (27,28).

Intranasal and External Radical Ethmoid/Frontal Sphenoidectomy

The early rhinologic surgeons were to some degree aware of the need for adequate sinus drainage and ventilation but they did not appreciate the need for retention of reversible hyperplastic mucosa. Most of the papers written until 1930 centered around the degree of turbinate excision, the extended procedures to incorporate the larger sinuses, and the best surgical approach. The concept of retaining mucosa was not understood and it was felt for many years that nasal mucosal flaps were adequate for relining the denuded sinuses. This thinking is still prevelent in many countries. In addition, it has been stated that the "modern" otolaryngologist has had inadequate training in ethmoidectomy and there may be more than a grain of truth to this statement. The developing endoscopic sinus surgeon will find it essential to understand the historical development of our current conservative philosophies.

Halle is credited with the early descriptions of radical intranasal ethmoidectomy and frontal and sphenoid sinusotomy. Mosher (1912) detailed the fine structure of the ethmoid labyrinth. He widely resected the middle turbinate and made the surgery more anatomic and safer. The resections he performed were still radical and he acquired many followers to his school of thought including Yankauer (1921) and Lederer (1953). Mosher initially was a radical surgeon of the old school. His techniques were based on his own anatomical studies and those of Parsons Schaeffer. The radical Mosher intranasal ethmoidectomy describes plunging into the agger nasi cells under the overhang of the middle turbinate. The ethmoid labyrinth was removed, starting anteriorly, by successive downward strokes of a curette carried along the orbital plate and fovea ethmoidalis. The middle turbinate was left intact as a landmark, until the sphenoid contents had been removed. The turbinates were then excised. Transantral ethmoidectomy was described when the antrum was diseased. This procedure gave inadequate visualization of the posterior lateral ethmoid cells and was not favored over the transnasal approach. In 1972, Eichel commented on Mosher's original ethmoidectomy and noted that in 1929 he had moved from the intranasal to external technique, which was then taken up by Ferris-Smith in 1934. During this time intranasal ethmoidectomy was banned in a number of centers owing to the seriousness of the complications.

External ethmoidectomy started at first as a radical and extended procedure and later became more conservative. The external radical ethmoid/frontal sphenoidectomy was first described by Jansen (1893) and then by Ritter (1906) (29,30). Lynch revived the operation in 1921 and Sewall made his contribution in 1926

(31). Sewall tied off the anterior and posterior ethmoid and the sphenopalatine arteries and later advocated the use of lateral nasal wall mucosal flaps to cover the exposed periorbita. Van Alyea (1941) commented on the periodic revival, every 15 to 20 years, of the Jansen–Ritter procedure. The radical operation was considered complete when the floor of the frontal sinus and the frontal sinus lining had been removed completely; the ethmoid cells all had been excised; the posterior wall of the frontal sinus, the fovea ethmoidales, and the roof of the sphenoid had been reduced to a continuous white bony plate; and the mucosa had been removed completely from the sphenoid sinus. The complications of the procedure were osteomyelitis, diplopia, blindness, meningitis, deformity, and anesthesia of the frontal region. Smith (1934) wrote in justification of this "complete" sinus operation for cases where advanced disease in the ethmoid labyrinth could not possibly be removed by an intranasal ethmoidectomy (32). Lynch (1926) wrote that the "modern or current external ethmoidectomy deserves less criticism as it is a less disfiguring procedure, depending upon how much bone is removed from the ascending process of the maxilla and frontal bone (33).

The incisions around the medial canthus of the eye all cause some degree of cosmetic disfigurement unless the incision is zigzagged or placed in an infraorbital skin crease. The approach to the anterior ethmoids through the lacrimal fossa or through the lamina papyracea has been described. The extent of the removal of the lamina papyracea has varied from just the lacrimal fossa (30%) back to the posterior ethmoid artery (100%). Despite the temporary diplopia often resulting from the disturbance of the local anatomy (globe, trochlea, medial and inferior rectus muscles), the operation offers the safest approach to the ethmoid sinuses. There is good visualization of the orbital contents, the lamina papyracea, the fovea ethmoidalis, and natural dehiscences in these structures can be identified. This approach has fluctuated in its popularity during this century but is generally considered to be the safest (with reference to the eye and brain) for the removal of advanced chronic hyperplastic polypoid sinusitis when previous multiple polypectomies and intranasal ethmoidectomies have been performed. It is probably the most successful approach in accessing all the ethmoid sinuses. There were numerous modifications of the external ethmoidectomy procedure. Extended incisions along the floor of the frontal sinus allowed removal of the floor, anterior wall, and brow for disease in this region (34).

Current External Approaches to the Ethmoid Labyrinth

The osteoplastic flap, still popular in Eastern North America, was designed totally to expose the frontal

sinuses and nasofrontal ducts. The underlying principle was the total removal of all the sinus mucosa, closure of the ducts, and encouragement of fibrous obliteration of the sinus by the placement of a free graft (35,36). In order to remove disease from the ethmoids, this procedure had to be combined with an external ethmoidectomy. Success rates are high and complications are few.

In Western North America the Boyden–Sewell frontoethmoidectomy is also popular. This is an external ethmoidectomy with enlargement of the nasofrontal duct and elimination of disease from both ends of the duct. An attempt is made to reline the duct with a septal or lateral nasal wall mucosal flap to prevent stenosis (37).

Both of these procedures are radical in terms of their alteration of the normal anatomy. Disease has to be removed from the ethmoid labyrinth in order to prevent failure. Radical frontal sinus surgery has continued to be practised. Unfortunately, the nasofrontal duct anatomy is altered, the duct's mucosa is removed with the Boyden–Sewell frontoethmoidectomy, and this results in postoperative duct stenosis and frontal recess scarring. It can take many years for complications to occur. These are recurrent attacks of acute/chronic frontal sinusitis and pyomucocele formation.

The current proponents of radical intranasal ethmoidectomy for advanced hyperplastic polypoid pansinusitis are often very experienced surgeons working in teaching institutions (38,39). They are involved in teaching programs and are performing an adequate number of the procedures to maintain their surgical skills and awareness of the anatomical peculiarities of this region. Those general otorhinolaryngologists performing only a few procedures a year should not expect to achieve the same success. Freidman and Kern (1979) reviewed 1000 consecutive intranasal ethmoidectomies and had a complication rate of 2.8% and no fatalities (40). Maniglia et al. (1981) reported on serious complications of ethmoidectomy with three cases of blindness and two cases of loss of ocular mobility. Intracranial complications occurred in the other eight. They pointed out that good visualization during surgery is of the utmost importance; a nasal septal reconstruction is often needed, and the ethmoidectomy is more complicated in patients who have had previous surgery, and especially in those where the middle turbinate had been removed (41). Eichel (1982) reported on a 12-year study and he had an 83% success rate in controlling nasal polyposis and a 92% revisional success rate. He concluded that intranasal ethmoidectomy may be the most important factor in controlling nasal polyposis and that the majority of patients gained long-standing remission from the disease (42). In a further review of revisional ethmoidectomy in 1985, Eichel described his technique, which was similar to Mosher's for the removal of disease, and commented on the ongoing argument as to whether the middle turbinate should be preserved or sacrificed. He reported a group of patients with a recalcitrant polyposis where the nasal mucosa appeared wet even after surgery (43). In 1982 Friedman et al. (44) proposed sphenoethmoidectomy for treating both asthmatic and nonasthmatic patients with chronic hyperplastic pansinusitis. In a further review (1986), Friedman (45) made a case for complete ethmoidal marsupialization, quoting a 1% complication rate and a 15% polyp recurrence rate. Stevens and Blair (1988) reviewed their 10-year experience of intranasal sphenoethmoidectomy. Over a 10-year period, 187 patients had 230 procedures. Sixty percent of the group had between 1 and 15 previous polypectomies. A complete sphenoethmoidectomy was performed with preservation of the base of the middle turbinate. A 3% complication rate was reported without any cases of death or blindness (46).

Development of Conservative Sinus Surgical Techniques

In 1951 Van Alyea said that the "successful therapeutic measures are those which spring from a sound knowledge of the anatomy, the physiology and the histopathology of the structures treated. The early rhinologists were not concerned about the preservation of functioning structures. In 1884 with the discovery of cocaine they began to completely disrupt nature's defense mechanisms and surgical techniques at the turn of last century were designed solely for the purpose of increasing the ease of dismantling the sinonasal complex. Anything that could be cut out, was, and for the next 40 years there was no satisfactory explanation for the failure of their methods."

Proetz developed the technique of displacement of thickened mucus from the sphenoid and posterior ethmoid sinuses and can be credited with the "rediscovery" of the cilia (47). As the pathophysiology of the nose was elucidated, rhinologists moved toward the conservative treatment of sinus disease. Jervey in 1939 makes reference to a variety of therapeutic measures. He discusses the role of suction and the local application of heat, the role of the infrared lamp and thermotherapy, the role of short-wave diathermy, and the importance of a good diet and a healthy climate. By this time sulfanilamide therapy was recommended for streptococcal infection and staphylococcus toxoid was used in selected cases (48). Childrey and Turnbull in 1939 instilled sulfanilamide in the maxillary antrum, which represents the first attempt at local antibiotic therapy in the sinuses (49,50). X-ray treatment for sinusitis was falling into disfavor. The radical sinus surgeons were still modifying their surgical experiments

to improve their results, the reporting of which was lacking in the literature of the day. "Some men make the same mistake for 50 years and they call that experience," stated Dr. Jacobi, quoted by Jervey, in 1929. Goodyear was questioning the reason for the total removal of the maxillary sinus lining in the Caldwell–Luc procedure. He felt that it was unreasonable to replace a diseased membrane by one composed of scar and a new epithelium. By observation he had established that not all Caldwell–Luc antra remained as open cavities and that many became infected and occluded with thick fibrous tissue. He questioned the importance of the inferior meatal window and its location (14).

Conservative Versus Radical Surgery

It is hard to determine exactly where the two extremes of a spectrum are when considering all the surgical procedures performed on the paranasal sinuses and nasal cavity. Van Alyea claimed the conservative procedure was one that stood the test of time. In 1951 he named conservative submucous resection of the septum and sinus irrigation as examples. After a review of the published literature of the first half of this century, it becomes clear that Van Alyea was a long way ahead of his time. His conservative thinking regarding surgery is very much in keeping with the current thoughts with regard to the philosophy behind CESS. He speaks of each sinus requiring special treatment techniques and says that the successful management of sinus disease requires a painstaking study and careful planning and in some cases a therapeutic regime covering a long period of time. He advocated the following concepts for conservative sinus surgery: conservative septoplasty, crushing or half-fracturing of an obstructing overaerated middle turbinate, conservative removal of thickened tissue from the sphenoethmoidal recess, conservative removal of ethmoid polyps, preservation of maxillary sinus lining during a Caldwell–Luc procedure, and preservation of the inferior turbinates with no submucous resection or cauterization.

Sinus Lavage

Proetz's method for displacement irrigation of the posterior ethmoids and sphenoid sinus has fallen into disfavor. It was a very wet experience for both the patient and physician! An alternative to inferior meatal puncture is irrigation through the natural ostium of the maxillary sinus. Myerson discussed the history of this technique. He described 24 types of cannulas in use in 1932 and described very accurately the technique for catheterization and sounding of the natural maxillary ostium. His technique was 80% successful in a series of 138 soundings. The natural osteal route to the maxillary sinus was favored over the inferior meatal route because of concern to avoid spreading infection to bone. Prior to the development of antibiotics, acutely inflamed maxillary sinuses were not sounded under any circumstances. In addition to the therapeutic advantages of antral lavage, experienced proponents of lavage gained a lot of information about the anatomy of the osteomeatal unit by palpation with the probe tip (51).

Van Alyea was well aware of the relationship between allergy, sinusitis, and polyps. He stressed the importance of attempting to control allergy in the treatment of chronic sinusitis. He was a strong advocate of irrigation of all sinuses and was particularly pleased with the results of frontal and sphenoid sinus irrigation, in the presence of disease. The techniques for frontal sinus irrigation are not commonly used today. Sasaki and Kirschner have described self-retaining triple lumen catheters for the frontal and maxillary sinuses, which may be left in place when repeated lavage is indicated (52). Irrespective of the technique of lavage employed, one has to consider patient acceptability of the procedure and the difficulty of clearing thick viscous mucus and mucopus from many chronically infected sinuses. This thinking is in keeping with a study by Flottes in 1960, who studied ostium patency of diseased maxillary sinuses and found that improving ostium patency with conservative treatment resulted in a cure of 16 out of 20 patients. Treatment failures occurred in those patients in whom ostium patency could not be established. In 1986 Melen, Fiber, Intrusion, Invasson, Jannert, and Lindaln studied 72 chronic maxillary sinuses in 66 patients with respect to maxillary ostium patency and nasal resistance. They found that patients with a functional maxillary ostium diameter greater than 2.5 mm were cured, whereas those with a small ostium averaging 0.9 mm had persistent disease. They concluded that improvement of ventilation of the maxillary sinus and cure of disease demanded either pharmacological or surgical treatment in order to improve the ostium patency (26). As can be seen from the above description of the development of intranasal sinus surgery, most of the procedures were based on the concepts of excision of disease, drainage, and permanent sinus aeration. Progress in the natural evolution of these concepts came from the understanding by Van Alyea (1942) of the reparative nature of chronically infected sinus mucosa and the development of better methods of visualizing the fine detail of the sinus mucosa.

DEVELOPMENT OF NASAL AND SINUS ENDOSCOPY

The development of the application of the endoscope has similarly affected the treatment of both nose and sinuses. Progress has been from its application in nasal diagnosis (nasal endoscopy), to examination of the sinuses with biopsy (sinus endoscopy or sinoscopy), and later to conservative or functional endoscopic sinus surgery (CESS or FESS).

Dionis (1714) described the first nasal speculum and Czermak (1858) succeeded in viewing the nasal pharynx using a small laryngeal mirror, which he called "rhinoscopy." Wertheim (1868) developed a "conchoscope" to look deeper inside the nose and named this "middle rhinoscopy." The discovery of cocaine, with its ability to vasoconstrict and anesthetize nasal mucosa, allowed Killian in 1896 to penetrate the middle meatus with the long flat blades of a nasal speculum. Hirschmann (1903) is credited with the first endoscopic examination of the sinonasal cavity using a modified cystoscope developed by Nitze in 1897 (53). He introduced Nitze's cystoscope into the middle meatus and from here Valentin and Zollner (1903) inspected the nasopharynx along the inferior meatus. Hirschmann (1901) introduced the cystoscope into the maxillary sinus through an enlarged tooth socket (sinoscopy) and Slobodnik examined the antrum through the natural ostium (Highmoroscopy). Sargnon (1908) entered the maxillary sinus via the anterolateral wall and extracted a foreign body through a small tube using the endoscope. In 1910 Imhofer removed a cotton tampon through an alveolar opening. Lack of enthusiasm for such instrumentation was largely a result of soiling and fogging of the optical system and inadequate distal illumination. The light sources of the day where less than adequate. One should note, however, that this excellent diagnostic tool had its early development about the time of the development of the great radical sinus surgical procedures. Spielberg (1922) developed an "antroscope" and Dennis and Mullin entered the antrum to make a diagnosis in cases where indications for the Caldwell–Luc operation were not absolute. Maltz (1925) asked Wolf of Berlin to construct an improved optical instrument and developed the term "sinoscopy" (54). Portmann (1925) and Botey (1926) developed the term "sinusopharyngoscopy" and "endo-rhinoscopy" and discussed examination of the sphenoid sinus. Zarniko (1925) found endoscopy to be "amusing" since most images were distorted and inaccurate.

During the 1930s, as progress was made in x-ray diagnosis, endoscopy fell by the wayside. It was rediscovered in the 1950s throughout Europe. Charsak (in Russia), Jimenez-Queseda (in Spain), and Von Riccabona (in 1955) employed Storz equipment. Despite its inadequate depth of field, Von Riccabona was able to examine 100 antra whose endoscopic findings were corroborated by ensuing radical surgery. Bauer (1955) and Wodak (1958) made attempts to correlate endoscopic and histologic findings from the nose and maxillary sinus as a basis for radical surgery. They had diffi culty examining the whole of the maxillary sinus and their findings were from the lateral wall.

A major breakthrough in instrumentation occurred with the development of fiber optics and glass wool light conductors allowing a distant cold light source and robot camera to be used. Draf (1973), Hellmich and Herberhold (1971), and Messerklinger (1971) continued their research into sinus disease and this resulted in Hopkins of England developing an endoscope with an air lens system. Hopkins along with Storz developed distal illumination using glass rods and Wolf and Lumina used glass fiber bundles. The result was a sixfold increase in distal illumination and a threefold increase in the size of the image. Photographic documentation of these improved images was developed by Timm (1964), Messerklinger (1972), Draf (1973), Terrier (1973), and Buiter (1976) (55–57).

Nasal endoscopy with a cold light source supplying a minimum of 150 watts of light is connected to the telescope by a fiberoptic or fluid-filled cable. This has replaced the traditional Vienna speculum and headmirror rhinologic examination. This technique requires a selection of telescopes with different fields of view. All telescopes have individual optical characteristics. This is the best way to map accurately any anatomical abnormality and pathology. The technique is optimal when the telescopes are hooked up to a microchip television camera and television (TV) monitor. This allows the patient and examiner to observe the anatomy and pathology of the intranasal examination together, and to review the findings on videotape. An endoscopic examination of the nasal airway demonstrates in greater detail the contents of the middle meatus, the middle turbinate size and position, the posterior nasal airway, and nasopharynx and mucosa detail. Specific details within the middle meatus that often cannot be seen by the traditional nasal examination and that are important for determining the type of endoscopic procedure are bulging of the uncinate process, the presence of intrameatal and intrasinal polypi encroaching into and obstructing the osteomeatal complex region, the width of the nasal airway at the anterior border of the middle turbinate, the posterior nasal airway patency, the posterior septal position, and the presence of other disease.

Sinus endoscopy developed in Europe in the 1970s prior to the introduction of the CT scanner. Radiology and sinus endoscopy were compared by Illum (1972), Jeppeson (1972), and Draf (1978) (56,58). Biopsies under direct vision were obtained, either through the canine fossa or inferior meatus, and in the early 1970s endoscopy began to spread throughout Europe. Illium and Jeppeson propagated sinoscopy in Scandinavia, Buiter in The Netherlands, and Terrier in Switzerland. Double entrance procedures were described by Hellmich and Herberhold in order to obtain biopsies and

this led to the development of the optical biopsy forceps. Draf developed small microbiopsy instruments integrated into the telescopes for excision of cysts and taking of biopsy specimens from the antrum. He extended these techniques into the frontal and sphenoid sinuses. Terrier, Baumann, and Pidoux (1976) established a new histomorphological classification for chronic maxillary sinusitis using endoscopic mucosal biopsy (59). Endoscopic biopsy techniques were carried forward to another level by Stammberger in 1986. Stammberger had studied as a junior resident under Messerklinger and at that time was involved in photographing the findings of the early experiments on mucus flow within the sinuses (60). They were able to photograph the intricate anatomy of the lateral nasal wall and show the infinite variability of the anatomical structures in normal and diseased states. This was at the time when accurate CT scanning of the lateral nasal wall and sinuses was becoming available in both Europe and North America.

At the present time the role of sinus endoscopy in the clinical setting for the diagnosis of chronic sinusitis is not clear. Maxillary sinus trephination to allow passage of a telescope and sheath is not an innocuous office procedure. It has a place for the biopsy of sinus mucosa and biopsy of sinonasal tumors for histological diagnosis. Frontal sinusotomy and endoscopic examination are useful methods of determining the extent of frontal sinus disease, especially around the superior os of the frontonasal duct and at the lateral extensions of the frontal sinus. This may be combined with sounding of the frontonasal duct from below with a Van Alyea cannula. This practice is unlikely to damage the frontonasal duct mucosa, but blind heavy instrumentation may. I feel that the best place to perform a full endoscopic sinonasal examination, including these rather specialized techniques, is in the operating room under local anesthesia and sedation.

DEVELOPMENT OF ENDOSCOPIC SINUS SURGERY

The term ethmoidectomy has been used loosely to describe all procedures, from conservative to radical, on the labyrinth and related sinuses. The first attempts at limited ethmoidectomy were those of Killian (1900). He described the uncinectomy in conjunction with widening the natural ostium of the maxillary sinus (60). Preservation of the middle turbinate during ethmoidectomy was considered necessary by Pratt (1925), Davison (1969), Eichel (1972), and Kern (1979) to control the size of the cavity in order to prevent dryness (43,61,62). Wigand (1981), Eichel (1972), and Friedman (1982) included opening the sphenoid and Wigand (1981), Ashikawa (1982), Messerklinger (1984), and

Stammberger (1985) opened the antrum in the presence of radiologic disease (63–66). Microscopic sinus surgery was introduced by Heermann (1958) who used the binocular microscope to excise polypi from the ethmoid labyrinth (67). Draf (1982) added the angled telescope to improve visualization. Wigand (1981) introduced the suction irrigation system to remove blood and improve visualization. Rigid endoscopic resections via the middle meatus were developed by Buiter and Strattman (1981), who described fontanellotomy as a means of creating a window into the antrum. Messerklinger and Stammberger had once again appreciated that the ethmoid sinuses were responsible for the development of chronic infection within the prechambers of the larger but ethmoid-dependent frontal, maxillary, and sphenoid sinuses. They described endoscopic ethmoidectomy starting with an uncinotomy to reveal the contents of the infundibulum. This was not a new approach but represented the first organized and photographed telescopic approach into the ethmoids. This method is now known as the Messerklinger technique. Stammberger (1985) developed techniques of endoscopic resection for anatomical obstructions within the osteomeatal complex, described by Naumann (1965), and of localized disease in the anterior lateral nasal wall (68–70). He took this knowledge further by demonstrating a safe anterior approach to the anterior bulla ethmoid cells and through the basal lamella into the posterior ethmoid cells. He described the telescopic approach into the sphenoid sinus through the common face with the posterior ethmoid cells; into the frontal sinus via the frontal recess; and into the maxillary sinus through the natural ostium within the middle meatus. This was the first comprehensive description of the organized telescopic dissection of the paranasal sinuses (63,64). Stammberger was responsible for teaching this anterior complete endoscopic dissection technique at many courses worldwide and this became known as "functional endoscopic sinus surgery." His intranasal concepts are currently taught widely in North America. New ideas for the development of safe endoscopic sinus surgery techniques using combined intranasal and external approaches are being developed. This is particularly true for frontal recess/duct/sinus disease, especially in revisional cases where landmarks are absent and scar has replaced healthy mucosa.

Wigand (1981) described the concept of "isthmus surgery" for extended ethmoidectomy into the larger but ethmoid-dependent sinuses. This involved the creation of windows into infected sinuses with the removal of irreversible mucosa and the preservation of reversible mucosa. This was another example of old knowledge being rediscovered and becoming accepted. Wigand described his technique for the removal of advanced disease from the anterior face of the sphenoid working forward along the skull base into the anterior ethmoids. This is now known as the Wigand endoscopic technique.

Theoretically, the increase in ventilation of the sinus or sinus cell by endoscopic individualized surgery should result in reduction in goblet cell numbers and resolution of symptoms. Lund has shown that this is not true in a certain group of patients with an inadequate inferior meatal antrostomy. There appears to be evidence that certain organisms such as *Hemophilus influenzae* are capable of immobilizing cilia as a result of toxin production. Doyle and Woodham (1990) have described the microbiology of chronic ethmoiditis and have demonstrated a high incidence of *Staphylococcus aureus* and coliforms in chronically infected ethmoid mucosa (71). From this work I believe that there is a role for postsurgical antibiotic and medical therapy of the chronically infected, but healing, sinus mucosa.

SUMMARY

This chapter has covered some of the high points in the history of the development of surgery for acute and chronic sinusitis. Sinus surgery had its roots in radical procedures and there has been a gradual change to conservative surgery in the past 100 years. The early development of sinus surgery was around the concept of drainage of an acutely infected sinus and the radical removal of its mucosa and mucoperiostium with aeration being a lesser consideration. Lives were saved, and surgical morbidity was a less important consideration. The range of disease, lack of antibiotics, and poor illumination and visualization made sinus surgery a difficult and dangerous proposition 100 years ago. Where do we stand today?

The last 10 years has seen a significant advance in our approach to the treatment of sinus disease. The change has been accelerated by the recent development of improved illumination and visualization via optical telescopes. This has allowed us to perform a more conservative and anatomical dissection based on the knowledge learned over the last 100 years.

Endoscopic diagnosis by telescopic examination and CT scan can help to determine the extent of sinus disease, the appearance of the anatomy, and the position of vital structures. This information is vital for surgical planning. The endoscopic examination performed in the clinic provides us with a lot of new information relating to the nasal airway and middle meatus. It helps us understand what is happening in the osteomeatal unit but does not tell us the state of the mucosa in each sinus cell. There is no way of determining preoperatively the state of the mucosa at a particular location in a sinus. The current CT scanners with reconstruction of images in different planes and three-dimensional (3-D) reconstruction with the C-arm during surgery help tremendously in the planning and performance of endoscopic surgery. The scanner, however, is not fool-proof and can underread the extent of the problem, especially in the fontanelle membranes of the medial walls of the antra.

Van Alyea focused on the concept of mucosal preservation and subsequent reversal following individualized conservative sinus surgery. Endoscopic sinus surgery has allowed us accurately to detect and remove irreversible disease, open sinus windows and clefts, and reexamine the result during the healing period. Individualized microendoscopic mucosal sinus surgery is now possible, but this is still based on a macroscopic visualization of the diseased mucosa through a brightly illuminated monocular telescope. Exactly what tissue should be removed and at what stage of the disease process is unknown. At the present time the individual cellular biochemistry of sinonasal mucosa is not fully understood. The local effect of internal and external environmental factors on sinus mucosa has to be established. They appear to bring about the reversible and irreversible changes in the mucosa we collectively call chronic sinusitis.

Current technical developments allow the accurate performance of endoscopic sinus surgery from the TV monitor. Woodham (1991) has described the added safety advantages of this technique, over conventional transtelescope viewing, using shorter wide angled endoscopes and an integrated TV camera system, which produces an excellent two-dimensional (2-D) monitor image. Loss of depth perception with 2-D images is a disadvantage of current endoscopic systems. The 3-D CT scanners used in the operating room will soon provide additional information that will improve the safety of the endoscopic dissection. Recent 3-D camera advances include a single camera universal adaptor that converts 2-D endoscopic TV images into realistic 3-D images. Working with white light, surgeons will have the benefit of realistic ''natural'' 3-D vision of the working area. It is predicted in the future that 3-D CT scanners will be married to 3-D camera systems. These advances will enhance learning the intricate anatomy of the sinonasal tract and will be especially valuable when training inexperienced surgeons. With the use of fine instruments, specific to microscopic dissection, and the technical improvements outlined above, the surgery will become safer. Stankiewicz (1987) has described the common complications of endoscopic sinus surgery (72–74; T. Greening, *personal communication*).

My current philosophy for the role of conservative endoscopic surgery (CESS) is based on individualized surgery to the affected sinuses by ''microectomies,'' meatostomies, and opening of narrow meatal clefts. Procedures to open the nasal airway include sep-toplasty and the resection of the leading edge of the middle turbinate, in certain cases. Macroscopic reversible mucosa is preserved and irreversible polypoid mucosa and scar are removed. Whether functioning mucosa can regenerate in this situation is uncertain.

The role of medical therapy for the treatment of chronic sinusitis, particularly following surgery, is still undetermined. Woodham and Doyle (1991) believe that there is an important role for postoperative antibiotics. This is in accordance with the bacterial sensitivities taken from tissue at the time of surgery. Postoperative antibiotics are given until the chronic bacterial infection has been eliminated from the sinus mucosa. This appears to take up to 12 weeks and the author's observations indicate that the mucopurulent postsurgical rhinorrhea parallels the thinning of the chronically infected mucosa (75).

Histopathological classifications for chronic sinusitis have not led to practical clinical classifications at this time. Indeed, the development of a working classification appears difficult to achieve. There is not a large series of results based on a classification of chronic sinusitis. Reporting of results often includes adjunctive endoscopic procedures. There appears to be a gradation of results depending on the duration and extent of the disease and whether previous radical surgery has been performed. Symptom improvement is a reasonable expectation for all patients. Cure is less well defined. Patients with early disease localized to one region should expect a cure. Some may still have allergic symptoms, but their facial discomfort and recurrent attacks of acute sinusitis will cease. Patients with primary advanced massive polypoid disease will be grateful of airway improvement and may achieve a cure with staged surgery if necessary. The problem cases are those who are requesting an endoscopic cure following previous multiple radical traditional resections. In these cases the majority of potentially reversing mucosa has likely been removed. This group should expect symptom improvement (75,76).

In conclusion, I have quoted Dr. Mosher's closing statement in his 1912 address to the American Rhinological Association: ''My ethmoidal operating has lacked definite plan and I easily became confused as to where I was and I was always in doubt as to how much had been accomplished at any given moment.''

This statement reminds us of the potential dangers when operating within the ethmoid labyrinth. We are removing benign disease, and the need for sound basic knowledge, good clinical judgment, and an organized surgical approach is of the utmost importance. Hopefully, the next 100 years will bring solutions to the many problems of the last 100 years, some of which still remain unsolved.

REFERENCES

1. Highmore N (1651). Cited by MC Myerson, ref. 52.
2. Schaeffer JP. *The nose, paranasal sinuses, naso-lachrymal passageways, and the olfactory organ in man.* Philadelphia: P Blakiston's Son & Co, 1920.
3. Mosher HP. A method of obliterating the naso-frontal duct and catheterizing the frontal sinus. *Laryngoscope* 1911;21:946.
4. Mosher HP. The applied anatomy and the intranasal surgery of the ethmoid labyrinth. *Trans Am Laryngol Assoc* 1912;34:25–39.
5. Mosher HP. The symposium on the ethmoid—the surgical anatomy of the ethmoidal labyrinth. *Am Acad Ophthalmol Otolaryngol* 1929;376–410.
6. Bryce G, Woodham JD. The cross-sectional osteology of the midface. *J Otolaryngol* 1988;17(1):4–11.
7. Van Alyea OE. *Nasal sinuses: an anatomic and clinical consideration.* Baltimore: Wilkins Co, 1951.
8. Ritter FN. *The paranasal sinuses—anatomy and surgical technique,* 2nd ed. St Louis: CV Mosby, 1978.
9. Lang J. *The clinical anatomy of the nasal cavity and paranasal sinuses.* Stuttgart: G Thieme Verlag, 1990.
10. Williams HL. Intranasal operation for chronic maxillary sinusitis. *JAMA* 1935;105:56–100.
11. Caldwell GW. Diseases of the accessory sinuses of the nose and an improved method of treatment for suppuration of the maxillary antrum. *NY Med J* 1893;58:526–528.
12. Luc H. My latest improvements in the radical treatment of chronic suppurations of the accessory cavities of the nose. *Ann Otol Rhinol* 1903;12(Sept):407–418.
13. Lothrop HA. Empyema of the antrum of Highmore—a new operation for the cure of obstinate cases. *Boston Med Surg J* 1897; 136:455–466.
14. Goodyear HM. Chronic antrum infection. *Arch Otolaryngol* 1934;20:542–548.
15. Sewall EC. External operation on the ethmosphenoid frontal group of sinuses under local anesthesia. *Arch Otolaryngol* 1926; 4(5):377.
16. Tilley H. Cited by PG Goldsmith. Accessory sinus disease in general practice. *Can Med Assoc J* 1943;48:426.
17. Bell RD, Stone HE. Conservative surgical procedures in inflammatory disease of the maxillary sinus. *Otolaryngol Clin North* 1976;9:175–186.
18. Murray JP. Complications after treatment of chronic maxillary sinus disease with Caldwell–Luc procedure. *Laryngoscope* 1983;93:282–284.
19. Sogg AJ. Intranasal antrostomy—causes of failure. *Laryngoscope* 1982;92:1038–1041.
20. Macbeth R. Caldwell–Luc Operation 1952–1966. *Arch Otolaryngol* 1968;87:630–636.
21. Freer OT. The antrum of Highmore; the removal of the greater part of its inner wall through the nostril, for empyema. *Laryngoscope* 1905;15:343–349.
22. Hempstead BE. End results of intranasal operation and maxillary sinusitis. *Arch Otolaryngol* 1939;30:711.
23. Hilding A. Experimental surgery of the nose and sinuses. *Arch Otolaryngol* 1931;16(9):9–18.
24. Messerklinger W. On the drainage of the normal frontal sinus of man. *Acta Otolaryngol (Stockh)* 1967;63:176–181.
25. Buiter CT. Nasal antrostomy. *Rhinology* 1988;26:5–18.
26. Melen I. Ostial and nasal patency in chronic maxillary sinusitis. *Acta Otolaryngol (Stockh)* 1986;102:500–508.
27. Lund VJ. The design and function of intranasal antrostomies. *J Laryngol Otol* 1986;110:35–39.
28. Lund VJ. *Inferior meatal antrostomy.* Thesis, Institute of Laryngology and Otology, London, 1985;1–17.
29. Jansen A. *Arch Laryng Rhine* 1893;1:135.
30. Ritter G. *Deutsch Med Wochenschr* 1906;32:1294.
31. Sewell EC. External operation of the ethmosphenoid frontal group of sinuses under local anesthesia. *Arch Otol* 1926;4:377.
32. Smith F. Management of chronic sinus disease. *Arch Otolaryngol* 1934;19:157.
33. Lynch RC. The technique of a radical frontal sinus operation which has given me the best results. *Laryngoscope* 1926;31: 377–411.
34. Skillern SR. Obliterative frontal sinusitis. *Arch Otolaryngol* 1936;23:268–284.
35. Montgomery WL. Surgery of the frontal sinus. *Otol Clin North Am* 1971;4:97–126.
36. Goodale RL, Montgomery WW. Experiences with osteointerior wall approach to frontal sinus. *Arch Otol* 1958;69:271–382.
37. Boyden GL. Surgical treatment of chronic frontal sinusitis. *Ann Otol Rhinol Laryngol* 1952;61:558–566.
38. Eichel BS. The intranasal ethmoidectomy procedure—historical, technical and clinical considerations. *Laryngoscope* 1972; 82:1806–1821.
39. Eichel BS. Surgical management of chronic paranasal sinusitis. *Laryngoscope* 1973;83:1195–1202.
40. Friedman HM, Kern EB. Complications of intranasal ethmoidectomy: a review of 1,000 consecutive operations. *Laryngoscope* 1979;89:421–432.
41. Maniglia AJ, Chandler R, Goodwin W, Flynn J. Rare complications following ethmoidectomies: a report of eleven cases. *Laryngoscope* 1981;91:1234–1244.
42. Eichel BS. The intranasal ethmoidectomy: a 12 year perspective. *Otolaryngol Head Neck Surg* 1982;90:540–543.
43. Eichel BS. Revision in ethmoidectomy. *Laryngoscope* 1985;95: 300–304.
44. Friedman WH, Katsantonis GP, Slavin R, et al. Sphenoethmoidectomy: its role in the asthmatic patient. *Otolaryngol Head Neck Surg* 1982;90:171–177.
45. Friedman WH. Sphenoethmoidectomy: the case for ethmoid marsupialization. *Laryngoscope* 1986;96:476–479.
46. Stevens HE, Blair NJ. Intranasal sphenoethmoidectomy: 10-year experience and literature review. *J Otolaryngol* 1988;17(5): 254–259.
47. Proetz AW. Displacement irrigation of nasal sinuses. *Arch Otolaryngol* 1926;4(1).
48. Jervey JW Jr. Conservative management of the sinuses. *South Med J* 1939;32:278–281.
49. Childrey JH. Use of sulfanilamide locally for sinal infection. *Arch Otolaryngol* 1939;986–987.
50. Turnbull FM. Intranasal therapy with sodium salt of sulfathiazole in chronic sinusitis. *JAMA* 1941;116(17):1899–1900.
51. Myerson MC. Natural orifice of the maxillary sinus. *Arch Otolaryngol* 1932;15:716–733.
52. Sasaki CT, Kirchner C, Goodwin J. Self-retaining catheters for continuous frontal and maxillary sinus lavage. *Otolaryngol Head Neck Surg* 1987;97(4):419–420.
53. Nitze M. Erste Mitteilung eines Cystokops. *Wien Med Wochenschr* 1879;29:649–652, 896–910.
54. Maltz M. New instrument: the sinuscope. *Laryngoscope* 1925; 35:805–811.
55. Messerklinger W. *Endoscopy of the nose.* Baltimore: Urban & Schwarzenberg, 1978.
56. Draf W. *Endoscopy of the paranasal sinuses.* New York: Springer Verlag, 1983.
57. Buiter CT. Nasal antrostomy. *Rhinology* 1988;26:5–18.
58. Illum P, Jeppeson F. Sinoscopy: endoscopy of the maxillary sinus. Technique, common and rare findings. *Acta Otolaryngol (Stockh)* 1972;73:506–512.
59. Terrier G, Baumann RP, Pidoux JM. Endoscopic and histopathological observations of chronic maxillary sinusitis. *Rhinology* 1976;14:129–132.
60. Killian G. Accessory sinuses of the nose and their relations to neighboring parts. Chicago: WT Keener & Co, 1904.
61. Pratt JA. The present status of the intranasal ethmoid operation. *Arch Otolaryngol* 1925;1:42–50.
62. Davison FW. Intranasal surgery. *Laryngoscope* 1969;79: 502–511.
63. Wigand ME. Transnasal ethmoidectomy under endoscopical control. *Rhinology* 1981;19:7–15.
64. Wigand ME. Endoscopic surgery of the paranasal sinuses and anterior skull base. Stuttgart: Thieme Verlag, 1990.
65. Ashikawa R, Ohkushi H, Ohmae T, Matsuda T. Clinical effects

of the nasal cavity (Takahshi's method). *Auris Nasus Larynx* 1982;9:91–98.

66. Stammberger H. Endoscopic endonasal surgery. New concepts in treatment of recurring rhinosinusitis. Part 1. Anatomical and pathophysiological considerations. *Otolaryngol Head Neck Surg* 1985;94:143–147.

67. Heermann J. Uber endonasale Chirurgie unter Verwendung des binocularen Mikroskopes. *Arch Ohr Nas Kehlkopfheilk* 1958; 171:295–297.

68. Stammberger H. Endoscopic endonasal surgery. New concepts in treatment of recurring rhinosinusitis. Part 2. Surgical technique. *Otolaryngol Head Neck Surg* 1985;94:147–156.

69. Stammberger H. Nasal and paranasal sinus endoscopy—a diagnostic and surgical approach to recurrent sinusitis. *Endoscopy* 1986;6:213–218.

70. Naumann HH. *International Congress Series 113*. Amsterdam: Excerpta Medica, 1965;80.

71. Doyle PW, Woodham JD. Evaluation of the microbiology of chronic ethmoid sinusitis. *J Clin Microbiol* 1991;29(11): 2396–2400.

72. Woodham JD, Doyle PW. Conservative endoscopic sinus surgery from the TV monitor using an integrated Nagashima endoscopic sinonasal system. *J Otolaryngol* 1991;20(6):448–451.

73. Woodham JD, Doyle PW. Surgical landmarks and resections for the safe performance of conservative endoscopic sinus surgery. *J Otolaryngol* 1991;20(6):451–454.

74. Stankiewicz JA. Complications in endoscopic intranasal ethmoidectomy: an update. *Laryngoscope* 1989;99(July):686–690.

75. Woodham JD, Doyle PW. Endoscopic diagnosis, medical treatment and a working classification for chronic sinusitis. *Otolaryngol* 1991;20(6):438–441.

76. Woodham JD. Conservative endoscopic sinus surgery for chronic sinusitis. *Br Columbia Med J* 1993;35(4):246–249.

CHAPTER 2

Embryology

Dale H. Rice

A thorough understanding of the embryology of the paranasal sinuses and midfacial structures is important for understanding the various diseases that can afflict this area. One cannot look at the embryology of a single area without taking into consideration regional embryology of the cranial–oral–facial region as well. These primary events occur between the fourth and eighth weeks of fetal life. Within the early developing brain, organization centers induce the formation of the cartilaginous and bony structures of the midface as well as the developing sensory organs. As the forebrain develops and enlarges, the olfactory bulbs begin to migrate anteriorly and take their superior position relative to the developing nasal and sinus structures. Since midfacial and nasal development occur simultaneously, each contributes to the other.

As the anterior foregut develops, an ectodermally derived limiting membrane develops at its anterior limit. The primitive forebrain lies above and the pericardial sac below. As the foregut tube further evolves, its most anterior part becomes the stomodeum. This anterior limiting membrane is called the oropharyngeal buccopharyngeal membrane (Fig. 1). As the maxillary processes migrate anterosuperiorly and the mandibular processes do so anteroinferiorly to the stomodeum, this structure becomes the buccal cavity. The buccopharyngeal membrane marks the separation of ectoderm of the developing mouth anteriorly and endoderm posteriorly. As the buccal pharyngeal membrane disintegrates, Rathke's pouch marks the superior attachment of the buccopharyngeal membrane (Fig. 2). It is ectodermally derived and will form the anterior contribution to the pituitary. At about the 26th day, Rathke's pouch is forming (1). At this point, there are three developing facial projections that define the nasal structure itself: the frontonasal process, the maxillary process, and the mandibular process (Fig. 3). The latter two are derived from the first branchial arch, while the

frontonasal process develops independently over the forebrain and contributes to the development of the forehead. The frontonasal process is ectodermally derived and contributes to the development of the nasal olfactory placodes, which are induced by their proximity to the developing olfactory nerves. Each of these placodes gives rise to medial and lateral nasal prominences, which then surround the nasal pit that will ultimately become the nares (Fig. 4). As the nasal pit deepens, it becomes the nasal sac (Fig. 5). As the cavity enlarges, the posterior limiting membrane, originally the nasal fin (Fig. 5), becomes the bucconasal membrane. Dissolution of this membrane that connects the primitive palate to the undersurface of the neurocranium forms the posterior choanae. The membrane usually dissolves at about 38 to 40 days of embryogenesis. Lack of dissolution of the bucconasal membrane is one of the theories of the origin of choanal atresia.

The frontonasal, maxillary, and mandibular prominences merge and eventually complete the development of the central facial structures. Fusion of the medial nasal prominence with the maxillary prominence contributes to the development of the upper maxilla and the philtrum of the upper lip. Simultaneously, intraorally the primary palate is derived from proliferation of the medial nasal process and forms the intermaxillary segment and the four maxillary incisors.

The nasopharynx and oropharynx are subsequently divided into separate anatomic compartments with the development of the primary and secondary palate. The latter is derived from the palatine shelf, which develops with the maxillary prominences and which changes from a vertical and lateral position to a medial and horizontal one. This change thus completes the development of the nasal floor separating the nasal cavity from the oral cavity.

With further development, the frontal prominence contributes to the forehead and nasal bridge while the

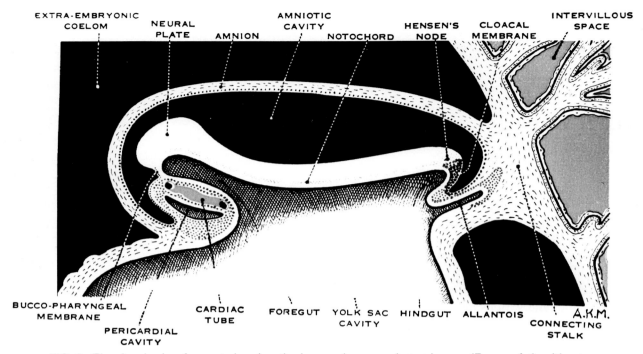

FIG. 1. The developing foregut showing the buccopharyngeal membrane. (From ref. 1, with permission.)

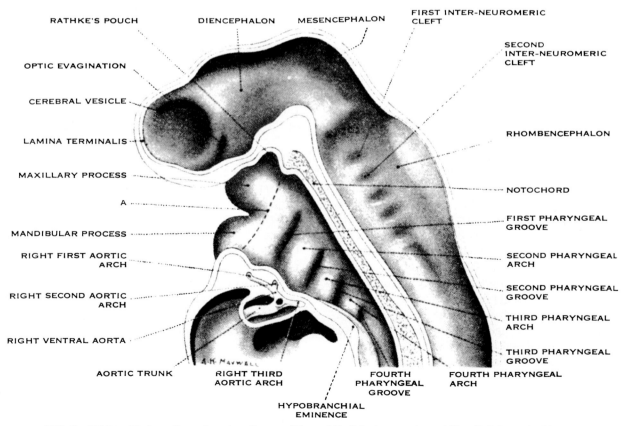

FIG. 2. Midsagittal section showing the position of Rathke's pouch and the disintegrated buccopharyngeal membrane. (From ref. 1, with permission.)

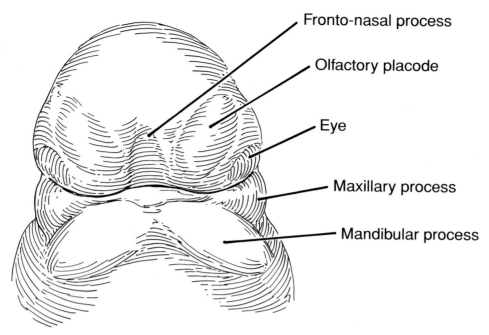

FIG. 3. Five-millimeter embryo showing beginning development of olfactory placode, frontonasal process, and maxilla.

two medial nasal prominences fuse to form the nasal tip and columella. The latter prominences develop into the alar cartilages. At this point, the anterior nares are occluded by epithelial plugs. Intranasally, the frontonasal process contributes to the development of the nasal capsule, which is the anlage for the developing nasal cartilaginous structures. This capsule will develop into two portions consisting of the mesethmoid (the nasal septal precursor) and the lateral ectethmoid (the conchae and lateral nasal wall) (Fig. 6). The frontonasal process grows posteriorly from under the cranium to the developing palate. It is joined by an exten-

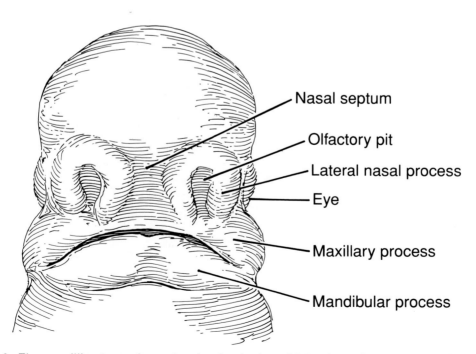

FIG. 4. Eleven-millimeter embryo showing beginning of lateral nasal processes and septum.

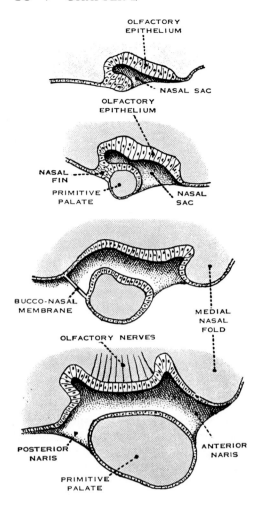

FIG. 5. Scheme to illustrate the formation of the nasal sac from the nasal pit and the eventual evolution of the olfactory epithelium as it connects to the olfactory nerves. Note position of the bucconasal membrane. (From ref. 1, with permission.)

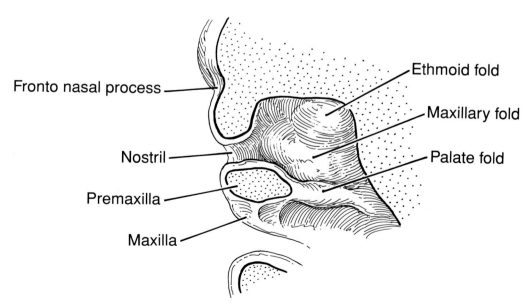

FIG. 6. Sagittal views of 12-mm embryo showing early development of lateral nasal wall.

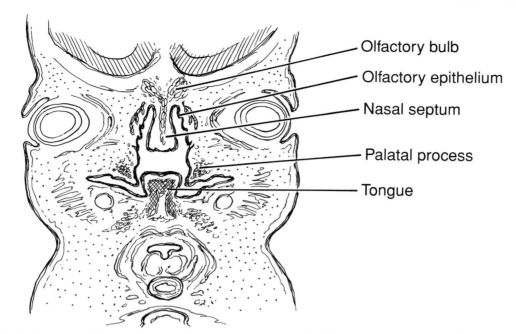

FIG. 7. Twenty-millimeter embryo showing development of the palatal processes, the nasal system. Note the sinuses themselves have not yet begun to develop.

Olfactory bulb
Olfactory epithelium
Nasal septum
Palatal process
Tongue

sion of mesoderm from the maxilla called the "tectoseptal" extension. These are the primordia of the septum. At about this time, the bucconasal membrane disintegrates to form the posterior choana. The septal cartilage, which arises from the mesethmoid, develops in a superior-to-inferior direction (Fig. 7). Simultaneously, the palatal shelves close, separating the oral cavity from the nasal cavity (Fig. 8). Ossification of the posterior part of the mesethmoidal cartilage forms the perpendicular plate of the ethmoid and the crista galli. More posteriorly and inferiorly, the vomer develops from the membranous ossification of connective tissue rather than from cartilage.

The nasolacrimal duct begins as a furrow between the maxillary and lateral nasal prominences. It connects the eye to the primitive nasal cavity. Initially, it is a solid tube of tissue that eventually canalizes to form a duct connecting the conjunctiva to the internal nasal cavity inferior to the attachment of the inferior turbinate. As the eye migrates from a lateral orientation relative to the developing nose, the nasal lacrimal duct assumes a more oblique rather than horizontal attitude. Complete patency of this duct may not occur until the first month postpartum. It may take even longer.

Development of the paranasal sinuses themselves begins at about this time. In the third to fourth month of fetal development, mucous membrane infiltrates the cartilaginous structures of the lateral nasal wall by the process of primary pneumatization. With further growth, secondary pneumatization occurs into the bony structures for which the sinuses eventually will be named (Fig. 9).

LATERAL NASAL WALL

Throughout this period of time, the lateral nasal wall increases its surface area. The original shallow grooves eventually develop into the inferior and middle meati with the formation of the like-named turbinates. The middle, superior, and, when present, supreme turbinates originally arise from the superior nasal septum, but continuing growth of the nasal cavity shifts them to the lateral wall. In the third trimester, there may be up to five turbinates above the inferior; but after birth, the superiormost of these coalesce and disappear (2). Thus the supreme turbinate decreases in identifiability with age. It has been reported to be present in 88% of fetuses, 73% of preadolescents, and 26% of adults (3). The agger nasi is an elevation superior to the inferior turbinate and anterior to the middle turbinate and marks pneumatization of the lacrimal bone. The olfactory sulcus is superior and anterior to the agger nasi and is limited superiorly by the mergence of medial and lateral nasal walls.

The middle meatus begins development in the late first trimester with the formation of the uncinate process. Somewhat later, the ethmoid bulla forms, leaving between them the infundibulum. The remaining anterior ethmoid air cells develop superior to the bulla over the ensuing weeks. Only the uncinate process, the ethmoid bulla, and the infundibulum are constant features. The remainder of the development in the middle meatus is quite variable. From the infundibulum will develop the maxillary sinus and the anterior ethmoid air cells, including those that pneumatize the ethmoid

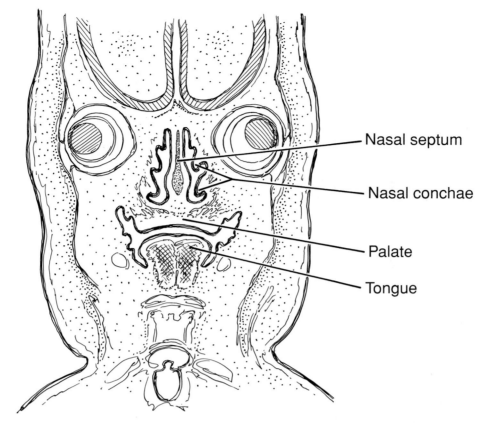

FIG. 8. Forty-six-millimeter embryo showing impending merger of the palatal processes with each other and the septum and the early development of the inferior and middle turbinates.

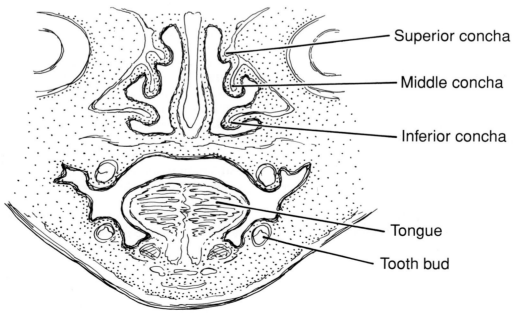

FIG. 9. Eighty-millimeter embryo showing further development of the lateral nasal wall.

bulla. In addition, the frontal sinus will form from the superior extent of the infundibulum as an outgrowth of the suprabullar ethmoid air cells.

MAXILLARY SINUS

The maxillary sinus begins as an outgrowth in the lateral wall of the ethmoid area of the nasal capsule in the third month of fetal life and is the first sinus to appear. This outgrowth begins immediately posterior to the developing uncinate process. The evagination forms in what is also known as the uncibullous groove (4). This outgrowth enlarges slowly throughout fetal life and the size of the sinus at birth is approximately 6 to 8 cm^3 (2). At birth, the maxillary sinus is fluid filled, making interpretation of plain film radiography difficult. By the fourth to fifth postnatal month, the maxillary sinus can be seen radiographically in a standard Water's projection. It appears as a triangular area medial to the infraorbital foramen. After birth, the rate of growth of the maxillary sinus is estimated to be 2 mm in vertical height and 3 mm in anterior/posterior dimension each year. Growth of the maxillary sinus continues rapidly until about 3 years of age and then more slowly until the seventh year. From 7 until about 12 years of age, there is another acceleration in growth, with pneumatization extending laterally as far as the lateral wall of the orbit, and inferiorly such that the floor of the sinus is level with the floor of the nasal cavity following the eruption of the secondary dentition. Thereafter, modest enlargement occurs until the late teens when the adult size is reached (5). Thus in the adult, the floor of the sinus is approximately 4 to 5 mm inferior to the floor of the nasal cavity (6).

In the adult, the maxillary sinus is approximately 15 mm in volume within the body of the maxilla. The average dimensions are 34 mm anteroposteriorly, 33 mm vertically, and 25 mm in width. The sinus is approximately triangular, with its base formed by the lateral wall of the nasal cavity and its apex at the zygomatic process. The roof of the sinus is the floor of the orbit and is approximately twice as wide as the floor, which is formed by the alveolar process of the maxilla.

The natural ostium of the maxillary sinus is located within the infundibulum, usually immediately inferior to the bulla ethmoidalis. Accessory ostia occur in 25% to 35% of individuals. The size and shape of the natural ostium vary depending on the anatomy of the ethmoid bulla and the uncinate process. Because of these bony limits, it is impossible to enlarge the natural ostium without removing bone as well as mucosa. This is not always true of accessory ostia, which may be located in the fontanelle, which lacks bone.

There are a number of variations involving the maxillary sinus with which the otolaryngologist–head and neck surgeon should be aware. Approximately 50% of maxillary sinuses have incomplete septi. In addition, true duplication of the maxillary sinus can occur in approximately 2.5% in anatomic studies. Accessory ostia occur in adults in a range of 25% to 50% but are reported to be less than 15% in children (6). In general, the maxillary sinuses are nearly symmetical, although true aplasia can occur, but is extremely rare. Hypoplasia, however, occurs in approximately 6% (7).

The floor of the maxillary sinus is the alveolar process of the maxilla. Most typically, the three molar tooth roots are most intimately related to the floor of the sinus, but in small sinuses, the first molar may not be and in enlarged sinuses, the premolars and even the canine may be.

ETHMOID SINUS

The anterior and middle ethmoid cells begin as evaginations in the lateral nasal wall in the middle meatus in the third fetal month. Somewhat later, the posterior cells evaginate the nasal mucosa in the superior meatus (4). All these cells enlarge gradually throughout fetal life. The ethmoid sinus has the greatest variation of the sinuses, largely because it can, and frequently does, extend beyond the ethmoid bone per se. The anterior cells actually originate in the frontal recess after it has grown from the middle meatus. At birth, the anterior sinus measures 4 mm high, 2 mm long, and 2 mm wide, while the posterior sinus measures 5 mm high, 4 mm long, and 2 mm wide. Like the maxillary sinus, the ethmoid sinuses are fluid-filled (2).

The ethmoid sinuses are difficult to visualize at birth—much more so than the maxillary sinus. They can, however, usually be visualized by 1 year of age in standard radiographs (8). In early development, the ethmoid cells tend to be spherical in shape but become flattened as they reach maximum development and encroach on adjacent cells. By the age of 12 years, the ethmoids have reached almost adult size—24 mm high, 23 mm long, and 11 mm wide for the posterior group (6). As these ethmoid cells pneumatize adjacent bones over the subsequent decade, the resulting sinuses are named for the bone invaded, rather than the cell of origin. Thus an ethmoid cell extending into the frontal bone is known as the frontal sinus. Others such as the agger nasi invade the lacrimal bone. By adulthood, the ethmoid bone is the lightest bone of the human skull because the pneumatization is so complete.

The surgeon needs to bear this in mind when operating on the ethmoid sinuses, particularly from an intranasal or transantral approach. Preoperative assessment of the radiographs will alert the surgeon to the relative thinness of the lamina papyracea and fovea ethmoidalis, as well as the relationship of various other structures to the ethmoid sinuses.

The ethmoid sinuses frequently encroach on adjacent structures. In 15% of patients, supraorbital extensions will occur into the frontal bone and in 1% of cases infraorbital extensions will occur into the maxilla. Posterior ethmoid cells may pneumatize part of the palate. Conchae bullosa are present in 12% of patients and may be from either anterior or posterior ethmoidal cells.

FRONTAL SINUS

The frontal sinus begins in the fourth fetal month, following the development of the frontal recess. The frontal sinus may arise from laterally placed anterior ethmoid cells within the frontal recess. In this situation, communication with the infundibulum is less direct. This situation is found in approximately 50% of specimens (9). A true nasofrontal duct only exists if the frontal sinus develops from an ethmoid cell within the ethmoid infundibulum. If it develops from the anterior part of the frontal recess, or from the frontal furrow, then only a nasofrontal ostium without a duct occurs. If the sinus arises directly from the ethmoid infundibular cells, the nasal connection tends to be more in alignment with the ethmoid infundibulum and directly up. The least common situation is when the frontal sinus arises as a direct extension of the entire frontal recess. In this situation, the communication between the frontal sinus and the middle meatus is large, although variable depending on the degree of impingement of adjacent anterior ethmoid cells. The sinus is small at birth and, at the time, essentially indistinguishable from anterior ethmoid cells. Early growth is slow, but the sinus is usually detectable independently by the end of the first year of life. Invasion of the vertical portion of the frontal bone begins at about the fifth year of life, and in most children over six, it can be demonstrated radiographically. By early adolescence,

the frontal sinus is large, although smaller than adult size, which is reached in late adolescence (6).

In 4% to 15% of patients, there will be failure of development of one of the frontal sinuses. In general, the sinus averages 28 mm in height, 27 mm in width, and 17 mm in depth.

Asymmetry between the frontal sinuses is more the rule than the exception as compared to the maxillary sinuses. Pneumatization may extend as far laterally as the temporal bones, but this is unusual.

SPHENOID SINUS

Before a discussion of the development of the sphenoid sinus begins, a consideration of the development of the sphenoid bone is important. The sphenoid takes origin principally in cartilage and is divided roughly into two principal components that persist until the seventh to eighth month of embryonic life. They are the presphenoid and postsphenoid. The presphenoid includes mainly the lesser wing, the body, and the tuberculum sella. The dorsum sella, the greater wings, and the pterygoid plates make up the postsphenoid part. Numerous ossification centers appear at about the ninth week of fetal life, the first two, one each in the lesser wings of the sphenoid lateral to the optic canals. Then two more appear in the presphenoid part of the body. The bony components of the postsphenoid ossify both in cartilage and in membrane. The first two ossification centers in the postsphenoid are in the cartilaginous greater wing between the foramen rotundum and ovale. The orbits part and those facing the infratemporal fossa take origin in membrane. In the postsphenoid part of the body, the first ossification centers are on either side of the sella.

The sphenoid bone at birth is comprised of three components (Fig. 10); a central portion consisting of the body and lesser wing and two lateral components each of which contains a greater wing and pterygoid plates. The craniopharyngeal canal that is connected

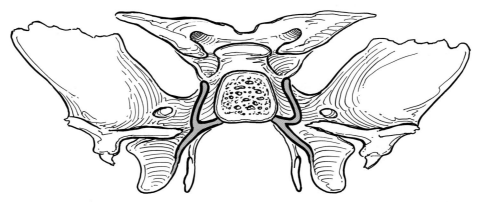

FIG. 10. Diagram showing the three principal components of the sphenoid bone found at birth.

to the hypothalamus and the pharyngeal primordium in the embryonic period may persist occasionally post-natally as an oblique septum between the pre- and postsphenoid. Additional septations may join the three principal components of the sphenoid seen at birth (Fig. 10) (10,11).

The sphenoid sinus can be identified in the fourth fetal month. The sphenoid sinus is an evagination of the posterior part of the nasal capsule. However, at birth, the sinus is represented largely as an evagination of the sphenoethmoidal recess. It remains small and does not start to grow until after the age of 3, when it begins to pneumatize the sphenoid bone itself. Growth is more rapid at this time and by the age of 7, the sinus has reached the level of the sella turcica.

Development may continue with involvement of the basisphenoid, or with arrest of development anywhere along this continuum. By adulthood, the average size is 20 mm in height, 23 mm in depth, and 17 mm in width. Asymmetry is frequent. With maximal development of the sphenoid sinus, the internal carotid artery and optic nerve may be covered only by mucosa in the lateral and superior walls.

There are basically three types of sphenoid sinuses in terms of pneumatization. The conchal type represents pneumatization that does not extend into the body of the sphenoid bone itself. This is present in only 2.5% of adults (10). In the presellar type, pneumatization extends only posteriorly to the sella turcica, but not beyond the vertical plane of the tuberculum sella. This occurs in 10% of adults. In the third or sellar type, pneumatization advances beyond the tuberculum sella in 90% of cases and is completely underneath the sella in 20% of cases and posterior to the sella in 10% of cases.

Pneumatization may extend laterally into the lesser and greater wings of the sphenoid and the basilar process of the occipital bone, but this is uncommon. Of the three single cavity sinuses, the sphenoid is most likely to have an irregular internal configuration. Incomplete septi and various recesses are common (12).

CONCLUSION

A thorough knowledge of embryology of the paranasal region is important for several reasons. First, this knowledge is quite useful in the accurate evaluation and management of congenital lesions. In addition, understanding the embryology and the embryologic anatomy aids in the understanding of the initiation and progression of inflammatory diseases, as well as the likely presenting symptoms and direction of spread of neoplastic diseases.

REFERENCES

1. Hamilton WJ, Mossman HW, eds. *Human embryology,* 4th ed. Baltimore: Williams & Wilkins, 1972;291–376.
2. Schaeffer JP. *The nose, paranasal sinuses, nasal lacrimal passages, & olfactory organ in man.* New York: McGraw-Hill, 1920.
3. Zimmerman AA. Development of the paranasal sinuses. *Arch Otolaryngol* 1938;27:793–795.
4. Libersa C, Laude M, Libersa JC. The pneumatization of the accessory cavities of the nasal fossa during growth. *Anat Clin* 1981;2:265–278.
5. Caffey J. *Pediatric x-ray diagnosis.* Chicago: Year Book Medical Publishers, 1967.
6. Van Alyea OE. *Nasal sinuses: an anatomic and clinical consideration,* 2nd ed. Baltimore: Williams & Wilkins, 1951.
7. Maresh MM. Paranasal sinuses from birth to late adolescence. *Am J Dis Child* 1940;60:58–75.
8. Shapiro R, Janzen AH. *The normal skull: a Rankin study.* New York: Paul B Hoeer, 1960.
9. Kasper KA. Nasal frontal connections. A study based on 100 consecutive dissections. *Arch Otolaryngol* 1936;23:322–343.
10. Gos CM. *Anatomy of the human body by Henry Gray.* Philadelphia: Lea & Febiger, 1975;179.
11. Lang J. *Clinical anatomy of the nose, nasal cavity & paranasal sinuses.* New York: G Thieme Verlag, 1989;88.
12. Hammer G, Radberg C. Sphenoidal sinus: anatomical and rhinologic study with reference to transsphenoidal hypophysectomy. *Acta Radiol* 1961;56:401–422.

CHAPTER 3

Anatomy and Histology

Paul J. Donald

ANATOMY

The secret to understanding the pathophysiology and management of sinus disease is the detailed comprehension of paranasal sinus anatomy. Surgical resections of all forms of sinus disease are clearly unsafe without an intimate familiarity with the anatomy and immediate relations of the sinuses. Since most of the sinuses develop as pneumatizations of solid bones, the extent of this process is highly variable between individuals. This is true even between sides of the same person. It is this high degree of variability that makes sinus surgery so difficult, especially considering the number of vital structures that abut them.

Before a detailed description of the nasal sinus anatomy is begun, a word of admonition is probably appropriate. With the rise in enthusiasm of endoscopic sinus surgery and the resultant plethora of subsequent complications it has engendered, it becomes patently and painfully obvious that the understanding of sinus anatomy among many practitioners is certainly less than optimal. Our forefathers in otolaryngology were traditionally well-versed in anatomy, a product of an enlightened time when subjects such as anatomy, pathology, and physiology formed the basis for the study of medicine in the undergraduate curriculum. The modern otolaryngologist, a victim of revisionist philosophy in modern basic medical education, begins specialty training with a rudimentary understanding of head and neck anatomy. The understanding of paranasal sinus anatomy with its high degree of variability and intimate relations to vital structures requires intensive study and comprehensive understanding. This is best acquired, as Vesalius stated, "not by books but by dissection do I propose to learn anatomy" and certainly not by weekend courses. This stinging invective is probably offensive to the young practitioner who may feel unnecessarily chided by my somewhat opinionated

vitriolic stance. Fortunately, in these modern times, there is a wealth of outstanding educational materials by which one can learn and appreciate the complexity of sinus anatomy. Superlative books of anatomy, videotapes, dissection courses, and self-instructional aids abound. These are an immense resource, but none can supplant the information and experience gained by dissection. A clear three-dimensional construct of the sinuses and their relations can only be definitively acquired by this modality of learning.

The embryology and development of the sinuses is comprehensively treated in the chapter, Embryology, by Rice. Only adult anatomy is described in this chapter.

The sinuses are the result of a mysterious process by which solid facial skeletal elements are invaded by respiratory mucosa and are thus pneumatized. The trigger for this process and its mechanism are a complete enigma.

The sinuses are lined by respiratory mucosa, which, although appearing histologically similar, has varying behavior when altered by a disease process. This is especially true of the frontal sinus. Whether this is a product of the anatomical conditions peculiar to each sinus or the result of the inherent nature of the mucosa itself remains unclear.

The sinuses are composed of the maxillary, ethmoid, frontal, and sphenoid sinuses (Fig. 1). The ethmoids are traditionally divided into anterior and posterior groups divided by the grand lamina of the middle turbinate. They are generally named for the bones they primarily pneumatize. The drainage ostia empty into the recesses of the lateral wall of the nose.

Maxillary Sinus

Although the current emphasis in the pathophysiology of sinus disease is on the ethmoidal sinuses, tradi-

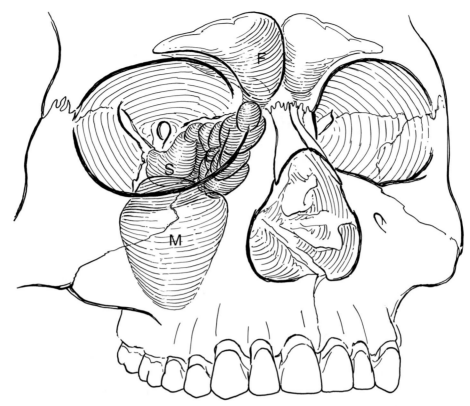

FIG. 1. Paranasal sinuses. M, maxillary; E, ethmoid; F, frontal; S, sphenoid.

tionally the maxillary sinus has been considered to be the keystone structure in most paranasal sinus disease processes. The maxillary sinus is the end result of pneumatization of the maxillary bone. To a variable and not necessarily symmetrical extent, the sinus occupies a key position in the central face.

Table 1 shows the average width and height of the

maxillary sinus through the various ages of development (1,2). According to Lang (1) the average length of the right sinus is 38.4 mm and the left 39.1 mm. The average width of the right is 26.2 mm and the left 26.9 mm (Fig. 2). The sinus sits as a six-sided box with its walls facing in six different directions (Fig. 3).

The maxillary bone and laterally articulating zygoma

TABLE 1. *Maxillary sinus measurements*

	Mean size		Minimal size		Maximal size		
Age	Width (mm)	Height (mm)	Width (mm)	Height (mm)	Width (mm)	Height (mm)	*n*
0–12 months	12	12.5	7	8	17	17	28
13–18 months	13	13.5	7	10	19	19	48
19–24 months	16	16	9	10	20	22	54
3 years	18	18	14	12	29	24	110
4 years	19.5	19.5	14	14	27	27	98
5 years	20.5	20	14	14	27	27	157
6 years	21.5	22	15	14	31	29	147
7 years	22.5	23	17	19	31	29	98
8 years	23	24	18	19	31	30	72
9 years	25	26.5	18	20	31	30	48
10 years	27	27	19	19	31	33	48
11 years	28	29	20	21	32	33	38
12 years	28	29	21	22	34	35	18
13 years	28	30	22	26	34	35	12
14 years	28.5	30	22	27	35	38	24
Roof segment in adults	26.4	40.4	10.1	29.3	39.8	56.9	50

From ref. 1, with permission.

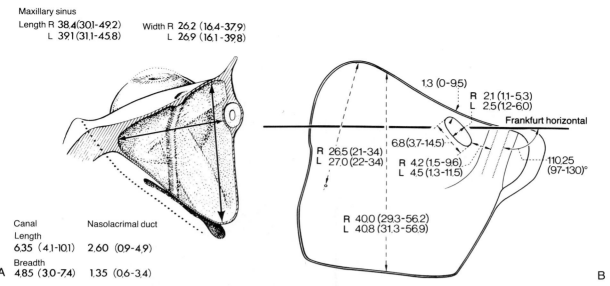

Maxillary sinus
Length R 38.4 (30.1-49.2)   Width R 26.2 (16.4-37.9)
       L 39.1 (31.1-45.8)   L 26.9 (16.1-39.8)

1.3 (0-9.5)

R 2.1 (1.1-5.3)
L 2.5 (1.2-6.0)

Frankfurt horizontal

R 26.5 (21-34)   6.8 (3.7-14.5)
L 27.0 (22-34)   R 4.2 (1.5-9.6)
                  L 4.5 (1.3-11.5)

110.25 (97-130)°

R 40.0 (29.3-56.2)
L 40.8 (31.3-56.9)

Canal   Nasolacrimal duct
Length
6.35 (4.1-10.1)   2.60 (0.9-4.9)
Breadth
A 4.85 (3.0-7.4)   1.35 (0.6-3.4)   B

FIG. 2. A: Cross-sectional view showing length and width of the sinus ostium. **B:** Parasagittal view showing height. Also shown are distances from the entry of posterosuperior alveolar nerve to orbital roof and average width of the sinus ostium. (From ref. 1, with permission.)

are pneumatized by the sinus. In general, the anterior walls, the roof, and occasionally the medial floor are thin. The posterior wall, lateral superior wall, and most of the floor are thick (Fig. 4). The floor of the sinus lays mainly over the alveolar ridge. This is a thick bone, mostly cancellous, that holds the upper dentition. It is pneumatized, often varying with skull configuration. To a variable degree, the medial floor overlies the hard palate. The sinus may even occasionally extend to within a few millimeters of the midline. The sinus's greatest pneumatization over the hard palate is midway in the anterior–posterior direction. The first molar tooth is the tooth that most commonly has a dehiscent root in the sinus floor. According to Lange (1), dehiscences are seen over the first molar in 2.2% of cases and over the second molar in 2%. Perforations of the antral floor may also be present over the second premolar as well as the third molar tooth. These osseous dehiscences produce a vulnerability to the nourishing neurovascular bundle of these teeth. In addition, this situation sets the stage for possible antral–oral fistula formation following dental extraction.

The pneumatization extends laterally into the body of the zygoma to a varying degree as well as posteriorly into the palatine bone (Fig. 5). The pneumatization of the zygoma is an important consideration in maxillectomy. Those patients with extensive pneumatization often require a resection that will include a considerable amount of the malar eminence producing a more severe type of cosmetic deformity. The vertical process of the palatine bone makes up a variable portion of the posterior–medial wall and sometimes a part of the posterior wall of the sinus.

Complete and incomplete septations of the sinus may exist and they may be in the vertical or horizontal plane (Fig. 6). A complete septation exists in about 1% to 2.5% of cases. Frontal lobulations descending from the sinus roof may be seen. Rugae in the floor of the sinus as well as bony ridges occurred in 56% of cases in Lang's (1) material. They averaged 7.8 mm high and 2.9 mm thick. In 10%, the ridges were more than 13 mm tall.

Separate or distinct duplication of the maxillary sinus may occur on either side. This type of duplication was seen in 6% of Lang's series (1), and for the most part the duplicated sinus emptied into the middle meatus posteriorly to the ethmoidal bulla and in another a posterior duplication emptied above the middle turbinate into the superior meatus. This probably represents a so-called Haller's cell, which is part of the ethmoid sinus bloc. Hypoplasia and rarely frank aplasia of the maxillary sinus may occur. In the hypoplastic sinus, the medial wall may be exceptionally thick (Fig. 7).

The floor of the sinus, as previously mentioned, descends to a varying degree into the alveolar ridge of the maxilla. This proceeds as the individual develops from childhood to adulthood. As it does so, it may descend below the level of the floor of the nose. The floor of the sinus is lower than the nasal floor in 26% of patients, at the same level in 28%, and above it in 6%. The next commonest scenario is the floor of the sinus below anteriorly and at the same level posteriorly. In the dentulous maxilla, there is usually a substantial amount of alveolar bone. Once the teeth are lost, the alveolar bone absorbs to a large degree, especially if a denture is not worn. The radiograph in Fig.

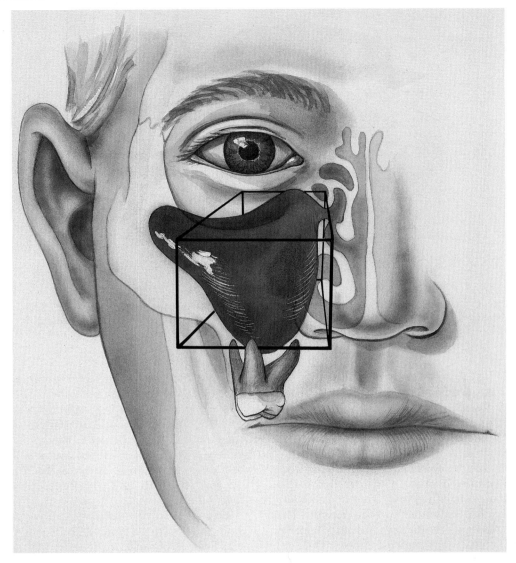

FIG. 3. Relationships of the maxillary sinus: the six-sided box concept (see text).

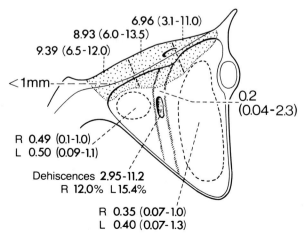

6.96 (3.1-11.0)
8.93 (6.0-13.5)
9.39 (6.5-12.0)
<1mm
0.2 (0.04-2.3)
R 0.49 (0.1-1.0)
L 0.50 (0.09-1.1)
Dehiscences 2.95-11.2
R 12.0% L 15.4%
R 0.35 (0.07-1.0)
L 0.40 (0.07-1.3)

FIG. 4. Transverse section showing orbital floor. Areas of orbital floor and percentage of dehiscence are illustrated.

8 shows an extreme case in which sensation in both jaws was lost from injury to both of the fifth nerves secondary to severe head trauma. A scant paper-thin layer of bone is all that remains of the maxillary alveolar ridge.

The curvilinear lateral wall of the sinus is very thin inferiorly. Traversing it are the anterior, posterior, and middle superior alveolar neurovascular bundles (Fig. 9), which supply the upper dentition. The nerves come from the infraorbital nerve and the arteries from the internal maxillary. The posterior superior alveolar nerve leaves the maxillary nerve just before it enters the infraorbital groove to become the infraorbital nerve, passes over the maxillary tuberosity in the infratemporal fossa, then enters the posterior alveolar canal to supply the distal teeth. It may take origin as one or two trunks. The middle branch is not constant and like the anterior–superior alveolar artery emanates from

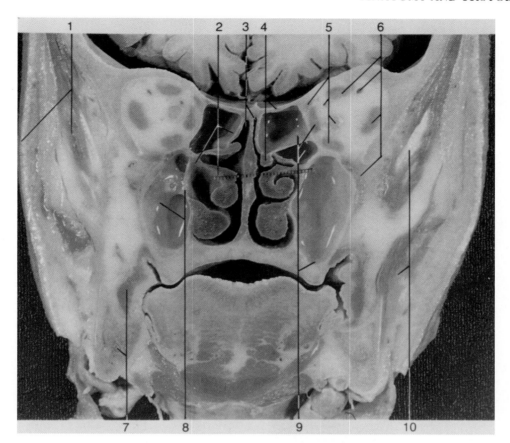

FIG. 5. Pneumatization of maxillary sinus over the hard palate. Note the difference in area of ethmoid exposed to maxillary sinus between sides. 1, Skin and temporalis muscle; 2, middle nasal concha with connections to the orbit and the sphenoidal plane, with a millimeter strip; 3, domes of the nasal cavity of unequal width; 4, sphenoidal plane and superior nasal concha; 5, superior oblique muscle, optic nerve, inferior rectus muscle, and ophthalmic artery; 6, superior rectus muscle, ophthalmic vein, lateral rectus muscle, and orbitalis muscle; 7, buccinator muscle and inferior alveolar nerve in an edentulous mandibula; 8, posterior wall of the maxillary sinus, and a large accessory ostium; 9, ethmoidal cells, medial rectal muscle, and a deep floor of the maxillary sinus; 10, tendon of the temporalis muscle and masseter muscle. (From ref. 1, with permission.)

the infraorbital, the former from the infraorbital groove and the latter from the infraorbital canal near the foramen. They travel in their own bony canals to supply the roots of the teeth. The neurovascular bundles track partly in bone and partially in the submucosa of the maxillary sinus lining. These vessels and nerves form loose interconnected arcades within the alveolar bone and supply the teeth.

Superiorly, the maxillary sinus wall merges with the malar process of the zygoma, the latter being extremely thick and strong. This bone emits the zygomaticofrontal and zygomaticofacial nerves, which have come from the zygomatic nerve, a direct branch of the maxillary in the pterygomaxillary fissure, and have entered the lateral orbital wall via the inferior orbital fissure. The lacrimal nerve is joined by a branch of the zygomaticofacial nerve, which carries off the autonomic fi-

bers from the vidian nerve destined for the lacrimal gland.

The roof of the maxillary sinus is the floor of the orbit. The roof slants inferiorly as one moves in a medial to lateral direction and the floor is convex into the cavity of the maxillary sinus to accommodate the curvature of the globe. The infraorbital nerve crosses the floor to exit the maxillary face via the infraorbital foramen. The canal for the infraorbital nerve is dehiscent in 14% of patients. (For details of the floor and infraorbital nerve, see the chapter, Fractures of the Zygoma, by Donald).

The anterior face of the sinus extends from the orbital rim to the teeth and is pierced superiorly by the infraorbital nerve. Its thinnest part is just above the canine tooth, the so-called canine fossa.

The posterior wall of the sinus is often comprised of

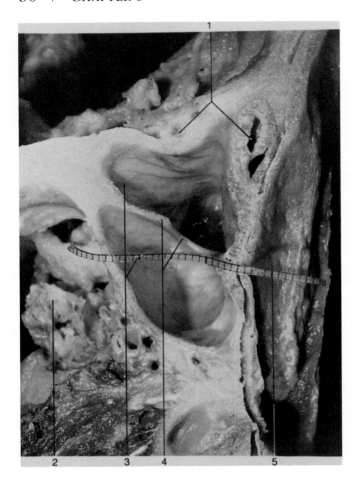

FIG. 6. Vertical septation of maxillary sinus, seen in horizontal section from below. (From ref. 1, with permission.)

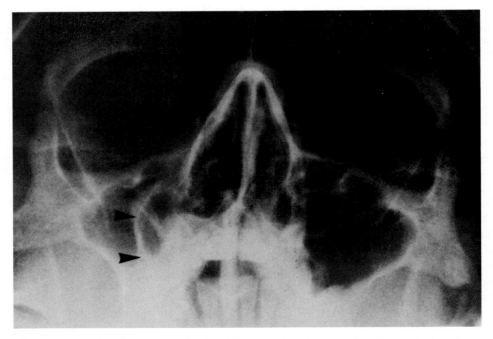

FIG. 7. Computer-assisted tomography (CAT) scan showing marked hypoplasia of maxillary sinus. *Arrows* point to displaced medial antral wall. (From ref. 3, with permission.)

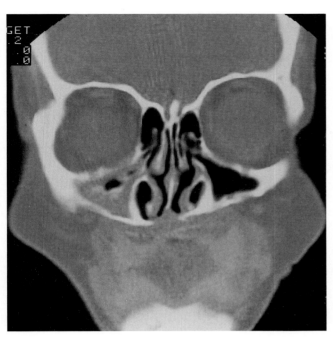

FIG. 8. Coronal CAT scan showing extremely thin bone of upper alveolar ridge.

skeletal elements other than the maxilla. The palatine bone inferiorly and occasionally the sphenoid make up this triangular shaped wall. The pterygoid plates articulate through a synostosis with the palatine bone inferiorly and then separate superiorly forming the pterygomaxillary fossa (Fig. 10).

The medial wall of the sinus, of all its confines, is the most complex. It forms the inferior aspect of the lateral wall of the nose. Contained within it is the nasolacrimal duct (described in detail in the chapter, Maxillary Fractures, by Donald). The exit of this duct is approximately 1 cm from the pyriform rim. The ostium of the maxillary antrum is traditionally described emptying into the posterior aspect of the hiatus semilunaris. In Lang's series, only 2% were located in the posterior quarter, 49% in the second quarter, 28% in the third quarter, and 22% in the anterior. A more recent investigation by Lang and Bressel (4) shows an equal distribution in each of the three most posterior quarters and none in the anterior (Fig. 11). According to Draf (5), the configuration of the ostium may be slit-like or triangular, especially in disease. Zuckerkandl (6) describes it as elliptical with its long axis in the sagittal plane, but in most instances, in the healthy individual, it is

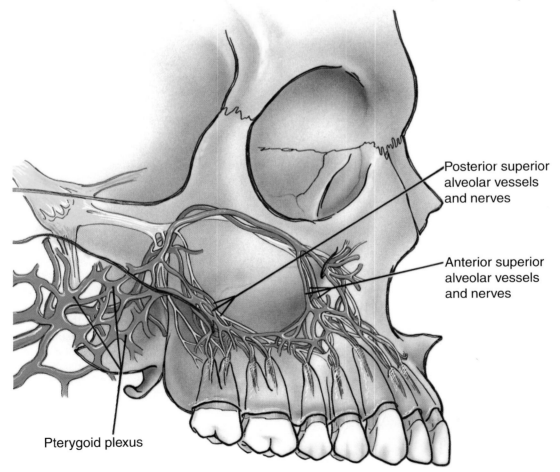

Posterior superior alveolar vessels and nerves

Anterior superior alveolar vessels and nerves

Pterygoid plexus

FIG. 9. Blood supply to the upper teeth via the maxillary sinus.

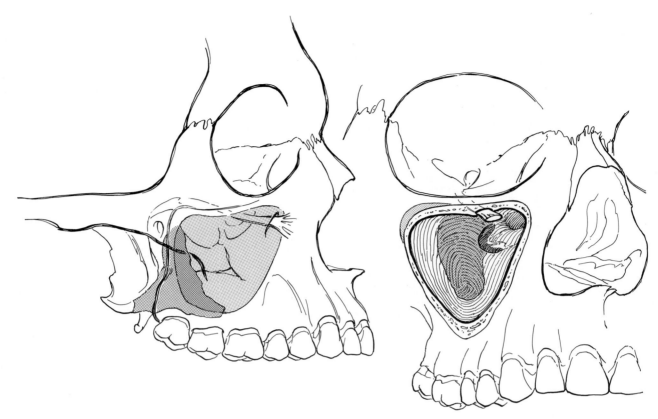

FIG. 10. Posterior wall of maxillary sinus.

round or oval in shape. The ostium, according to Zuck-erkandl (6), usually measures from 7 to 11 mm long and 2 to 6 mm high. The material in Lang's dissection revealed diameters as listed in Fig. 11. The ostium is considered a duct or canal if it is longer than 3 mm. Simon (7) classified the maxillary antral egress as a

canal in 83% of cases and an ostium in 17%. The percentage of osteal declination in an anterior–inferior versus a posterior–inferior direction is illustrated in Fig. 11.

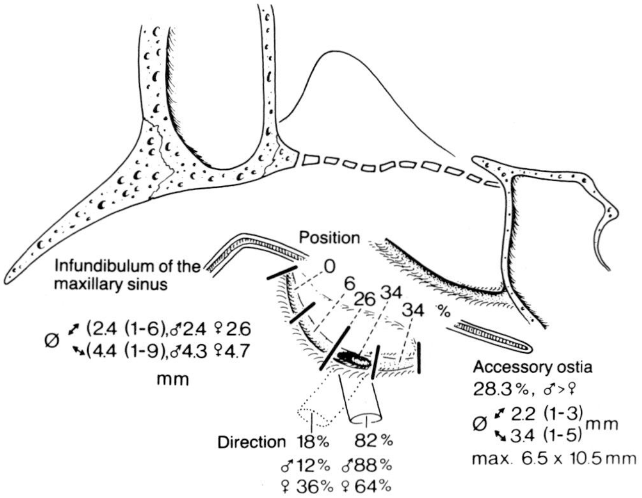

The bony osteal size is usually quite substantial but the mucosal covering may narrow it markedly. Mucosal bands may cross it, producing what appears to be two ostia. As illustrated in Fig. 11, Lang (1) found accessory ostia in 28% of cases. Other authors have reported an incidence as low as 15% and as high as 40% (8,9). These ostia are usually small holes in thin membranes that cover natural bony dehiscences in the middle meatus called fontanelles. The mucosa in some patients can be seen to move in and out with respiration. The primary ostia are located an average of 1.6 mm from the superior extent of the sinus and approximately 4 mm posterior to the nasolacrimal duct (see the chapter, Frontal and Ethmoid Complex Fractures, by Donald). Bolger et al. (10) have shown that the wall of the duct is in common with the edge of the natural sinus ostium and Calhoun et al. (11) found the average distance to the duct to be 9 ± 3 mm with a range from 1.8 to 18 mm. Thus the duct is clearly in jeopardy when the back biter is used in endoscopic sinus surgery.

The anatomical relations of the maxillary sinus provide the mechanism of manifestation of the manifold disease processes that afflict the sinuses. The relation-

FIG. 11. Lateral wall of nose illustrating maxillary sinuses and declinations, ostia sizes and declinations. (From ref. 1, with permission.)

ship of the floor of the sinus to the maxillary teeth and roof of the oral cavity has already been described.

The lateral and anterior walls are related to the soft tissues of the middle one-third of the face. The fat pad of Bichat lies adjacent to the lateral sinus wall with posterosuperior extensions into the infratemporal fossa. It is covered by a facial layer and is notably prominent in infants. This prominence is thought to aid the infant in sucking and is sometimes called the suctorial pad. Subcutaneous fat, a few facial mimetic muscles, and the skin of the face form the remainder of the immediate relations of this wall.

The posterior wall is related to the overlying pterygoid plates inferiorly and posterosuperiorly to the pterygomaxillary space. The medial and lateral pterygoid muscles take origin on the plates and are intimately related to the posterior wall of the sinus. The internal maxillary artery passes through both heads of the lateral pterygoid muscle to gain the pterygomaxillary space. The maxillary branch of the trigeminal nerve enters the space via foramen rotundum, leading from the floor of the middle cranial fossa. Medial and inferior to it, the vidian nerve enters this space through the pterygoid canal, a foramen in the sphenoid bone traversing the anterior wall of the foramen lacerum. This nerve carries parasympathetic fibers from the greater superficial petrosal nerve and sympathetic fibers from the internal carotid artery plexus. Its parasympathetic fibers synapse within the sphenopalatine ganglion, which is subtended from the maxillary nerve. The nerve beyond this point becomes a mixed nerve, carrying sensory and autonomic fibers to the nasal cavities, nose, ocular adnexa, and face.

The superior wall of the sinus is related to the globe. The details of this relationship are most clearly outlined in the chapters, Sinusitis by Gluckman and Fractures of the Zygoma by Donald. The antral roof—and thus the orbital floor—is the thinnest wall of the orbit and the most vulnerable to trauma. It is obliquely crossed in its lateral one-third by the infraorbital canal containing the infraorbital nerve. The medial aspect of the roof is the floor of one or more ethmoid cells. The contribution to these cells is wider behind than anteriorly.

Ethmoid Sinuses

The ethmoid bloc is the most complex of the sinuses. It often appears to be the pivotal sinus in the pathophysiology of sinus inflammatory disease. The ethmoid labyrinth is well suited to its name. A series of air cells comprised of thin plates of bone lined with respiratory mucosa, each with its own individual ostium, makes up the complex. The cells occupy the area between the orbit and the lateral wall of the nose and between the anterior cranial fossa superiorly and the maxillary sinus inferiorly. The ethmoid bone has a curious configuration. Figure 12 illustrates in diagrammatic form the various components of this fascinating structure. Most of the bony plates are thin and lightweight. The lateral wall of the sinus, the lamina papyracea, is a paper-thin bone that also makes up most of the medial wall of the orbit. The medial wall of the sinus forms the lateral wall of the nose and provides the attachment of the middle turbinate. A horizontal plate of bone (the cribriform plate) connects the ethmoid bloc of one side to its fellow on the opposite side. There are two central vertically disposed midline processes. The superior process is the crista galli; and the inferior is the perpen-

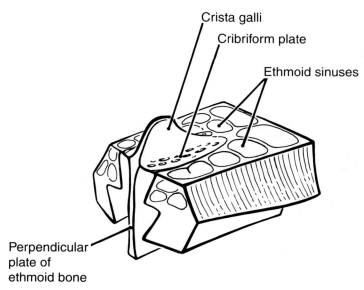

Crista galli

Cribriform plate

Ethmoid sinuses

Perpendicular plate of ethmoid bone

FIG. 12. Block diagram illustrating the ethmoid complex.

dicular plate of the ethmoid, which makes a substantial contribution to the nasal septum.

The sinuses are roughly divided into an anterior and posterior group, depending on which meatus they empty into. The anterior group empties into the middle meatus and the posterior into the superior meatus.

The bloc measures 4 to 5 cm in length and 2.5 to 3 cm in height. The width is narrower anteriorly, usually around 0.5 cm; and wider posteriorly, about 1.5 cm. The labyrinth of each side may have as few as 4 cells, but as many as 17. The usual number of cells is between 7 and 11 (12). In Van Alyea's dissections, 72% of specimens fell into this latter group.

Anterior cells tend to be smaller and the posterior ones larger. The cell of Onodi is a large posterior ethmoid cell that invades the anterior–superior aspect of the sphenoidal sinus. It is sometimes mistaken for the sphenoidal sinus itself, but invariably there will be a sphenoidal sinus below it.

The cells have been classified according to their location in relation to fixed anatomical features. An understanding of the anatomy of the lateral wall of the nose is integral to this classification (Fig. 13). There are three turbinates that are constant—inferior, middle, and superior—and one that is inconstant—the supreme turbinate. A supreme turbinate was found in 67% of skulls in Van Alyea's series (12) and there were 38% of speci-

mens with ostia emptying into the supreme meatus. Beneath each turbinate is a meatus named after the overlying turbinate. Each turbinate is comprised of a thin hollow conchal bone covered in a thick mucosa. In the submucosal tissue is a rich network of cavernous blood vessels whose histology is similar to the corpora cavernosa of the genitalia.

The inferior meatus is the site of egress of the nasolacrimal duct. The superior meatus is the exit point of the ostia of the posterior and the supreme meatus is the exit point of the ostia of the postreme cells. Most of the complexity of the lateral wall of the nose is concentrated in the middle meatus. With the middle turbinate removed, the anatomy becomes apparent (Fig. 14). The middle turbinate attachment forms an inverted V-shape starting from superior to inferior in the anterior–posterior direction (13). A J-shaped curvilinear groove called the hiatus semilunaris extends from the point of exit of the frontonasal duct to a flattened-out area posterior to the limit of the middle turbinate. At the anterior limit of the hiatus semilunaris is the infundibulum of the frontonasal duct. The level of this structure is the midpupillary line. Beneath the hiatus semilunaris is a stout, flat, strong piece of bone called the uncinate process, an important anatomical landmark. Superior to the hiatus is the ethmoidal bulla, a laterally bulging bubble-like piece of bone with exiting foramina

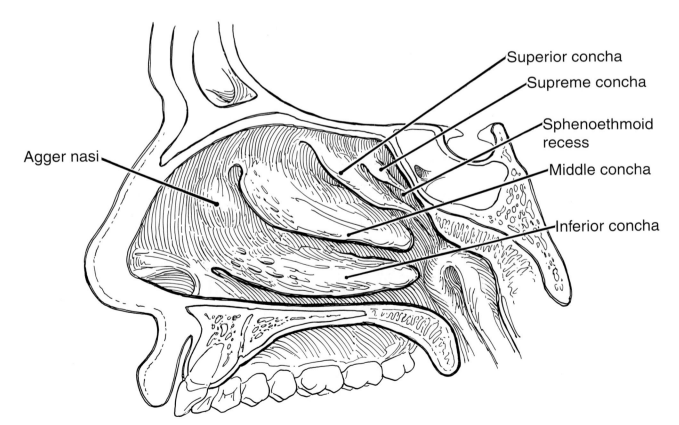

FIG. 13. Lateral wall of the nose.

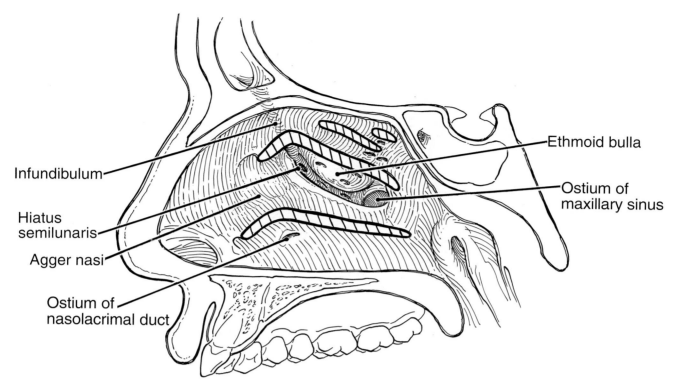

FIG. 14. The turbinates are removed and the meatus exposed.

of the "bullar cells" pock-marking its surface. In 30% of Lang's material, the bulla was not aerated and was a solid bone. In such instances, this was called the lateral torus by Grünwald (14). The bullar cells may be highly developed and extend behind the posterior cells to encroach on the sphenoid sinus or extend anteriorly to involve the infundibulum.

Posterior to the superior meatus, and to a much less degree the middle meatus, is the sphenoethmoidal recess. This is a common drainage area for the sphenoidal sinus and the posterior ethmoid cells (Fig. 15). The air cells have been classified by Mosher (15) and Van Alyea (12) into various groups in order to provide some order and ease of understanding of their arrangement and location. Table 2 describes Van Alyea's classification. This taxonomy assigns the various cellular groups according to their points of exit.

A few of the cell groups require special consideration. The agger nasi groups are located anteriorly to the uncinate process. Van Alyea stated that this group is the most anteriorly located and most consistent of all the cells. They are bounded posteriorly by the uncinate process and the bone anteroinferiorly to it, and laterally by the lacrimal bone and the ascending process of the maxilla (16). It lies just anterior and anterosuperiorly to the anterior attachment of the middle turbinate. Although in the early 1900s investigators reported these cells to be present in 40% to 50% of cases, in modern times they are reported to be present in almost 100% of cases (17–19). The word "agger" means "ridge" and as such is described by Mattox and Delaney (13) to represent a vestigial turbinate. Indeed, Arey (20) describes the origin of the conchae (hence turbinates) from the so-called turbinals. The agger nasi is said to arise from the "nasoturbinal," which is a rudimentary structure compared to the others. The number and extent of cells are highly variable and may even invade the nasal bones and frontal process of the maxilla. The cells usually number between one and four.

The middle concha itself is often highly pneumatized. A very large air cell may cause excessive ballooning of the middle turbinate and cause nasal obstruction. This called a concha bullosa (Fig. 16).

Usually there are one to four bullar cells that empty into the hiatus semilunaris or into a groove above the bulla called the suprabullar furrow.

An inconstant number of cells of highly variable size are grouped around the egress from the frontal sinus. These are called the frontoethmoidal cells, the frontal recess cells, and, those that then also course over the roof of the orbit, the orbital ethmoid cells. As described by Van Alyea (12), these are suprainfundibular and suprabullar in location. These cells usually drain into the infundibulum and the area of the frontal recess, which is the expanded fluted end of the frontonasal duct or ostium.

There are instances in which the ethmoid cells expand over the orbital roof and create a situation in

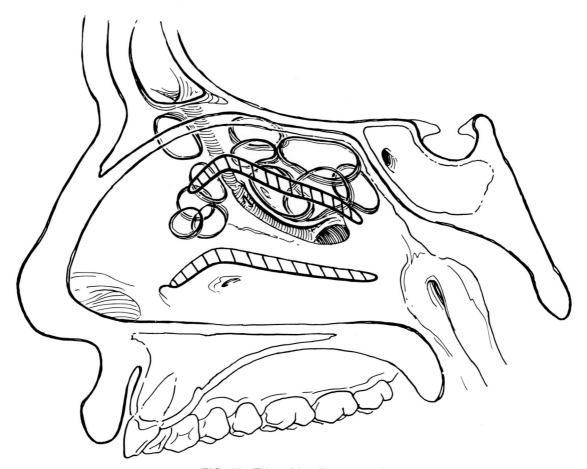

FIG. 15. Ethmoid cells exposed.

which they interpose themselves between the orbital roof and the frontal sinus floor. Indeed, the roof of the orbital ethmoid is often made up by the horizontal process of the frontal bone. Extensive development of the orbital cells precludes adequate exenteration by either endoscopic surgery or traditional intranasal eth-

TABLE 2. *Classification of ethmoidal cells*

I. Middle meatus
   A. Infundibular cells
      1. Agger nasi cells
      2. Terminal (tip) cells
      3. Suprainfundibular cells
      4. Inferior
   B. Bullar cells
      1. Bullar cells
      2. Suprabullar
      3. Haller's cells
II. Superior meatus
   A. Posterior cells
   B. Onodi cells
III. Supreme meatus
   A. Postreme cells

Adapted from ref. 12.

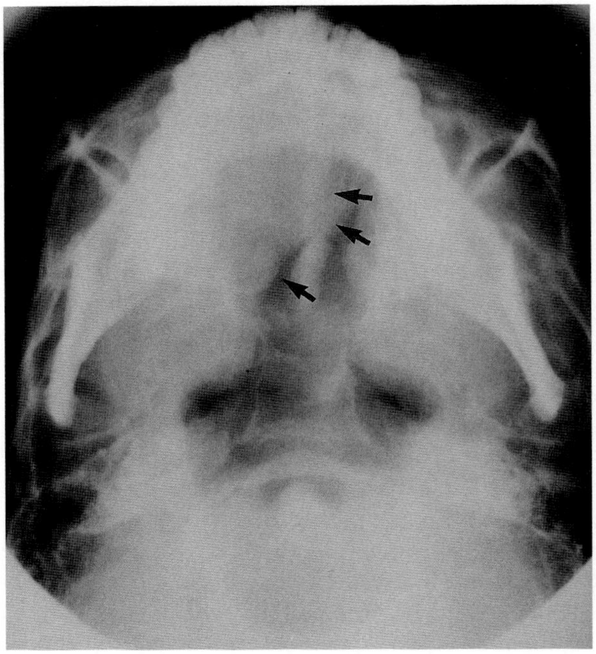

FIG. 16. Radiograph of concha bullosa. *Arrows* indicate fluid level within this massive air cell.

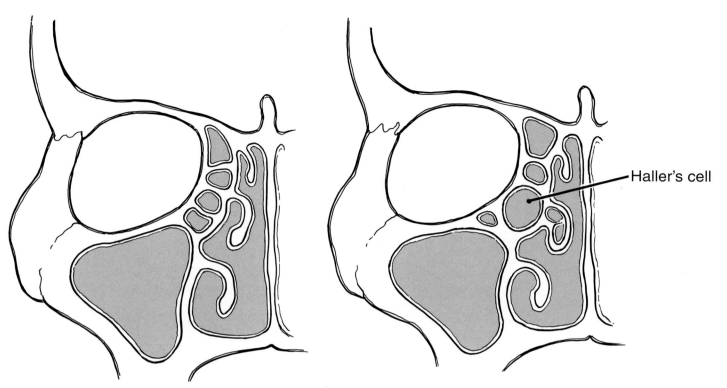

FIG. 17. Haller's cell within the attachment of the middle turbinate to the lateral nasal well *(arrow).*

moidectomy (21). The orbital cells can bulge into the lumen of the frontal sinus or even the region of the frontonasal duct, causing obstruction.

The posterior cells by definition drain into the superior meatus between the superior and middle turbinates. They usually number between two and six and tend to be larger than the anterior cells. Van Alyea (16) found the number to vary between 0 and 9 in his material. The drainage of these cells tends to be in the more anterior aspect of the meatus in a groove near the attachment of the superior turbinate (14).

The postreme cells empty into the supreme meatus above the superior turbinate and are commonly absent or number as many as only two or three. Van Alyea (12) found such cells in only 43% of his material. However, he did find one specimen with no posterior cells, but one immense postreme cell emptying into the superior meatus.

There are two groups of cells that deserve special consideration: the Haller's cells and the cell of Onodi. The Haller's cell (Fig. 17) arises from the attachment of the middle turbinate to the lateral wall of the nose. It abuts against the medial wall and floor of the orbit. It may extend inferiorly into the maxillary antrum and actually presents a more flattened widened bone between it, the antrum, and the overlying ethmoid bloc. The cells may be located in either or both of the anterior and posterior parts of the orbit. The Haller's cells

are often lateral to the infundibulum into which they drain.

The cell of Onodi is an enlarged expanded posterior ethmoidal cell that is located anterior and superior to the sphenoidal sinus. It has been found in 9% to 12% of anatomic material examined (16). This cell is separated from the sphenoid sinus below by a horizontal plate of bone. According to Lang, the Onodi cell comes about by virtue of the relationships of the ethmoid to the sphenoid bone during fetal life. As the anteriorly located ethmoid bone grows posteriorly and covers over the sphenoid bone in some cases, subsequent pneumatization creates the aforementioned relationship. This cell or surrounding cells surround the optic nerve and may extend to the anterior wall of the sella turcica (Fig. 18). The bone over the nerve is usually only about 0.5 mm thick. In 4% of cases, the wall is dehiscent (20).

Sphenoid Sinus

The sphenoidal sinus is a usually paired and asymmetrically developed pneumatization of the body of the sphenoid bone (Fig. 19). The sinus is in the geometric center of the head and is absent in only 1% to 1.5% of cases (14). Congdon (22) in 1920 divided the degree of pneumatization of the sphenoid sinus into three types: conchal, presellar, and postsellar (Fig. 20). The conchal type occurs when the sinus is very small, is situ-

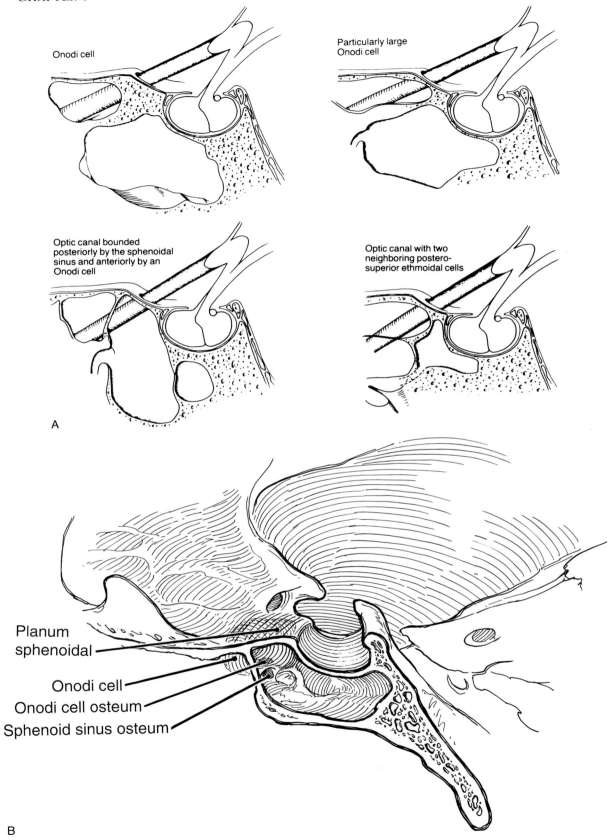

FIG. 18. A: Various types and configurations of Onodi cells that surround the optic nerve. **B:** Onodi cell relationship to sphenoidal sinus. (From ref. 1, with permission.)

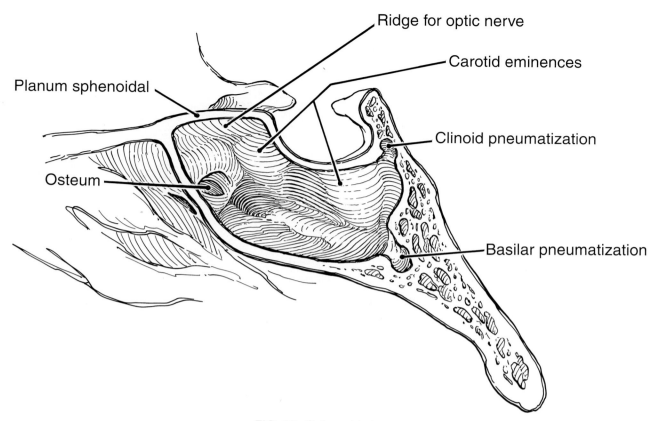

Planum sphenoidal

Ridge for optic nerve

Carotid eminences

Clinoid pneumatization

Osteum

Basilar pneumatization

FIG. 19. Sphenoid sinus.

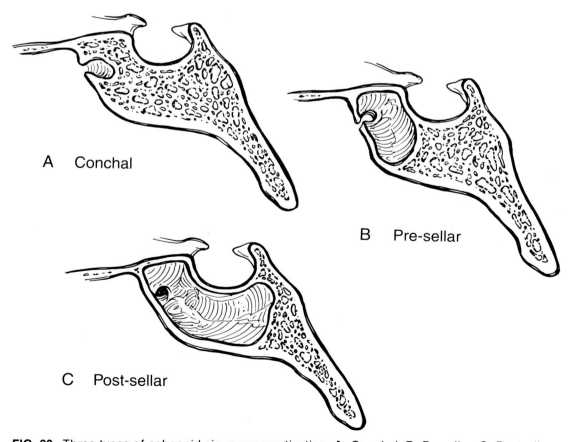

A   Conchal

B   Pre-sellar

C   Post-sellar

FIG. 20. Three types of sphenoid sinus pneumatization. **A:** Conchal. **B:** Presellar. **C:** Postsellar.

ated well in front of the sella turcica, and is separated from it by a significant thickness of bone. Presellar pneumatization has no indentation of the sella into the sphenoid sinus, whereas the sellar and postsellar does. In fact, in marked cases of postsellar pneumatization the bone between the brain stem and sinus can be exceedingly thin. Congdon found conchal pneumatization in only 9 (5%) of 181 specimens he dissected, presellar in 43 (23.5%), and postsellar in 121 (67%). There were 8 (4.5%) sinuses that were considered to be intermediate between conchal and presellar in type. Hammer and Radberg (23) reported the conchal type in 2.5%, presellar in 11%, "sellar" in 59%, and mixed types in 27%.

Schaeffer (24) reported the average volume of the sinus as 7.4 cm^3 and Dixon (25) with variations between 0 and 14 cm^3. According to Lang (1), the adult sinus averages 13.5 mm wide superiorly, 16.9 mm in the middle, and 18.7 mm in its lowest segment. The length averaged 19.4 mm in the upper part, 4.8 mm in the middle, and 18.5 mm in the lower. There was a high degree of variation found in each region dependent on the pattern of pneumatization and the presence or absence of an Onodi cell.

The intersinus septum of the sphenoid sinus is usually off the midline. A midline sinus is present in only 27% of cases. In 43% the sinus begins in the midline but deviates from the vertical, assuming an "S," "C," or other configuration as a posterior progression is made. Only 25% of cases have a completely vertical septum.

Accessory septations or grooves were found in 30% of 212 specimens dissected by Congdon (22) and 30% of 300 sphenoid sinuses examined by Cope (26). These septations are thought to arise from the synchondroses of the major fetal components of the sphenoid bone. These connections run in a transverse and longitudinal direction. A ridge or septum may arise as a vestige of the craniopharyngeal canal. During embryonic life, this was the connection of the hypophyseal diverticulum to the buccal ectoderm. As the two separate during development, this may persist as a ridge or septum between the presphenoid and basisphenoid of the developing bone (1,27). The separate sinuses created by these septations drain into the principal sinus (Fig. 21).

The well-pneumatized sphenoid sinus may have a multiplicity of recesses—areas of pneumatization that spread into contiguous bony structures. The septal recess, also called the sphenovomerine bulla, is a pneumatization of the rostrum of the sphenoid that spreads even into the vomer. This creates a central air cell in the posterior septum. The ethmoidal recess is a direct extension into the posterior ethmoid, most often into its posteroinferior part (1). Further ethmoidal extensions can extend into the orbit and maxilla. Extensions either superiorly or inferiorly to the optic nerve are

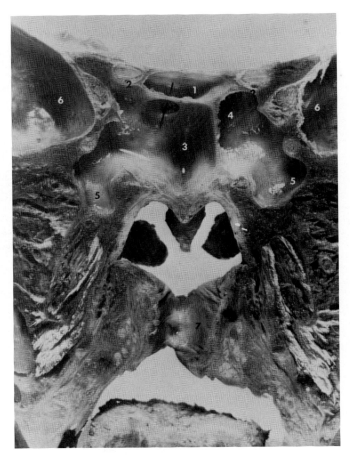

FIG. 21. Coronal section of head through sphenoidal sinus. 1, Accessory sphenoid sinus with ostium emptying into main sinus; 2, optic nerves; 3, sphenoid sinus proper; 4, pneumatization just above the origin of pterygoid plates. 5, pterygoid extension of sphenoid sinus; 6, greater wings of sphenoid; 7, congenital cleft of soft palate. (From ref. 29, with permission.)

among the most dangerous. Moreover, the optic nerve may be devoid of bone in these regions (Fig. 19). Pneumatization of the orbital process of the palatine bone can occur as an extension of the sphenoidal sinus. This is an uncommon situation and can occur also from an ethmoid cell or even as an extension of the maxillary sinus.

An inferolateral recess has been described as far as the greater wing of the sphenoid and even into the posterolateral wall of the orbit (28). The extension can reach as far as the foramen rotundum, foramen ovale, and the petrous apex (Fig. 22) (1,28). The pterygoid recess is very commonly seen. The sphenoid sinus extends laterally into the bone at the root of the pterygoid plates. It descends into the plates to various depths. This extension can reach as far as the eustachian tube.

The important features of the lateral sphenoidal sinus wall are extensively described in the chapter by Pearson. The bulges produced by the optic nerve, in-

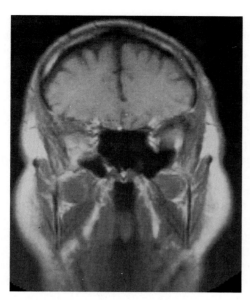

FIG. 22. CAT scan in coronal plane showing inferolateral sphenoid sinus recess reaching into the greater wing of the sphenoid. (From ref. 30, with permission.)

ternal carotid artery, vidian nerve, pituitary gland, and abducent and maxillary nerves are illustrated in the chapter by Pearson (Fig. 9).

The sphenoid sinus ostium usually empties into the sphenoethmoidal recess. The opening was round in 70% of specimens examined by Lang and averaged 3.4 mm in diameter (1). Ostia of pinhead size were seen 18% of the time. The opening was elliptical in 30% of cases. The opening usually is located in the upper one-third of the anterior wall of the sphenoid sinus, usually within a few millimeters of the cribriform plate. Rarely, it may empty at the level of the sinus floor. In Van Alyea's specimens, 30% were within 1 to 2 mm of the nasal septum and 50% were 3 mm or more beyond (12). This was vitally important at the time this monograph was published because of the common practice of sinus cannulation in the treatment of inflammatory disease. Rarely, the sinus may empty into an Onodi cell or other posterior ethmoid cell, and even more rarely in the root of the pterygoid process or the orbital process of the palatine bone.

Frontal Sinus

The frontal sinus is a pneumatization of the frontal bone that originates either by the development of a frontoethmoidal air cell that invades the frontal bone or as an upward extension of the infundibulum of the middle meatus of the nose. The development of the frontal sinus is relatively late. It is merely a dimple in the frontal bone at birth, pea-sized at three to four years of age, and generally does not extend higher than the eyebrows by 12 to 14 years of age. It is not fully

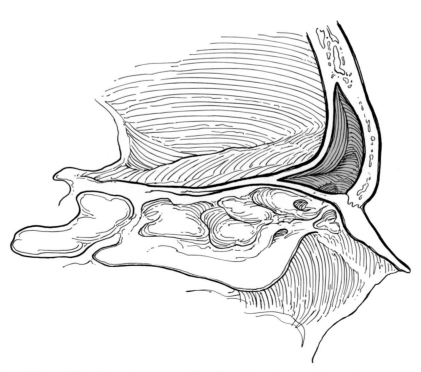

FIG. 23. Lateral view of the sinus demonstrating the triangular configuration and illustrating the feathered-out recesses that exist at the extremities of the sinus.

developed until age 16 to 18 in men and 12 to 14 in women (31). After the age of 6 to 8 years, the growth of the sinus exceeds that of the frontal bone itself. Arashi et al. (31) have demonstrated that the width and height of the sinus expand at approximately the same rate. The size of the frontal sinus is highly variable, ranging from a couple of cubic centimeters in volume to occupying most of the area of the frontal bone (Fig. 23). According to Millosslawski (32), the height varies from 5 to 66 mm with an average height of 24.3 mm. Lang and Haas (33) measured the lateral distance of the lateral wall from the midline and it was found to be 29 mm with a variation between 17 and 49 mm.

The configuration of the sinus is roughly triangular with the apex superior and the base inferior (Fig. 23). Most of the floor is made up by the orbital roofs. That portion of the floor that is located near the midline overlaps, in part, the fovea ethmoidalis and overlies the anterior ethmoidal sinus (Fig. 24). The most anterior aspect of the sinus floor is directly above the root of the nose and contains hardened, thickened bone. The orbital roof is thin, as is the posterior wall of the frontal sinus. Riding in the midline of the posterior wall and

facing anteriorly into the anterior cranial fossa is a thickened triangular ridge into which inserts the superior sagittal sinus (Fig. 25A). Arising in the frontal vein emanating from the foramen caecum, the sinus slowly enlarges in size as it ascends along the frontal spine on the inner surface of the calvarium. If this sinus is torn during frontal sinus fracture, it can be ligated along its length up to about the level of the coronal suture with little risk of developing neurological sequelae. Ligation beyond this point may produce quadriplegia or death (Fig. 25B).

The anterior wall of the sinus, especially inferiorly, is by far the strongest. There is a definite trilayered structure similar to the rest of the calvarium with an anterior and posterior table and intervening diploë to all of the walls of the sinus, although the diploë is scant in the posterior walls and floor (Fig. 26).

The extremities of the sinus become feathered out into very narrow crevices (Fig. 23). In some sinuses, this makes subsequent mucosal removal very difficult. This is especially true where the posterior wall and the floor of the sinus meet. The posterior wall curves from a vertical into a horizontal disposition to a varying degree depending on how much pneumatization of the

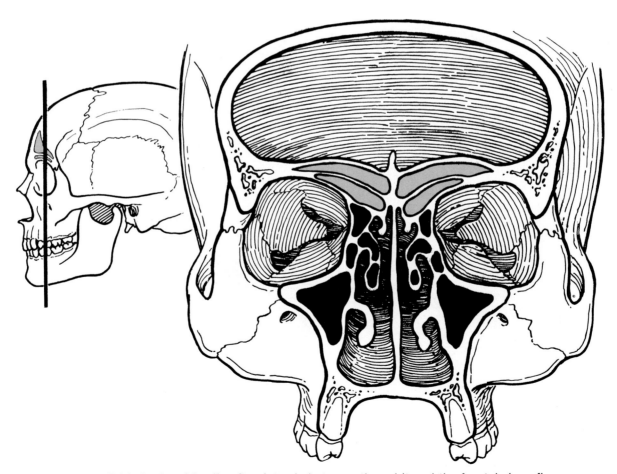

FIG. 24. Orbital ethmoid cells often intrude between the orbit and the frontal sinus floor.

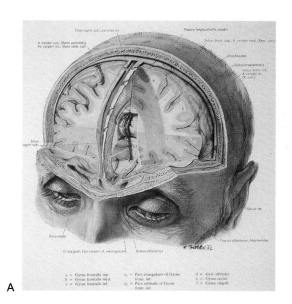

A

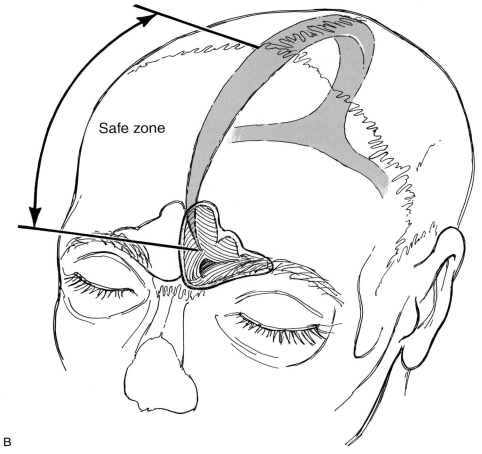

Safe zone

B

FIG. 25. A: Dissection of the anterior cranial fossa demonstrating the intimate relationship of the posterior wall of the frontal sinus to the superior sagittal sinus. B: Area of safety for ligation of the superior sagittal sinus.

orbital roots has occurred. Pneumatization all the way to the lesser wing of the sphenoid to the optic canal has been described (34). Witt (35) found that 40% of the skulls in his collection had duplication of the orbital roof, 23% of which were bilateral.

Frontal bullar cells are found in approximately 10%

to 20% of cases (1). These are superiorly extending ethmoid cells that pneumatize the orbital roof and project to a varying degree into the frontal sinus.

The sinus wall usually has a midline septum separating the cavity into two sides. Aplasia of the left frontal sinus was found by Novak and Mehls (36) in 3.6% of

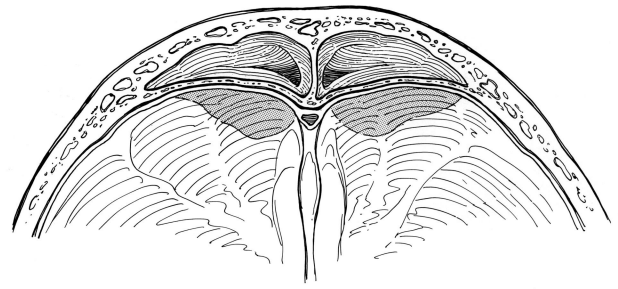

FIG. 26. Horizontal section of calvarium illustrating the paranasal sinuses. Note the thick arch configuration of the anterior frontal sinus wall and the thin posterior wall.

men and 2.8% of women. Complete aplasia of the sinus is found in 12% to 17% of Europeans. Curiously, aplasia is seen in 35% of other races, and in 52% of Eskimos (1). More than two frontal sinuses are very uncommon, found in 1.5% of sinuses by Boege (37), 10% by Onodi (38), and 3% in the material examined by Jovanovic (39). However, incomplete septations of various lengths extending from the roof of the sinus are not uncommon. These give the sinus its scalloped configuration.

The frontonasal duct leads from the anteromedial extent of the frontal sinus floor into the infundibulum of the middle meatus. The floor in this region funnels into the duct. The ducts are found on either side of the intersinus septum. Van Alyea in his review (12) indicated that the frontal sinus egress was in the form of an ostium rather than a duct that leads into the infundibulum in approximately 80% of cases. Lang (1), on the other hand, found the converse to be true. In his material, he found a duct in 77% of cases and an ostium in only 23%. The duct width averages 5.1 mm at its widest and 2 to 6 mm at its most narrow. The length of the duct averaged 6.2 mm, with a range of 3.2 to 14.9 mm. The duct may be associated with an ethmoidal or frontoethmoidal air cell on its way to the middle meatus.

HISTOLOGY

Although there are clear morphological similarities between the histology of the nasal cavities and the paranasal sinuses, there are numerous distinct differences. The nose and the sinuses are lined with a pseu-

dostratified columnar ciliated epithelium. The epithelium is comprised of a layer of basal cells, columnar cells, and goblet cells, all of which abut against the basement membrane (Fib. 27). The latter two reach the epithelial surface, whereas the basal cells do not. The columnar cells have both cilia and microvilli on their luminal surface. The goblet cells may or may not have microvilli, depending on their stage of secretion.

Salivary glands of the seromucinous type are seen submucosally under the basement membrane but are much more common in the nasal septum and turbinate mucosa and rare in the sinuses.

The mucosa of the nasal cavity is much thicker than that of the sinuses. It varies in histology with geographic location and anatomic variations with the nose. Dry squamous epithelium is found at the nares with hair follicles at the nasal verge. Seromucinous glands are more numerous in the mucosa near the choanae. Mucosa tends to be thin and dry over bony excrescences and outcroppings that are characteristically notable over the nasal septum and in the nasal valve area (40). A more plushy thick mucosa is found over the turbinates, especially their ends and in niches and recesses of the nose. Seromucinous glands are found in the sinuses almost exclusively around the sinus ostia and rarely on the walls (41,42).

Sinus mucosa is much thinner than that lining the rest of the nasal cavity. Epithelium tends to be lower; there are generally few goblet cells; and seromucinous glands are extremely scarce. The basement membrane is attenuated or not readily discernible and the laminae propria are often absent. The basic cells are columnar ciliated epithelial cells. They average 5 μm long and

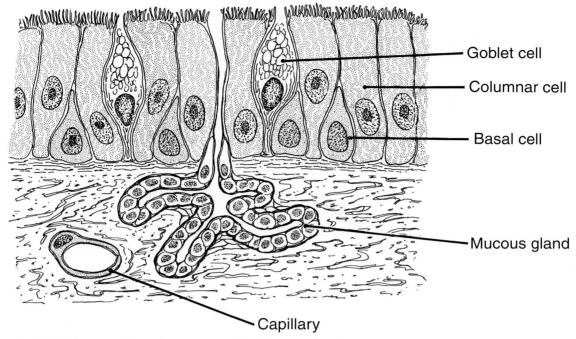

- Goblet cell
- Columnar cell
- Basal cell
- Mucous gland
- Capillary

FIG. 27. Drawing of cellular components of the nasal and sinus mucosa. Note that all cells reach the basement membrane.

0.2 μm thick and carry between 100 and 150 cilia on each luminal cell surface. Microvilli are much smaller, averaging around 1.5 μm long and 0.08 μm in diameter (Fig. 28) (43). Goblet cells are shorter except during the active phase of secretion. During rest, the cell surface is covered completely with microvilli and mea-

sures 1.5 μm in length and 0.08 μm in diameter (43). As mucus granules aggregate and coalesce, they rise to the cell surface, the microvilli disappear, and the mucus droplet begins to protrude from the cell surface (Fig. 29), connected to it only by a thin stalk. The cell then ruptures, discharges its contents, and

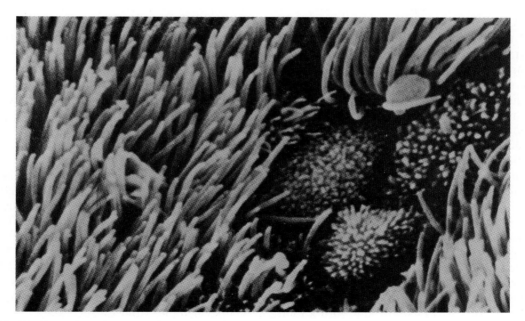

FIG. 28. Scanning electron micrograph of nasal mucosa showing cilia interspersed with patches of microvilli. (×8000). (From ref. 43, with permission.)

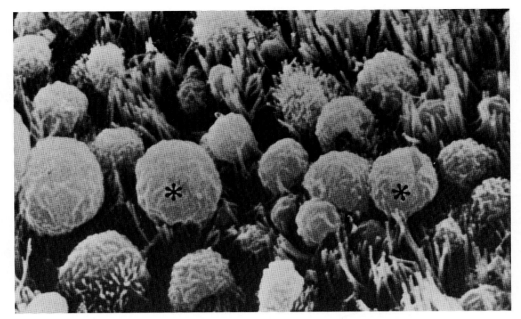

FIG. 29. Scanning electron micrograph of nasal mucosa depicting goblet cells. The *asterisks* denote mucus-secreting stage of cells. (×8000). (From ref. 43, with permission.)

then collapses only to be reborn as its cycle begins again.

The seromucinous glands are simple tubular or branched, somewhat flattened glands. They empty into a relatively short excretory duct that contains some goblet cells and into the lumen of the nose or sinus as a single or bifurcated duct. The glands are usually 100 to 200 μm thick, 0.6 to 1.2 mm long, and 0.8 to 1.5 mm wide (44).

Sinus mucosa is quite uniform in thickness for each sinus; 0.2 to 0.7 mm in the frontal and sphenoidal sinuses and 0.3 to 0.8 mm in the maxillary and ethmoid sinuses (42). In normal sinuses, the epithelium varies between 25 and 50 μm in thickness. The basement membrane is scant, the subepithelial layer is sparse and densely adherent to the underlying periosteum, making a true mucoperiosteum. In the narrow recesses of the sinuses, especially the extremities of the frontal sinuses, the mucosa is very thin with epithelial cells taking on a cuboidal character. The cells tend to be more widely dispersed and more loosely arranged than in the nose. There are fewer desmosomal contacts and there are long finger-like cytoplasmic interconnections between cells (45).

The density of seromucinous glands is strikingly different in the nasal mucosa compared to that in the sinuses. There are fewer than 50 in the frontal and sphenoidal sinuses and 50 to 100 in the ethmoid and maxillary sinuses. In marked contrast, the nasal mucosa has a density of 7 to 10 glands/mm² with a total of about 36,000 glands on the septum and turbinates (46,47). In addition, the serous glands have less zymo-

gen and fewer organelles. The mucous glands have smaller droplets, but with an increased tendency to coalesce and blend (45). Goblet cell density is markedly diminished as well when compared to the nasal cavity. Goblet cells are most dense in the ethmoid sinuses, but still 15 times less dense than in the nose (43). This fact was alluded to as far back as 1934 by Lotta and Schall (48). There are 9700 goblet cells/mm² in the maxillary sinus and 6000 cells/mm² in the frontal sinus (49). In the ethmoid sinuses, both seromucinous glands and goblet cells are far less dense in the posterior cells than the anterior cells. According to Tos et al. (44), some posterior cells have no goblet cells at all. This accounts for a much higher volume of mucous output from the nose than the sinuses. The capillaries of sinus mucosa have fewer fenestrae than nasal mucosa and thus have a lesser tendency to lose fluid and perhaps render the sinuses more prone to infection (45).

Although alluded to in the past, Torjussen et al. (50) were the first to describe metaplasia in nasal and sinus mucosa. The mucosa can go through the metaplastic steps of a pure stratified cuboidal epithelium, a mixed cuboidal and stratified squamous epithelium, and a true stratified squamous epithelium (Fig. 30). In the metaplastic process, one stage in the aforementioned sequence will naturally precede the next. These findings are encountered in normal individuals (43) but are also evident in increased numbers in individuals who have been chronically exposed to irritants such as dryness, chemical fumes, and tobacco smoke. Individuals are born with a set number of mucous glands, but portions of these will be replaced with the metaplastic process

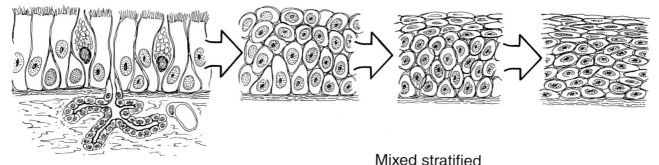

Pseudostratified ciliated columnar epithelium

Stratified cuboidal epithelium

Mixed stratified cuboidal stratified squamous epithelium

Stratified squamous epithelium

FIG. 30. Stages of metaplasia of respiratory mucosa in nose and sinuses.

that seems to increase with age. Over the age of 40 years, approximately 30% of people will have foci of metaplasia (43). Loss of pseudoepitheliomatous cell cilia is also a normal part of the aging process. The goblet cells in aging epithelium tend to produce less mucus in a process called "microapocrine secretion."

The natural process of metaplasia proceeds to the production of foci of stratified squamous epithelium. The surface electron micrographs are characteristic (Fig. 31). The flattened polygonal epithelial cells are surrounded by raised ridges called terminal bars. At points where a cell has been desquamated, there appears a groove-like structure called a linear bar. In dysplastic epithelium, a more disorganized pattern is seen

with distorted cilia and cells with pleomorphism and loss of nuclear polarity. These were found in patients exposed to nickel processing over many years and some of these had progressed to frank invasive squamous cell carcinoma (51). In this cohort of patients, a marked increase in frequency of metaplastic epithelium is seen as well.

The mucus has a gel and a sol layer with the narrow sol layer covering the cilia, facilitating their movement, and the gel layer on top to which foreign material will stick. The mucus blanket sweeps from the nares to the choanae and in the sinus cavities toward their ostia. The only exception to this is the frontal sinus in which the mucus blanket sweeps from the ostium, arcs over

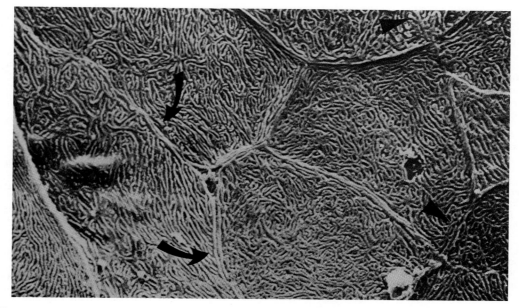

FIG. 31. Scanning electron micrograph of stratified squamous epithelium: the end product of mucosal metaplasia. The polygonal cells demonstrate numerous microridges. *Arrows* denote terminal bars and *arrowheads* indicate linear bars. (×2400). (From ref. 51, with permission.)

the roof of the sinus, and progresses along the floor to empty into the lateral aspect of the frontal sinus ostium (49).

REFERENCES

1. Lang J. *Clinical anatomy of the nose, nasal cavity & paranasal sinuses*. New York: G Thieme Verlag, 1989;62–69.
2. Menger W, Kocoglu V. Paranasale Sinustiden im Saüglings-und Kindesalter und ihr Beziehung zu den Bronchiteden. *Med Welt (Stuttg)* 1969;31:1686–1693.
3. Zizmor J, Noyek AM, eds. *An atlas of otolaryngologic radiology*. Philadelphia: Saunders, 1978;149.
4. Lang JS, Bressel AH. Über den Ductus nasofrontalis bzw. das ostium des sinus frontalis und die vorderen siebbein zellen. *(in preparation)*.
5. Draf W. *Endoscopy of the paranasal sinuses*. Berlin: Springer Verlag, 1983.
6. Zuckerkandl E. *Normal und Pathologische Anatomie der Nasenhöhle und iher pneumatischen Anhänge*. Braumüller Thien, 1882;134–135.
7. Simon E. Anatomy of the opening of the maxillary sinus ostia. *Arch Otolaryngol* 1939;29:640–649.
8. Rice DH, Schaefer SD. *Endoscopic paranasal sinus surgery*. New York: Raven Press, 1988;21.
9. Messerklinger W. *Endoscopy of the nose*. Baltimore: Urban & Schwartzenberg, 1978;11–12.
10. Bolger WE, Parsons DS, Mair EA, Kuhn FA. Lacrimal drainage system injury in functional endoscopic sinus injury. *Arch Otolaryngol* 1992;18:1179–1184.
11. Calhoun KH, Rotzler WH, Stiernburg CM. Surgical anatomy of the lateral nasal wall. *Otolaryngol Head Neck Surg* 1990;102:156–160.
12. Van Alyea OE. *Nasal sinuses: an anatomic and clinical consideration*, 2nd ed. Baltimore: Williams & Wilkins, 1951.
13. Mattox DE, Delaney RG. Anatomy of the ethmoid sinus. *Otolaryngol Clin North Am* 1985;18:3–14.
14. Grünwald L. Deskriptive und topor graphische Anatomie der Nase und ihrer Nebenhälen. In: Denker A, Kahler O, eds. *Die Krankheiten der Luftwege und der Mundhöhle*. Berlin: Springer/München: Bergmann, 1925;S1–95.
15. Mosher NF. Symposium of the ethmoid. The surgical anatomy of the ethmoid labyrinth. *Trans Am Acad Ophthalmol Otolaryngol* 1929;34:376–410.
16. Van Alyea DE. Ethmoid labyrinth: anatomic study with consideration of the clinical significance of its structural characteristics. *Arch Otolaryngol Head Neck Surg* 1939;29:881–901.
17. Kuhn FA, Bolger WE, Tisdal RG. The agger nasi cell in frontal recess obstruction: an anatomic, radiologic and clinical correlation. *Operative Techniques Otolaryngol Head Neck Surg* 1991;2:226–231.
18. Bolger E, Butzin CA, Parsons DS. Paranasal sinus bony anatomic variations and mucosal abnormalities: CT analysis for endoscopic sinus surgery. *Laryngoscope* 1991;101:56–64.
19. Zinreich S, Kennedy DW, Galyler BW. Computed tomography of nasal cavity and paranasal sinuses: an evaluation of anatomy for endoscopic sinus surgery. *Clear Images* 1988;1:2–10.
20. Arey LB. *Developmental anatomy*, 6th ed. Philadelphia: Saunders, 1958;528.
21. Wigand ME. *Endoscopic surgery of the paranasal sinuses and anterior skull base*. New York: Thieme Medical Publishers, 1990;41.
22. Congdon ED. The distribution and mode of origin of septa and walls of the sphenoid sinus. *Anat Rec* 1920;18:97.
23. Hammer G, Radberg C. Sphenoidal sinus: an anatomical and roentgenological study with reference to transsphenoidal hypophysectomy. *Acta Radiol* 1961;56:401–422.
24. Schaeffer JP. *The nose, paranasal sinuses, nasolacrimal passageways and olfactory organ in man*. Philadelphia: Blackston, 1920;125–129.
25. Dixon FW. A comparative study of the sphenoid sinus (a study of 16 skulls). *Ann Otol* 1937;46:687–698.
26. Cope YZ. The internal structure of the sphenoid sinus. *J Anat* 1917;51:127–136.
27. Goss CM, ed. *Gray's anatomy*, 29th American ed. Philadelphia: Lea & Febiger, 1975;179.
28. Peele JC. Unusual anatomical variations of the sphenoid sinuses. *Laryngoscope* 1957;67:208–237.
29. Ritter FN. *The paranasal sinuses: anatomy and surgical technique*. St. Louis: CV Mosby, 1978;83.
30. Donald PJ. Cranial facial surgery for head and neck cancer. In: Johnson JT, ed. *AAO instructional volume 2*. St. Louis: CV Mosby, 1989;230.
31. Yuge A, Takio M, Masami T. Growth of frontal sinus with age—an x-ray tomographic study. In: Meyers E, ed. *New dimensions in otorhinolaryngology—head & neck surgery*, vol 2. New York: Excerpta Medica, 1985;326–327.
32. Millosslawski M. Die sinus frontales. Diss. Moskau 1903. (Cited after Jber Anat: Jena 1905.)
33. Lang J, Haas R. Nerve befunde zur bodenregion der fossa cranialis anterior. *Verb Anat Ges (Jena)* 1979;73:77–86.
34. Flesch M. Varietäten—Beobachtungen aus dem Präpariersaale zu Würzberg in den Winter—sesmestern 1875/76 und 1876/77 *Verh Phys Med Ges Wurzb* 1979;13:1–38.
35. Witt E. Ausbreitung der stirnhöhlen und Siebbinzellen über die orbita. *Med Diss Rostock* 1908.
36. Novak R, Mehls G. Die aplasien der sinus maxillares und frontales unter besenderer Berucksichtigung der pneumatisation bei spalttragern. *Anat Anz* 1977;142:441–450.
37. Boege K. Zur anatomie der Stirnhohlen (sinus frontalis). Diss Konigsherg; Pr. *Jber Fortsch Anat Entw. Gesch* 1903;8(III):33.
38. Onodi A. *The anatomy of the nose and its accessory sinuses: an atlas for students and practitioners*. (Translated from the 2nd edition by St Clair Thompson.) London: Lewis, 1895.
39. Jovanovic S. Supranumerary frontal sinuses on the roof of the orbit: their clinical significance. *Acta Anat (Basel)* 1961;45:33–142.
40. Wigand ME. *Endoscopic surgery of the paranasal sinuses and anterior skull base*. New York: Thieme Medical Publishers, 1990;1–3.
41. Edelstein DR, Bushkin SC. Applied nasal physiology. In: Anand VK, Panje WR, eds. *Practical endoscopic sinus surgery*. New York: McGraw-Hill, 1993;18–19.
42. Batsakis JG. Pathology of the nose and paranasal sinuses: clinical and pathological considerations. In: Goldman JL, ed. *The principles and practices of rhinology*. New York: Wiley, 1987;27–28.
43. Boysen M. The surface structure of human nasal mucosa: I. Ciliated and metaplastic epithelium in normal individuals. A correlated study by scanning transmission electron and light microscopy. *Virchows Arch B Cell Pathol* 1982;40:279.
44. Tos M, Morgensen C, Novatny Z. Quantitative histology of the normal ethmoid sinus. *ORL J Otorhinolaryngol Relat Spec* 1978;40:172–180.
45. Toppozada HH, Talat MA. The normal maxillary sinus mucosa. An electron microscopic study. *Acta Otolaryngol (Stockh)* 1980;89:204.
46. Tos M. Distribution of mucus-producing elements in the respiratory tract: differences between the upper and lower airway. *Eur J Respir Dis* 1983;64 (Suppl 128):269.
47. Tos M, Morgensen C. Mucus production in the nasal sinuses. *Acta Otolaryngol Suppl (Stockh)* 1979;360:131.
48. Lotta JS, Schall RF. The histology of the epithelium of the paranasal sinuses under various conditions. *Ann Otol Laryngol Rhinol* 1934;43:945–949.
49. Tos M, Morgensen C, Novatny Z. Quantitative histology of the normal frontal sinus. *Arch Otolaryngol* 1980;106:143.
50. Torjussen W, Solberg LA, Hogetveit AC. Histopathologic changes of nasal mucosa in nickel workers: a pilot study. *Cancer* 1979;49:963–974.
51. Boysen M, Ruth A. The surface structure of the human nasal mucosa. II. Metaplasia, dysplasia and carcinoma in nickel workers. A correlated study by scanning, transmission electron and light microscopy. *Virchows Arch B Cell Pathol* 1982;40:295–309.

CHAPTER 4

Physiology

Dale H. Rice and Jack L. Gluckman

The nose and paranasal sinuses are anatomically closely related; however, while the function of the nose is fairly well understood, almost nothing is known about the function of the paranasal sinuses.

In lower primates and other animals, nasal function, particularly olfaction, may be essential for day-to-day survival. In humans, however, this is less important although impaired nasal breathing and olfaction may affect other organ systems and of course the quality of life. The three major functions of the nose are olfaction, respiration, and protection.

The exact function of the paranasal sinuses remains an enigma with multiple possibilities being suggested, but none being particularly convincing. Examples include contributing to the resonance of the voice; warming and humidifying of inspired air; and helping to dampen pressure changes within the nose (e.g., during sneezing). It has been suggested that they may form a type of shock absorber for the brain, but this seems unlikely as it would depend on the degree of pneumatization of the sinuses. The sinuses do contribute mucus to the nasal cavity although this seems an insignificant amount compared to the total volume from the nose itself. However, the ostia of the frontal, maxillary, and anterior ethmoid sinuses appear well positioned to supply the mucus where it is most needed, that is, in the middle meatus.

OLFACTION

The sense of smell is mediated via the stimulation of olfactory receptor cells by volatile chemicals. These receptors are located in neuroepithelium closely related to but not confined to the cribriform plate. The olfactory receptors lie in pseudostratified columnar epithelium. Within this epithelium are the following types of receptor cells:

1. Bipolar olfactory neuron, which is a primary sensory neuron with an olfactory knob from which several olfactory cilia extend.
2. Basal cell, which replaces the bipolar neuron cells every 7 weeks.
3. Sustentacular cell, which acts as a support cell supplying nutrients for the bipolar neuron cells.
4. Microvillar cell, for which there is no clearly defined role except perhaps as an aid in olfaction.
5. Bowman's glands, which provide a serous component to the mucous layer covering the olfactory epithelium.

The exact mechanism of olfaction is somewhat vague. Multiple theories have been proposed but none have really been supported scientifically (1,2). There is some suggestion that different odors produce different patterns of activity across the olfactory mucosa. Whatever the explanation at the molecular level, depolarization of the bipolar neuron occurs, resulting in an action potential that is transmitted along the olfactory nerve, and the information is processed centrally in the olfactory tubercle, pyriform cortex, amygdaloid nucleus, and hypothalamus. Of interest is the fact that the olfactory receptor cells are the only nerve cells capable of regeneration, allowing theoretically at least the possibility of regeneration after severe injury.

In addition, the maxillary branches of the trigeminal nerve are important for the perception of noxious odors and therefore also play a protective role against toxic and/or pungent odors.

PROTECTION

The nose and paranasal sinuses play an important role in protecting the body from any harmful substances in the air we breathe. To accomplish this, a number of mechanisms are employed.

Filtration

The coarse vibrissae, situated like guardians of the anterior nares, provide the initial filtration of the inhaled air. Likewise the anterior nares are protected by keratinized squamous epithelium interspersed with sweat and sebaceous glands, which further aid in expelling any unwanted foreign material.

Sneeze Reflex

This reflex is a classic local response to noxious and irritating substances in the air and is extremely effective in forceful expulsion of the irritant. This is a primitive neuromuscular physiologic response mediated via the afferent fibers of trigeminal nerve with efferent fibers to the mucosal blood vessels and glands causing copious secretions and nasal congestion. The phrenic nerve activates the inspiration, which is followed by forceful expiration. In addition, the palate is raised and the superior constrictor contracts, as do the diaphragm and abdominal muscles, forcing the nasopharynx open and hence the sneeze.

Mucous Blanket

The *mucous blanket* is probably the most important protective mechanism utilized by the nose and the paranasal sinuses. This blanket consists of an outer and inner layer. The *outer layer* is highly viscous, elastic, and tenacious and, lying on top of the cilia, is able to trap the inspired particles. The *inner layer* is less viscous and occupies the space in which the cilia lie, that is, between the outer mucous layer and the cell surface. The cilia are able to function easily in this layer.

The mucus is produced by the mucous and serosanguinous glands present in the nose and paranasal sinuses. It consists of 96% water and 3% to 4% glycoproteins. Approximately 600 to 1800 cc of mucus is produced per day (3). Most of the inhaled particles greater than 2 μm in diameter are entrapped in this blanket with only particles less than 1 μm being able to pass through the nose and directly into the lungs. The vast majority of the inhaled particles are trapped in the mucous blanket in the anterior one-third of the nose.

The mucus contains immunologically active substances, most of which are secreted by the goblet cells (4–9) (Table 1), which act on the entrapped particles. It also contains mast cells, polymorph leukocytes, and eosinophils.

The secretion of the mucus by the nasal and paranasal sinus glandular cells is regulated predominantly by parasympathetic nerve fibers, which reach the glands

TABLE 1. *Components of nasal secretion*

Glycoproteins	IgA (monomeric)
S-IgA	IgM
Secretory piece	IgE
Lysozyme	Histamine
Lactoferrin	Prostaglandin
IgG	D$_2$
	Leukotriene C$_4$

from the superior salivary nucleus via the greater petrosal nerve and the sphenopalatine ganglion and also by the sympathetic nerve fibers that affect the vascular supply. In addition, the neuropeptides, particularly substance P, have an effect on the mucous membranes causing hypersecretion, vasodilatation, and extravasation of plasma with its immunologically active proteins.

Ciliary Action

The speed and direction of the flow of mucus vary in the different sinuses and are dependent on the ciliary action in each sinus. The mucous blanket of the nose is cleared approximately every 10 to 20 min in the nose and 10 to 15 min in the paranasal sinuses (10). Three types of mucociliary flow have been described as (a) smooth, moving at 0.84 cm/min, (b) jerky, at 0.3 cm/min, and (c) mucostatic, at less 0.3 cm/min. The normal ciliary beat frequency is 10 to 15 per second. Each beat consists of a rapid propulsive stroke followed by a slow recovery stroke. During the propulsive stroke the tips of the cilia are in contact with the outer viscous layer of the mucous blanket while the slow recovery stroke remains entirely within the inner serous layer.

Morphologically the cilia are long, thin organelles that project from the luminal surface of the columnar epithelial cells. They are approximately 0.7 μm long and 0.3 μm thick and are composed of microtubules. The number of cilia on the cell surface varies between 50 and 300, depending on the area of the nose, that is, occupying approximately 10% of the cell surface anteriorly to virtually 100% more posteriorly (11). The energy for the ciliary function comes from adenosine triphosphate produced in the mitochondria at the base of the cilia.

The cilia function best in a humid environment; however, when the relative humidity drops below 50%, or when the temperature drops below 18°C, ciliary activity is impaired. It also may be impaired in areas where opposing mucosal surfaces come into direct contact with each other (e.g., swollen ostium) (Fig. 1).

While the mucociliary system is functioning well, it prevents bacterial infection and protects the mucosa from injury and drying. However, when damaged, virus and bacteria may penetrate the blanket with resultant damage to the underlying cells (12). Since most

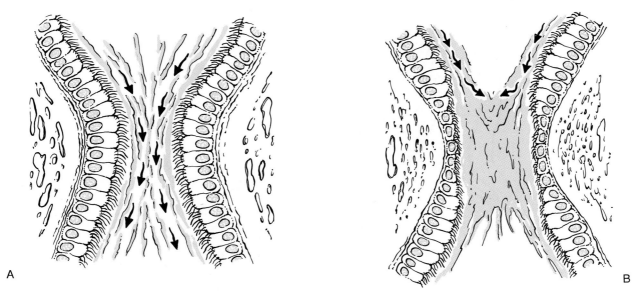

FIG. 1. Diagram showing how the apposition of mucosal surfaces can halt mucous flow.

viral upper respiratory infections resolve sponta-neously, cellular and ciliary recovery ensues, and the system overcomes the infection. Chronic infection re-sults if the system fails to recover (e.g., severe infec-tion), when there is impaired sinus drainage, or when

the mucous blanket is unable to be moved (e.g., in the presence of prolonged ciliary stasis). Likewise, normal sinus drainage is dependent on the amount of mucus produced, the effectiveness of the ciliary beat, the con-dition of the ostia, and the status of the ethmoidal clefts

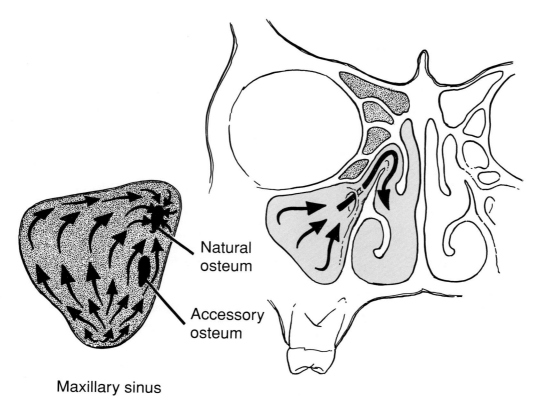

Natural osteum

Accessory osteum

Maxillary sinus

FIG. 2. Diagram showing spiral pattern of flow of the mucous blanket in the maxillary sinus toward the natural ostium.

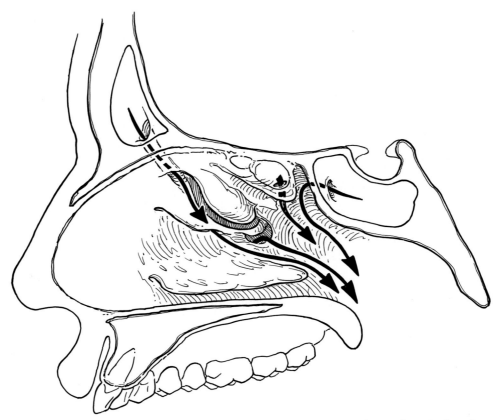

FIG. 3. Diagram showing the normal flow of mucous from the anterior and posterior sinuses.

into which the respective sinus ostia open. Nasal activity (e.g., sniffing) may enhance the movement of the mucus out of the sinuses.

Mucous Flow in the Paranasal Sinuses

Normal mucous flow occurs in a fairly predictable way. In the *maxillary sinus* the flow begins at the floor of the sinus and moves toward the natural ostium in a spiral pattern (Fig. 2). These secretions then empty into the very narrow ethmoidal infundibulum. Mucous transport in the *ethmoid sinuses* is generally directly toward the individual ostia with rare exceptions. All cells of the ethmoid anterior to the basal lamella drain into the middle meatus while all cells posterior and superior to the basal lamella drain via the superior meatus into the sphenoethmoidal recess (Fig. 3). The *frontal sinus* behaves quite differently and is the only sinus in which there is at least a partial retrograde flow of mucus. Mucus flows initially into the sinus superiorly

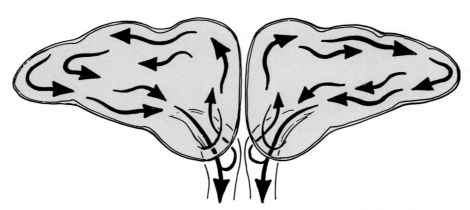

FIG. 4. Diagram showing circular flow of mucous blanket in frontal sinus.

along the medial wall, then continues laterally along the roof and returns to the ostium via the floor and lower portions of the anterior and posterior walls. It only then exits via the frontal recess into the infundibulum (Fig. 4). In the *sphenoid sinus* there is a relatively direct although slightly spiral transport of mucus toward the natural ostium, which then empties into the sphenoethmoidal recess (Fig. 5).

Once in the nose, drainage from the anterior sinuses runs along the uncinate process to the inferior turbinate, then into the nasopharynx, generally passing anteriorly and inferiorly to the eustachian tube orifice. The posterior sinus secretions travel from the sphenoethmoidal recess into the nasopharynx posteriorly and superiorly to the eustachian tube. This close association with the eustachian tube explains the frequency of eustachian tube symptoms in patients with chronic sinusitis or other upper respiratory afflictions.

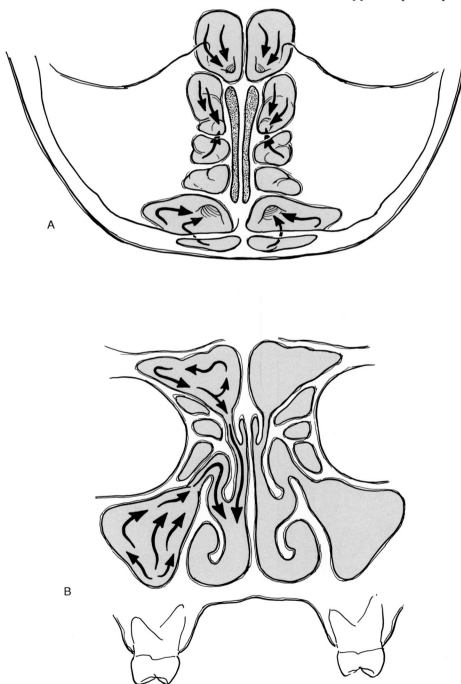

FIG. 5. A: Diagram showing convergence of mucous flow from maxillary, frontal, and anterior ethmoids. **B:** Diagram showing mucous flow of sinuses as viewed in the axial plane.

Of note, in the nasopharynx where the respiratory epithelium of the nasal cavity abuts the squamous cell epithelium of the pharynx, the active cilia-based transport of the mucus ceases and the mucus may be retained for a short period before gravity and the swallowing mechanism move it on. This is particularly noticeable in patients with thick tenacious secretions and can be extremely annoying to the patient.

Isolated mucosal swelling that does not block the sinus ostium will not usually affect mucous transport. Mucosal surfaces that come into close or direct contact with each other may block mucous flow depending largely on the cohesion and viscosity of the gel layer (Fig. 1). If the surface tension is sufficient to bridge the gap, mucous flow will cease. If surface tension is below that which will cause cohesion, then flow will continue.

The natural ostium of the maxillary sinus in the adult is usually 1 to 3 mm in size and empties into the middle meatus in the area of the infundibulum. If the ostium is smaller than 2.5 mm in size, the sinus is predisposed to infection. Accessory ostia are frequently found but are usually bypassed by the normal mucociliary flow and only occasionally drain mucus. If mucus accumulates within the sinus in the dependent position, the flow will be impaired as the viscosity of the mucus is more than the working cilia can overcome. In this situation the mucus may be retained until it flows out by gravity, a change in position, or intervention with aspiration.

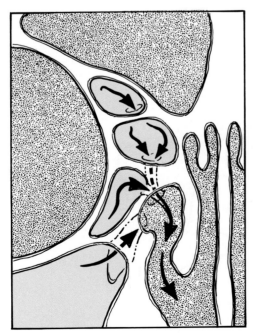

FIG. 6. Diagram showing ostiomeatal complex where minimal obstruction can inhibit the flow from all the anterior ethmoids and the frontal and maxillary sinuses.

The ethmoid cells are the lynchpin in the drainage of the anterior sinuses. Physiologic or anatomic obstruction in the infundibulum or frontal recess can secondarily obstruct the maxillary or frontal sinuses, which may appear to a casual observer more seriously involved than the ethmoids themselves (Fig. 6).

RESPIRATION

The nose is essential to normal efficient respiration. It plays a role in warming and humidification of inspired air as well as acting as a resistor, which seems important for pulmonary function. The normal resting respiratory rate is 12 to 24 times per minute, resulting in an airflow of approximately 15 to 30 liters/min. The flow within the nasal cavity is turbulent, resulting in prolonged contact with the mucosa, rendering warming and humidification more efficient. Oral respiration is unphysiologic and is used only for short periods of time during increased demands. Air inspired in this way will obviously not be adequately warmed or humidified.

Humidification

The nose and paranasal sinuses have the unique ability to maintain the humidity of the inspired air at 85% almost irrespective of the environmental humidity (13). This is important to prevent drying of the lower respiratory tract during respiration. In very dry climates or situations, however, the nose may not be able to accomplish this important task, with a resultant thick, tenacious postnasal drip. The moisture for this process comes predominantly from transudation with very little from secretion by the goblet cells.

Temperature Regulation

The rich vasculature of the nasal cavity permits warming of the inspired air, which also facilitates the alveolar exchange during respiration. During the passage of air through the nose, the air can be heated from 25 to 37°C.

Control of Airflow (Airway Resistance)

The nose acts as a variable resistor and may account for 40% of total airway resistance. The most significant of the high-resistance areas is the *nasal valve*. This is anatomically defined as that anterior area bordered by the nasal septum, upper lateral cartilage, anterior aspect of the inferior turbinate, and floor of the nose. This is responsible for at least half of the nasal resistance to airflow (14). Contrary to popular opinion, it is not just the angle of the upper lateral cartilage to the septum, but the relationship of all these anatomic boundaries that plays a role. The narrowing of this area changes the airflow from laminar to turbulent, which permits improved filtering, humidifying, and warming.

Another area of resistance is further posterior in the nose and is created by the relationship of the nasal septum and the turbinates and of course is aggravated by anything that may cause turbinate hypertrophy (e.g., allergy, autonomic dysfunction).

Another resistor mechanism is the dilator naris muscle, which, by causing flaring of the nasal alae, can result in improved airflow. This is not noted in a normal nose in a patient in good health but in a diseased state (e.g., hypoxia and hypercapnia) can be important (15).

Another cause of altered resistance is the *nasal cycle*. In the normal nose, a cycle exists of one nasal passage being widely open with increased secretion from both serous and mucous glands, while the other nasal passage is obstructed with nearly complete cessation of secretion. These sides switch every 1 to 5 hr on average. The explanation for this cycle is unknown but is due to engorgement of the turbinates. It is particularly apparent during sleep and is position dependent, with the dependent side being obstructed and the upper side patent. This reverses when the patient changes position. The cyclic engorgement and decongestion are present in about 80% of normal people, many of whom are unaware of its presence (16). Keuning (17) studied 17 young adults with normal nasal cavities on rhinoscopy, noting regular nasal cycles in seven ranging from every 2 to 7 hr. In six others there were no patency reversals and in the rest there were irregular cycles. The factors that control the cycle are unknown but are dependent on the presence of the nasal septum; that is, as the congested tissue impinges on the septum, it results in a negative feedback with resultant decongestion and congestion on the opposite side. At all times during this cycle, the total nasal resistance remains constant with no sensation of nasal obstruction.

While the relationship of sinus function to nasal function remains somewhat obscure, it is known that sinus ostium patency is dependent not only on the size of the bony aperture but also on the thickness of the mucosa. Therefore even a minimal change in the thickness of the mucosa can produce a profound effect on the size of the ostium. Thus any kind of nasal vasomotor response either normal, as in the nasal cycle, allergic, or inflammatory can obstruct the sinus ostium. The functional integrity of the sinuses is therefore directly dependent on nasal breathing.

Vascular Mechanisms of Resistance

To maintain normal resistance, the complex system of blood vessels in the mucosa constrict and dilate de- pending on internal and external stimuli. These vessels are small arteries and arterioles, the peripheral capillaries, and the sinusoidal vessels. These vessels are under sympathetic and parasympathetic control via various mediators. This vasomoter response is influenced by hormones, emotions, the environment, and multiple drugs.

RHINOMANOMETRY

Rhinomanometry assesses nasal resistance by measuring the nasal air pressure and airflow, that is, the pressure divided by the airflow. Unfortunately, one of the difficulties encountered is that the nasal flow rate is not constant because of the turbulent flow. The most effective technique of rhinomanometry is the one utilizing a facial mask with a pressure transducer in the nasopharynx. The reading in the nasopharynx is then compared with the atmospheric pressure and the flow rate determined by the flowmeter in the mask. Posterior rhinomanometry with the pressure transductor in the oral cavity and anterior nozzle rhinomanometry are less satisfactory and informative in the clinical setting. There is some controversy as to the exact role of rhinomanometry in the clinical setting, although there seems to be good correlation with the symptom of nasal obstruction. Thus there is potentially some practical application by evaluating patents pre- and post-treatment to determine the efficacy of the treatment (18).

REFERENCES

1. Mozell DG. Electrophysiology of the olfactory system. *Ann NY Acad Sci* 1964;116:38–428.
2. Laffort P, Patte F, Etcheto M. Olfactory coding on the basis of physiochemical properties. *Ann NY Acad Sci* 1974;237:193–208.
3. Tos M. Mucous elements in the nose. *Rhinology* 1976;14:155–162.
4. Richmore JT, Marshall ML. Cytology of nasal secretions: further diagnostic help. *Laryngoscope* 1976;86:516–518.
5. Tomasi TB, Tan EM, Soloman A, Pendergast RA. Characteristics of the immune system in certain external secretions. *J Exp Med* 1965;121:101–134.
6. Agshael GD, Druce HM, Barasiuk JN, Kaliner MA. Pathophysiology of rhinitis. I. Assessment of the sources of protein in methacholine-induced nasal secretions. *Am Rev Respir Dis* 1989;138:413–420.
7. Meredith SD, Raphael GD, Barasiuk JN, Bako SM, Kaliner MA. The pathogenesis of rhinitis. III. The control of IgG secretion. *J Allergy Clin Immunol* 1989;84:920–930.
8. Fleming A. On a remarkable bacteriolytic element found in tissues and secretions. *Proc R Soc Lond [Biol]* 1992;93:306–317.
9. Masson PI, Heremans JF, Dive CH. An iron binding protein common to many external secretions. *Clin Chim Acta* 1966;14:735–739.
10. Hilding AC. The role of the respiratory mucosa in health and disease. *Minn Med* 1967;50:915–919.
11. Mygiend N, Bretlau P. Scanning electron microscopic studies of the human nasal mucosa in normal persons and in persons

with perineal rhinitis. II. Secretion. *Acta Allergy* 1974;29: 216–280.

12. Green RN. The role of viral infection in the etiology and pathogenesis of chronic bronchitis and emphysema: the consideration of a naturally occurring animal model. *Yale J Biol Med* 1968;40: 461–476.

13. Hair CE, Fischer MD, Preslar MJ. Humidification of air by nasal mucosa. *Laryngoscope* 1969;79:375–381.

14. Phillips P, McCaffrey TV, Kern E. In: Blitzer A, Lawson W, Friedman W, eds. *Physiology of the human nose in surgery of the paranasal sinuses,* chap. 2. Philadelphia: Saunders, 1991.

15. Brancatisano TP, Dodd DS, Engel LA. Nasal resistance. *Respir Physiol.* 1986;64:177–189.

16. Hasegawa M, Kern EB. The human nasal cycle. *Mayo Clin Proc* 1977;52:28–34.

17. Keuning J. On the nasal cycle. *Rhinol Int* 1968;6:99–136.

18. McCaffrey TV, Kern EB. Clinical evaluation of nasal obstruction. *Arch Otol* 1979;105:542–545.

CHAPTER 5

Microbiology

Dale H. Rice

The microbiology of the upper respiratory tract has been well studied, particularly in recent years. This has come about partly because of improved techniques in aerobic and anaerobic culturing methods. The density and diversity of the normal flora vary greatly from site to site in the upper respiratory tract, being more dense in the oral cavity than the nose and the sinuses. Nasal mucus has a bacterial concentration ranging from 10^3 to 10^6 bacteria per milliliter with a 5:1 ratio of anaerobes to aerobes (1,2). Interestingly, in one study it was noted that the lowest bacterial count did not occur during antibiotic therapy, but 3 days later (2). Presumably, the mucous membranes of the upper respiratory tract are sterile prior to birth but become colonized during passage through the vaginal canal (3).

In the anterior naris the most common colonization is by *Staphylococcus epidermidis* and diphtheroid species. With this said there are, however four basic categories of organisms: (a) coagulase-positive, gram-positive cocci; (b) coagulase-negative, gram-positive cocci; (c) lipophilic and nonlipophilic gram-positive rods (diptheroids); and (d) Enterobacteriaceae. In one report (2) there was noted to be an inverse relationship between coagulase-negative staphylococci and lipophilic *Corynebacterium*. The staphylococcus carrier rate itself is highest in newborn infants ranging from 52% to 100% and then declines gradually with age (4,5). The anterior naris is also an important reservoir for *Mycobacterium leprae* from which it is transmitted to others. The nose is in fact the main site for the organism to lodge and multiply. Topical treatment with a bactericidal agent makes lepromatous lepers noninfectious and is important to control transmission of this disease (6).

The indigenous microorganisms of any animal develop in an orderly sequence called ecological succession, which eventually results in a relatively stable bacterial population in a given body site. The most important factor in determining the floral composition at a given site is the local environment. That environment is determined by the conditions at the site, which include such factors as moisture, temperature, the oxidation–reduction potential, the P_{O_2}, P_{CO_2}, pH, ionic composition, local nutrients, other microbial competition, and adherence affinities. These conditions and their permutations allow for the development of unique ecological niches for various microorganisms. One of the most significant factors in colonization of a particular site is the adherence affinity of the bacteria in question. Once attached, the given bacteria tend to be difficult to remove and thereby have a major competitive edge over transient invading microorganisms.

In addition to the above mentioned factors, microbial interactions also play a major role in maintaining the particular ecology of a site. This interaction has been well known for over 100 years when Pasteur and Joubert noted in 1877 that in urine inoculated with "common bacteria" and then with the anthrax bacillis the ultimate result was the death of the anthrax bacillis (7). Although many of the mechanisms for these interactions are not known, there are four recognized possibilities: (a) production of an inhibiting substance, (b) creation by mixed cultures of an unfavorable growth environment, (c) creation of ecologic competition for nutrients, and (d) interference related to a host-mediated defense (8).

All these cofactors are influenced in the nose and sinuses by two other factors. The first factor is the presence of lysozyme, lactoferrin, and other immunologically active proteins, including immunoglobulin A (IgA), which are found in the normal nasal mucus, and the second is the action of the cilia itself in both propelling microorganisms into the nasopharynx, as well as preventing nasopharyngeal bacteria from migrating retrograde into the nasal cavity itself (9).

BACTERIAL SINUSITIS

Sinusitis is an inflammation of the mucous membranes of the paranasal sinuses, nearly always resulting from stasis of secretions. Stasis may be secondary to physical obstruction, to infection, or to allergy. The accumulated mucus provides an excellent culture medium for bacteria. An antecedent viral upper respiratory infection is probably the most common cause of bacterial sinusitis, although this is not well established. In approximately 10% of cases, maxillary sinusitis will be of dental origin (10). Sinusitis accounts for approximately 1 million work-days lost in the United States annually and chronic sinusitis is the most common chronic disorder afflicting Americans. The definitions of acute, subacute, and chronic sinusitis are largely subjective and in the case of subacute have little practical meaning. Acute sinusitis can be viewed as a single episode of bacterial infection that resolves within 2 to 3 weeks. Persistence beyond that time, particularly in the face of active appropriate treatment, signals chronic sinusitis.

The bacteriology of acute sinusitis has been studied by way of sterile direct sinus puncture since 1949 (11). Over the ensuing decades, the findings from sinus puncture studies from a variety of institutions have been in relatively good agreement (12,13). The most frequently identified species of aerobic bacteria in acute sinusitis are *Streptococcus pneumoniae, Hemophilus influenzae, S. pyogenes, S. viridans,* γ-hemolytic streptococcus, *Pseudomonas* species, and *Staphylococcus aureus.* The vast majority of cases are currently caused by *S. pneumoniae* and *H. influenzae,* with these two alone accounting for greater than 70% of cases (14). A significant minority of acute infections, approximately 7%, are caused by anaerobic bacteria. Prominent among them are anaerobic streptococci, *Bacteroides,* and *Fusobacterium. Moraxella catarrhalis* accounts for approximately 4% of infections with an increasing percentage producing β-lactamase. *Staphylococcus aureus* is an unusual cause of acute sinusitis but is important because of its virulence and its resistence to the usual therapy. In one study a significant percentage of patients with sphenoid sinus involvement grew out *S. aureus* (29%). Because of this, if it is known that the sphenoid sinus is involved an appropriate antibiotic should be used (15).

In a histological study it was shown that acute bacterial infection of the sinus mucosa begins in the mucosal secretions rather than the tissues (16). Next, the bacteria spreads into the glandular cells, which are clearly the point of least resistance, and from there reach the deeper mucosal layers below the epithelial cells, facilitating penetration into the deeper tissues. Thus it is recommended that in the initial treatment plan restoration of the mucosal defense system should be a primary consideration. In addition, antibiotics should be given at levels that provide a minimum inhibitory concentration in the secretions as well as in the mucosa.

While it has always been stated that the normal paranasal sinuses are sterile, recent study has shown that this is probably not the case. In one study, 12 asymptomatic adults undergoing elective surgery underwent aseptic aspiration of the maxillary sinus (17). In all 12 patients, aerobic bacteria were isolated with seven anaerobic species being isolated as well. Another study had the same findings (18). Thus the sinuses do in fact contain a bacterial flora in low concentrations. These bacteria may proliferate to cause acute infection under conditions that defeat the normal mucociliary defense mechanisms. Supporting this concept is the fact that the organisms found in these studies in normal sinuses are the same as those most commonly identified in acute sinusitis. Thus if one wishes to culture in acute sinusitis, it must be done quite carefully. Ideally, this study should be done under sterile conditions, which are essentially impossible when it involves the maxillary sinus. Any cultures of the maxillary sinus must by nature traverse the nasal or the oral cavity. Despite that, the ideal specimen would still be a direct aspirate of the sinus contents or a piece of the lining mucosa obtained under sterile conditions. Cultures of material at the sinus ostium are not nearly as satisfactory. In a classic study, Axelsson and Brorson (19) found that nasal and sinus cultures agree only 64% of the time. A Gram stain should be ordered on every specimen. This serves several purposes. First, many patients in this situation will already be on antibiotic therapy, which may prevent growth on culture. In addition, occasionally a tentative diagnosis can be made from the morphology of the organisms. Small gram-positive cocci in chains suggest streptococci, while large gram-positive cocci suggest staphylococci. Multiple organisms suggest a mixed aerobic–anaerobic infection. The specimen should be cultured for both aerobic and anaerobic bacteria and the culture should be transported immediately to the laboratory. The season of the year may influence the culture results with *Hemophilus influenzae* dominating in late winter and early spring while *Streptococcus pneumoniae* shows no seasonal variation (20).

CHRONIC SINUSITIS

If the mucociliary defense mechanisms are sufficiently damaged or if the initial therapy is inadequate, the patient may develop chronic sinusitis. Once established, this condition is best thought of as one of structural damage rather than a pure infectious process that can be cured with antimicrobial agents. Experience has shown that even prolonged treatment with appropriate antibiotics is usually not effective, while intervention aimed at reestablishing the mucociliary system will be effective.

Anaerobic organisms are well known to play a more prominent role in chronic sinusitis. Anaerobic bacteria were first described by Pasteur in 1861. Thereafter, interest in these organisms appeared about every 30 years. However, this interest would wane on each occasion largely because of the difficulty and expense in culturing these organisms at that time. In the late 1960s, technological advances developed at the Virginia Polytechnic Institute sparked a new anaerobic renaissance (21). The anaerobic organisms most commonly found are the same as those most commonly found in acute sinusitis, namely, the anaerobic streptococci, *Bacteroides* species, and *Fusobacterium*. In a now classic study, Frederich and Braude (22) in 1974 studied 83 patients with chronic sinusitis where the cultures were obtained in the operating room under sterile conditions. Of the 83 patients studied, 24 had pure cultures of anaerobic organisms with streptococci being the most common followed by *Corynebacterium* and *Bacteroides*. Su et al. (23) felt that culturing the mucosa itself was more accurate than culturing the secretions and speculated that the normal flora of the sinus might be the true etiologic factor following breakdown of the mucociliary system.

Little evidence is available concerning the bacteriology of the ethmoid sinus because of the difficulty getting direct cultures. In one study of 105 children, mucosal cultures were taken directly from the ethmoid bulla during endoscopic ethmoidectomy (24). The most common organisms isolated were α-hemolytic streptococci, *Staphylococcus aureus*, *Moraxella catarrhalis*, *Streptococcus pneumoniae*, and *Hemophilus influenzae* non-type B. The patients studied all had, of course, chronic sinusitis. Multiple organisms were found in 61 while 40 showed no growth.

VIRUSES

Viruses have not been well studied in sinusitis probably for several reasons. First, they are difficult to study directly. Second, for all practical purposes, there is no effective antiviral therapy. Third, the vast majority are self-limiting and need no significant active intervention.

On the other hand, it must be remembered that viruses are the most common cause of acute upper respiratory tract infections and they usually involve the nose and paranasal sinuses. Viruses are not considered to be part of the normal flora of the sinuses, although they may be on rare occasions cultured from asymptomatic individuals (25). It is widely felt that bacterial sinusitis is frequently preceded by a viral upper respira-

tory tract infection. In one study, acute sinusitis was observed to occur after 0.5% of upper respiratory tract infections (26). In addition, several virus families have been isolated in sinus aspirates from patients with acute sinusitis (27). The most commonly cultured viruses include rhinovirus, influenza virus, and parainfluenza virus. Studies of patients with upper respiratory tract infections caused by rhinoviruses showed sinus abnormalities on magnetic resonance imaging (MRI) consisting of mucosal thickening and fluid accumulation, an appearance no different from what would be seen in bacterial sinusitis (28). Viruses can be isolated in up to 15% of aspirates from patients with the clinical signs and symptoms of acute sinusitis (29).

MYCOSIS

Mycotic infections are rare in the general population. These infections have increased importance in patients who are immunocompromised for any of a variety of reasons. These include patients with uncontrolled diabetes, patients with acquired immunodeficiency syndrome (AIDS), patients on immunosuppressant therapy, and patients on prolonged courses of broad-spectrum antibiotics. The majority of true fungal infections of the nose and sinuses are caused by either the Phycomycetes *(Mucor, Rhizopus)* or *Aspergillus*. A wide variety of other mycotic pathogens have been reported but are much less common. Because these infections often occur in the already debilitated patient, early recognition and aggressive management are important to a favorable outcome.

These fungal pathogens are common saprophytes found in dust and soil and on plants. Thus exposure is commonplace.

Fungal sinusitis most commonly occurs in the patient with severe leukopenia (white cell count less than 1000/ml) or in diabetic acidoses (30). Rhinocerebral mucormycosis occurs most commonly in the uncontrolled diabetic who accounts for 70% of cases (31). These fungi appear to thrive in an acidic environment rich in glucose. Thus the ketoacidosis not only favors the mycotic growth but also results in diminished phagocytic activity and delays leukocyte aggregation. Mucormycosis is clinically quite similar to aspergillosis. There are three separate species that may be involved and these are *Rhizopus, Mucor,* and *Absidia*.

Differentiation of these is clinically unnecessary as the presentation and treatment are the same. Like aspergillosis, this disease originates in the nose and paranasal sinuses and may also directly invade the orbit and brain as well as vascular structures. These particular pathogens have a predilection for arterial wall invasion, leading to an arterial thrombosis and tissue necro-

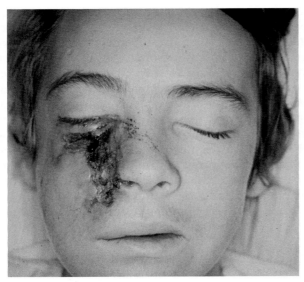

FIG. 1. Photograph of 19-year-old uncontrolled diabetic with mucormycosis of the right maxillary sinus. Advancing vascular thrombosis and tissue necrosis lead to the soft tissue cheek necrosis seen.

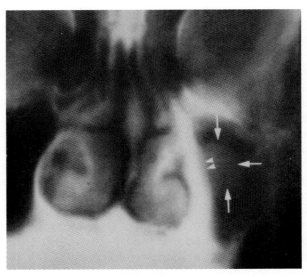

FIG. 3. Polytomagram showing *Aspergillus* fungal ball on medial wall of left maxillary sinus (*three single arrows*).

sis (Figs. 1 and 2). Early signs include a blood-tinged rhinorrhea or black necrotic crusting intranasally, particularly on the turbinates. On potassium hydroxide examination, the organism is seen to have broad nonseptate branched hyphae.

Aspergillosis is the most common fungal infection of the sinuses (32) and affects men and women equally with no racial predisposition. It may be clinically indistinguishable from mucormyocosis. However, histologic examination of potassium hydroxide-mounted specimens reveal hyphae of small size with uniform

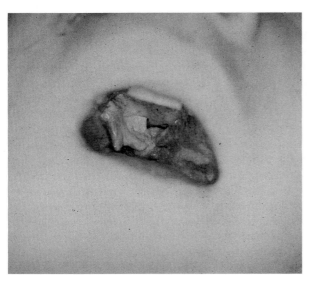

FIG. 2. Intraoral photograph of the same patient as in Fig. 1, showing necrosis of the right hard palate.

septation and acute dichotomous branching. The indolent form of aspergillosis may occur in otherwise healthy individuals. This is usually confined to a single maxillary sinus with symptoms often similar to acute recurring sinusitis (Fig. 3). This is not a true infection as the mucous membranes are not invaded, and the fungal elements merely reside within the sinus. Systemic fungal therapy is not indicated for this disease. Invasive aspergillosis is usually rapidly progressive. There is a progressive gangrenous mucoperiosteitis leading to soft tissue and bony destruction. The infection may spread to invade the orbit or the anterior cranial fossa. The vascular system as well may be invaded. Early signs and symptoms may be relatively nonspecific. The patient may complain of unilateral nasal obstruction or rhinorrhea. Examination may show only crusting of the anterior turbinate and the roof of the nasal cavity. However, this crust covers a necrotic anesthetic mucosa. This should be biopsied immediately and stained with potassium hydroxide (33). Histologic demonstration of mucosal invasion is necessary to make the appropriate diagnosis.

Rhinosporidiosis is a chronic granulomatous disease occurring commonly in India and the Sudan and sporadically throughout the world. The organism is considered to be a fungus and usually involves the nasal, palatal, and conjunctival mucosa (34). It presents with an erythematous nasal lesion that bleeds on touching. It may be unilateral or bilateral and is otherwise indolent and painless.

The treatment for fulminant mycotic infections has several parts. Perhaps the most important is aggressive correction of the underlying medical problem. The second is the systemic administration of specific antifun-

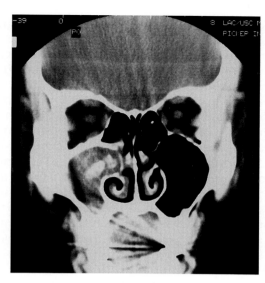

FIG. 4. Coronal CT scan of right maxillary allergic fungal sinusitis. Note heterogeneous density of intrasinus material, a common finding.

gal therapy, generally amphotericin B. Third is the local debridement of necrotic tissue in an effort to slow and perhaps prevent the spread. Following debridement, local irrigation of the cavity with an antifungal agent such as betadine may be helpful.

Both *Aspergillus* and *bipolaris* species, and on rare occasions others, may illicit an allergic response in the sinuses. This leads to a chronic progressive inflammatory response that may even cause bone expansion and destruction. Despite this, however, there is no tissue invasion by the fungal elements and it is thus not a true fungal infection, but merely an intense allergic reaction to these fungal elements (Fig. 4). Treatment requires extensive debridement and aeration of the sinuses but does not require systemic therapy with amphotericin B or other agents and the patients involved are not immunocompromised. Irrigation of the sinuses with a topical antifungal agent as well as either topical or systemic steroid treatment will speed recovery.

OTHER INFECTIONS

A number of other infections may involve the nose and paranasal sinuses but are quite uncommon. Nasal involvement by tuberculosis is extremely rare in the absence of pulmonary disease. When it does occur, it is characterized by rhinorrhea, pain, and obstruction. The lesion itself is erythematous, edematous, and nodular with an associated exudate. Perforation of the cartilaginous septum may occur, but the nasal floor and bony septum are rarely involved. Diagnosis is made by biopsy and by culture.

Syphilis may also involve the nasal cavity. It rarely will involve the sinuses alone. Nasal involvement usually is seen in tertiary syphilis rather than in the early stages. Most typically involved are the bony and cartilaginous nasal septum. Congenital syphilis may also involve the nose and is characterized by marked rhinitis with nasal obstruction and mucopurulent rhinorrhea. In either case, perforation of the septum may lead to saddle nose deformity. A biopsy will reveal a nonspecific lymhoplasmacytic perivascular inflammatory cell infiltrate and special stains are needed to demonstrate the *Treponema pallidum* organism.

Rhinoscleroma is endemic to subtropical countries such as Central and South America. In the United States it is seen most frequently in the southwestern and western regions. The organism is *Klebsiella rhinoscleromatis*. The infection generally begins in the anterior nasal cavity as a firm submucosal plaque that grows into nodules that lead to nasal obstruction. On biopsy the lesion shows a chronic granulomatous reaction with Mikulicz's cells.

Leprosy is endemic to warm climates and in medically deprived patients. The etiologic agent is *Mycobacterium leprae*. It may involve the skin and the mucosa of the upper respiratory tract. The nasal cavity and sinuses are most likely to be involved in lepromatous leprosy, which is the disseminated form and occurs in patients with a low resistance to the organism. In this situation the bacteria can be found in all tissues of the body. Lesions in the nose appear as red granular ulcers and may result in septal perforation.

ANTIBIOTICS

The various penicillins are bactericidal because their mode of action is the inhibition of the synthesis of the bacterial cell wall. Penicillin has one of the widest dosage margins of safety of any drug used today. Since the penicillins are excreted by the kidneys, renal impairment will lead to higher than normal blood levels and perhaps to neurotoxicity from increased concentrations in the cerebrospinal fluid. Penicillins cross the blood–brain barrier satisfactorily for therapeutic purposes particularly when the meninges are inflamed. The penicillins are very effective against pneumococcal and streptococcal infections in particular, as well as the usual anaerobic bacteria found in the upper aerodigestive tract. These factors, in addition to its low cost, make it the antibiotic of choice for many routine acute infections. On the other hand, penicillin has several disadvantages. The first is its sensitivity to destruction by gastric acid. For that reason it is best given on an empty stomach, even in the penicillin V form. Second, penicillin may cause hypersensitivity reactions in up to 5% of patients. The most common hypersensitivity reaction is a rash that may or may not preclude future use of the drug, but it is probably wise to avoid it if other reasonable choices are available. Anaphylactic reactions occur in about 1 in 10,000 patients and may be fatal. Anaphylaxis may occur even in patients without a previous history of a reaction. However, fatal reactions are more common when the drug is given parenterally and for that reason oral administration is preferred when satisfactory dose levels can be achieved. The third and perhaps major disadvantage of penicillin, from a practical standpoint, is its inactivation by bacteria that produce β-lactamase. This enzyme attacks the β-lactam ring in the molecule of penicillin and its derivatives such as ampicillin, amoxicillin, carbenicillin, and ticarcillin.

Fortunately, a number of penicillin derivatives have been developed that are resistant to β-lactamase hydrolysis. These drugs include methicillin, oxacillin, cloxacillin, dicloxacillin, and nafcillin. All of these, except methicillin, come in oral preparations. Of these, when given in the fasting state, dicloxacillin achieves the highest serum levels after oral administration. The main indication for the use of these drugs is against penicillin-resistant staphylococcal infections. Furthermore, these drugs carry the same risk as conventional penicillin in allergic patients.

Another group of penicillins, the amino-penicillins, were developed to increase the spectrum of activity against gram-negative organisms, in particular, *Hemophilus influenzae, Proteus mirabilis,* and *Escherichia coli.* These drugs include ampicillin, amoxicillin, bacampicillin, cyclacillin, and hetacillin. Unfortunately, the amino-penicillins are inactivated by β-lactamase and thus are ineffective against many staphylococcal infections. Of these drugs, only ampicillin is destroyed by gastric acid so the others may be given at mealtimes while ampicillin should be given 1 hour before or 2 hours after a meal. An increasing percentage of *Hemophilus influenzae* infections have made these drugs less appealing choices in the treatment of sinusitis than they had been in the past.

The cephalosporins, like the penicillins, inhibit cell wall synthesis and are thus bactericidal. The first generation cephalosporins are active against a wide spectrum of gram-positive cocci including penicillin-resistant staphylococci and against many gram-negative bacilli, particularly *E. coli, P. mirabilis,* and *Klebsiella.* Unfortunately, for head and neck infections, they are often ineffective against *Hemophilus influenzae.* The first generation cephalosporins include cephalothin (Keflin), cefazolin (Ancef, Kefzol), cephapirin (Cefadyl, Cefatrexil), cephradine (Velosef, Anspor), cephalexin (Keflex), and cefadroxil (Duracef, Ultracef). The second generation cephalosporins were developed to increase their activity against *Hemophilus influenzae* and the *Bacteroides* species. These drugs include cefaclor (Ceclor), cefamandole (Mandol), and cefoxitin

(Mefoxin). Of these second generation cephalosporins only cefaclor is available in an oral form. The third generation cephalosporins were developed to increase their activity against *Pseudomonas* as well as *Hemophilus* and *Bacteroides.* Unfortunately, these same drugs have decreased activity against staphylococci compared to their predecessors. These drugs include cefotaxime (Claforan) and moxalactam (Moxam). The cephalosporins are most useful against penicillin-resistant *Staphylococcus aureus* infections. The same infections however, can, be treated with drugs in the antistaphylococcal penicillin class. However, in patients who have had a rash reaction to penicillin, the cephalosporins may be a safer choice. In any patients with a history of an anaphylactic reaction, cephalosporins should probably not be used unless there is no good alternative, as cross-sensitivity occurs in up to 10% of patients. Cefaclor is the only available oral drug among all the cephalosporins that is effective against *Hemophilus influenzae* including ampicillin-resistant strains. It is thus an excellent choice for sinusitis when *S. aureus* or ampicillin-resistant *H. influenzae* bacteria are suspected. If there is an intracranial complication secondary to sinusitis, cephalosporins should not be used as they cross the blood–brain barrier very poorly except for moxalactam.

Loracarbef (Lorabid) is a synthetic β-lactam antibiotic of the carbacephem class of oral antibiotics. It differs from cephalosporins only slightly chemically. Loracarbef is bactericidal by inhibiting cell wall synthesis. The absorption orally is much improved on an empty stomach than when administered with food. Loracarbef is excreted in the urine completely unmetabolized. It is effective against most staphylococci and streptococci, including β-lactamase-producing staphylococci, but is inactive against methicillin-resistant staphylococci. It is also effective against a number of gram-negative aerobes including *E. coli, H. influenzae,* and *M. catarrhalis.* In addition, it has significant effect against a number of important anaerobic organisms in head and neck infections, including *Fusobacterium, Peptococcus, Peptostreptococcus,* and *Propionibacterium.*

The erythromycins inhibit bacterial protein synthesis and are therefore, in general, bacteriostatic. Erythromycins are the least expensive and have the fewest side effects of the penicillin substitutes for penicillin-allergic patients. In addition, they are nearly as effective against streptococci and pneumococci as penicillin and are effective against most strains of staphylococci, even those that produce β-lactamase.

Erythromycin is also effective against many strains of *Hemophilus influenzae* but is more effective when combined with a sulfonamide such as sulfisoxazole. The latter combination is sold under the name of Pediazole. It is especially useful against ampicillin-resistant

Hemophilus influenzae. Ten to fifteen percent of patients will experience significant gastrointestinal distress with some of the erythromycin preparations. This can be minimized by using the estolate (Ilosone) form with mealtimes as it is not affected by the presence of food in the stomach. In addition, the ethylsuccinate (EES, Pediamycin, Wyamycin-E) form is even enhanced by the presence of food.

Clindamycin and lincomycin suppress protein synthesis and are therefore bacteriostatic. Although lincomycin, erythromycin, and chloramphenicol are not structurally related, they all bind at the identical site on the bacterial ribosome, so that the effect of one inhibits the action of another if they are used concurrently. Clindamycin is effective against all gram-positive coccal infections, including those caused by β-lactamase-producing staphylococci. It also has a broad activity against anaerobic organisms. The oral use of clindamycin has been followed by gastroenteritis and diarrhea with the most serious manifestation being that of pseudomembranous colitis, a rare disorder characterized by severe diarrhea, dehydration, and sometimes death. Thus if diarrhea occurs with the use of this drug, it should be discontinued immediately. Lastly, clindamycin only poorly crosses the blood–brain barrier.

The tetracyclines inhibit protein synthesis in the same manner as the aminoglycosides and are therefore bacteriostatic. When first introduced, the tetracyclines were effective against a broad spectrum of infectious diseases including many of the organisms involved in sinusitis. However, over the years many strains of these organisms have become resistant to the point that tetracycline should not be used unless cultures have demonstrated sensitivity. In addition, tetracycline is absorbed poorly when administered with calcium, magnesium, and aluminum ions and therefore should not be administered with antacid preparations or with the consumption of milk products.

Imipenem is a carbopenem that is chemically closely related to the penicillins, cephamycins, and cephalosporins. It has a broad spectrum of activity against many gram-positive and gram-negative aerobic and anaerobic organisms. Exceptions, however, include *Pseudomonas cepacia* and methicillin-resistant *Staphylococcus aureus.* It is available only in the intravenous form.

The sulfonamides are bacteriostatic by competitively inhibiting the incorporation of *p*-aminobenzoic acid (PABA) into tetrahydropteroic acid. This in turn inhibits folic acid synthesis. They are active against a broad spectrum of gram-positive and gram-negative bacteria. Resistance, however, is common. Trimethoprim is a dehydrofolate reductase inhibitor used to potentiate the activity of the sulfonamides by the sequential inhibition of folic acid synthesis. It is active against most gram-positive and gram-negative organisms. Exceptions include *Pseudomonas aeruginosa* and *Bacteroides* species. The combination of trimethoprim and sulfamethoxazole (Bactrim, Septra) is active against *S. aureus, S. pyogenes, Streptococcus pneumoniae, E. coli,* and *Proteus mirabilis.*

Clavulanate and sulbactam are β-lactamase inhibitors. When combined with an antibiotic sensitive to β-lactamase, the antibiotic's spectrum is extended. Thus amoxicillin plus calvulanate (Augmentin) is active against *Hemophilus influenzae, Moraxella catarrhalis,* staphylococci, *E. coli, K. pneumoniae, Proteus* species, and *Bacteroides* species. Adding sulbactam to ampicillin (Unasyn) produces a similar result.

CONCLUSION

The bacteriology of acute and chronic sinusitis is reasonably well known. This knowledge will allow one to choose an appropriate antibiotic for both acute and chronic sinusitis. Care must be taken to give the antibiotic in the proper dose for the proper length of time.

More unusual infections require a high index of suspicion for their possibility. Special studies may need to be performed to establish the correct diagnosis and allow for appropriate treatment.

REFERENCES

1. Gorback SL, Bartlett JG, Tally FP. *Biology of anerobes.* Kalimazoo, MI: Upjohn Company, 1981.
2. Aly R, Miabach HI, Strauss WG, et al. Effect of system making antibiotics on nasal bacterial ecology in man. *Appl Microbiol* 1970;20:24.
3. Sommers HM. The indigenous microbiota of the human host. In: Youmans GP, Paterson PT, Sommers HM, eds. *The biologic and clinical basis of infectious diseases.* Philadelphia: Saunders, 1980;83–94.
4. Williams REO. Healthy carriage of *Staphylococcus aureas:* Its prevelance and importance. *Bacteriol Rev* 1963;27:56.
5. Cunlife AC. Incidence of *S. aureus* in the anterior naris of healthy children. *Lancet* 1949;2:411.
6. Prabhakar MC, Appa Rao AV, Krishna DR, et al. How non-infectious are the non-infectious lepromatous leprosy patients? *Lepr India* 1983;55:576.
7. Florey HW. The use of microorganisms for therapeutic purposes. *Yale J Biol Med* 1946;19:101.
8. McCabe WR. Role of the reticuloendothelial system and bacterial interference in embryonated eggs. *J Lab Clin Med* 1968;72:318.
9. Goldman JL. Bacteriological and cytological criteria for diagnosis in nasal and sinus diseases: basis and interpretation. *Trans Ophthamol Otolaryngol* 1954;4:68.
10. Waldman RH. Sinusitis. In: Waldman RH, Kluge RM, eds. *Infectious diseases.* New York: Medical Examination Publishing, 1984.
11. Urdal K, Verdal P. The microbial flora in 81 cases of maxillary sinusitis. *Acta Otolaryngol* 1949;37:20–52.
12. Rantanen T, Arvilomni H. Double blind trial of doxycycline in acute maxillary sinusitis: a clinical and bacteriological study. *Acta Orolaryngol (Stockh)* 1973;76:58–62.
13. Jousimies-Somer HR, Savolainen S, Ylikoski JS. Bacteriologi-

cal findings of acute maxillary sinusitis in young adults. *J Clin Microbiol* 1988;19:19–25.

14. Gwaltney JM Jr, Scheld WM, Sande MA, Sydnor A. The microbial etiology and antimicrobial therapy of adults with acute community acquired sinusitis: a 15-year experience at the University of Virginia and review of other selected studies. *J Allergy Clin Immunol* 1992;90:457–461.

15. Lew D, Southwick FS, Montgomery WW, Weber AL, Baker AS. Sphenoid sinusitis: a review of 30 cases. *N Engl J Med* 1983;309:1149–1154.

16. Lundberg C. Bacterial invasion of the sinus mucosa. *Acta Otorhinolaryngol Belg* 1983;37:589.

17. Brook I. Aerobic and anaerobic bacterial flora of normal maxillary sinuses. *Laryngoscope* 1981;91:372.

18. Daley CL, Sand M. The runny nose: infection of the paranasal sinuses. *Infect Dis Clin North Am* 1988;2:131.

19. Axelsson A, Brorson JE. The correlation between bacteriological findings in the nose and maxillary sinus in acute maxillary sinusitis. *Laryngoscope* 1973;83:2003.

20. Chapnick JS, Bach MC. Bacterial and fungal infections of the maxillary sinus. *Otolaryngol Clin North Am* 1976;9:43.

21. Gorbach SJ, Bartlett JG. Anaerobic infections. *N Engl J Med* 1974;290:1289.

22. Frederich J, Braude AI. Anaerobic infection of the paranasal sinuses. *N Engl J Med* 1974;290:135.

23. Su W, Liu C, Hung SY, et al. Bacteriological study in chronic maxillary sinusitis. *Laryngoscope* 1983;93:931.

24. Muntz HR, Lusk RP. Bacteriology of the ethmoid bulla in children with chronic sinusitis. *Arch Otolaryngol Head Neck Surg* 1991;117:179–181.

25. Bannatyne RM, Clausen C, McCarthy L. Cumitech 10. In: Duncan IBR, ed. *Laboratory diagnosis of upper respiratory tract infections*. Washington, DC: American Society of Microbiology, 1979.

26. Dingle JH, Badger GF, Jordan WS Jr. *Illness in the home: a study of 25,000 illnesses in a group of Cleveland families*. Cleveland: Western Reserve University Press, 1964.

27. Gwaltney JM Jr, Sydnor A Jr, Sande MA. Etiology and antimicrobial treatment of acute sinusitis in adults. *Ann Otol Rhinol Laryngol* 1981;90:68–71.

28. Turner BW, Cail WS, Hendley JO, Hayden FG, Doyle WJ, Sorrentino JB, Gwaltney JM Jr. Physiologic abnormalities in the paranasal sinuses during experimental rhinovirus colds. *J Allergy Clin Immunol* 1992;90:474–478.

29. Malow JB, Creticos CM. Non-surgical treatment of sinusitis. *Otolaryngol Clin North Am* 1989;22:809–818.

30. Berlinger NT. Sinusitis in immunodeficient and immunosuppressed patients. *Laryngoscope* 1985;95:29–33.

31. Forma JL. Rhinocerebral mucormycosis. In: Gates GA, ed. *Current therapy in otolaryngology—head and neck surgery 1984–1985*. Philadelphia: BC Decker, 1984.

32. McGuirt WF, Harrill JA. Paranasal sinus aspergillosis. *Laryngoscope* 1979;89:1563–1568.

33. McGill RJ, Simpson G, Healy GB. Fulminant aspergillosis of the nose and paranasal sinuses: a new clinical entity. *Laryngoscope* 1980;90:748–754.

34. Schlech WF, Gorden GA. Symposium on granulomatous disorders of the head and neck: fungal and parasitic granulomas of the head and neck. *Otolaryngol Clin North Am* 1982;15:493–513.

CHAPTER 6

Pathology

Regina Gandour-Edwards

The diversity of tissues that comprise the nasal cavity and paranasal sinuses is one of the most complex in the human body. The lining includes squamous and respiratory mucosa, as well as specialized olfactory epithelium. The submucosa includes numerous seromucinous or minor salivary glands, blood and lymphatic vessels, peripheral nerves, and connective tissue. These mucosae and soft tissues are adherent to underlying bone and hyaline cartilage. This complex array of tissue types gives rise to numerous pathologic lesions of diverse differentiation.

The intent of this brief chapter is to provide a general overview of sinonasal pathology for the otolaryngologist. Numerous excellent references, listed at the end of this chapter, are suggested for an encyclopedic approach and for in-depth discussion of specific entities (1–5).

Lesions of the sinonasal region are a challenge for both otolaryngologist and pathologist and include several lesions that have similar or overlapping morphology. Modern pathologic techniques including immunohistochemistry and/or electron microscopy are commonly utilized for diagnosis. Immunohistochemistry has become a powerful tool for pathologic diagnosis and has proved effective in the classification of the undifferentiated and/or small cell lesions of the sinonasal tract (6). It is important to appreciate, however, that currently no one antibody can determine whether a lesion is benign or malignant. Standard pathologic criteria of architecture, nuclear configuration, and mitotic rate remain the essential morphologic features for diagnosis. A general overview of the commonly utilized antibodies for immunohistochemical diagnosis is summarized in Table 1.

The transfer of technology from basic research to clinical application is advancing rapidly. Molecular probes including both in situ hybridization and polymerase chain reaction methodology are being utilized, for example, in the study of human papillomavirus in squamous papilloma and carcinoma and Epstein–Barr virus in nasopharyngeal carcinoma. Flow cytometry has become an important method for phenotyping lymphomas of the sinonasal tract. Current and future studies will utilize techniques such as DNA ploidy analysis and probes for biologic markers including tumor suppressor genes, oncogenes, and as yet unidentified entities.

To optimize diagnosis and patient care, it is essential that the surgeon and pathologist maintain a dialogue of mutual respect and vigilant communication. A preoperative or prebiopsy consultation with the pathologist will ensure that the tissue is properly allocated and processed for special studies if indicated. Individual pathology laboratories will have preferred media and fixatives for immunohistology, electron microscopy, flow cytometry, and so on. Provision of the pertinent clinical history and precise anatomic location is mandatory. An intraoperative consultation including frozen section and/or touch preparations may be indicated to ensure that adequate, representative tissue has been obtained for the diagnostic workup. Intraoperative frozen section is *not* the optimum technique for definitive diagnosis, because of the potential for sampling error or interpretive error due to freezing artifact (7,8).

SINONASAL POLYPS

Sinonasal polyps are inflammatory swellings of the mucosa rather than true neoplastic growths. The majority occur in the ethmoid recesses and upper lateral nasal wall near the middle turbinate and may be single, multiple, and bilateral. Some are caused by allergy or

TABLE 1. *Common antibodies utilized in sinonasal tract pathology*

Cytokeratins	Epithelial tissues (e.g., squamous and glandular mucosa), carcinomas, papillomas
Vimentin	Mesenchymal tissues (e.g., connective tissue, muscle), sarcomas
Human muscle actin	Smooth/skeletal muscle, rhabdomyosarcoma, leiomyoma
Leukocyte common antigen	Lymphocytes, plasma cells
L26	B-cell lymphocytes, B-cell lymphoma
UCHL	T-cell lymphocytes, T-cell lymphoma
S-100	Neural crest tissues (e.g., melanoma, olfactory neuroblastoma)
HMB-45	Melanoma
Chromagranin A	Neurosecretory granules (e.g., olfactory neuroblastoma)
CD 68	Macrophages, histiocytes; malignant fibrous histiocytoma
Factor VIII	Endothelial cells (e.g., hemangioma, angiofibroma)

cystic fibrosis but many are of obscure etiology. The pathologic mechanism of sinonasal polyps is under investigation and current theories favor a connective tissue dysfunction due to immunoglobulin E (IgE)-mediated response in the lamina propria, which results in fluid retention below the epithelial surface. The presence of specific locally produced IgE bound to the corresponding allergen at this site and the presence of IgE, probably locally produced, within the fluid add support to this hypothesis (9). Grossly, polyps are soft, polypoid, translucent masses up to several centimeters in diameter. Histologically, the surface mucosa is typically intact and covered by respiratory epithelium with

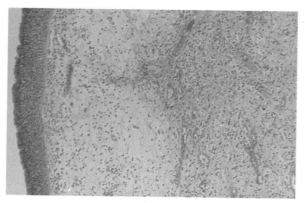

FIG. 1. Sinonasal polyp (H&E, ×40). Intact respiratory-type epithelium and edematous stroma.

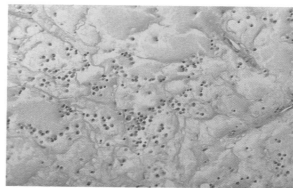

FIG. 2. Sinonasal polyp (H&E, ×100). Edematous stroma with eosinophils.

increased mucous goblet cells and/or areas of squamous metaplasia (Figs. 1 and 2). The basement membrane is frequently thickened and eosinophilic. The stroma is edematous and myxomatous with scattered fibroblasts and variable vascularity. Chronic polyps may have a fibrotic stroma. Seromucinous glands are usually absent. The inflammatory cell infiltrate is variable, consisting of a mixture of eosinophils, lymphocytes, plasma cells, and tissue mast cells. Neutrophils are not prominent unless there is concurrent infection. Sinonasal polyps with stromal atypia have been described particularly in younger patients. The stroma contains large, variable stromal cells that are felt to be reactive myofibroblasts. The lesion may be confused with botryoid type embryonal rhabdomyosarcoma (10). The antrochoanal polyp is a sinonasal inflammatory polyp arising from the maxillary sinus antrum, often from the lateral sinus wall. These are typically solitary, unilateral lesions and the gross appearance is similar to common sinonasal polyps. They present in the nasal choanae, often extending from one side to the other, causing bilateral nasal obstruction. The microscopic appearance is also similar; however, there are typically fewer mucinous glands and eosinophils and they have a more fibrous and vascular appearance than standard polyps (11).

HETEROTOPIC GLIA

Heterotopic glial tissue or nasal gliomas generally present at birth or within the first few years of life and develop as a failure of normal embryonic development. Approximately 30% present intranasally high within the nasal vault or along the lateral wall of the nasal fossa or middle turbinate. They may be confused grossly with nasal polyps. Radiographic studies are necessary to exclude communication with the cranial cavity (encephalocele). Microscopically, ill-defined nests of astrocytes and neuroglial fibers are surrounded

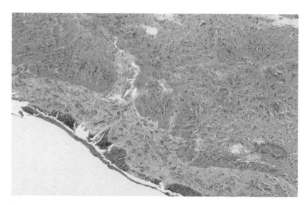

FIG. 3. Heterotopic glia (H&E, ×40). Intact mucosa with dense, pink bundles of glial tissue.

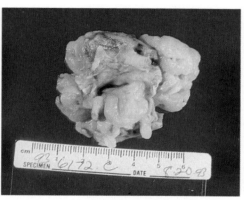

FIG. 5. Inverted papilloma. Gross photograph of inverted papilloma from the nasal cavity.

by fibrous tissue. Neurons are rarely present (Fig. 3). Surgical excision is curative (12).

SINONASAL PAPILLOMA (SCHNEIDERIAN PAPILLOMA)

The so-called Schneiderian membrane is formed from invaginating ectoderm of the olfactory plates. The histology is identical to and continuous with nasopharyngeal mucosa, which is of endodermal origin (13). Sinonasal papillomas are benign tumors derived from Schneiderian epithelium and composed of columnar or ciliated respiratory epithelium with varying degrees of squamous differentiation. Papillomas are relatively uncommon, representing only 0.4% to 4.7% of all sinonasal tumors (14). They are generally unilateral and comprise three histologic types: septal (exophytic or fungiform) papilloma, inverted papilloma, and cylindrical cell (oncocytic or columnar cell) papilloma.

Septal papillomas occur almost exclusively on the nasal septum, while the inverted and cylindrical cell types occur along the lateral nasal wall and less fre-

quently in the paranasal sinuses. Septal papillomas, which constitute 50% of all sinonasal papillomas (15,16) have a characteristic exophytic, cauliflower-like appearance. Histologically, they are composed of papillary fronds of thick squamous, transitional, and/or respiratory epithelium with delicate fibrovascular cores (Fig. 4). Surface keratinization is uncommon and this feature assists in separating these lesions from verruca vulgaris (keratinizing papillomas) of the nasal vestibule. Septal papillomas are distinguished from papillary malignancies by their cellular and nuclear uniformity and absence of mitoses.

Inverted papillomas comprise 47% of sinonasal papillomas (17) and are typically large, polypoid masses (Fig. 5). They characteristically arise from the region of the middle turbinate and often secondarily extend into the maxillary and ethmoid sinuses. Histologically, they are composed of epithelial nests that grow in an endophytic or "inverted" pattern (Figs. 6 and 7). The epithelium may be squamous and/or columnar admixed with goblet cells and mucin-containing microcysts. Surface keratinization is seen in perhaps 10% to 20%

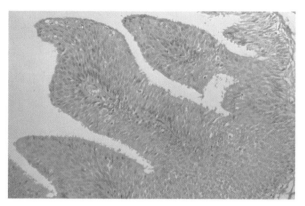

FIG. 4. Septal papilloma (H&E, ×100). Uniform papillae with fibrovascular cores covered by hyperplastic, squamous cells arising from the nasal septum.

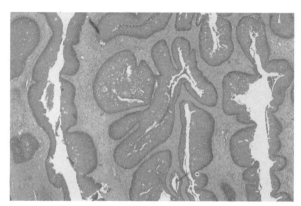

FIG. 6. Inverted papilloma (H&E, ×40). Hyperplastic squamous cells growing into underlying ducts in an "inverted" pattern.

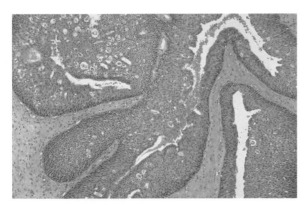

FIG. 7. Inverted papilloma (H&E, ×100). Uniform squamous cells with a smooth, "pushing" border.

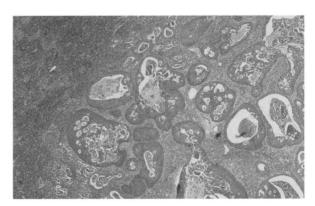

FIG. 9. Metachronous carcinoma (H&E, ×100). Metastatic carcinoma in a cervical lymph node.

of tumors; and mitoses are occasionally present in basal or parabasal areas. The nuclei are uniform. Although inverted papillomas are histologically benign, they have seemingly unlimited growth potential and local aggressiveness. Infiltration of underlying bone and cartilage is often seen and extension to the nasopharynx, orbit, and cranial cavity has been reported (18). Recurrence is common unless aggressive surgery is performed.

Cylindrical cell papillomas are rare and contribute only 3% of sinonasal papillomas. Histologically, they are characterized by dense pink, oncocytic epithelium and abundant mucin-filled cysts.

Human papillomavirus (HPV) has been detected in a minor subset of sinonasal papillomas and is implicated as an etiologic agent. Studies utilizing in situ hybridization and polymerase chain reaction techniques have detected subtypes HPV 6, 11, and 16. To date, there is no definite association of a specific HPV subtype with a histologic type nor with recurrence or malignant transformation (19–27).

Synchronous and metachronous carcinomas have been reported in cylindrical cell papilloma and inverted papilloma at rates of 4% to 24% (28). Criteria for malignancy includes nuclear pleomorphism, increased mitoses, and abnormal mitoses. One of our recent cases involved an 88-year-old woman with a 6-year history of recurrent papilloma in the maxillary sinus and nasopharynx who developed both pulmonary and cervical metastases (Figs. 8 and 9).

SQUAMOUS CELL CARCINOMA

Squamous cell carcinoma is characterized by a disorganized, invasive growth of large, epithelial cells with intercellular bridges and cytoplasmic keratin. Adjacent or overlying atypia of the surface mucosa is typically present. Squamous cell carcinoma is graded into well, moderately, and poorly differentiated types (Figs. 10 to 12) by the degree of resemblance to normal squamous tissue. Specific criteria include definition of intercellular bridges, amount of keratinization, nuclear pleomorphism, mitotic rate, and degree of cell cohesion (sheets versus small nests).

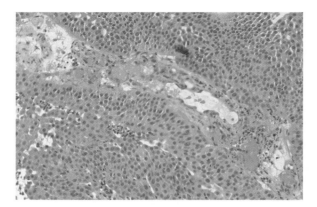

FIG. 8. Metachronous carcinoma (H&E, ×100). Invasive carcinoma developing in an inverted papilloma in the maxillary sinus.

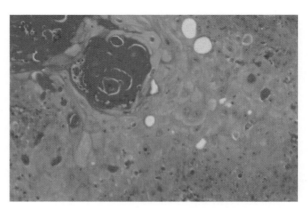

FIG. 10. Squamous cell carcinoma (H&E, ×100). Well-differentiated histology with abundant keratin and intercellular bridges.

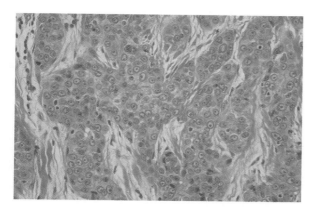

FIG. 11. Squamous cell carcinoma (H&E, ×100). Moderately differentiated histology with larger nuclei, less keratin, and increased nuclear pleomorphism.

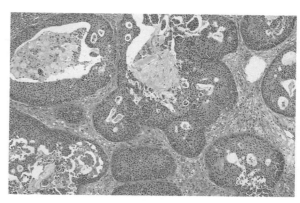

FIG. 13. Nonkeratinizing squamous cell carcinoma (H&E, ×100). Invasive tumor in the maxillary sinus composed of nonkeratinizing squamous cells and numerous microcysts.

Nasal Vestibule

The nasal vestibule is lined by hair-bearing skin; and the squamous cell carcinomas are similar to those of other cutaneous sites. Squamous cell carcinoma is the most common malignant tumor of the nasal vestibule; and the typical histology is well differentiated and keratinizing. It most often affects the anterior septum and columella and has a propensity for aggressive spread along the periosteum of the premaxilla and maxilla (29).

Sinonasal Mucosa

In the sinonasal region, squamous carcinoma is seen as friable, fungating growths. Fifty-eight percent occur in the antrum, 30% in the nasal cavity, 10% in the ethmoid, and 1% in the frontal and sphenoid sinuses (30). Invasion into surrounding bony walls and adjacent vital cavities is common. Risk factors include radiation exposure, tobacco smoking, wood dust exposure, and exposure to the carbonyl extraction processes used in nickel refining (31–34).

Squamous cell carcinoma is the most common malignancy originating from this respiratory mucosa. The majority (approximately 80%) are poorly differentiated and keratinizing with a papillary, exophytic, or inverted growth pattern. The well differentiated, nonkeratinizing types have also been called transitional carcinoma, cylindrical cell carcinoma, or columnar Ringertz carcinoma (Fig. 13).

Nasal Cavity

In the nasal cavity, the majority (85%) of squamous carcinomas occur in the lateral wall and floor (35). Carcinomas of the septum are felt to be rare (36). Lymph node metastasis develops in a minority, approximately 15%, of patients. The lymphatic drainage is predominantly to the submental and submandibular lymph nodes but also includes the facial, superficial parotid, and deep cervical chains. These midline lesions, however, can metastasize to bilateral and/or contralateral sites. Systemic metastases are less common (10%) (37); T, M, N classification has not been established for nasal cavity malignancy.

Paranasal Sinuses

Eighty percent of paranasal sinus squamous cell carcinomas occur in the maxillary antrum (38). Bony invasion of the sinus wall is common. T classification of maxillary sinus carcinoma has been defined (Table 2). Regional lymph node metastasis is uncommon if the tumor is confined to the sinus walls. Once invasion of the facial soft tissues or oral cavity occurs, metastases are more frequent. However, the initial lymphatic

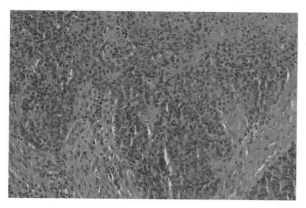

FIG. 12. Squamous cell carcinoma (H&E, ×100). Poorly differentiated histology with scant cytoplasm, no keratin, and smaller nests of tumor.

TABLE 2. *T classification of maxillary sinus carcinoma (39)*

T1	Tumor limited to the antral mucosa with no erosion or destruction of bone
T2	Tumor with erosion or destruction of the infrastructure (inferior–anterior structure as defined by Ohngren's line[a]) including the hard palate and/or the middle nasal meatus
T3	Tumor invades any of the following: skin of cheek, posterior wall of maxillary sinus, floor or medial wall of orbit, anterior ethmoid sinus
T4	Tumor invades the orbital contents and/or any of the following: cribriform plate, posterior ethmoid or sphenoid sinuses, nasopharynx, soft palate, pterygomaxillary or temporal fossae, base of skull

[a] Ohngren's line is defined as the plane passing through the inner canthus and the mandibular angle, which divides the upper jaw into the superoposterior structure (suprastructure) and inferoanterior structure (infrastructure). The suprastructure includes the posterior bony wall and posterior half of the superior bony wall. The other bony walls belong to the infrastructure.

drainage of the antrum is to retropharyngeal lymph nodes, which are not easily palpable.

NASOPHARYNGEAL CARCINOMA

As implied from the name, nasopharyngeal carcinoma arises from the nasopharyngeal epithelium, particularly the lateral wall. Secondary involvement of the nasal cavity and/or paranasal sinuses, however, occurs. Nasopharyngeal carcinoma is essentially a squamous cell carcinoma that is histologically classified as keratinizing, nonkeratinizing, or transitional cell or undifferentiated carcinoma. The tumor was previously referred to as "lymphoepithelioma." Nasopharyngeal carcinoma is rare in the United States but accounts for 18% of all cancers in China (40). There is a strong association with Epstein–Barr virus (41,42). The clinical presentation typically includes an obstructive nasopharyngeal mass and cervical metastases. The primary tumor is often submucosal and may be small and subtle.

The tumors are classified by the World Health Organization system based on histopathology (43). Type I, the keratinizing type, represents 25% of cases and is identical to conventional squamous cell carcinoma. Type II, the nonkeratinizing type, is the least common (15%), with sheets of epithelial cells resembling transitional cell carcinoma of the bladder. Type III, the most common variant, is the undifferentiated type (60%) and consists of syncytial nests of large pink cells with pleomorphic nuclei and prominent nucleoli. The cell margins are indistinct and mitoses frequent. The cell nests are surrounded by a dense infiltrate of nonneoplastic lymphocytes.

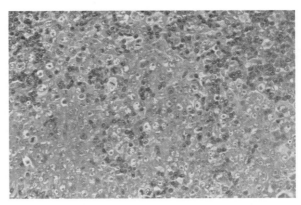

FIG. 14. Nasopharyngeal carcinoma (H&E, × 100). Irregular nests of large, pink tumor cells have indistinct cell borders and are surrounded by a dense infiltrate of lymphocytes.

Immunohistochemistry is often helpful in the separation of the undifferentiated type from lymphoma. Nasopharyngeal carcinoma will stain with cytokeratin and epithelial membrane antigen and will not react with leukocyte common antigen (44) (Figs. 14 to 16).

Nasopharyngeal carcinoma is treated with radiation therapy. The keratinizing type tends to remain localized but to have a 5-year survival rate of only 10% to 20% because of its radioresistance. The undifferentiated type is the most radiosensitive and has a 5-year survival rate of 60% despite a 10% to 20% rate of lymph node metastasis. The nonkeratinizing type is variably radioresponsive with a 5-year survival rate of 35% to 50% (45).

OLFACTORY NEUROBLASTOMA

Olfactory neuroblastoma or esthesioneuroblastoma is an uncommon tumor that arises from the olfactory

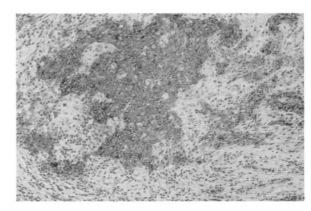

FIG. 15. Nasopharyngeal carcinoma (× 100). Immunohistochemistry with anti-low-molecular-weight cytokeratin antibody. The tumor cells are reactive and stain brown with the dimethylaminoazobenzene (DAB) chromogen.

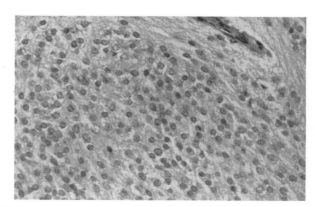

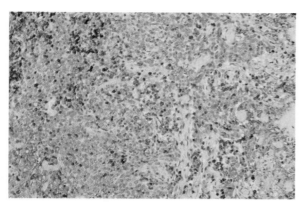

FIG. 16. Nasopharyngeal carcinoma (×100). Immunohistochemistry with anti-leukocyte common antigen antibody. The tumor cells are negative *(blue)* and the surrounding lymphocytes are positive *(brown)*.

FIG. 18. Olfactory neuroblastoma (H&E, ×100). Uniform, small neuroblasts with pink neuronal extensions.

TABLE 3. *Olfactory neuroblastoma grading (Hyams') (49)*

Grade I	Lobular architecture, uniform round neuroblasts, well-defined neurofibrillary component, frequent pseudorosettes (Homer–Wright rosettes), variable calcification
Grade II	Less defined neurofibrillary component, scattered mitoses
Grade III	Increased cellularity, individual cell pleomorphism, increased mitoses, necrosis
Grade IV	Necrosis is common, nuclei are hyperchromatic and anaplastic, cytoplasm indistinct, calcification uncommon

epithelium (membrane) of the upper nasal cavity, which is the most common site of presentation (46). Rare cases have presented in the lower lateral nasal cavity and maxillary antrum and were felt to arise from ectopic olfactory epithelium (47). The neoplastic cell is the olfactory bipolar neuron. The role of the sustentacular or supporting cells of the olfactory membrane is obscure (48). Grossly, the tumors are glistening, soft, and polypoid and frequently extend into the paranasal sinuses and nasopharynx. Microscopically, the tumor consists of clustered masses of small cells with round uniform nuclei representing the primitive neuroblasts (Figs. 17 and 18). A variable amount of pink, fibrillar tissue is admixed and represents neural fibrils, which are felt to be cytoplasmic extensions from the neuroblasts. Four histologic grades have been defined (Table 3).

The diagnosis of olfactory neuroblastomas often requires ancillary studies such as immunohistochemistry for chromagranin A and synaptophysin. Electron mi-

croscopy demonstrates dense core neurosecretory granules and neuronal processes (50) (Figs. 19 and 20).

Treatment is surgical, followed by radiation therapy. Three-year survival varies with clinical stage (Table 4): >90% in stage A, >80% stage B, and <50% for stage C. The majority of tumors are locally aggressive and invade adjacent structures such as the orbit and cranial

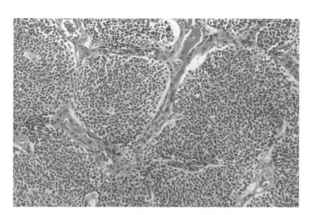

FIG. 17. Olfactory neuroblastoma (H&E, ×40). Grade I olfactory neuroblastoma with defined, round nests of uniform neuroblasts.

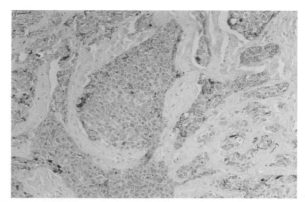

FIG. 19. Olfactory neuroblastoma (×100). Immunohistochemistry with anti-chromagranin A antibody. The neuroblasts react strongly, demonstrating the presence of neurosecretory granules.

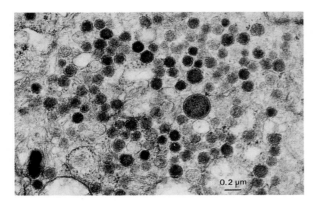

FIG. 20. Olfactory neuroblastoma (electron micrograph). The numerous, round, dense structures are dense core neurosecretory granules.

TABLE 4. *Kadish staging olfactory neuroblastoma (51)*

Stage A	Tumor confined to nasal cavity
Stage B	Tumor involves nasal cavity and one or more paranasal sinuses
Stage C	Tumor extends beyond sinonasal tract

cavity. The metastatic rate to regional lymph nodes, lungs, and bone is 20% to 40% (51).

SINONASAL UNDIFFERENTIATED CARCINOMA

Sinonasal undifferentiated carcinoma is a recently identified aggressive, undifferentiated carcinoma of the nasal cavity and paranasal sinuses. The tumor presents as a large, fungating mass in the nasal cavity with extension to multiple paranasal sinuses. Microscopically, medium sized, pleomorphic cells are arranged in nests and sheets with large, irregular nuclei and a small to moderate amount of pink cytoplasm. Mitotic figures are abundant. Vascular channels distended with tumor having central necrosis are commonly seen (Figs. 21 and 22). With immunohistochemistry, the cells are re-

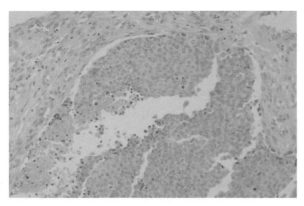

FIG. 21. Sinonasal undifferentiated carcinoma (H&E, ×100). A nest of large, undifferentiated tumor cells within a vascular space.

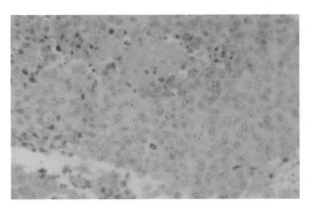

FIG. 22. Sinonasal undifferentiated carcinoma (H&E, ×250). Necrosis in center of tumor cell nest.

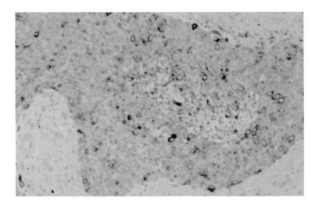

FIG. 23. Sinonasal undifferentiated carcinoma (×250). Immunohistochemistry with anti-low-molecular-weight cytokeratin antibody. The tumor cells are strongly reactive.

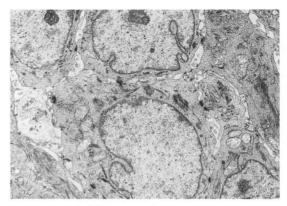

FIG. 24. Sinonasal undifferentiated carcinoma (electron micrograph). The cells have primitive cell junctions and no neurosecretory granules or neuronal processes. This assists in distinguishing these tumors from high grade olfactory neuroblastoma.

active with cytokeratin and negative for neuroblastic, lymphoma, or rhabdomyosarcoma antigens (Fig. 23). Electron microscopy demonstrates primitive epithelial cells with no neurosecretory granules (52) (Fig. 24).

Sinonasal undifferentiated carcinoma is important to separate from other sinonasal tumors such as olfactory neuroblastoma because of its more aggressive course. A large series of patients has not yet been analyzed but cervical lymph node metastases have been reported and recently occurred in one of our patients (53).

ADENOID CYSTIC CARCINOMA

Adenoid cystic carcinoma is composed of small, basal type duct-lining cells and myoepithelial cells arranged in a characteristic cribriform pattern. It is the most common malignant tumor of minor salivary (seromucinous) glands and accounts for approximately 37% of all epithelial tumors in the sinonasal tract (54). Adenoid cystic carcinomas have been reported throughout the sinonasal tract; however, the most common locations are maxillary antrum (47%), nasal cavity and adjacent sinus (21%), and nasal cavity (11%) (55). The tumors grow slowly and commonly present as polypoid masses with bony invasion. The disease is characterized by slow but relentless progression over years with sometimes late (10- to 15-year) recurrences and distant metastases. Adenoid cystic carcinoma characteristically spreads along perineural spaces including those of the maxillary division of the trigeminal nerve and may traverse the foramen ovale to the gasserian ganglion Figs. 25 and 26). Histologically, three patterns have been described—tubular, solid, and cribriform—and tumors are classified by which pattern dominates (e.g., >50% of the tumor). The cribriform type is the most common and is considered the "classic" pattern. Nests of cells demonstrate multiple circular spaces filled with bluish mucinous material or pink,

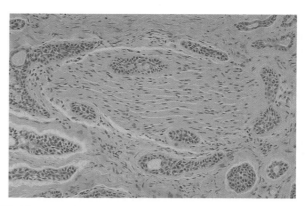

FIG. 26. Adenoid cystic carcinoma (H&E, ×100). Invasion of the perineural sheath of the trigeminal nerve.

hyalinized material (Fig. 27). The tubular pattern consists of cells arranged in individual ducts or tubules while the solid pattern, as expected from the name, has nests or sheets of basaloid cells with little cystic formation (Fig. 28).

Perzin et al. (56) found a correlation between these

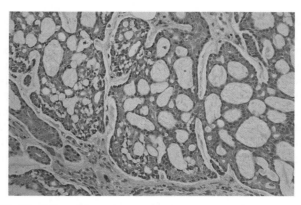

FIG. 27. Adenoid cystic carcinoma (H&E, ×40). The classic "Swiss cheese" appearance of cribriform pattern.

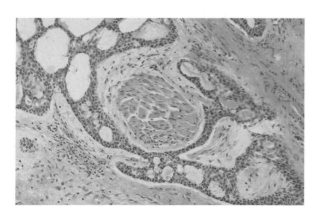

FIG. 25. Adenoid cystic carcinoma (H&E, ×100). The tumor frequently surrounds peripheral nerves.

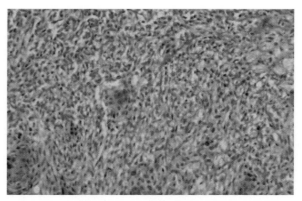

FIG. 28. Adenoid cystic carcinoma (H&E, ×100). The solid nests of basaloid cells characterize the solid pattern, which has a poorer prognosis.

histologic patterns and survival rates as follows: tubular, 8 years: cribriform, 9 years; and solid, 5 years. Recurrence rates were as follows: tubular, 59%; cribriform, 89%; and solid, 100%. Lymphatic spread is low (i.e., 13% to 16%); however, hematogenous metastasis is high (40%) with lung and bone representing the most common sites of distant spread (57).

SINONASAL ADENOCARCINOMA

Sinonasal adenocarcinoma refers to adenocarcinomas that arise from the surface respiratory mucosa and/or seromucinous (minor salivary) gland tumors (58). They are also called mucinous, "colonic type," or enteric adenocarcinomas and have been categorized into papillary, sessile, and alveolar-mucoid types. The tumor occurs predominantly in men and is associated with wood dust exposure. Sinonasal adenocarcinomas typically arise from the middle turbinate or ethmoid sinus and less commonly from the antrum. Grossly, the tumors are polypoid or poorly defined and friable with hemorrhagic and gelatinous foci. The papillary type arises from surface mucosa and consists of multiple fronds of cytologically malignant cells on fibrovascular cores. This histologic pattern is considered low grade and has the best prognosis of the group. The sessile type is felt to arise from minor salivary ducts and contains goblet cells and glands that bear a striking resemblance to colonic adenocarcinoma (Figs. 29 and 30). Argentaffin and Paneth cells are sometimes present. The alveolar-mucoid variant arises from seromucinous glands and remains within the lamina propria. It contains signet ring cells, numerous goblet cells, and nests of tumor cells suspended in mucinous pools reminiscent of a "colloid carcinoma" pattern. An admixture of sessile and alveolar-mucoid patterns has been described. Only rare reports of colonic adenocarcinoma metastatic to the sinonasal tract have been published. The clinical course is similar to adenoid cystic

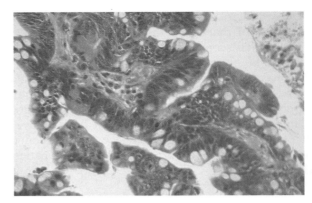

FIG. 30. Sinonasal adenocarcinoma (H&E, ×100). The tumor surface has goblet cells and resembles primary adenocarcinoma of the colon.

carcinoma with local invasion and low rate of nodal and systemic metastases (59).

NASOPHARYNGEAL ANGIOFIBROMA

Nasopharyngeal angiofibroma or juvenile angiofibroma is a relatively rare, benign tumor that typically occurs in the nasopharynx with rare examples in the paranasal sinuses. The nasal cavity and/or paranasal sinuses may be involved secondarily. Angiofibroma occurs almost exclusively in men, and the typical patient is an adolescent (60). Grossly, the tumors are nodular, rubbery, deep red to tan, noncircumscribed masses. Microscopically, varying sized vascular channels lined by plump, uniform, endothelial cells are embedded in a fibrous stroma of vascular and fibrous tissue of spindle or stellate fibroblastic cells. The vascular spaces are irregular and "staghorn" in shape and their walls have no elastic tissue and little or no smooth muscle (Figs. 31 and 32). Scattered mitoses may be

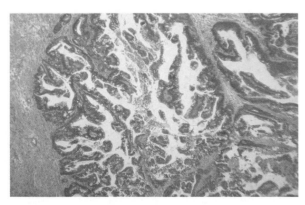

FIG. 29. Sinonasal adenocarcinoma (H&E, ×40). Invasive tumor in the nasal cavity with a sessile appearance.

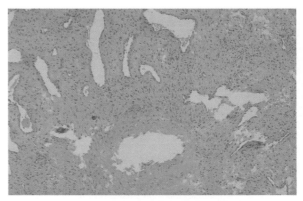

FIG. 31. Nasopharyngeal angiofibroma (H&E, ×40). Multiple irregular vascular spaces are embedded in cellular, fibrovascular stroma.

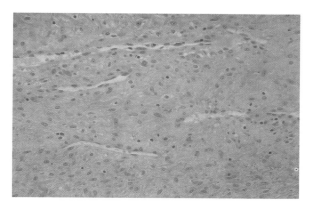

FIG. 32. Nasopharyngeal angiofibroma (H&E, × 100). The tumor vessels lack a smooth muscle wall.

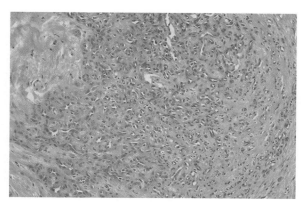

FIG. 34. Capillary hemangioma (H&E, × 100). The individual vessels are lined by uniform endothelial cells.

present; however, there is no significant pleomorphism or necrosis.

The pathogenesis remains obscure and the tumors are felt to arise from the nasopharyngeal fibrovascular tissue near the base of the pterygoid plates (61). No definitive evidence of hormonal imbalance has been demonstrated. Treatment is surgical excision, often with preoperative vascular embolization to control perioperative bleeding. Recurrence rates without intracranial extension are low and prognosis is generally excellent. Malignant degeneration is exceedingly rare and almost exclusively limited to patients who have received prior radiation therapy (62).

CAPILLARY HEMANGIOMA OF THE SINONASAL TRACT

The capillary hemangioma of the sinonasal tract is also called pyogenic granuloma, hemangioma of granulation tissue type, and lobular capillary hemangioma. These benign vascular proliferations are thought by some to be reactive rather than truly neoplastic (63).

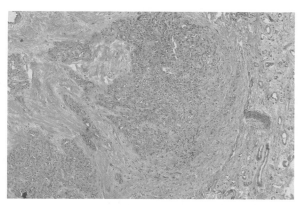

FIG. 33. Capillary hemangioma (H&E, × 40). The lesion has a pseudolobular appearance on low power and was excised from the nasal cavity.

In the sinonasal tract, they occur most often in the anterior portion of the nasal septum known as Little's area or Kiesselbach's triangle and in the tip of the turbinates. The etiology is unclear, but the lesions are associated with trauma and pregnancy. Hemangiomas are benign and rarely recur. Grossly, smooth, polypoid masses are seen measuring up to 1.5 cm. Surface ulceration is common.

Microscopically, the vessels are arranged in clusters or lobules with a central, slightly larger, vessel surrounded by those of smaller caliber. The endothelial lining cells are frequently prominent and tufted in appearance (Figs. 33 and 34). Mitoses and increased cellularity are present in more active lesions; however, true nuclear pleomorphism and abnormal mitotic figures are absent (64). Accompanying granulation tissue and inflammation are common as well as overlying squamous metaplasia.

SINONASAL HEMANGIOPERICYTOMA

Hemangiopericytoma is an uncommon soft tissue tumor of controversial etiology. Most investigators feel that the tumor arises from pericytes, which are spindle cells that surround blood vessels and are thought to have smooth muscle and baroreceptor functions (65,66). Fifteen to twenty percent of hemangiopericytomas occur in the head and neck, with >50% of these occurring in the sinonasal tract. The majority appear to arise in the paranasal sinuses with secondary involvement of the nasal cavity. Grossly, they are red-tan to gray-tan, polypoid masses high in the nasal cavity (67).

Microscopically, hemangiopericytomas are circumscribed, densely cellular sheets of uniform spindle cells surrounding thin walled, irregular endothelium-lined spaces. The vascular spaces are classically described as having a staghorn or antler-like configuration. Reti-

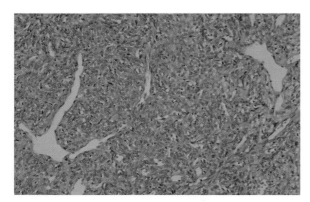

FIG. 35. Sinonasal hemiangiopericytoma (H&E, ×100). Irregular, "staghorn" vessels are surrounded by densely packed spindle cells. (Courtesy of Philip J. Vogt, MD.)

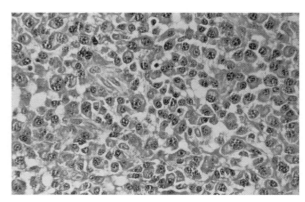

FIG. 37. Extramedullary plasmacytoma (H&E, ×250). Sheets of pleomorphic and binculeate plasma cells are present in this nasal lesion.

culin fibers outline individual cells (Figs. 35 and 36). The vascular spaces do not react with endothelial cell markers (Factor VIII or *Ulex europaeus*). Considerable histologic variation is reported such as a fibrosis, hyalinization, and/or a myxoid degeneration. Occasional mitoses are present but significant mitotic activity and necrosis are not typical features.

The majority of sinonasal hemangiopericytomas behave indolently, with a 60% recurrence if inadequately treated surgically. Malignant hemangiopericytomas are characterized by cellular anaplasia and increased mitoses. Only 10% have distant metastases to the lung. Lymph node metastases are rare. The tumors are considered to be radioresistant (68).

EXTRAMEDULLARY PLASMACYTOMA

Extramedullary or solitary plasmacytomas are defined masses of atypical/neoplastic plasma cells. Upper, respiratory mucosa is a common site with the majority of these occurring in the sinonasal tract. Grossly, the

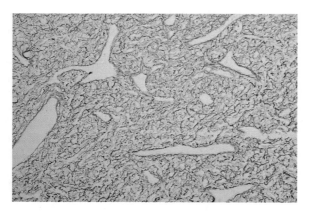

FIG. 36. Sinonasal hemangiopericytoma (reticulin, ×100). The spindle cells are individually outlined by reticulin fibers. (Courtesy of Philip J. Vogt, MD.)

lesions may be polypoid or submucosal masses. Microscopically, sheets of oval cells with basophilic cytoplasm and eccentrically placed nuclei are characteristic. The nuclear chromatin pattern is distinctive with multiple dense chromatin masses arranged in a cartwheel pattern (Fig. 37). Varying numbers of less differentiated cells may be present with increased large, pleomorphic, and/or binucleate nuclei and mitotic figures. Amyloid deposits may be present.

It is unusual for patients to have increased serum or urine levels of immunoglobulins; however, immunohistochemistry typically demonstrates monoclonal immunoglobulins in plasmacytoma. The lesions are usually treated with radiotherapy and a 50% 10-year survival rate has been reported. Some patients, however, have local recurrences and others eventually develop multiple myeloma (69).

SINONASAL LYMPHOMA

Sinonasal lymphomas account for only 3% to 5% of upper respiratory tract lymphomas, with the majority occurring in Waldeyer's tonsilar ring (70). Malignant lymphomas are currently divided into Hodgkin's and non-Hodgkin's types, although advancing molecular biology continues to shape our understanding and classification of these tumors. Lymphomas are also currently classified by their B- or T-cell phenotype utilizing immunohistochemistry and flow cytometry for surface marker analysis. Non-Hodgkin's lymphoma is the most common type seen in the sinonasal tract, with Hodgkin's type occurring rarely.

Both B-cell and T-cell lymphomas occur in the sinonasal tract, as well as a minority portion of nonclassifiable phenotypes. Studies report variable proportions of B- and T-cell lymphomas (71,72); however, it is clear that the T-cell phenotype is more common in the nasal cavity than other Waldeyer's ring sites or other extra-

FIG. 38. Nasal B-cell lymphoma (H&E, ×100). Sheets of large, individual, pleomorphic cells with large nuclei and scant cytoplasm.

nodal sites. Interestingly, both B- and T-cell lymphomas of the sinonasal tract have demonstrated associated Epstein–Barr virus antigens in Asian and non-Asian populations (73,74).

Sinonasal B-cell lymphomas tend to be diffuse, monomorphous infiltrates of large cleaved and/or immunoblastic cells, which invade throughout the mucosa and soft tissues. The T-cell lymphomas are also diffuse, large cells but frequently demonstrate necrosis and angioinvasion (75). A newly defined subset of aggressive nasal cavity lymphomas mark with the natural killer (NK) cell antibody (CD56) (76). As may be expected, the T-cell lymphomas and NK cell lymphomas are more aggressive and have a poorer prognosis than the B-cell lymphomas.

The biopsy diagnosis and immunophenotyping of sinonasal lymphomas require adequate fresh tissue. Pre-biopsy consultation with the pathologist is essential for optimum tissue handling. The angioinvasive T-cell sinonasal lymphomas may have features of polymorphic reticulosis and/or Wegener's granulomatosis, which

are all included in the differential diagnosis of midline necrotizing lesions. Recent studies have found that a majority of lesions previously classified as polymorphic reticulosis are indeed T-cell lymphomas (77,78) (Figs. 38 and 39).

Radiation therapy is the primary therapy with reported 5-year disease-free survival of 90% in stage T1-2 patients and 50% for stage T3-4 patients. T staging utilizes the AJC system for epithelial tumors (79).

RHABDOMYOSARCOMA

Rhabdomyosarcoma is the most common soft tissue sarcoma in children and young adults as well as the most common soft tissue sarcoma of the head and neck (80). Sinonasal rhabdomyosarcomas constitute a minor component of these tumors and commonly present with a polypoid configuration, which is described histologically as botryoid or "grape-like" in appearance (Fig. 40). Four histologic subtypes are described: embryonal, alveolar, pleomorphic, and mixed. The embryonal variant is the most common with sheets of large round and spindle cells with abundant eosinophilic cytoplasm called rhabdomyoblasts (Fig. 41). Cross-striations resembling those found in skeletal muscle fibers are often present. Mitoses and necrosis are commonly seen. Immunohistochemical stains for human muscle actin (HMA), desmin, and/or myoglobin are confirmatory (81) (Fig. 42). Electron microscopy reveals primitive bundles of actin and myosin filaments with Z banding (Fig. 43).

The alveolar subtype consists of poorly defined groups of single, small, dense, round cells with irregular nuclei and scant cytoplasm (Fig. 44). This histology is included in the poorly differentiated "small round blue cell tumors of childhood." An alveolar pattern with cell clusters resembling lung alveolar tissue is variable and the primitive cells may appear in solid

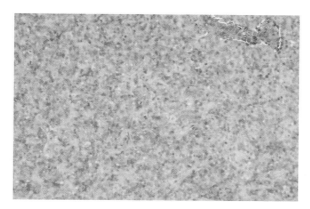

FIG. 39. Nasal B-cell lymphoma (×100). Immunohistochemistry with anti-B-cell antibody (L26). The lymphoma cells are strongly reactive.

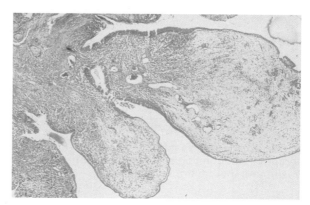

FIG. 40. Rhabdomyosarcoma (H&E, ×40). Botryoid or "grape-like" architecture of embryonal rhabdomyosarcoma of the nasal cavity.

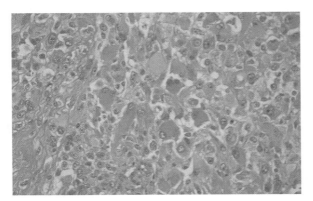

FIG. 41. Embryonal rhabdomyosarcoma (H&E, ×100). Rhabdomyoblasts are large pleomorphic cells with abundant pink cytoplasm.

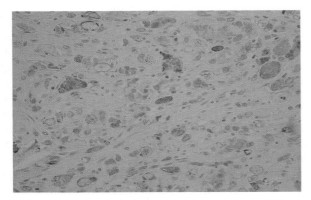

FIG. 42. Embryonal rhabdomyosarcoma (×100). Immunohistochemistry with anti-human muscle actin antibody. The rhabdomyoblasts are strongly reactive.

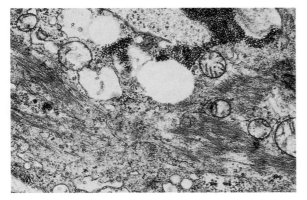

FIG. 43. Embryonal rhabdomyosarcoma (electron micrograph). Rhabdomyoblasts with dense bundles of thick (myosin) and thin (actin) myofilaments.

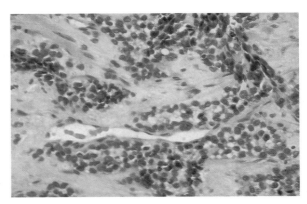

FIG. 44. Alveolar rhabdomyosarcoma (×100). The alveolar type of rhabdomyosarcoma is characterized by small, round cells with scant cytoplasm. These have a poorer prognosis than the embryonal type.

sheets or trabecular nests. Mitoses and necrosis are common.

The pleomorphic histology is uncommon, particularly in the head and neck, and consists of large pleomorphic cells with multinucleate and bizarre nuclear features. Prognosis is strongly linked to histology with the alveolar variant having a less favorable course than the embryonal type at all stages. Rhabdomyosarcoma metastasizes to regional lymph nodes as well as hematogenously to bone, lung, and brain. Overall 5-year survival is as follows: stage I, 83%; stage II, 70%; stage III, 52%; and stage IV, 20% (82).

Staging has been developed by the Intergroup Rhabdomyosarcoma Study Group (Table 5).

MALIGNANT FIBROUS HISTIOCYTOMA

Malignant fibrous histiocytoma is the most common soft tissue sarcoma of late adult life and uncommonly occurs in the head and neck (83). The sinonasal tract is one of the most common upper respiratory locations (84). The tumor appears as a varying sized nodule and

TABLE 5. *Intergroup rhabdomyosarcoma study staging (82)*

Stage I	Localized disease, with tumor completely resected
Stage II	Grossly resected tumor with microscopic residual disease and negative regional lymph nodes; microscopic residual disease and positive regional lymph nodes; or regional lymph nodes involved or extension of tumor into adjacent viscera without microscopic residual disease
Stage III	Incomplete resection or biopsy of primary tumor with gross residual disease
Stage IV	Metastatic disease present at time of diagnosis

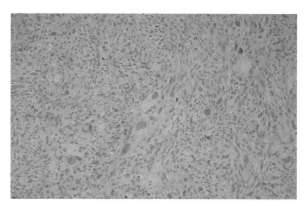

FIG. 45. Malignant fibrous histiocytoma (H&E, ×40). Pleomorphic spindle cells and multinucleate giant cells are arranged in a storiform or cartwheel pattern.

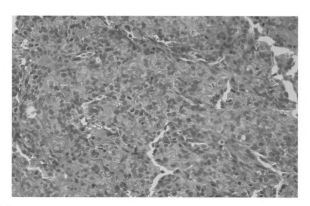

FIG. 47 Osteosarcoma (H&E, ×100). Large pleomorphic spindle cells are embedded in a dense, pink matrix of osteoid.

may present as a large, destructive mass. These sarcomas are typically of high grade histology with a cellular mixture of large, pleomorphic spindle or fibroblast-like cells and giant, multinucleated histiocyte-like cells (Figs. 45 and 46). Malignant fibrous histiocytoma is graded as other sarcomas by the degree of pleomorphism, necrosis, and mitotic rate. Histologic subtypes include storiform-pleomorphic (most common), myxoid, inflammatory, angiomatoid, and giant cell types. The storiform-pleomorphic type is seen most commonly in the head and neck and has a fascicular or cartwheel architecture of spindle and giant cells. The myxoid variant has a slightly better prognosis than the other types. Prognosis is generally poor with metastases to lung, lymph nodes, liver, and bone. Lymph node metastases occur in approximately 15% of cases. The storiform-pleomorphic type has a recurrence rate of 66% and metastatic rate of 42%.

OSTEOSARCOMA

Only 6% of osteosarcomas occur in the head and neck region with the majority occurring in the mandible

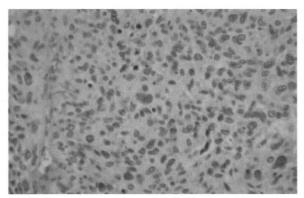

FIG. 46. Malignant fibrous histiocytoma (H&E, ×100). The individual spindle or fibroblast-like cells are mixed with larger histiocyte-like cells.

(85). The maxilla is the second most common head and neck site, however, and cases in the maxillary and ethmoid sinuses have been reported. The tumors present as poorly defined, destructive masses and grossly may be firm, gritty, fleshy, or fibrous. The histology is that cellular sheets of large spindle and pleomorphic cells admixed with osteoid (Fig. 47). Osteoid has a dense, pink, and often lace-like appearance and is essential for diagnosis. Fibrous and chondroblastic elements may be present; however, the presence of osteoid classifies the sarcoma as osteosarcoma or osteogenic sarcoma.

Radical surgery followed by adjunctive radiation and/or chemotherapy is the recommended therapy. The prognosis for sinonasal osteosarcomas is generally poor with reported recurrence rates of 80% usually occurring within the first postoperative year. Metastases to lungs and brain typically occur within the first 2 years and reduce survival to zero (86,87).

MELANOMA

Sinonasal mucosal melanomas comprise 0.6% to 2.5% of all malignant melanomas and arise from melanocytes, which have migrated from the neural crest (88). The majority of these tumors occur in the nasal cavity especially along the nasal septum, lateral wall, and inferior and middle turbinates. Grossly, the tumors are sessile or polypoid and may be pink, brown, or black. Mucosal ulceration is common.

Microscopically, the tumor cells are typically large and pleomorphic with epithelioid or spindle morphology. The growth pattern may be papillary, solid, organoid, and/or mixed (Figs. 48 and 49). Dense brown cytoplasmic melanin granules may be seen and confirmed by a Fontana stain. A significant number (10% to 30%) of sinonasal melanomas are amelanotic and require immunohistochemistry with S-100 or HMB-45 antibodies to confirm the diagnosis (Figs. 50 and 51).

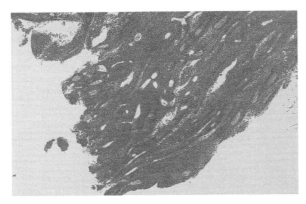

FIG. 48. Sinonasal melanoma (H&E, ×40). This distinct papillary architecture is not uncommon in sinonasal melanomas and may be confused with other papillary lesions, including benign papillomas.

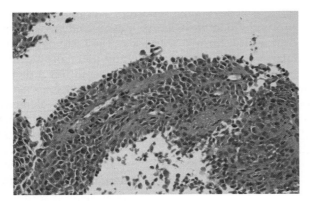

FIG. 49. Sinonasal melanoma (H&E, ×100). The individual cells have dark but otherwise uniform nuclei and no cytoplasmic melanin pigment.

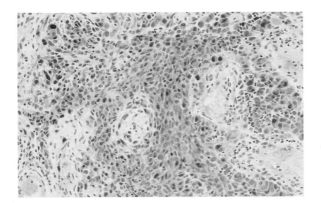

FIG. 50. Melanoma (×100). Immunohistochemistry with anti-S-100 antibody decorates the melanoma cells.

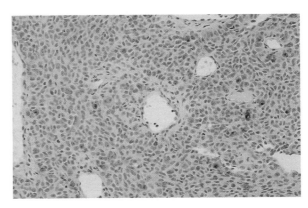

FIG. 51. Melanoma (×100). Immunohistochemistry with anti-HMB-45 antibody stains a small but significant number of the melanoma cells.

S-100 is a calcium regulatory protein found in cells of neural crest origin while HMB-45 was developed from a melanoma cell line. Rarely, electron microscopy is necessary is demonstrate melanosomes or premelanosomes.

Reported 5-year survival rates for nasal and paranasal sinus mucosal melanomas are 11% to 30% and generally worse than for cutaneous melanomas. Nasal cavity melanomas demonstrate 50% recurrent rate. Factors such as size, location, pigmentation, and histology have not shown prognostic significance. Regional lymph node metastases and distant metastases occur in approximately 20% of patients (89).

REFERENCES

1. Barnes EL. *Surgical pathology of the head and neck.* New York: Marcel Dekker, 1985.
2. Hyams VJ, Batsakis JG, Michaels L. *Tumors of the upper respiratory tract and ear. Atlas of tumor pathology, second series fascicle 25.* Washington DC: AFIP, 1988.
3. Barnes EL, Peel RL. *Head and neck pathology. A text/atlas of differential diagnosis.* New York: Igaku-Shoin, 1990.
4. Shanmugaratnam K. *Histologic typing of tumours of the upper respiratory tract and ear,* 2nd ed. Berlin: Springer-Verlag, 1990.
5. Wenig BM. *Atlas of head and neck pathology.* Philadelphia: Saunders, 1993.
6. Mills SE, Fechner R. Undifferentiated neoplasms of the sinonasal region: differential diagnosis based on clinical, light microscopic, immunohistochemical and ultrastructural features. *Semin Diagn Pathol* 1989;6:316–328.
7. Gandour-Edwards R, Donald P, Wiese D. Intraoperative frozen section diagnosis in head and neck surgery. Experience at a university medical center. *Head Neck* 1993;15(1):33–38.
8. Gandour-Edwards R, Donald P, Lie JT. The clinical utility of intraoperative frozen section diagnosis in head and neck surgery. A quality assurance perspective. *Head Neck* 1993;15: 373–376.
9. Freinkiel S, Chagnon F, Small R, Rocyhon L, Cohen C, Black M. The immunologic basis of nasal polyp formation. *J Otolaryngol* 1985;14:89–91.
10. Campagno J, Hyams VJ. Nasal polyposis with stromal atypia. *Arch Pathol Lab Med* 1976;100:224–226.
11. Batsakis JG, Sneige N. Choanal and angiomatous polyps of the sinonasal tract. *Ann Otol Rhinol Laryngol* 1992;101(7):623–625.

12. Wenig BM. *Atlas of head and neck pathology*. Philadelphia: Saunders, 1993;14–15.

13. Geschickter CF. Tumors of the nasal and paranasal sinuses. *Am J Cancer* 1935;24:637–660.

14. Lampertico P, Russell WO, MacComb WS. Squamous papilloma of upper respiratory epithelium. *Arch Pathol* 1963;75:81–90.

15. Hyams VJ. Papillomas of the nasal cavity and paranasal sinuses. A clinicopathologic study of 315 cases. *Ann Otol Rhinol Laryngol* 1971;80:192–206.

16. Norris HJ. Papillary lesions of the nasal cavity and paranasal sinuses. Part I. Exophytic (squamous) papillomas. A study of 28 cases. *Laryngoscope* 1962;72:1784–1797.

17. Norris HF. Papillary lesions of the nasal cavity and paranasal sinuses. Part II. Inverting papillomas. *Laryngoscope* 1963;73:1–17.

18. Barnes EL. Diseases of the nose, paranasal sinuses, and nasopharynx. In: Barnes EL, ed. *Surgical pathology of the head and neck*. New York: Marcel Dekker, 1985;412.

19. Syrjanen S, Happonen RP, Virolainen E, Siivonen L, Sryjanen K. Detection of human papillomavirus (HPV) structural antigens and DNA types in inverted papillomas and squamous cell carcinomas of the nasal cavities and paranasal sinuses. *Acta Otolaryngol (Stockh)* 1987;104(3–4):334–341.

20. Klemi PJ, Joensuu H, Siivonen L, Virolainen E, Syrjanen S, Syrjanen K. Association of DNA aneuploidy with human papillomavirus-induced malignant transformation of sinonasal transitional papillomas. *Otrolaryngol Head Neck Surg* 1989;100(6):563–567.

21. Judd R, Zaki SR, Coffield LM, Evatt BL. Sinonasal papillomas and human papillomavirus: human papillomavirus 11 detected in fungiform schneiderian papillomas by in situ hybridization and the polymerase chain reaction. *Hum Pathol* 1991;22(6):550–556.

22. Judd R, Zaki SR, Coffield LM, Evatt BL. Human papillomavirus type 6 detected by the polymerase chain reaction in invasive sinonasal papillary squamous cell carcinoma. *Arch Pathol Lab Med* 1991;115(11):1150–1153.

23. Furuta Y, Shinohara T, Sano K, et al. Molecular pathologic study of human papillomavirus infection in inverted papilloma and squamous cell carcinoma of the nasal cavities and paranasal sinuses. *Laryngoscope* 1991;101(1 Pt 1):79–85.

24. Sarkar FH, Visscher DW, Kintanar EB, Zarbo RJ, Crissman JD. Sinonasal schneiderian papllomas: human papillomavirus typing by polymerase chain reaction. *Mod Pathol* 1992;5(3):329–332.

25. Furuta Y, Takasu T, Asai T, et al. Detection of human papillomavirus DNA in carcinomas of the nasal cavities and paranasal sinuses by polymerase chain reaction. *Cancer* 1992;69(2):353–357.

26. Kashima HK, Kessis T, Hruban RH, Wu TC, Zinreich SJ, Shah KV. Human papillomavirus in sinonasal papillomas and squamous cell carcinoma. *Laryngoscope* 1992;102(9):973–976.

27. McLachlin CM, Kandel RA, Colgan TJ, Swanson DB, Witterick IJ, Ngan BY. Prevalence of human papillomavirus in sinonasal papillomas: a study using polymerase chain reaction and in situ hybridization. *Mod Pathol* 1992;5(4):4.

28. Benninger MS, Roberts JK, Sebek BA, Levine HL, Tucker HM, Lavertu P. Inverted papillomas and associated squamous cell carcinomas. *Otolaryngol Head Neck Surg* 1990;103(3):457–461.

29. Goepfert H, Guillamondegui OM, Jesse RH, Lindberg RD. Squamous cell carcinoma of the nasal vestibule. *Arch Otolaryngol* 1974;100:8–10.

30. Lewis JS, Castro EB. Cancer of the nasal cavity and paranasal sinuses. *J Laryngol Otol* 1972;86:255–262.

31. Hayes RB, Raatgever JW, de Bruyn A, Gerin M. Cancer of the nasal cavity and paranasal sinuses, and formaldehyde exposure. *Int J Cancer* 1986;37(4):487–492.

32. Hayes RB, Kardaun JW, de Bruyn A. Tobacco use and sinonasal cancer: a case-control study. *Br J Cancer* 1987;56(6):843–846.

33. Vaughan TL, Davis S. Wood dust exposure and squamous cell cancers of the upper respiratory tract. *Am J Epidemiol* 1991;133(6):560–564.

34. Barton RT. Nickel carcinogenesis of the respiratory tract. *J Otolaryngol* 1977;6:412–422.

35. Hyams VJ, Batsakis JG, Michaels L. *Tumors of the upper respi-

36. Wenig BM. *Atlas of head and neck pathology*. Philadelphia: Saunders, 1993;57.

37. Barnes EL. Diseases of the nose, paranasal sinuses, and nasopharynx. In: Barnes EL, ed. *Surgical pathology of the head and neck*. New York: Marcel Dekker, 1985;423.

38. Verbin RS. Diseases of the nose, paranasal sinuses, and nasopharynx. In: Barnes EL, ed. *Surgical pathology of the head and neck*. New York: Marcel Dekker, 1985;424.

39. Hermanek P, Sobin LH. *TNM classification of tumors*, 4th ed. Berlin: Springer-Verlag, 1987;27–29.

40. Hyams VJ, Batsakis JG, Michaels L. *Tumors of the upper respiratory tract and ear. Atlas of tumor pathology, second series fascicle 25*. Washington DC: AFIP, 1988;62.

41. Pearson GR. Epstein–Barr virus and nasopharyngeal carcinoma. *J Cell Biochem Suppl* 1993;17F:150–154.

42. Raab-Traub N. Epstein–Barr virus and nasopharyngeal carcinoma. *Semin Cancer Biol* 1992;3(5):297–307.

43. Shanmugaratnam K. *Histologic typing of tumours of the upper respiratory tract and ear*, 2nd ed. Berlin: Springer-Verlag, 1990;32–33.

44. Madri JA, Barwick KW. An immunohistochemical study of nasopharyngeal neoplasms using keratin antibodies: epithelial versus nonepithelial neoplasms. *Am J Surg Pathol* 1982;6:143–149.

45. Shanmugaratnam K, Chan SH, de-The G, et al: Histopathology of nasopharyngeal carcinoma: correlations with epidemiology, survival rates, and other biological characteristics. *Cancer* 1979;44:1029–1044.

46. Shah JP, Feghali J. Esthesioneuroblastoma. *Am J Surg* 1981;142:456–458.

47. Church LE, Uhler IV. Olfactory neuroblastomy. *Oral Surg* 1959;12:1040–1047.

48. Chaudry AP, Haar JG, Koul A, Nickerson PA. Olfactory neuroblastoma (esthesioneuroblastoma). *Cancer* 1979;44:564–579.

49. Hyams VJ, Batsakis JG, Michaels L. *Tumors of the upper respiratory tract and ear. Atlas of tumor pathology, second series fascicle 25*. Washington DC: AFIP, 1988;241–245.

50. Taxy JB, Bharani NK, Mills SE, Frierson HR Jr, Gould VE. The spectrum of olfactory neural tumors: a light-microscopic, immunohistochemical and electron microscopic analysis. *Am J Surg Pathol* 1986;10:687–695.

51. Kadish S, Goodman M, Wang CC. Olfactory neuroblastoma. *Cancer* 1976;37:1571–1576.

52. Frierson HF, Mills SE, Fechner RE, Taxy JB, Levine PA. Sinonasal undifferentiated carcinoma. An aggressive neoplasm derived from schneiderian epithelium and distinct from olfactory neuroblastoma. *Am J Surg Pathol* 1986;10:771–779.

53. Deutsch BD, Levine PA, Stewart FM, Frierson HF Jr, Cantrell RW. Sinonasal undifferentiated carcinoma: a ray of hope. *Otolaryngol Head Neck Surg* 1993;108(6):697–700.

54. Osborn DA. Morphology and the natural history of cribriform adenocarcinoma (adenoid cystic carcinoma). *J Clin Pathol* 1977;30:195–205.

55. Gnepp DR. Diseases of the nose, paranasal sinuses, and nasopharynx. In: Barnes EL, ed. *Surgical pathology of the head and neck*. New York: Marcel Dekker, 1985;432–433.

56. Perzin KH, Gullane P, Clairmont AC. Adenoid cystic carcinoma arising in salivary glands: a correlation of histologic features and clinical course. *Cancer* 1978;42:265–282.

57. Spiro RH, Huvos AG, Strong EW. Adenoid cystic carcinoma of salivary gland origin. *Am J Surg* 1974;128:512–520.

58. Gnepp DR, Heffner DK. Mucosal origin of sinonasal tract adenomatous neoplasms. *Mod Pathol* 1989;2(4):365–371.

59. Barnes L. Intestinal-type adenocarcinoma of the nasal cavity and paranasal sinuses. *Am J Surg Pathol* 1986;10(3):192–202.

60. Barnes EL. Diseases of the nose, paranasal sinuses, and nasopharynx. In: Barnes EL, ed. *Surgical pathology of the head and neck*. New York: Marcel Dekker, 1985;416.

61. Fu Y-S, Perzin KH. Non-epithelial tumors of the nasal cavity, paranasal sinus and nasopharynx. A clinico-pathologic study I. General features and vascular tumors. *Cancer* 1974;33:1275–1288.

62. Batsakis JG, Klopp CT, Newman W. Fibrosarcoma arising in

a "juvenile" nasopharyngeal angiofibroma following extensive radiation therapy. *Am Surg* 1955;21:786–793.

63. Hyams VJ, Batsakis JG, Michaels L. *Tumors of the upper respiratory tract and ear. Atlas of tumor pathology, second series fascicle 25*. Washington DC: AFIP, 1988;134–136.

64. Kapadia SB, Heffner DK. Pitfalls in the histopathologic diagnosis of pyogenic granuloma. *Eur Arch Otorhinolaryngol* 1992; 249(4):195–200.

65. Compango J, Hyams VJ. Hemangiopericytoma-like intranasal tumors. *Am J Clin Pathol* 1976;66:672–683.

66. Compagno J. Hemangiopericytoma-like tumors of the nasal cavity: a comparison with hemangiopericytoma of soft tissues. *J Laryngoscopy* 1978;88:460–469.

67. Hyams VJ, Batsakis JG, Michaels L. *Tumors of the upper respiratory tract and ear. Atlas of tumor pathology, second series fascicle 25*. Washington DC: AFIP, 1988;147.

68. Eichorn JH, Dickersin GR, Bhan AK, Goodman ML. Sinonasal hemangiopericytoma: a reassessment with electron microscopy, immunohistochemistry, and long-term follow-up. *Am J Surg Pathol* 1990;14:856–866.

69. Kapadia SB, Desai U, Cheng VS. Extramedullary plasmacytoma of the head and neck. A clinicopathologic study of 20 cases. *Medicine (Baltimore)* 1982;61:317–329.

70. Hyams V, Batsakis JG, Michaels L. *Tumors of the upper respiratory tract and ear. Atlas of tumor pathology, second series fascicle 25*. Washington DC: AFIP, 1988;209.

71. Ferry JA, Sklar J, Zukerberg LR, Harris NL. Nasal lymphoma. A clinicopathologic study with immunophenotypic and genotypic analysis. *Am J Surg Pathol* 1991;15(3):268–279.

72. Campo E, Cardesa A, Alos L, et al. Non-Hodgkin's lymphomas of nasal cavity and paranasal sinuses. An immunohistochemical study. *Am J Clin Pathol* 1991;96(2):184–190.

73. Kanavaros P, Lescs MC, Briere J, et al. Nasal T-cell lymphoma: a clinicopathologic entity associated with peculiar phenotype and with Epstein–Barr virus. *Blood* 1993;81(10):2688–2695.

74. Arber DA, Weiss LM, Albujar PF, Chen YY, Jaffe ES. Nasal lymphomas in Peru. High incidence of T-cell immunophenotype and Epstein–Barr virus infection. *Am J Surg Pathol* 1993;17(4): 392–399.

75. Fellbaum C, Hansmann ML, Lennert K. Malignant lymphomas of the nasal cavity and paranasal sinuses. *Virchows Arch A Pathol Anat Histopathology* 1989;414(5):399–405.

76. Wong KF, Chan JK, Ng CS, Lee KC, Tsang WY, Cheung MM. CD56 (NKH1)-positive hematolymphoid malignancies: an aggressive neoplasm featuring frequent cutaneous/mucosal involvement, cytoplasmic azurophilic granules, and angiocentricity. *Hum Pathol* 1992;23(7):798–804.

77. Liang R, Todd D, Chan TK, et al. Nasal lymphoma. A retrospective analysis of 60 cases. *Cancer* 1990;66(10):2205–2209.

78. Ho FC, Choy D, Loke SL, et al. Polymorphic reticulosis and conventional lymphomas of the nose and upper aerodigestive tract: a clinicopathologic study of 70 cases and immunophenotypic studies of 16 cases. *Hum Pathol* 1990;21(10):1041–1050.

79. Tran LM, Mark R, Fu YS, Calcaterra T, Juillard G. Primary non-Hodgkin's lymphomas of the paranasal sinuses and nasal cavity. A report of 18 cases with stage IE disease. *Am J Clin Oncol* 1992;15(3):222–225.

80. Enzinger FM, Weiss SW. *Soft tissue tumors*, 2nd ed. St. Louis: CV Mosby, 1988;448–488.

81. Eusebi V, Ceccarelli C, Gorza L, Schiaffino S, Bussolati G. Immunocytochemistry of rhabdomyosarcoma: the use of four different markers. *Am J Surg Pathol* 1986;10:293–299.

82. Wharam MD, Beltangady MS, Heyn RM, et al. Pediatric orofacial and laryngopharyngeal rhabdomyosarcoma. An Intergroup Rhabdomyosarcoma Study report. *Arch Otolaryngol Head Neck Surg* 1987;113(11):1225–1227.

83. Enzinger FM, Weiss Sw. *Soft tissue tumors*, 2n ed. St Louis: CV Mosby, 1988;269–300.

84. Barnes L, Kanbour A. Malignant fibrous histiocytoma of the head and neck. *Arch Otolaryngol Head Neck Surg* 1988;114: 1149–1156.

85. Garrington GE, Scofield HH, Cornyn J, Hooker SP. Osteosarcoma of the jaws. *Cancer* 1967;80:377–391.

86. Fu Y-S, Perzin KH. Non-epithelial tumors of the nasal cavity. paranasal sinus and nasopharynx. A clinico-pathologic study II. Fibrous dysplasia, ossifying fibroma, osteoblastoma, giant cell tumor and osteosarcoma. *Cancer* 1974;33:1289–1305.

87. Caron AS, Hajdu SI, Strong EW. Osteogenic sarcoma of the facial and cranial bones. *Am J Surg* 1971;122:719–725.

88. Barnes EL. Diseases of the nose, paranasal sinuses, and nasopharynx. In: Barnes EL, ed. *Surgical pathology of the head and neck*. New York: Marcel Dekker, 1985;437–439.

89. Hyams VJ, Batsakis JG, Michaels L. *Tumors of the upper respiratory tract and ear. Atlas of tumor pathology, second series fascicle 25*. Washington DC: AFIP, 1988;248–251.

CHAPTER 7

Radiology

Dale H. Rice

Computed tomography (CT) and magnetic resonance imaging (MRI) are now the modalities of choice for studying the paranasal sinuses. Plane films still have a limited role in the screening of patients with sinus infections and minor trauma but will not be discussed further in this section beyond the following. At this point in time, only four plane film projections are routinely employed in preliminary examinations. These consist of the Caldwell, the Waters, the submentovertex, and lateral views. In the Caldwell view, the patient is positioned face toward the x-ray cassette with the orbitomeatal line perpendicular to the cassette and the x-ray beam angled 15 degrees caudally. When properly done, this view will place the petrous pyramids in the lower third of the orbits. The Caldwell view is the best projection for the frontal and ethmoid sinuses. In the Waters view, the patient also faces the cassette, but the orbitomeatal line is angled 37 degrees to the plane of the cassette. In this case, the x-ray beam is perpendicular to the cassette, centered on the anterior nasal spine of the patient. The idea is to drop the petrous pyramids below the maxillary sinuses to avoid their obscuring sinus detail. The Waters view is the best projection for evaluation of the maxillary sinuses. The submentovertex view was first described by Schuller and Pfeiffer (1). The orbitomeatal line in this projection is parallel to the x-ray film cassette. The x-ray beam is directed perpendicular to the orbitomeatal line and centered just anteriorly to the plane of the external auditory meatus at slightly varying distances, depending on the radiologist's preference. This protection is best for the sphenoid and ethmoid sinuses as well as for the nasal cavity. The lateral view is done with the patient facing in a direction parallel to the x-ray cassette with the nose then rotated 5 degrees toward the cassette to avoid superimposition of the posterior walls of the maxillary sinuses. The x-ray beam is perpendicular to the cassette and is centered near the outer can-thus of the eye with the orbitomeatal line parallel to the cassette. The lateral view is best for the frontal sinuses and maxillary sinuses.

PLANE FILM ANATOMY

Plane films by their nature are limited in detail assessment compared to CT scans and MRI, the major disadvantage being the superimposition of three dimensions into two. Because of this, detail is inherently less clear. Consequently, the extent of both soft tissue disease and bone destruction will consistently be underestimated. On the other hand, because of the decreased cost, ready availability, low radiation dose, and ease of examination, these plane films are often preferential initial studies.

ETHMOID SINUSES

The ethmoid sinuses are best evaluated on plane film examination with the Caldwell view (Fig. 1). The disadvantage is that all the ethmoid cells are superimposed on each other as well as structures in the skull posterior to them. This makes evaluation of individual ethmoid cells difficult or impossible, rendering interpretation of minimal inflammatory or neoplastic disease quite difficult. In the ideal situation the air density of the ethmoid sinus should be similar to the air density around the inferior turbinate if, in fact, that area is disease-free. On the other hand, the lamina papyracea and the fovea ethmoidalis should be relatively clearly delineated, although not nearly to the degree that they are in the coronal CT scans. The anterior margin of the lamina papyracea, which articulates with the lacrimal bone, is poorly seen. Occasionally, a small indentation or groove is seen on the upper medial orbital wall. This bony canal houses the anterior ethmoid artery and vein

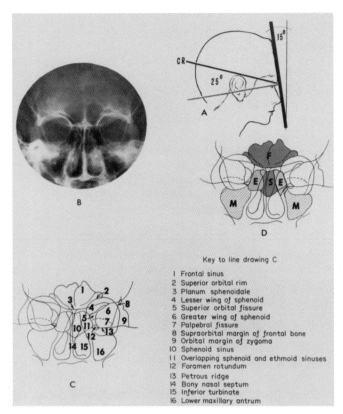

FIG. 1. Caldwell view of paranasal sinuses. (From ref. 2, with permission.)

Key to line drawing C

1 Frontal sinus
2 Superior orbital rim
3 Planum sphenoidale
4 Lesser wing of sphenoid
5 Superior orbital fissure
6 Greater wing of sphenoid
7 Palpebral fissure
8 Supraorbital margin of frontal bone
9 Orbital margin of zygoma
10 Sphenoid sinus
11 Overlapping sphenoid and ethmoid sinuses
12 Foramen rotundum
13 Petrous ridge
14 Bony nasal septum
15 Inferior turbinate
16 Lower maxillary antrum

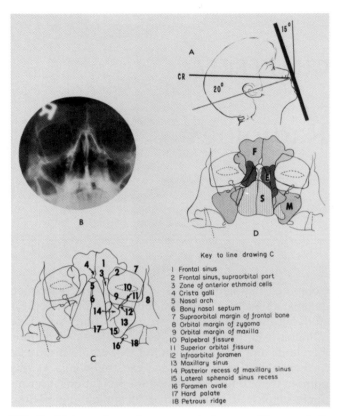

FIG. 2. Waters view of paranasal sinuses. (From ref. 2, with permission.)

Key to line drawing C

1 Frontal sinus
2 Frontal sinus, supraorbital part
3 Zone of anterior ethmoid cells
4 Crista galli
5 Nasal arch
6 Bony nasal septum
7 Supraorbital margin of frontal bone
8 Orbital margin of zygoma
9 Orbital margin of maxilla
10 Palpebral fissure
11 Superior orbital fissure
12 Infraorbital foramen
13 Maxillary sinus
14 Posterior recess of maxillary sinus
15 Lateral sphenoid sinus recess
16 Foramen ovale
17 Hard palate
18 Petrous ridge

along with the terminal branches of the nasociliary nerve and marks the level of the floor of the anterior cranial fossa. The ethmoidal maxillary plate can also often be seen and marks the posterior–inferior boundary between the ethmoid and maxillary bones. Also visible, if present, are the supraorbital ethmoid cells representing pneumatization into the orbital plate of the frontal bone. These are usually symmetrical and, if not, opacification or destruction on that side should be suspected.

Only the most anterior ethmoid cells can be visualized on the Waters view with the middle and posterior ethmoid cells hidden by the nasal fossa. On the submentovertex view, the palate, nasal septum, turbinates, and anterior floor of the frontal sinus are superimposed on the ethmoids, preventing a detailed evaluation. In summary, for plane film evaluation of the ethmoid sinuses the Caldwell view is the preferential view to use.

MAXILLARY SINUSES

Unlike the ethmoids, the maxillary sinuses are best evaluated using the Waters view (Fig. 2). In the vast majority of patients the maxillary sinuses are symme-

tric in size and configuration with only minor variations being common. On the other hand, hypoplasia of one or both can occur as well as the complete absence of one or both. When hypoplasia does occur, the roof of the hypoplastic sinus has a greater medial to lateral downward slope. This is unimportant except that on plane films this feature may simulate an orbital floor blowout fracture. The distinction is readily made, however, since the hypoplastic sinus also usually has a clearly thicker lateral bony wall secondary to the decreased pneumatization of the maxilla. Certain diseases such as fibrous dysplasia, brown tumors, Paget's disease, and giant cell tumors may encroach on the sinus cavity as well, but these are generally easily identified. The Waters projection also gives an excellent view of the inferior orbital rim, although much of the orbital floor itself is more oblique to the plane of the film so that small fractures or depressions may be obscured. Both the superior and inferior orbital fissures can be seen on the Waters view as well. The body of the zygoma can be seen on the Waters view but the base view is necessary for evaluation of the zygomatic arches when evaluating possible fractures. A common mistake with the Waters view is projecting the soft tissue shadow of the upper lip across the lower border of the maxillary sinus. This can be mistaken for a soft

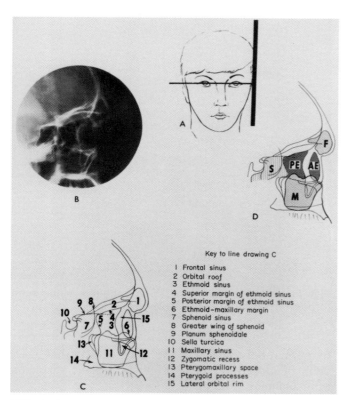

FIG. 3. Lateral view of paranasal sinuses. (From ref. 2, with permission.)

Key to line drawing C

1 Frontal sinus
2 Orbital roof
3 Ethmoid sinus
4 Superior margin of ethmoid sinus
5 Posterior margin of ethmoid sinus
6 Ethmoid-maxillary margin
7 Sphenoid sinus
8 Greater wing of sphenoid
9 Planum sphenoidale
10 Sella turcica
11 Maxillary sinus
12 Zygomatic recess
13 Pterygomaxillary space
14 Pterygoid processes
15 Lateral orbital rim

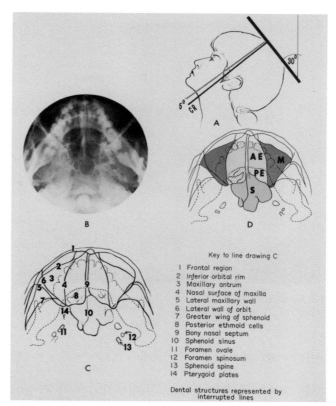

FIG. 4. Submentovertex or base view of paranasal sinuses. (From ref. 2, with permission.)

Key to line drawing C

1 Frontal region
2 Inferior orbital rim
3 Maxillary antrum
4 Nasal surface of maxilla
5 Lateral maxillary wall
6 Lateral wall of orbit
7 Greater wing of sphenoid
8 Posterior ethmoid cells
9 Bony nasal septum
10 Sphenoid sinus
11 Foramen ovale
12 Foramen spinosum
13 Sphenoid spine
14 Pterygoid plates

Dental structures represented by interrupted lines

tissue density within the sinus. Soft tissue swelling of the cheek, particularly if unilateral, can mimic clouding of the maxillary sinus on the Waters view.

In the lateral view (Fig. 3) the choroid processes of the mandible project over the inferior–posterior aspect of the maxillary sinuses and they simulate soft tissue masses or a fractured bony segment. Additionally, the orbital floor can be seen as two separate lines representing anteriorly the lowest and flattest area of the floor and more posteriorly the region of the orbital apex. The lateral view also best shows the inferior extension of the maxillary sinus and its relationship to the hard palate and tooth roots. This relationship changes during childhood and adolescence to adult age. The infratemporal portion of the maxillary sinus wall is poorly seen on both the Caldwell and Waters views. It is best evaluated with the lateral radiograph. The submentovertex view as well shows the curved nature of the wall (Fig. 4).

FRONTAL SINUSES

Since the frontal sinuses develop independently, asymmetry is quite common. When unilateral or bilateral aplasia or hypoplasia does occur, the smaller fron-

tal sinus usually consists of a single centrally concave recess, which contains little air compared to the amount of overlying bone and frequently appears as if it were opacified on plane films. The larger sinuses frequently have scalloped margins with partial septations that project into the sinus lumen. Regardless of the size of the frontal sinuses, however, they never violate the orbital contour in the normal state. The margin of the frontal sinus is outlined by a thin dense rim called the mucoperiosteal line, which separates the sinus from the adjacent frontal bone. This margin is important in trying to differentiate between a completely opacified frontal sinus versus an aplastic sinus. If no margin is seen on any of the projections, aplasia is probable. Most information about the frontal sinus is obtained from the Caldwell and Waters views where the bulk of the sinus is best projected. It is important to realize that on the lateral view only the near medial anterior and posterior tables are well seen, while on the submentovertex view, the caudal portions of the sinus walls are better seen than the cephalic portions, which are curving away from the x-ray beam. The European fifth view (Fig. 5), a hyperextended base view, will protect the profile of the posterior wall of the frontal sinus through the primary palate. This is especially useful in evaluating the posterior wall in cases of fracture.

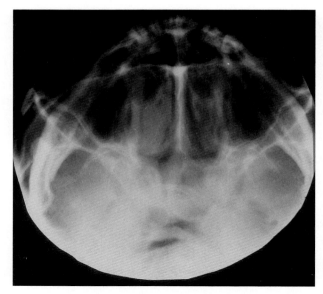

FIG. 5. European fifth view or hyperextended base view. (From ref. 3, with permission.)

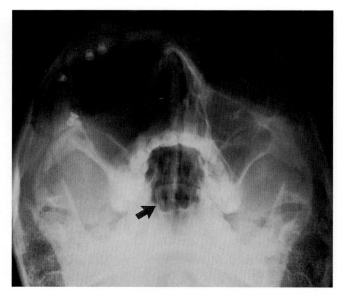

FIG. 6. Maltz view demonstrating sphenoid sinus seen through open mouth (see *arrow*).

SPHENOID SINUSES

The sphenoid sinuses are difficult to evaluate by routine films largely because they are deep within the skull, surrounded by numerous other bones, regardless of the projection, that interfere with interpretation. This is compounded by the extreme variability in their pneumatization. Approximately 50% of people have only a central sinus cavity while the other 50% will have lateral recesses in addition. Generally, the sphenoid can be otherwise reasonably well evaluated by a combination of the lateral and submentovertex views. However, the best projection to appreciate the frontal perspective of the sphenoid sinus is the Maltz view, which is simply the Waters view taken through an open mouth. The mandible is thrown out of field, no longer obscuring the sphenoid (Fig. 6). The lateral view is particularly useful for evaluating the planum sphenoidale, the sellar floor, and the posterior wall of the sinus. The submentovertex view, on the other hand, also shows lateral extensions of the sinus that are not appreciable on the lateral projection. These extensions can also be seen on the Caldwell and Waters views. In the Caldwell view, these lateral extensions are viewed through the orbit, while on the Waters view, they can be seen projecting through the maxillary sinus.

Normal mucosal thickness on plane films is 1 to 2 mm. Polyps appear as radiodensities with a smooth contour with some surrounding air shadow if singular, but since polyps often occur in multiples they can appear as a multibosselated radiodensity. The commonest incidental finding on sinus radiographs is probably the smooth domed maxillary cyst. It is usually asymptomatic, has uniform density, and is surrounded

by normal bone (Fig. 7). Any sinus density that is accompanied by bone erosion must raise the suspicion of malignancy (Fig. 8).

COMPUTED TOMOGRAPHY

Computed tomography (CT) is particularly suited for evaluating dense cortical bone and for fine bone detail in planning sinus surgery. CT is also now widely accepted as the most sensitive technique for identifying normal and abnormal adjacent soft tissue structures. Four to five millimeter thick contiguous sections are taken in the axial and/or coronal planes, depending on the disease process under examination. For maximum visualization of bone and adjacent bone- and air-containing structures, a wide window setting is ideal. Win-

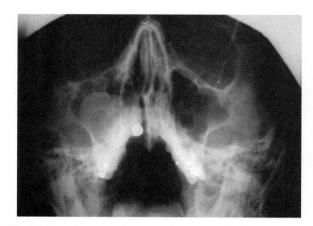

FIG. 7. Simple retention cyst in right maxillary sinus.

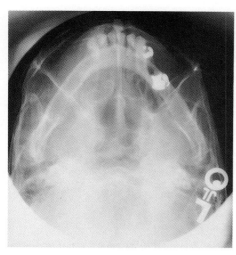

FIG. 8. Base view showing bone erosion of medial maxillary sinus wall secondary to malignant neoplasm (see *arrow*).

dow settings should be in the range of 2000 to 4000 HU. For closer examination of the mucosa, a narrow window is used, similar to that for lung parenchyma in the range of 140 to 400 HU. For inflammatory lesions, the examinations are performed without intravenous contrast. For the routine evaluation, in patients with inflammatory diseases, the coronal scan is sufficient. Exceptions are made for more detailed evaluation of the nasofrontal duct and the posterior walls of the frontal and sphenoid sinuses, where a combination of axial and coronal scans is more useful.

For the evaluation of neoplastic diseases, intravenous contrast used in both axial and coronal planes should be obtained.

Magnetic resonance imaging (MRI) is most useful in evaluating neoplastic diseases of the paranasal sinuses. This is especially true when one must separate tumor from obstructive mucosal disease. In general, the T1 weighted image gives better soft tissue detail, while T2 weighted images give an increased signal to both neoplastic and inflammatory processes. For the best detail, a sinus coil should be used.

INFLAMMATORY DISEASE

Normal sinus mucosa is so thin that it is not visualized on CT scans or on MRI. Thus if no mucosa is visible between the air and the bone, it can generally be assumed to be normal. The differential diagnosis of soft tissue thickening on CT scan or MRI includes inflammatory disorders of either infectious or nonin-

fectious source, fibrosis, or neoplasms. For the evaluation of acute or chronic inflammatory disorders, coronal CT scan is the preferred imaging technique. The amount of soft tissue thickening seen in the sinus can vary from 1 to 2 mm to complete opacification. In this setting the amount of thickened mucosa as compared to the amount of collected fluid is quite variable. CT scan is well suited to evaluate the thickening or thinning of bone in response to acute or chronic infection. This is easier to assess in the maxillary and sphenoid and frontal sinuses than in the ethmoid sinuses. Usually the sinuses should be viewed at wide window settings so sinus disease is not obscured and misinterpreted as an aplastic sinus. An improper setting can completely miss a diseased sinus.

When one is considering sinus surgery in the patient with chronic inflammatory disease, coronal CT imaging is the study of choice. Areas of mucosal thickening and obstruction are well demonstrated not only in the region of the osteomeatal complex but in the other sinuses as well. For these patients, soft tissue thickening in the middle meatus is the most frequent finding with other changes depending on the chronicity and severity of the disease and the specific sinuses involved (Fig. 9). In general, with CT scans, the inflamed mucosa is characterized by enhancing tissue along the sinus walls while low-density areas, most often in the central part of the larger sinuses, are indicative of secretions (Fig. 10). With MRI, inflamed mucosa is characterized by high signal intensity on both T1 and T2 weighted images. MRI may even demonstrate the herniation of swollen, edematous maxillary sinus mucosa through the ostium into the middle meatus.

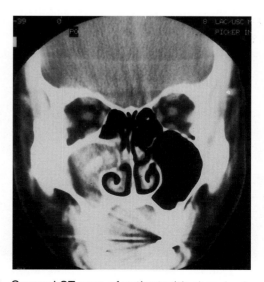

FIG. 9. Coronal CT scan of patient with chronic sinusitis.

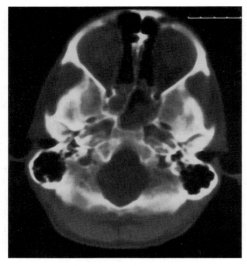

FIG. 10. Axial CT scan of sphenoid sinusitis in patient with AIDS.

Air–fluid levels are most common in the maxillary and frontal sinuses and are easily seen on coronal CT scans. Mucosal thickening can also be detected in barotrauma, which is most common in the frontal sinus, followed in frequency by the ethmoid sinus and the maxillary sinus. This mucosal thickening results from bleeding within the mucosa or directly into the sinus itself. CT scanning is also effective in detecting the complications of inflammatory sinus disease. Orbital cellulitis or abscesses are readily demonstrated on CT scan, particularly in the axial projection. This is generally characterized by a diffuse increase in density in the medial orbital wall between the lamina papyracea and the medial rectus muscle (Figs. 11 and 12). Frontal bone osteomyelitis may also be readily demonstrated. CT scan is also effective at detecting intracranial complications other than perhaps early meningitis. It is,

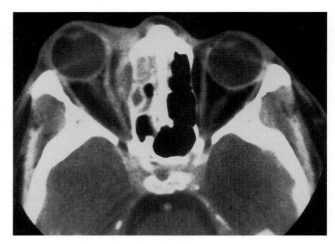

FIG. 12. Axial CT scan or subperiosteal abscess secondary to ethmoid sinusitis.

however, excellent at demonstrating epidural and subdural empyemas, as well as brain abscesses and cavernous sinus thrombosis. Epidural and subdural empyemas are demonstrated as extracerebral collections of low-density fluid, usually lenticular shaped if epidural, or crescentic shaped if subdural. The capsule of the empyema usually enhances. Both of these are commonly secondary to frontal sinusitis, which will also be demonstrated. Most brain abscesses are located at or near the corticomedullary junction and are commonly in the frontal or temporal lobes. They will appear as a low-density area, often with rim enhancement (Fig. 13).

Mucous retention cysts are found in approximately 10% of patients (4). Since the mucous retention cyst results from the obstruction of a seromucinous gland in the wall in the sinus mucosa, the wall of the resulting

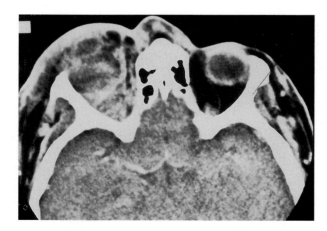

FIG. 11. Axial CT scan of orbital cellulitis. Note diffuse involvement of orbital structures.

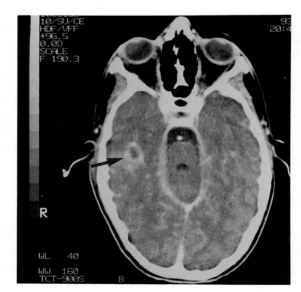

FIG. 13. CT scan of brain abscess showing rim enhancement.

cyst is the epithelium of the duct and gland itself (5). These mucous retention cysts can occur in any of the sinuses but are far more common in the maxillary sinus. Serous retention cysts can also occur and result from the accumulation of serous fluid in the submucosal layer of the mucosa and thus are not true cysts. These tend to occur in the floor of the maxillary sinus.

Benign cysts of the paranasal sinuses usually manifest as hemispheric densities projecting from the sinus wall into the lumen on CT scan or MRI. On the CT scan they appear as water dense lesions with no bony changes. On MRI, however, they give off a bright signal on both T1 and T2 weighted images. They most often occur on the floor and lateral wall of the maxillary sinus (Figs. 14 and 15).

Polyps result from increased swelling of the normal mucosa, but the exact pathogenesis has not been clearly elucidated. Small intrasinus polyps may not be distinguishable from mucous retention cysts. In the clinical setting polyps are more likely to present in the nasal cavity after prolapsing through the sinus ostium, the majority coming from the ethmoid sinuses. At this point, the polyps are usually large and numerous, and there is opacification of a large percentage of the sinuses. An important exception is the antrochoanal polyp, which represents 4% to 6% of all nasal polyps. These are generally unilateral, solitary lesions manifested by unilateral nasal airway obstruction. Only approximately 8% of these patients will have other polyps, while 15% to 40% will have a history of allergy (6). Interestingly, the majority of antrochoanal polyps occur in younger age groups and tend to recur if incompletely removed. On CT scan, the majority of inflammatory or allergic polyps tend to have a mucoid attenu-

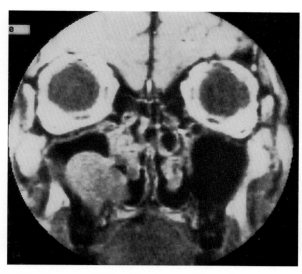

FIG. 15. Coronal MRI of large maxillary sinus polypoid lesion in Fig. 14. Note better demonstrated ethmoid disease in coronal projection.

ation (10 to 18 HU) with mucosal enhancement occasionally seen at the polyp surface. Long-standing polyps typically have more collagen and fibrous tissue, with a resulting higher attenuation of 20 to 35 HU. In the usual setting of multiple polyps in the sinuses and in the nasal cavity, it may be difficult on CT scan to distinguish this mass-appearing lesion from a neoplasm. The CT scan appearance of a central sinus density separated from the sinus wall by a zone of lower attenuation could be seen in either intrasinus hemorrhage, allergic fungal sinusitis, or polyps (7).

Mucoceles are the most common expanding lesions of the paranasal sinuses and are lined by cuboidal epithelium, which surrounds the mucoid secretions. They develop from an obstruction of a sinus ostium, from a compartment of a septated sinus, or as an entrapment within a frontal sinus fracture line. The wall of the lesion is the sinus mucosa and the sinus cavity expands as the bony walls are remodeled to accommodate the enlarging cyst. They occur most commonly in the frontoethmoid region followed at a distant second by the maxillary sinus (8). On CT scan, a mucocele usually appears as an expanded sinus cavity filled with a homogeneous material of mucoid attenuation. One or more sinus walls are remodeled but may be either of normal thickness or thin or eroded. In the latter circumstance, only the sinus mucosa and the periosteum of the bone confine the mucous secretions. If there is an inflammatory component signifying a mucopyocele, the sinus mucosa is seen as a thin zone of enhancement just inside the bony sinus walls (9). The most common location is the frontoethmoid suture, but the symptoms elicited will depend on the sinus involved and the wall being expanded. On CT scan, the majority of muco-

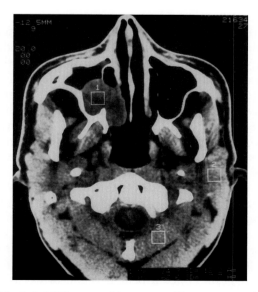

FIG. 14. Axial CT scan of large maxillary sinus polypoid lesion.

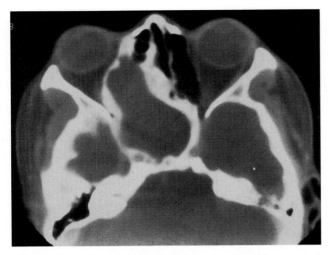

FIG. 16. Axial CT scan of large sphenoethmoid mucocele presenting as decreasing visual acuity.

celes have a homogeneous appearance. They do not enhance. MRI has the ability to differentiate fluid-filled structures from benign and malignant tumors, because fluid-filled structures give a high signal on both T1 and T2 weighted images (Figs. 16 and 17).

With a frontal sinus mucocele, on CT scanning one will see a loss of the normal scalloping septa with expansion of the sinus cavity and thinning of the bone. Often the first symptom, as with ethmoid mucoceles, is displacement of the eye.

Postoperative scanning is not routinely recommended after surgery for inflammatory disease. The clinical status of the patient is paramount in evaluating success and failure. However, in patients with persistent symptoms and normal intranasal examination, repeat coronal scanning will serve to evaluate the status

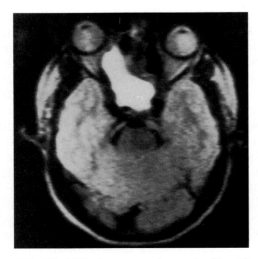

FIG. 17. MRI of same lesion as in Fig. 16.

of the sinuses. This can be very helpful in detecting small areas of residual disease that need attention. Occasionally, it will show complete resolution of the preoperative disease and cause one to investigate further for additional causes of similar symptoms.

Fungal diseases have a quite varied appearance in the sinuses. The maxillary and ethmoid sinuses are most frequently involved with the sphenoid occasionally involved and the frontal rarely. The surrounding bone may undergo a wide variety of changes in isolation or in combination. With mycetoma or allergic fungal sinusitis, intrasinus concretions can plainly be seen (10). (See the chapter by Donald, Fungal Infections, Fig. 5.) While a large variety of fungal diseases have been reported, the most common are aspergillosis and mucormycosis if the infection is invasive and aspergillosis or *Bipolaris* in allergic fungal sinusitis.

A cholesteatoma rarely can occur within a sinus. In the frontal bone cholesteatomas probably arise from a congenital rest and may not be connected to the sinus at all. Those that occur within a paranasal sinus generally involve the maxillary, probably as a result of squamous metaplasia of the sinus mucosa, secondary to chronic infection. These may also appear as the sinus counterpart of cholesterol granuloma (11). On CT scan, a cholesteatoma is an expansile lesion that has soft tissue, has mucoid-like attenuation, and may be indistinguishable from a mucocele.

NEOPLASTIC DISEASE

A significant problem in imaging sinonasal neoplasms is the fact that many, if not all, of them are accompanied by surrounding chronic inflammatory disease, making accurate delineation sometimes quite difficult. When imaging these tumors, one must be particularly aware of critical areas of potential extension that might significantly alter the operative or radiation therapy approach. These areas include, in particular, the floor of the anterior and middle cranial fossa, the pterygopalatine fossa, the orbits, the palate, and the infratemporal fossa, as well as extension into the subcutaneous tissue of the face. While CT scanning does not require contrast medium for the evaluation of inflammatory diseases, it definitely does for the evaluation of neoplastic lesions. Even with contrast, the separation of tumor from surrounding inflammatory tissue is often quite difficult. One should bear in mind that, in imaging these lesions, unless there is bone involvement, it may not be possible to separate out a neoplastic from a non-neoplastic lesion. Bone destruction suggests aggressive tumor behavior while bone remodeling suggests either a benign lesion or occasionally some of the lower grade malignant lesions. Some carcinomas like squamous cell carcinoma enhance very little on contrast CT scan and make separation from inflammatory lesions even more difficult.

Neoplastic lesions in bone are easily detected on CT scan. The aneurysmal bone cyst, while it is neither an aneurysm nor a true cyst, is easily detected on CT scan. It may be unilocular or multilocular with a "soap bubble" or "honeycomb" radiolucency. The peripheral bone margins demonstrate bone remodeling and destruction. The several odontogenic cysts are also easily detected. The primordial cyst arises from degeneration of the enamel structures and the cyst fills a place normally occupied by a tooth, since the enamel forms before the calcified dental structures (12). The dentigerous cyst is considerably more common. Most occur in the second and third decades of life and arise in an unerupted tooth after the crown of the tooth has developed. It appears as a cystic lesion into which the crown of the tooth projects. It may be either unilocular or multilocular and resorption of roots of neighboring teeth is common. Radiographically, the cysts must be distinguished from a normal dental follicle. If the pericoronal space exceeds 2.5 mm in width, there is a high chance that the unerupted tooth may become a dentigerous cyst (13).

The periapical or radicular cyst is the most common cyst of the jaws and arises from erupted infected teeth and usually is the sequela to a preexisting periapical granuloma. It is more common in the maxilla than the mandible. The odotogenic keratocyst is an uncommon lesion associated with Marfan's syndrome and the basal cell nevus syndrome. It tends to occur in the second and third decades of life, affecting the mandible two to four times more than the maxilla, and generally occurs in the posterior aspect of the jaws. These cysts are invasive. The ameloblastoma is the most common tumor that arises from the epithelial components from the embryonic tooth, but still this tumor comprises only 1% of all jaw cysts and tumors. It typically occurs in the third and fourth decades of life in the premolar area. On CT scans, these tumors tend to have a nonenhancing, nonhomogeneous appearance showing a multiloculated lytic lesion with no mineralized component.

Computerized tomography and magnetic resonance imaging are the modalities of choice for assessing location and extent of tumors of the paranasal sinuses. The most common benign tumors, ignoring polyps, are the inverted papilloma and the osteoma.

Osteomas are often discovered as incidental findings but may, with progressive enlargement, cause symptoms (Figs. 18 and 19). They are most frequently located in the frontoethmoid suture and may be divided into cortical and cancellous types. If they continue to expand, they will cause displacement of adjacent bone, often with displacement of the globe. Expansion intracranially may occur.

The CT scan appearance in fibrous dysplasia is de-

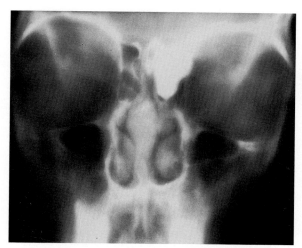

FIG. 18. Coronal CT scan of frontoethmoid osteoma.

pendent on the amount of fibrous tissue that develops within the newly formed osteoid and calcified cartilage. There is generally a uniform opacification of the entire sinus cavity and adjacent bone, often with expansion of the involved sinus cavity (Fig. 20). The ossifying fibroma, on the other hand, is generally a well circumscribed lesion that tends to be more aggressive in behavior. Both lesions tend to occur in adolescents, usually women. All osseous and fibro-osseous lesions are well seen with either CT scan or MRI.

The inverted papilloma is an uncommon epithelial tumor, usually occurring in the nasal cavity. It appears to arise from the inferior or middle turbinate on the lateral nasal wall (Fig. 21). With progressive growth, however, it can expand into the maxillary and ethmoid sinuses and is occasionally associated with squamous cell carcinoma (Fig. 22). It is well demonstrated by CT scan and MRI, although MRI will more accurately separate out obstructive mucosal disease (Figs. 23 and 24).

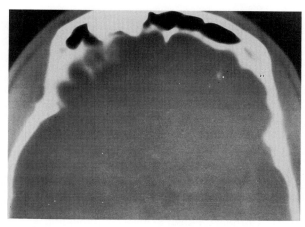

FIG. 19. Axial CT scan of frontal osteoma.

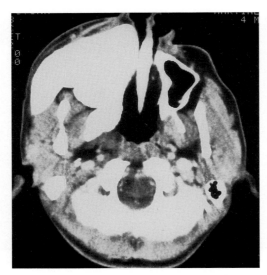

FIG. 20. Fibrous dysplasia of maxilla.

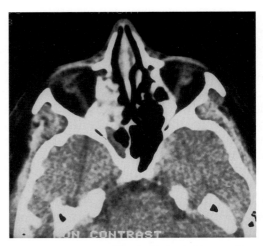

FIG. 22. Axial CT scan of inverted papilloma discovered to have squamous cell carcinoma within a pathologic examination.

Malignant tumors of the paranasal sinuses comprise less than 1% of all malignancies and approximately 3% of malignant lesions of the upper aerodigestive tract. CT scanning and MRI are paramount in the evaluation of malignant tumors for optimum treatment planning. Approximately 80% appear to arise within the maxillary sinus (Figs. 25 and 26), while most of the remainder arise from the ethmoid sinuses (Fig. 27). For the evaluation of malignant tumors with CT scanning, contrast enhancement may or may not add to the information obtained. CT scanning is best for evaluating extension of a tumor through bone into the surrounding tissues, such as the orbit, pterygomaxillary fossa, in-

fratemporal fossa, or intracranial cavity (Figs. 28 and 29). MRI is particularly useful in evaluating malignant neoplasms because of its ability to separate tumor tissue from thickened mucosa or retained mucus. CT scanning often does this poorly, while MRI usually will show the presence of obstructed mucosal disease separate from the tumor itself. Furthermore, MRI may show tumor extension into adjacent structures better than the CT scan (Fig. 30).

The addition of gadolinium contrast has done much to delineate the difference between inflammation and tumor. Tumors generally tend to show a much brighter signal with contrast than inflammatory tissues, as well as surrounding soft tissue. The tissue that is the excep-

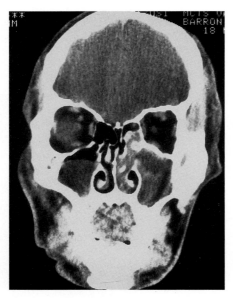

FIG. 21. Coronal CT scan of inverted papilloma with secondary obstruction of ethmoid and maxillary sinuses.

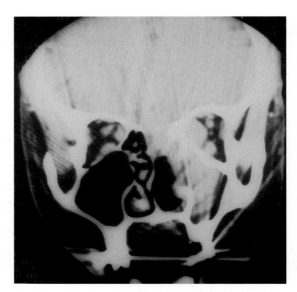

FIG. 23. Coronal CT scan of inverted papilloma invading orbit despite prior resection and radiation therapy.

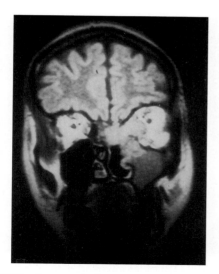

FIG. 24. MRI of same lesion as in Fig. 14. This lesion proved fatal from intracranial spread despite continued benign diagnosis on histologic examination.

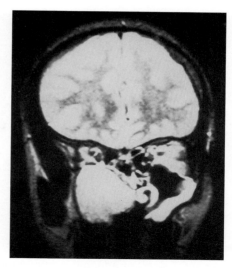

FIG. 26. Coronal MRI of osteogenic sarcoma.

tion to that rule is fat. With new fat suppression software programs, tumor can clearly be differentiated from this tissue. The presence of fibrosis and edema are still confounding factors, despite gadolinium.

Metastatic lesions to the paranasal sinuses are infrequent with only about 100 cases formally reported in the literature. The renal cell carcinoma is the most common, followed by the lung and the breast. In general, the presence of distant metastases to the paranasal sinuses implies a very poor prognosis. The single exception is the situation of a primary renal cell carcinoma with a solitary paranasal sinus metastasis. In this situation the successful excision of both the primary and the metastasis may result in good survival (14). On

CT scan, metastatic lesions from these distant primaries show bone-destroying aggressive soft tissue masses that enhance minimally with contrast. There is no reliable way to tell a metastatic lesion from a primary paranasal sinus carcinoma. The only exceptions potentially are those lesions from renal cell carcinoma and melanoma, which do tend to enhance and also tend to remodel as well as destroy the sinus walls. Furthermore, the metastatic prostatic carcinoma may give a purely osteoblastic metastasis. The most important radiographic indication of metastases in this setting is the presence of more than one lesion if, in fact, that occurs. This, however, is an uncommon situation.

MRI is generally far superior to CT scan is differentiating tumor from adjacent inflammatory disease. The T2 weighted MRI is able to separate these two because

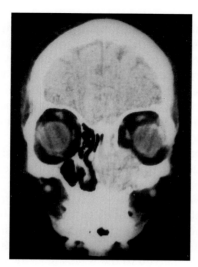

FIG. 25. Coronal CT scan of small cell carcinoma arising within maxillary sinus.

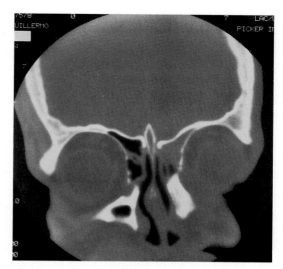

FIG. 27. Coronal CT scan of Burkitt's lymphoma of right ethmoid.

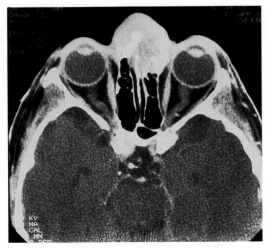

FIG. 28. Axial CT scan of adenoid cystic carcinoma of ethmoid sinus showing invasion of left orbit.

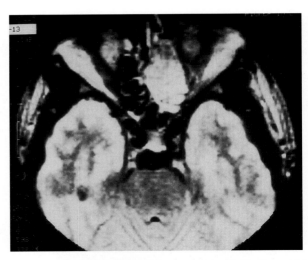

FIG. 30. Axial MRI of leiomyosarcoma of left ethmoid invading orbit with benign mucosal disease demonstrated anterior to tumor.

of the high water content in inflammatory mucosa and in secretions. Tumors, in contrast, are highly cellular and have an intermediate intensity signal (15). MRI is especially good at distinguishing tumors with a rich vascular network such as the angiofibroma. Dynamic scanning identifies the highly vascular nature of these tumors with a combination of T1 proton density and T2 weighted sequences. The MRI will reveal multiple flow void channels representing the major tumor vessels (16,17). In general, carcinomas have an intermediate intensity signal with a fairly homogeneous internal architecture. Occasionally, localized areas of hemorrhage or necrosis can be seen. MRI is particularly good at detecting extension of the tumor beyond the confines of the sinus itself. Malignant melanoma, like most of the other carcinomas, presents as a homogeneous mass

of intermediate signal intensity on MRI except for a few that will have a high T1 weighted signal intensity because of the presence of paramagnetic melanin. The MRI gives consistent findings on the evaluation of cystic lesions. The cyst fluid has an intermediate signal on T1 weighted images and a high signal on T2 weighted images. If there is a tooth involved, it will give no signal on any imaging sequence. In this regard, the MRI appearance is similar to that of a noninvasive antral aspergilloma. The ameloblastoma gives a nonhomogeneous mixed signal intensity with intermediate intensity on T1 and proton density weighted images with variable and intermediate and high signal intensities on T2 weighted images.

TRAUMATIC INJURIES

High-resolution CT scanning has revolutionized imaging for facial trauma. CT scanning's sensitivity to bone allows it to exactly delineate the location and extent of every fracture. This is particularly true if both axial and coronal scans are obtained. This ability to assess fractures accurately has occurred parallel with the advancing armamentarium of the craniofacial reconstructive surgeon for primary repair.

A noncontrast CT scan is the modality of choice for the most complete evaluation of the facial skeleton, soft tissues, brain, and dural spaces in the trauma patient (18). A combination of axial and coronal CT scans provides the most complete diagnostic information (19). In the CT evaluation of naso-orbital fractures, because of the posterior displacement, careful attention should be given to the bones near the optic canal, especially in planning the operative repositioning of these displaced bones. In CT evaluation of all these

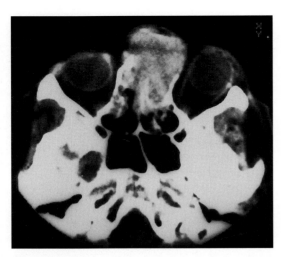

FIG. 29. Axial CT scan of plasmocytoma of left ethmoid showing encroachment on orbit and extension into right ethmoid.

fractures, care should be taken to note whether the fractures are displaced or nondisplaced, whether there is a rotation of the fractured fragment around either a vertical or horizontal axis, or displacement without rotation, and the degree of complexity of these fractures. The axial and/or coronal CT scans are particularly important in evaluating areas such as the orbital floor and the anterior and posterior tables of the frontal sinus. No single projection can adequately evaluate all these areas. Medial orbital wall fractures can be particularly difficult to evaluate if there is no significant displacement. Orbital emphysema can be a strong clue to their presence, as can the identification of fat within the ethmoid sinus.

All midface trauma should include assessment of the orbits, skull base, and frontal sinuses. This is optimally done with CT scans.

The Le Fort I fracture is a low midface fracture involving the maxillary antra bilaterally and the nasal cavity above the level of the hard palate. This fracture tends to be less common and more horizontal than Le Fort II and III fractures. Because the fracture line is in the axial plane, it may be difficult to detect on axial CT scan, particularly if minimal displacement is present. The Le Fort II fracture, or pyramidal fracture, extends from the nasion obliquely across the ethmoid bones through the medial wall of the orbit. The fracture also extends across the orbital floor and rim involving the medial portion of the orbital process of the maxilla before extending inferiorly and posteriorly across the anterior and lateral walls of the maxillary sinus inferior to the zygomatic process and arch, which usually remain intact (Fig. 31). The pterygoid plates may be disrupted at a more superior level than they are for Le Fort I fractures with the fracture plane extending

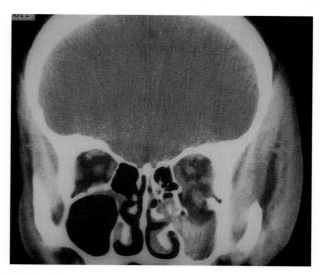

FIG. 32. Coronal CT scan showing orbital floor fracture with displacement of bone and soft tissue inferiorly.

across the inferior orbital fissure. On CT scan, a Le Fort II fracture will involve the ethmoid sinuses, medial orbital wall, and medial aspect of the orbital floor. The absence of suprazygomatic involvement differentiates the Le Fort II fracture from the Le Fort III fracture.

The Le Fort III fracture, or cranial facial disjunction, totally separates the midface from the skull base. Typically, a combination of midface fractures is seen in conjunction with Le Fort III fractures. The classic fracture extends across the nasofrontal suture through the inferior extensions of the frontal bone (frontomaxillary processes) and ethmoid air cells to reach the orbital floor. The orbital floor fracture extends posteriorly into the inferior orbital fissure and the pterygoid plates and then laterally into the lateral orbital wall and zygomatic arches. The lateral orbital involvement may resemble a zygomaticomaxillary fracture, although the typical tripod fracture lacks both the medial extension of the Le Fort III fracture and the posterior extension into the inferior orbital fissure. Many injuries are combinations of these fractures and left to right asymmetry is frequent. Orbital floor fractures are best seen in the coronal scans (Fig. 32).

For the evaluation of zygomaticomaxillary (tripod) fractures, CT scanning is ideal. The zygomaticofrontal fracture is usually best visualized in the coronal plane (Figs. 33 and 34), while the temporal and sphenoid fractures are generally best appreciated in the axial plane. Some of these fractures may extend along the lateral orbital wall to cause orbital apex fractures. These may require thin section CT scans for more critical assessment of the optic canal and superior orbital fissure.

Nasoethmoid fractures often occur together. Small low-velocity forces many produce simple nasal frac-

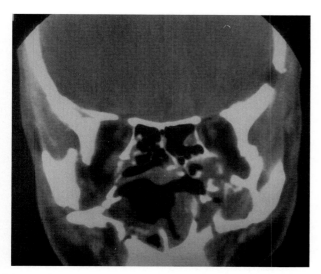

FIG. 31. Coronal CT scan showing severe Le Fort II fracture with depressed orbital floor.

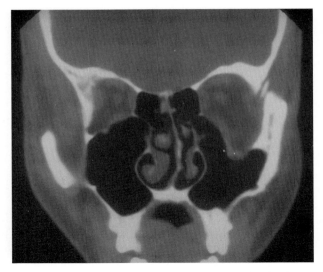

FIG. 33. Coronal CT scan showing depressed left trimalar fracture with secondary exophthalmos.

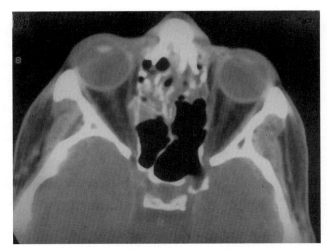

FIG. 35. Axial CT scan showing nasoethmoid complex fracture.

tures but high-velocity trauma invariably causes a comminution of the entire nasoethmoid complex (Fig. 35) CT scanning, because of its sensitivity to bone, is able to show these fractures quite well despite the thin ethmoid septa and the usual opacification of the sinuses from related hemorrhage. Nasoethmoid fractures may be a component of a Le Fort II fracture or may occur in isolation. The axial CT scan will also prove useful in assessing the presence or absence of traumatic telecanthus as well as injury to the medial canthal ligament system. The orbital floor and the cribriform plate are best assessed with coronal CT, while most of the rest of the components of the nasoethmoid fracture are readily assessed with axial scanning.

Fractures of the frontal sinus deserve special men-

tion. These fractures need to be carefully assessed because complications can be either acute or long delayed. These fractures occur in two major types: anterior table fractures and combined anterior and posterior table fractures. High-resolution CT scan documents well both anterior and posterior table injuries. Fractures to the anterior table are almost always comminuted, while combined anterior–posterior table fractures may be either linear or comminuted. Associated fractures of importance are supraorbital rim fractures medial to the supraorbital notch and nasoethmoid complex fractures. These latter fractures generally occur only in comminuted fractures of the sinus walls. Isolated anterior table fractures rarely involve the ostia of the frontal sinuses, which generally lie posterior and medial in the floor of the sinus (Fig. 36). This is true even when the anterior table is severely comminuted

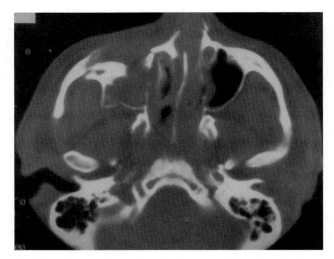

FIG. 34. Severe right trimalar fracture showing displacement of the anterior and posterior walls of the maxilla.

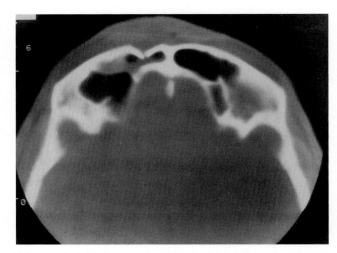

FIG. 36. Axial CT scan showing isolated, depressed anterior table fracture.

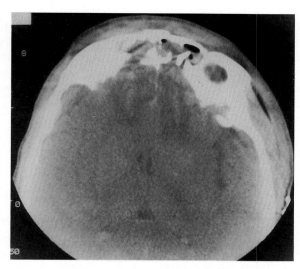

FIG. 37. Axial CT scan showing comminuted fracture of anterior and posterior tables of frontal sinus.

and displaced. On the other hand, anterior table fractures accompanied by a unilateral supraorbital rim fracture will have comminution of the sinus floor with damage to the nasofrontal orifice. Furthermore, anterior table fractures with accompanying nasoethmoid complex fractures will generally show damage to both nasofrontal ducts.

Linear fractures of the anterior and posterior tables are usually nondisplaced or minimally displaced. If the fractures are transverse, the nasofrontal drainage system will be undamaged. Vertical linear fractures, however, may extend into the nasofrontal drainage system, but in general the injuries in that area will be minimal and the drainage system will remain patent. Comminuted fractures of the anterior and posterior tables usually do involve the floor of the frontal sinus and cause circumferential damage to the nasofrontal drainage system (Fig. 37). These fractures may also be associated with nasoethmoid complex fractures, in which case the drainage system will always be significantly injured.

Fractures of the sphenoid bone, whether associated with extensive skull base or facial fractures, may be difficult to detect. In most cases there is little or no bony displacement and fracture detection frequently relies on displaying minimal bone discontinuity on CT scan. These fractures may cause injury to the optic nerve or structures in the superior orbital fissure. For complete assessment, both axial and coronal scans may be needed. If there is lateral displacement of the sphenoid wall on the coronal image, there is significant possibility of injury to contents within the cavernous sinus or to the internal carotid artery itself. In this instance, angiography may be worthwhile.

True blowout fractures are uncommon as these re-

quire the sudden application of force to the relatively incompressible soft tissues of the orbit without direct injury to the orbital rim. In this situation the medial floor or medial wall of the orbit is usually involved. These fractures are best assessed with coronal CT scans. CT scan is useful in assessing these fractures as it not only will show fatty prolapse into the maxillary sinus, but it may also be able to show the presence of hemorrhage or edema within the orbit, which might affect muscle function and resemble entrapment when in fact there is none (see the chapter by Donald, Fractures of the Zygoma).

The intimate association of the sinuses with the orbit calls for critical assessment of the orbit during the CT evaluation of facial and sinus trauma. The superior, medial, and inferior walls of the orbit also form the wall of a paranasal sinus. Zygomaticomaxillary fractures involve the lateral orbital wall and rim and usually involve, in addition, the zygomatic recess of the maxillary sinus. These may also involve orbital floor fractures. Nasoethmoid complex fractures often involve the lamina papyracea.

MRI plays a small role in the evaluation of facial trauma but can be helpful in differentiating blood from inflammatory reactions and edema fluid. MRI is more accurate in doing this if the study is performed at least 48 hr after the injury, allowing time for the blood to break down into methemoglobin. This can be distinguished by its high T1 weighted signal intensity from edema and infection, which have intermediate to low T1 weighted intensities (20). MRI is also particularly sensitive to displacement of soft tissue through bony defects and this can be particularly helpful in evaluating the anterior and medial skull base.

IMAGING THE POSTOPERATIVE PARANASAL SINUSES

Imaging the postoperative sinuses can be particularly treacherous unless one knows the operative procedure performed and the disease that prompted the procedure. These problems are best managed by routinely obtaining the baseline postoperative imaging study 4 to 6 weeks following the procedure. This is particularly important when dealing with neoplasms. In this setting again, CT is the best single study to use and, depending on the situation, should be in either the coronal or the coronal and axial planes; contrast may or may not be desirable depending on the exact situation, but it is more likely to be desirable when evaluating neoplasms. In noncontrast studies, inflammatory reactions usually have a lower attenuation value than neoplasms, whereas the opposite is true on contrast enhanced studies. However, enough variations exist to make this differentiation less confident than it might be.

In evaluating neoplastic diseases, MRI is better at differentiating recurrent tumor from sites of active infection but may not differentiate scar as readily. In addition, early bone changes will be undetected. MRI, however, is exquisitely sensitive to inflammatory processes, where one expects a low to intermediate signal intensity on T1 and proton density weighted images and a high signal intensity on T2 weighted images. Neoplasms, on the other hand, typically give an intermediate signal intensity in all imaging and sequences. Some assistance may be gained using gadolinium contrast. Either CT scanning or MRI can be used to evaluate the progress in an osteoplastic frontal sinus obliteration. Over time the fat gradually undergoes fibrosis until the fibrosis represents one-third to one-half the volume of the original fat. Importantly, however, throughout this process no volume loss occurs so the sinus remains obliterated. Generally, the bone flap can readily be detected with the proper window settings on CT scan showing the ragged uneven appearance caused by the beveling of the bone cut. This should not be mistaken for osteomyelitis, which appears more as bone demineralization, erosion, or sequestration accompanied by swelling and cellulitis of the overlying soft tissues with evidence of infection in the fat. On MRI, infection gives a high T2 weighted signal within the fat as well as generally in the surrounding forehead tissues.

CT scanning is particularly important in evaluating chronic inflammatory disease in the ethmoid sinuses after prior surgery; unfortunately, CT scans cannot reliably differentiate fibrosis from infection without the use of contrast, where inflammation typically enhances and fibrosis does not. The differences in attenuation, however, may not be sufficient to establish a definitive diagnosis. This may be distinguished more easily with T2 weighted MRI.

Postoperative evaluation of craniofacial resections can be particularly tricky. The anterior dura adjacent to the defect becomes thickened and it enhances on contrast studies and this appearance may persist indefinitely. In addition, the cranial contents and the supporting paracranial flap may bulge slightly downward into the upper nasal ethmoid cavity, simulating a tumor mass on axial CT scan. This can occasionally be resolved with coronal studies.

CONCLUSION

Modern imaging techniques allow for very precise study of the paranasal sinuses. For bone detail and inflammatory disorders, CT is usually the best study. For neoplasms, MRI may be the single best study, but CT will give valuable information about the adjacent bone. Similarly, MRI is exquisitely sensitive to mucosal inflammation where this etiology of mucosal thickening is in doubt.

REFERENCES

1. Merrill B. Atlas of roentgenographic positions, 3rd ed. St Louis: CV Mosby, 1967.
2. Dolan KD. Radiographic anatomy of the nasal sinuses. *Otolaryngol Clin North Am* 1971;4:13–24.
3. Donald PJ. Frontal sinus and nasofrontoethmoidal complex fractures. A self-instructional package from the American Academy of Otolaryngocology–Head and Neck Surgery, Alexandria, 1980.
4. Fascenelli FW. Maxillary sinus abnormalities: radiographic evidence in an asymptomatic population. *Arch Otolaryngol* 1969; 90:190.
5. Zizmore J, Noyek AM. Inflammatory disease of the paranasal sinuses. *Otolaryngol Clin North Am* 1973;6:459.
6. Batsakis JG. The pathology of head and neck tumors: nasal cavity and paranasal sinuses, Part V. *Head Neck Surg* 1980;2:410.
7. Naul LG, Hise JH, Ruff T. CT of inspissated mucous in chronic sinusitis. *Am J Neuroradiol* 1987;8:574.
8. Zizmore J, Noyak AM. Cysts, benign tumors, and malignant tumors of the paranasal sinuses. *Otolaryngol Clin North Am* 1973;6:487.
9. Torjussen W. Rhinoscopical findings in nickel workers with special emphasis on the influence of nickel exposure and smoking habits. *Acta Otolaryngol (Stockh)* 1979;88:279.
10. Kopp W, Fotter R, Steiner H, et al: Aspergillosis of the paranasal sinuses. *Radiology* 1985;156:715.
11. Dodd GD, Jing B-S. Radiology of the nose, paranasal sinuses, and nasopharynx. Baltimore: Williams & Wilkins, 1977; 131–133.
12. Barnes L, Verbin RS, Gnepp DR. Diseases of the nose, paranasal sinuses and nasal pharynx. In: Barnes L, ed. *Surgical pathology of the head and neck,* vol I. New York: Marcel Dekker, 1985.
13. Stafne EC, Gibilisco JA. *Oral roentgenographic diagnosis,* 4th ed. Philadelphia: Saunders, 1975.
14. Bernstein JM, Montgomery WW, Balogh K. Metastatic tumors to the maxilla, nose and paranasal sinuses. *Laryngoscope* 1966; 76:621.
15. Som PM, Shapiro MD, Biller HF. Sinonasal tumors and inflammatory tissues: differentiation with MRI. *Radiology* 1988;167:803.
16. Som PM, Lanzieri CF, Sacher M, Extracranial tumor vascularity: determination by dynamic CT scanning. II. The unit approach. *Radiology* 1985;154:407.
17. Lufkin R, et al. Magnetic resonance imaging of vascular tumors of the head and neck. *Clear Imaging* 1987;1:14.
18. Brant-Zawadzki MN, Minagi H, Federle MP. High resolution CT with image reformation in the maxillofacial pathology. *Am J Roentgenol* 1982;138:477.
19. Zilkha A. Computed tomography in facial trauma. *Radiology* 1982;144:545.
20. Zimmerman RA, Bilaniuk LT, Hackney DB. Paranasal sinus hemorrhage: evaluation with MRI imaging. *Radiology* 1987;162:499.

PART II

Inflammatory Disease

CHAPTER 8

Basic Allergy and Immunology

Paul J. Donald

The three chapters following this are written by individuals who have a wealth of experience in the management of the patient who suffers from nasal and sinus allergy. The chapter by Murphy, dealing with inhalant allergy, is written by a well-trained, highly experienced otolaryngologist in private practice, who, over a 20-year span because of his location in the Yakima Valley of central Washington State, has treated innumerable patients with allergic diatheses. The chapter by Borges and Heiner on food allergy is written by a senior professor of pediatric allergy in academic practice at UCLA. In contrast, the chapter by Trevino, also dealing with the highly controversial area of food allergy, is authored by an otolaryngologist in private practice with a broad clinical experience who is a part-time attending physician on the professorial staff of the Department of Otolaryngology–Head and Neck Surgery at LSU, Shreveport. The purpose of presenting two chapters devoted to the topic of food allergy is to demonstrate the conflict of information that exists concerning the nature and management of these allergic diatheses as they affect the nose and sinuses.

The present chapter is devoted to a brief overview of the nature of the basic mechanisms involved in the allergic response. It is only fair to say at this point that although frankly demonstrable allergy as established by standard sensitivity and hematologic tests is manifest in many patients with rhinosinusitis, there is a large cohort of patients with the clinical picture that we recognize as allergic in type in whom no allergy can be demonstrated. This presents a real puzzle to the clinician who is sure that an allergy exists but cannot prove it.

One of the commonest disease processes to confront the otolaryngologist in his daily practice is otolaryngic allergy. In fact, nearly 10% of the population suffers from allergic reactions to extrinsic allergens. Allergic rhinitis is a key component in a large percentage of patients who develop acute and chronic sinusitis. Without recognition and effective management of the allergic diathesis, the inflammatory disease will elude control.

Much of our understanding of the molecular basis for the allergic process has come from the science of immunology (1). Currently, this is probably the most rapidly developing of the basic sciences related to medicine. Physicians who graduated from medical schools two decades ago or more usually find this complex but fascinating field extremely confusing and very difficult to comprehend. In an attempt to better understand the molecular–biologic and pathophysiologic basis for the allergic response, some explanation of the basic pathways and interreactions of the immune system are presented.

It is estimated that there are as many cells belonging to the immune system in humans as there are brain cells (2)—some 100 billion (3). In the upper aerodigestive tract, the mast cells that contain so many of the biologically active substances that are responsible for the allergic reaction number about 32 billion (4,5).

Historically, the allergic reaction has been known for over 150 years. The classical symptoms of allergic rhinitis were described as early as 1819 by John Bostock of England (6). He identified the fact that his own "summer catarrh" of sneezing, itchy eyes, and nasal congestion occurred only during the summer months. In 1828, he associated his symptoms with the cutting of hay and deduced his problems were related in some way to substances emanating from the hay. He thus coined the term "hay fever" (6).

Although the prime target cell of the allergic reaction—the mast cell—was described in 1877 by Paul Ehrlich, the significance of degranulation and the release of ''vasoactive amines'' were not described until the 1940s (7).

In 1921, Prausnitz and Kustner described the passive transfer of a small amount of serum of an individual afflicted with allergic rhinitis to the skin of a nonsensitized individual. They pricked the serum in and discovered that it produced a weal. They thus demonstrated an ''allergic factor'' within the blood of the affected donor. The actual symptoms of allergic rhinitis were clearly described as far back as 1872 (5). In 1923 the syndrome was dubbed atopy and ascribed to a ''reaginic antibody'' (7).

In the 1960s, Bennich and Johansson in Sweden, independently of one another, identified a protein component of myeloma protein called ''ND protein.'' In conjunction with L. Wide, they identified this substance as the globulin IgE and established it as the factor responsible for the production of allergic symptoms. This then was the so-called reaginic antibody that Prausnitz and Kustner had demonstrated by their passive transfer test over 40 years before.

THE LYMPHOCYTE

The lymphocyte is the principal cell in the immune process. The various types of lymphocytes take origin in a common pluripotential stem cell (Fig. 1). Lymphocytes are labeled as either B cells, T cells, or nul cells. B cells are those responsible for the humoral or antibody-mediated immune response. They will, upon antigenic stimulation, release specific immunoglobulin once initially sensitized by the particular antigen that is idiosyncratic to it. The T cells are involved in a host of immunological tasks and are responsible for the cell-mediated response. The nul cells are a heterogeneous population and contain the natural killer (NK) cells and the antibody-dependent cellular cytotoxicity (ADCC) cells.

The B cells (so called from their original identification in the bursa of Fabricius in chickens) take origin in the bone marrow and liver. They make their first appearance in about the seventh week of intrauterine life. When first developing, the small immature B pre-lymphocyte has a small amount of surface IgM but it is not until further differentiation and maturation takes place, at around the eighth week, that the surface receptors for Fc and C3 characteristic of a mature B lymphocyte occur. Curiously, each B lymphocyte is idiosyncratic for only one specific antigen and becomes monoclonal in that regard. In addition, some B lymphocytes assume the role of memory cells that do not divide but respond as affector cells when later challenged by the same antigen to which they were initially sensitized. These memory cells affect the maturation of B cells to plasma cells and their elaboration of humoral antibody.

T cells are the active cells of cell-mediated immunity. They are found in the paracortical areas of lymph nodes and because they are thymus dependent are given the ''T'' designation. T cells are divided into a number of classes. Helper T cells allow B cells to produce antibody. Antigens that require helper T cells to activate the immune system are called T-cell-dependent antigens. There is another class of antigens that do not require T cells for activation. They are called T-cell-independent antigens. They can directly stimulate the B cells totally independently of the helper cells. Helper cells also can influence other T cells to be active in cell-mediated immunity.

On the other hand, another population of T cells, called suppressor T cells, assumes the role of blocking either the humoral or the cellular response. They are stimulated to balance the possible ''overenthusiastic'' helper cell response by a further class of helper cells designated as CD4 or ''suppressor-inducer'' cells. This produces an autoimmunoregulatory circuit.

The third class of T cells (Fig. 1) are the ''business end'' of the line: the effector T cells. One of their principal functions is their cytotoxic property. They have an ingenious method of identifying cells requiring elimination. In order to be effective, they not only have to recognize the specific antigen on the cell surface that marks the cell for destruction, but they must also recognize the major histocompatibility complex (MHC) antigen on the cell surface as well. The latter ''tells'' the cytotoxic T cell that the target is indeed a cell (and

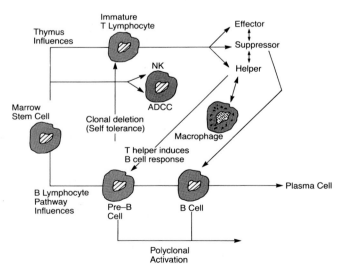

FIG. 1. Diagram illustrating the major pathways of development of the lymphocyte series. The upper path shows the development and differentiation of the T cells. The lower pathway shows the B cells. The nul cell population is thought to develop from the early T cell line. (Adapted from ref. 8.)

not free antigen) and the antigen marks the cell for elimination.

The nul cell population begins to develop in the B-cell line. However, they express markers for CD2, 3, and 8, which are normally restricted to T cells. The first group is the so-called natural killer cells. These are large granular lymphocytes that fix to affected cells by specific glycoproteins that they recognize on the cell surface. When this binding occurs, the NK cell releases its granules, causing lysis of the target cell. The most notable of the compounds secreted in these granules is perforin, which has a molecular structure similar to C9 and causes the formation of large cell membrane pores and subsequent cell death. They are stimulated to proliferate by interleukin 2 and possess these receptors on their cell surface. They produce interferon γ (IFN-γ) and must be related to T cells in some way (1). The other prominent cell in the nul cell line is the ADCC cell or "K" cell. This cell has an Fc IgG receptor on its cell surface. When this cell comes into contact with a target cell possessing an IgG antibody bound to an epitope on its surface, it combines with this antibody at the Fc site and the ADCC cell releases a series of cytotoxic substances that kill the target cell (Fig. 2). The curious thing is that this so-called K cell is not sensitized to the target cell but simply binds to the IgG on its cell surface.

TYPES OF IMMUNE REACTION

There are six basic types of immunity that have been identified (Table 1). Gell and Coombs classified the first four reactions and also described the fifth. The

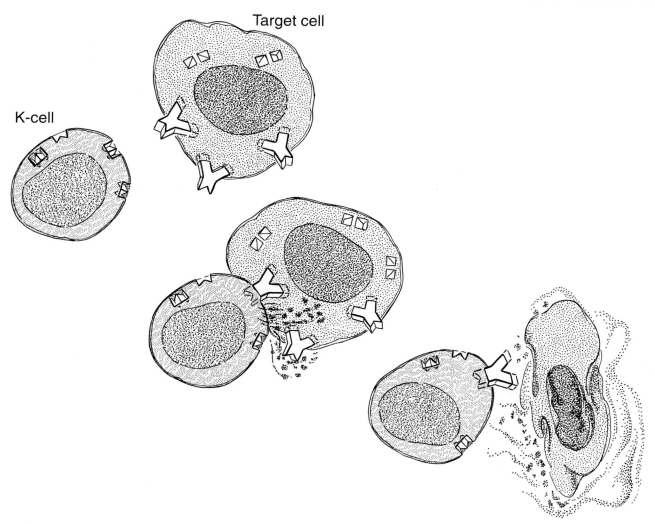

FIG. 2. Action of the ADCC cell of the nul cell line. The K cell attaches to a target cell that is primed by the presence of immune globulins on its surface. The lymphocyte attaches to the Fc end, resulting in degranulation and the release of cytotoxic materials causing death of the target cell.

TABLE 1. *Types of immunity*

Type I	Anaphylactic
Type II	Cytotoxic
Type III	Immune complex
Type IV	Delayed hypersensitivity
Type V	Stimulating antibody
Type VI	Antibody-dependent cell-mediated cytotoxicity

Type I, or anaphylactic hypersensitivity, is the variety most commonly identified with allergic rhinitis and described as atopy. The reaction involves the attachment of sensitized IgE antibodies to mast cells to which the antigen binds. This humorally mediated phenomenon is immediate and the resulting release of compounds from the mast cell results in the smooth muscle contraction, arteriolar dilatation, and the mucus outpouring that we commonly associate with allergy.

Type II reactions are cell mediated. Antibody binds to a cell membrane and in so doing precipitates the complement cascade up to C8 or C9 resulting in that cell's death. It may also promote phagocytosis of that cell. This type of reaction is often seen in autoimmune disease.

Type III hypersensitivity occurs through the activation of immune complexes. Immune complexes are a combination of a precipitating antibody and antigen that fuse either in the circulating blood or in the tissues. The antigen often exists in excess as, for example, in the case of persistent infection. The complexes deposit themselves in a target tissue and set up an inflammatory focus (the "Arthus" reaction). When complement is fixed, "anaphylatoxins" will be released as products cleaved from C3 and C5 (i.e., C3a and C5a), which in turn will degranulate mast cells (1). With a small amount of antigen excess, complexes are localized relatively close to the point of entry of the antigen. In the cases of moderate or marked antigen excess, there is the formation of soluble complexes that travel throughout the body either to be deactivated by macrophages in the liver or to be deposited in a host of other body tissues to cause localized inflammation and the potential for widespread tissue injury.

Type IV or cell-mediated immunity is the delayed-type hypersensitity we see as exemplified in the standard PPD TB test. With the introduction of antigen, a preprimed memory T cell, along with an antigen-containing cell possessing Class II MHC molecules on its surface, promotes the formation of blast cells and subsequent T cells (Fig. 3). These release a number of factors that attract and activate macrophages. They also stimulate cytotoxic T cell precursors to become killer cells. This produces the usual indurated and ulcerative process seen in positive skin tests to bacterial antigens.

Type V reactions are mediated through an IgG antibody. In the normal situation, certain target cells have surface receptors that have a steric attraction to specific antibodies produced by self. When they combine, there is the stimulation of specific intracellular tasks

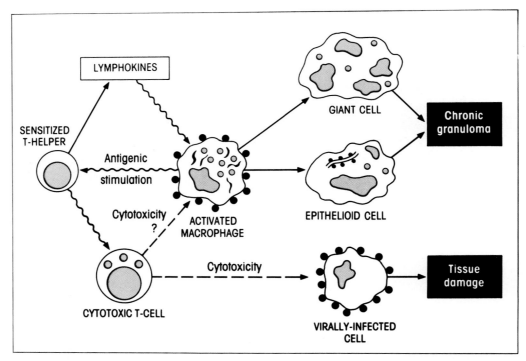

FIG. 3. The basic mechanism of Gel and Coombs, Type IV hypersensitivity. (From ref. 1, with permission.)

such as the production and secretion of hormone. An example of the Type V hypersensitivity is that seen in Grave's disease. There is the production of autoantibodies in excess that resemble TSH, which cause overstimulation of the thyroid.

The Type VI hypersensitivity reaction is discussed by some (8) as a separate entity and by Roitt (1) as a subtype of Type II reaction. This involves the so-called K lymphocyte of the nul cell series called the ADCC cell. The target cell has bound IgG that attaches to the K cell. This cell in turn then releases cytotoxic substances. It is important to understand that the T cells themselves are not sensitized in any way. The target cells show the $C\alpha2$ and $C\alpha3$ receptor portion of the Fc fragment of the IgG. The target cell now "loaded" awaits the arrival of a K cell, which will attach and release its cytotoxic materials.

IMMUNOGLOBULINS

The basic immunoglobulin structure as depicted in Fig. 4 is composed of two pairs of identical polypeptide chains arranged in a Y-type configuration. There are two light chains and two heavy chains. They are bound together by three disulfide bonds. The compound has a molecular weight of 200,000. The antibody has two distinct regions: the Fab fragment (fragment antigen-binding) and the Fc fragment (fragment crystallizable). The Fab fragment contains the position at which the antibody combines with the antigen and the Fc contains the site that binds to the target cell. The N terminal portion of the polypeptide chain on the Fab side has an enormous number of different molecular configurations, whereas the C terminal side on the Fc fragment has remarkable uniformity among different antibodies. Depending on the chemical configuration of the heavy chain constant areas (Fig. 5), the immunoglobulins of humans are classified into types G, A, M, D,

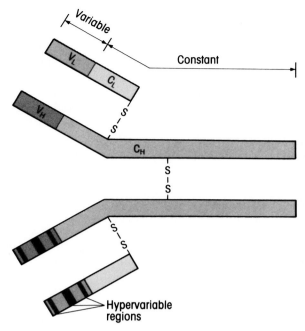

FIG. 5. Illustration of the light (L) and heavy (H) chain portions of the immunoglobulin molecule. The constant and variable regions of the structure are designated by uppercase letters (C) for constant and (V) for variable. (From ref. 8, with permission.)

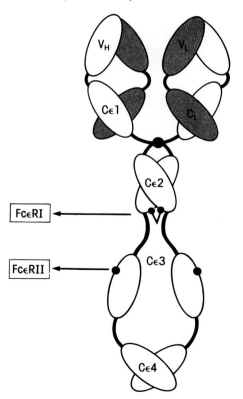

FIG. 6. Binding sites on the IgE molecule for the receptor sites on the mast cell surface (high-affinity receptors at the $C\epsilon2$ domain on the Fcϵ RI locus and the low-affinity sites at the $C\epsilon4$ domain on the Fcϵ RII locus). (From ref. 8, with permission.)

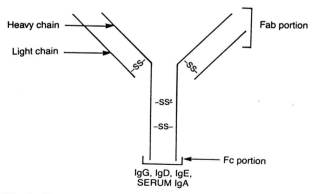

FIG. 4. The basic immunoglobulin structure. (From ref. 8, with permission.)

and E. Thus they are dubbed IgG, IgA, IgM, IgD, and IgE.

The immunoglobulin responsible for the atopic state is IgE (9). In the normal nonallergic individual, it is found in extremely low concentrations in the serum: 0.7 to 450 ng/ml compared to 8 to 16 mg/ml for IgG. It has the shortest half-life of all the immunoglobulins at 2.3 days (10). The highest concentration of IgE is found adherent to mast cells at the portals of entry of offending pathogens, especially the upper aerodigestive tract. The binding is at the so-called high-affinity receptor Fcε RI sites located in the Cε3 domain of the IgE molecule (Fig. 6). There are also low-affinity receptor sites located in the Cε2 domain at the Fcε RII locus that adhere to inflammatory cells and B lymphocytes.

IgE is found in skin, respiratory secretions, and serum. Its levels are age dependent with a low to nonexistent level around the time of birth and slowly rising between the ages of two and nine years. During the teens, levels become stabilized in the normal individual, then decrease after age 60 to 70. In the atopic child, there may be an elevated IgE even at birth, but if not, rising IgE levels become manifest soon thereafter. It is synthesized in lymphoid tissues of the gut and respiratory systems.

Control of IgE synthesis is not well understood but appears to be mediated by B cells under the control of a balance between helper T and suppressor T cell activity. The principal cell of importance appears to be the population of suppressor T cells. A number of studies have shown a depression of suppressor T cells in atopic individuals (11,12). One of the current thoughts in the mechanism of action of desensitization of the atopic individual to allergens is not only the production of specific IgG blocking antibody but also the stimulation of suppressor T cell numbers.

IgA is an immunoglobulin that is unrelated to the atopic condition. However, it has an important role in the immune defense in the mucosa of the nose and paranasal sinuses. Immunoglobulin A is found in nasal mucus, saliva, tears, sweat, colostrum, pulmonary secretions, and the gastrointestinal and urinary tracts. This antibody is active against microorganisms at their potential portals of entry into the body. IgA is secreted by the plasma cells aggregated at these sites. The antibody is active in its dimeric form. The dimer comes together in the plasma cell by the joining together of two monomeric forms through their Fc fragments by virtue of a cysteine-rich linkage polypeptide of molecular weight (MW) 15,000 called the J chain (Fig. 7). The dimeric form is secreted into the extracellular fluid and picked up by a glandular epithelial cell via an attach-

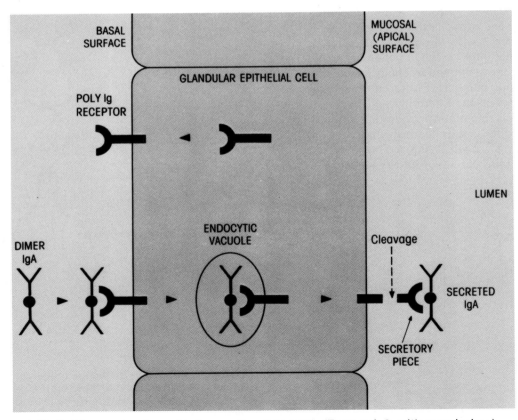

FIG. 7. The mechanism of IgA secretion (see text). (From ref. 8, with permission.)

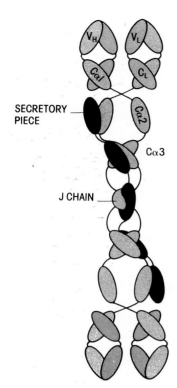

FIG. 8. J chain joining the two IgA molecules together to make the active dimeric form.

ment to a polyimmunoglobulin g receptor protein on its basal surface (Fig. 8). This polyimmunoglobulin is the secretory component precursor that will eventually endow the dimer with its characteristic activity. This complex enters the cell by endocytosis and migrates to the luminal surface of the cell. As it is secreted, a portion of the secretory component precursor is split off. The residual single polypeptide chain left attached to the dimeric IgA with a gram molecular weight (GMW) of 60,000 is called secretory piece. The antibody acts by precluding the adherence of invading microorganisms to the mucosal surfaces. In addition, aggregates of IgA can bind to polymorphonuclear leukocytes and stimulate the activation of the so-called alternative complement pathway.

THE MAST CELL

In the anaphylactic type of allergic reaction, the key cell is the mast cell. The mast cell is similar to the basophil but is tissue bound rather than circulating. Its precise origin is unclear, but it probably takes its genesis from a mesenchymal stem cell rather than from the bone marrow. It is a large cell about four times the size of an eosinophil. It is seen in concentrations of 1 to 10 $\times$ 10^6 cells/g tissue (13,14) and are specifically aggregated in bronchial tissues (being found even in the

bronchial lumen), gastrointestinal mucosa, nasal mucosa, and skin. They are seen within the epithelium and deeper in perivenular areas. Within skin, they are found in the dermal–epidermal junction as well as the deeper aforementioned perivenular sites. The mast cell has a plethora of large, dense intracytoplasmic granules, measuring about 0.6 μm in diameter, that are the sites of the various vasoactive and bioactive secretion products characteristic of this cell (Fig. 9). The cell membrane is of a double-layer configuration with a ruffled border. The membrane possesses 50,000 to 300,000 active receptor sites for the Fc fragment of IgE and C3b as well as C3a and C5a. The configuration of this membrane differs at different anatomical sites. Their constitution in the gastrointestinal tract is distinct from that in the nasal mucosa.

In the classical IgE-mediated anaphylactic reaction, sensitized mast cells with IgE molecules bristling from their cell surfaces come into contact with the offending antigen. The antigen is at least bivalent and connects at two sites, one on a single Fab site on one IgE antibody and the other to an adjacent Fab site on a second IgE molecule (Fig. 10). A series of events ensues that results in the degranulation of the mast cell with the release of potent bioactive substances.

The commonest scenario is for the antigen to fix to two sterically adjacent antibodies. Once this hapten attaches, there is a cell membrane change in the mast cell and mobilization of intracellular Ca^{2+}. There is then a triggering of a series of complex biochemical reactions, producing "fusogens" that result in fusion of the intracytoplasmic granules, and degranulation then ensues. In addition, there is stimulation of the production of arachidonic acid metabolites formed from the cyclo-oxygenase and lipoxygenase pathways. The divalent connection of the antigen to the mast cell surface is the most common, but trimer and tetramer attachments occur to a lesser degree and are even more potent stimulators of the mast cell degranulation pathway.

In addition to the IgE-mediated process, the mast cell has receptor sites for C3b and the small split-products of the complement cascade C3a and C5a. These latter two, the so-called anaphylatoxins, have receptor sites on the mast cell and will cause degranulation. Similarly, a number of compounds can directly stimulate mast cell mediator release. Certain enzymes, polycations, radiocontrast media, and opiates are a few examples of these (16).

This comes about from the mediators liberated from the mast cell such as histamine, serotonin, heparin, eosinophil- and neutrophil-activating factor, and platelet-activating factor (PAF). In addition, substances are synthesized such as leukotrienes LTB_4, LTC_4, and LTD_4, PGD_2, and thromboxanes, as well as a possible rise in cyclic AMP (Table 2).

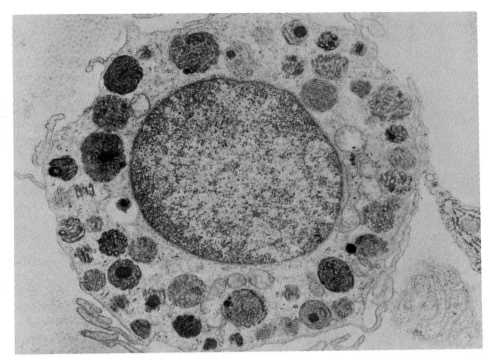

FIG. 9. Electron micrograph of mast cell from human lung. Note ruffled border and the large intracytoplasmic granules. (From ref. 15, with permission.)

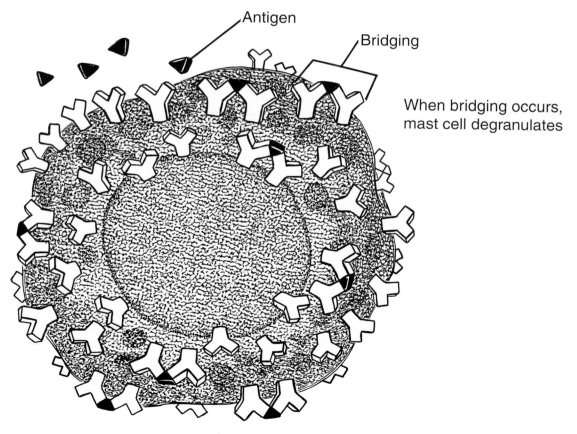

FIG. 10. Antigen bridging two adjacent Fab sites of IgE molecules on mast cell surface. Mast cell then degranulates with the release of powerful vasoactive substances.

TABLE 2. *Synthesized substances*

Mediator	Molecular weight	Function
Histamine	111	Increased vascular permeability, smooth muscle contraction, stimulation of suppressor T cells, prostaglandin generation, H1 chemotaxis and inactivation of eosinophils, H2 inhibition of neutrophil chemotaxis and activation, elevation of cAMP (H1) and cGMP (H2)
Serotonin	182	Contraction of smooth muscle, increased vascular permeability
PAF	400	Release of platelet amines, platelet aggregation, sequestration of platelets
Arachidonic acid metabolites Cyclo-oxygenase PGD		Increased vascular permeability, contraction of smooth muscle, increase of cAMP, inhibition of platelet aggregation
Lipoxygenase Leukotriene C, D, E (SRS-A)		Contraction of smooth muscle, increased vascular permeability, generation of PGs
Leukotriene B		Chemotaxis of neutrophils
ECF-A	360–390	Eosinophil and neutrophil chemotaxis and deactivation
EDF-oligopeptides	1300–2500	Eosinophil and neutrophil chemotaxis and deactivation
Neutrophil chemotactic factor	750,000	Neutrophil chemotaxis and deactivation
Heparin	60,000	Anticoagulation, antithrombin III interaction, inhibition of complement activation
Chondroitin sulfate		Platelet factor IV interaction
Chymase	29,000	Proteolysis with chymotryptic specificity
Tryptase	140,000	Proteolysis with tryptic specificity, cleavage of C3, Hageman factor, and kinin from kininogen
Arylsulfatase A	60,000	Hydrolysis of various sulfate esters
N-acetyl-β-D-glucoseaminidase	158,000	Cleavage of glucosamine residues
β-Glucuronidase	300,000	Cleavage of glucuronide conjugates

From ref. 17, with permission.

THE ALLERGIC REACTION

The patient with nasal and paranasal sinus allergy is the victim of a familial disease. In almost all cases, a positive history for atopic diseases can be obtained. The pattern for genetic inheritance is not clearly understood but is thought to be polygenic in type. A combination of a specific HLA histocompatibility type in concert with the IgE regulator gene determines the pattern (18). In some individuals, the specificity is so narrow that if they are never exposed to the precise agent to which they are allergic, then the condition will never become manifest.

On first exposure to an antigen, sensitized B cells (so-called memory cells) are stimulated to undergo blast formation and, in concert with helper and suppressor T cells, mature to plasma cells and produce antigen-specific IgE. The IgE fixes to the specific receptor sites on the mast cell surface via its Fc end. The host is exposed to the exciting antigen and it is absorbed. Since in inhalant allergy, most commonly seen in allergic rhinosinusitis, the allergen comes into contact with the mucosa of the upper aerodigestive tract, the site of reaction is in the submucoa and around the deep perivenular areas. Circulating antigen spans two adjacent Fab sites on the antibody protruding from the mast cell surface (Fig. 8). The adherence of antigen stimulates mast cell granules to coalesce and discharge a host of bioactive substances into the tissues and circulating blood.

The substances cause bronchoconstriction, an outpouring of nasal mucus, engorgement of the nasal and sinus mucous membrane, the appearance of eosinophils, and the hypersecretion of tears.

This syndrome is obviously the symptom complex associated with the clinical entity we recognize as allergic rhinitis. There are other symptoms produced by these bioactive substances that are often not so readily identified with allergy such as facial flushing, headache, and feelings of fatigue and tiredness. When classic hay fever symptoms occur in a patient on a seasonal basis with a positive family history, a minimal amount of mental exercise readily reveals the diagnosis. Perennial allergy, especially when some of the more vague symptoms are manifest, especially generalized fatigue and inanition, which according to Krause (7) is one of the commonest symptoms of the allergic diathesis, is commonly passed off as a depression or other psychological ailment. The symptoms of facial congestion, dental pain, facial pain and tenderness, and nasal congestion, which mimic acute sinusitis, may all occur purely on the basis of allergy. These patients usually do not manifest purulent nasal secretions, facial erythema, fever, or an elevated white blood cell (WBC) count. Interruption of the symptom-producing complex by either withdrawing the offending allergen, blocking the antibody–antigen reaction (by desensitization), or inhibiting mast cell degranulation (by the use of cromolyn sodium), or impeding the effect of those substances produced by mast cells (decongestants and antihistamines) will often promptly thwart the allergic reaction.

This highly complex sequence of biomolecular events produces among other disease processes the symptom complex we recognize as allergic rhinitis. Moreover, it sets the stage for the development of acute and chronic sinusitis.

REFERENCES

1. Roitt A. Hypersensitivity. In: *Essential immunology,* 7th ed. Oxford: Blackwell Scientific Publications, 1991;255.
2. Koshland DE. Editorial. *Science* 1987;283:1023.
3. Fischbach GD. Mind & brain. *Sci Am* 1992;267:48.
4. Murphy S. Asthma concepts. In: Krause FH, ed. *Otolaryngic allergy & immunology.* Philadelphia: Saunders, 1989;66.
5. King HC. Inhalant allergy. In: Krause FH, ed. *Otolaryngic allergy & immunology.* Philadelphia: Saunders, 1989;72.
6. Bostock J. Of the catarrhus aestivus, or summer catarrh. *Med Chir Trans* 1828;14:437.
7. Krause FH. Interface: immunology–allergy–otorhinolaryngology. In: Krause FH, ed. *Otolaryngic allergy & immunology.* Philadelphia: Saunders, 1989;40–47.
8. Rabin BS. Structure & physiology of the immune system. In: Krause FH, ed. *Otolaryngic allergy & immunology.* Philadelphia: Saunders, 1989;3–9.
9. Nemirovsky MS. Mucosal immune response. In: Pollquin J, Ryan A, Harris J, eds. *Immunobiology of the head & neck.* San Diego, CA: College Hill Press, 1984;122–123.
10. Rose B, Marquort D. Nasal allergy. In: Pollquin J, Ryan A, Harris J, eds. *Immunobiology of the head & neck.* San Diego, CA: College Hill Press, 1984;157–214.
11. Buckley RH, Becker WG. Abnormalities in the regulation of human IgE synthesis. *Immunol Rev.* 1978;41:288.
12. Beer DI, Asband ME, McCaffery RP, et al. Abnormal histamine induces suppressor-cell function in atopic patients. *N Engl J Med* 1982;306:454.
13. Patterson NA, Wasserman SI, Said JW, et al. Release of chemical mediators from partially purified human lung mast cells. *J Immunol* 1976;117:1356.
14. Mikhail GR, Miller-Milinskor A. Mast cell population in human skin. *J Invest Dermatol* 1964;43:249.
15. Ryan AF. Cells and tissues of immunity. In: Pollquin J, Ryan A, Harris J, eds. *Immunology of the head & neck.* San Diego, CA: College Hill Press, 1984;14.
16. Chenosith DE, Wasserman SI, Ryan AF. Nonspecific immune response: the role of accessory stems in the expression and regulation of specific immunity. In: Pollquin J, Ryan A, Harris J, eds. *Immunobiology of the head & neck.* San Diego, CA: College Hill Press, 1984;122–123.
17. Poliquin JF, Ryan AF, Harris JP, eds. *Immunobiology of the head & neck.* San Diego, CA: College Hill Press, 1984;65.
18. Austen FK. Disorders of immune mediated injury. In: Wilson JD, Braunwald E, Isselbacher KJ, et al., eds. *Harrison's textbook of medicine,* 12th ed. New York: McGraw-Hill, 1991;1423.

CHAPTER 9

Allergy in the Clinical Office

Michael J. Murphy

ALLERGY IN THE NOSE AND ITS SINUSES

Nasal allergy is an immunologically mediated response that is common in humans, frequently overlooked, and a potential factor in nasal and sinus obstruction, which may be contributory to nasal disease.

Allergy is an exuberant response on the part of a susceptible individual to organic, natural, or artificial antigens in the environment. Just as the fair-skinned individual overresponds to the sun, the allergic individual's nasal mucosa responds exuberantly to airborne agents such as dust, pollen, danders, molds, and other irritants. The reaction, being immunologically mediated, once started, is a generic inflammatory response within nasal and sinus mucosa. To understand nasal allergy it is necessary to explore the population at risk, offending agents, methods of diagnosis, and management of the phenomenon.

THE ALLERGIC INDIVIDUAL

Allergy, which means overreaction, is not a disease per se. The allergic process, by causing increased swelling and hypersecretion, may promote factors that contribute to a disease process. Allergic sensitivity affects approximately 18% or one in six of the general population (1).

Symptoms associated with allergy occur generally between 6 months and 50 years of age. In childhood, there is a 2:1 male predominance. Symptoms are more likely to occur during growth spurts. Hormonal factors are operative. Susceptible females usually become symptomatic during puberty, and by the twenties, the sex differential is lost. Affected women are more likely to become symptomatic during pregnancy, menstrual periods, or at the time of menopause.

Allergy is a genetically predisposed condition with multiple family members being so affected. Fre-

quently, the allergic symptoms are not stated as such but are referred to as "chronic bronchitis" or "chronic sinus condition."

The allergic person must be immunologically competent to initiate the response. There has to be a period of exposure to allow the formation of immunoglobulin E (IgE) antibodies against the specific allergens. The exposure period is generally 6 months. This is why children begin to have allergic symptoms at approximately 6 months of age, and offending agents are predominantly perennials such as dust, molds, or other environmentally noxious agents such as cigarette smoke. Pollen allergy generally is not a problem until approximately 5 to 6 years of age because the accumulative exposure has not been sufficient, until that age, to initiate the formation of antigen-specific antibodies. This explains why younger children have a predominance of symptoms during the fall, winter, and early spring when dust and molds are more abundant. They remain relatively symptom free during the warmer months of the year.

THE ALLERGIC REACTION

Allergic rhinitis is an immunologic process that involves the production of immunoglobulins in the class of IgE. The process by which this antibody is formed and its role in the inflammatory process are as follows. An antigen enters the nasal cavity and alights on the permeable mucous membrane. It migrates into the submucosal region, which is rich in vascular tissue and macrophages. The macrophage entraps the antigen and transports the exogenous material to T-lymphocytes that encode the antigenic material and stimulate the production of antibodies to the allergen in B-lymphocytes. B-lymphocytes then migrate to the tissue and IgE, antigen specific, will be secreted into the interstitial tissues. After this immunoglobulin has been pro-

112 /

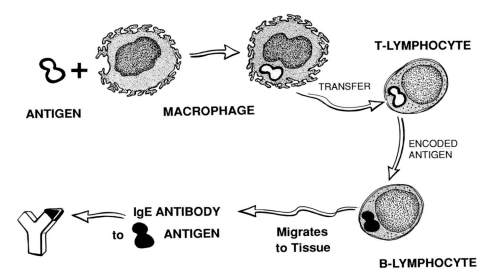

FIG. 1. Schematic of IgE-specific antibody formation.

duced, subsequent rechallenge by the specific antigen causes binding of two IgE antibodies to the exogenous material that then lock onto a mast cell receptor site (Fig. 1). The mast cells are abundant in nasal tissue. The linkage of the antigen and antibodies onto the mast cell stimulates degranulation and extrusion of the granules into the interstitial tissue. The chemical mediators within the granules are released. These chemical mediators lead to the symptoms and signs of allergic rhinitis.

Histamine, preformed in the mast cell granule, when released, causes an immediate (within minutes) bio-

chemical process that locally affects tissue, producing an increase in epithelial and endothelial permeability, plasma protein leakage, hypersecretion, itching, and sneezing. A plethora of other substances are similarly released: platelet-activating factor, eosinophilic chemotactic factor, arachidonic acid, kallikreins, and others (Fig. 2). These substances induce a biochemical cascade of reactions that lead to delayed responses (hours) that propagate the inflammatory reaction. These reactions lead to the symptoms of nasal inflammation, congestion, rhinorrhea, pruritus, and sneezing. Pharmacologic therapy is directed against these

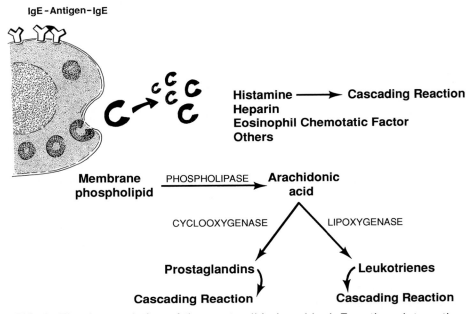

FIG. 2. The degranulation of the mast cell induced by IgE–antigen interaction.

biochemical reactions. Concurrent with these reactions, the body must have the potential to invoke a supressor system to dampen and eventually inactivate these effects. Otherwise, there would be a runaway response leading to systemic anaphylaxis. The allergic individual may be one who has an overproduction of specific IgE, one with a diminished T-lymphocyte suppressor system regulating the IgE production, or a diminished suppressor system for the chemically mediated cascading response (2–4).

THE DIAGNOSIS OF ALLERGY

The diagnosis of allergy is based on a detailed history, thorough physical examination, and appropriate laboratory studies. Symptoms of allergy—congestion, rhinorrhea, and pruritus—are nonspecific. It is when they are associated with a known exposure to some external antigen that the clue of a possible allergic response is suspected. Often, however, the patient does not go to the physician's office for the management of allergy but, rather, for control of chronic cough, sinusitis, or headache where association with an external agent is not obvious. Presenting symptoms and signs may actually be infection, such as a sinusitis, and suspicion of allergy as a contributing factor may only arise after repeated visits, noting the infectious process occurs during the same season of the year following the peak of an offending pollen. Because the allergic response leads to tissue swelling, this reaction may lead to possible osteomeatal obstruction of the sinuses, which could result in retained secretions and progress to subsequent infection. Seasonal regularity of such events should alert the physician that possible allergic mechanisms are operative. Control of subsequent infections can occur with effective management of the allergic state. Perennial allergens such as dust, danders, molds, smoke, and other airborne irritants similarly can lead to changes that would predispose the susceptible individual to infections. A meticulous gleaning of historical information is necessary to characterize the exogenous antigens. This will be covered in a subsequent section.

Physical findings of pale to violaceous swollen nasal tissue with anterior and posterior rhinitis are not always encountered. There may be superimposed infections or changes altered by the use of over-the-counter (OTC) medications. Chronic use of vasoconstrictive nasal sprays are especially problematic in masking the physical findings of allergy.

AIRBORNE ANTIGENS

To evaluate the timing of symptoms relative to airborne antigen exposure, one must have a knowledge of the offending antigens within a particular geographic location.

The concept of "peak" in an allergic season is important. The IgE-mediated response requires a certain amount or dose of antigen to trigger clinical symptoms. The allergic person requires less antigen than the normal individual. There is a minimal inducing concentration that is necessary to initiate clinical symptoms. The concentration of inhalants in the air varies for specific reasons with availability of the antigen depending on the biologic clock or physical factors of the originator of the pollen. The peak or maximal concentration period is that time when the concentration is the highest of any specific antigen. This time frame corresponds to a period when susceptible individuals would be most likely to be symptomatic from these antigens. The level of specific antigen at other times may be insufficient to initiate an allergic response.

There are other factors that also determine pollen density. Rain has a tendency to wash pollen from plants and thus lower the amount of available pollen to be dispersed in the wind. In dry areas, or during dry periods within a given location, pollen that is not attached will tend to recirculate and reoffend the sensitized patient from one windy period to another. This effect may be cumulative. This is why arid areas, which seemingly do not have a high biomass of available pollen, have very high pollen counts because of the recirculation that occurs. This also explains the cleansing effect of a rainstorm.

The Pollens

Pollen is a part of the germ tissue of plants. Some are macroscopic and are distributed by insects. Others are microscopic and are spread by the wind. It is the latter, because of their small size, that can be transmitted through air to the respiratory mucosa and can offend sensitized patients. The three major groups are trees, grasses, and weeds. The pollen calendar is determined by biologic factors. These factors are usually related to climatic conditions, primarily the amount of sunlight and thermo units available. The seasons may be brief or prolonged depending on the geographic area. In general, trees pollinate in late winter to early spring (peaking at Easter), the grasses pollinate in late spring to early summer (peaking at Memorial Day), and the weeds pollinate in late summer to early fall (peaking at Labor Day). Pollen may be present from any of these groups for protracted periods of time, but usually symptoms occur during peak density periods of pollination.

Trees

The pollen from the large deciduous trees such as elm, birch, poplar, cottonwood, oak, and ash are the usual offending agents to the tree-pollen-sensitive patient. These trees pollinate from small flowers formed after the emerging buds. The level of pollen is dependent on the wind velocity and the temperature that induces its formation. As the temperature rises this enhances the flower production and leads to heightened levels of pollen. The density of pollen is exponentially related to wind velocity. The greater the wind velocity the greater the pollen count. One would naturally anticipate allergic symptoms to be especially problematic on warm, windy days. After the flower pods have been fertilized, they form seeds, which terminates the pollination process. Simple observation of the state of the deciduous trees in a given location will alert the observer to the presence of tree pollen being an offending agent. Pollen counts are frequently part of the news service in many locations and are available from reference laboratories in many locations throughout the country.

The conifers, which produce macroscopic pollen that is typically present in late spring, are not thought to be major sources of allergenic airborne pollen. However, in the mountain areas of the West and East where these trees predominate, they can be problematic because of the high density of pollen that can be available on gusty, windy days. They are also frequent offenders around the home environment because many yards include shrubbery arborvitae, juniper, or other evergreens, which are frequently disturbed in the "spring cleanup." Close proximity to the pollen under these circumstances allows it to be an irritant or activator of the allergic process.

Grass

The grasses emerge as a potent pollen in late spring. The first peak of pollen production occurs with the first cutting of hay by the farm community. This is the period of time when grass blades have matured and the pollen pods have formed. Like trees, this pollen is spread by wind. The pollen phase is determined by thermo units available to form the grass blades and tufts. In some locations, such as southern Texas, grass is essentially a perennial pollinating plant. In more northern regions of the United States, the season is generally from May to the first of July.

Grass, because of its universal dispersement over the landscape in both arid and wet environments, is present in almost all locations on the earth. Another factor that determines time of pollination is elevation. At higher elevations, the cooler evenings do not provide sufficient thermo units for development of the plant until a later date. This may lead to significant grass pollen symptoms even into late summer in such locations.

Weeds

The weed group includes many plant species that are universally distributed over the landscape. Because of the diversity of the group there are many modes of fertilization and propagation of the pollens. Some, such as dandelions, are distributed by insects. Others, such as ragweed, are spread by the wind. The peak is generally late August to early September. This process is completed at the time of a killing frost, which terminates the biologic activity of the plant. The most notorious of the offending agents is short ragweed, which is present east of the Rockies. Other subspecies of ragweed are distributed throughout the United States.

House Dust

House dust is perennial but, like the other airborne agents, has a peak season. Dust as an antigen is heterogeneous. It is composed of numerous particles such as the breakdown products of fabrics, parts of house mites, bedding material, furniture stuffing, and fractional particles of organic and inorganic substances. Dust density increases with circulation of air. The peak of the dust season is when there is confinement to a dwelling where air is being recirculated for heat or air conditioning. Dust density is further enhanced by low humidity. Low humidity allows particles to become electrostatically charged leading to enhanced disbursement because of repulsion of dust particles. It is for this reason, in the northern climates, that the highest density of house dust generally occurs in the dead of winter.

The density of dust can be reduced by maintenance of the furnace and its conduits, the reduction of surfaces to trapped dust, and frequent cleaning.

Molds

Molds, like dust, are ubiquitous and lead to exposures that are both seasonal and situational. The offending agent is the microscopic mold spore. The spore is the germ seed of the mold or fungus mycelium, and because of its small size, there is a high correlation between its presence and extrinsic asthma. On a seasonal basis, mold spore density is frequently associated wit the presence of nasal polyps.

Situationally, molds thrive on decayed matter in a damp, reasonably cool environment. Such an environment can be cellars, bathrooms, kitchens, or other sources where retained moisture is allowed to condense. Molds are also part of the smut associated with plant matter. Often overlooked sources of molds are houseplant soil and refrigeration drip pans.

Out-of-home environment molds are an active part

of the biologic environment. In certain parts of the country the distribution of spore production is seasonal. In general, they propagate when there is a damp environment with cool evenings and daytime temperatures of 40°F or higher. These conditions are met in late winter to early spring and late fall to early winter. Spores within the soil are dispersed by the wind. Symptoms of congestion following a dust storm on a dry, windy day would lead one to be suspicious of mold sensitivity. Allergic symptoms following mowing the lawn are usually caused by mold spores. In the process of cutting the grass, the soil is dispersed and mold spores are liberated into the environment causing symptoms in the susceptible individual.

Danders

The danders are the hair, saliva, and excrements of animals—dogs, cats, cattle, sheep, and so on. The domestication of dogs and cats has made their frequent potent perennial allergens available to the susceptible individual, and, like house dust, these allergens are dispersed into the environment during periods when air is being recirculated by the heating/cooling system. Avoidance of danders can be simplified if they are an identified problem. Some older homes in which the base of the plaster included animal hairs, such as horse hair to give body and support to the plaster, may be a source of dander exposure.

Chemicals

Our environment is awash with noxious fumes. These may have deleterious effects on the susceptible individual, perhaps not always on an immunologic basis but, clearly, often irritative. The passive effect of cigarette smoking is well described. Other noxious fumes such as general pollution, wood burning, and household chemicals frequently play a role in susceptible individuals.

Many individuals do not suspect chemical irritants as a problem in their symptom complex because of familiarity with products and failure to associate chemical irritants in those products with their symptoms. Ninety percent of the cosmetics contain formaldehyde as a base stabilizer or disinfectant. In the susceptible individual application of cosmetics can easily produce or contribute to symptoms.

THE LABORATORY DIAGNOSIS OF ALLERGY

As in other fields of medicine, diagnosis of allergic rhinitis can usually be made after obtaining a careful history that will connect exposure to symptoms, corre-

lated by physical findings. The purpose of laboratory testing is to confirm the individual's sensitivity to offending agents. The patient who complains of congestion, rhinorrhea, and itchy eyes after being exposed to cigarette smoke, by definition, is allergic to the smoke. Tests will only confirm that impression. If they fail, there is a problem with the test, not the diagnosis.

In patients with nasal polyps or pansinusitis, allergy may be suspected. Nonspecific factors such as elevated eosinophil count may be present. A nasal cytogram, with presence of eosinophils, may point to the presence of allergy but does not define offending agents. Such tests are nonspecific. Specific tests for allergy are important in providing specific data to assist the patient in avoidance therapy. It is also essential data to be gathered prior to instigation of immunotherapy.

Methods of Testing

The classic test for confirmation of allergy is the passive transfer test. This is not practical on a clinical basis and currently *in vitro* and *in vivo* tests are performed to confirm offending antigens.

In vivo test includes prick testing with a specific antigen, intradermal testing with a specific antigen, or provocative testing by inhalation of an offending antigen onto the nasal mucous membrane. All tests must be interpreted in conjunction with the patient's historic symptom complex.

Skin prick testing is a qualitative and quantitative test in which a small prick is placed in the skin into the dermal layer and antigen is applied to the site. The response is measured by a wheal-flair dermal reaction. This is an immediate phase response mediated by histamine. The magnitude of the response is measured as $0+$ to $4+$. A $4+$ reaction is a large reaction including pseudopod extensions. The back is the favorite location to apply these tests. The reaction in the skin is possible because of the presence of IgE-specific antibody within dermal tissue to allow coupling with specific antigen and to release endogenous histamine from the mast cells. There is a high correlation between intradermal reaction and the nasal mucous membrane susceptibility to a similar offending antigen.

The intradermal testing is a modification of the above. The biochemical reaction to the antigen is the same. By delivering the same volume of substance but varying the amount of antigen, it is possible to identify qualitatively and quantitatively the allergic response to a specific agent by measurement of the size of the wheal. Intradermal testing by this method is referred to as serial dilution. This is used as a determinant of the starting point for rapid desensitization.

Nasal provocative testing is an accurate biologic

gauge for a sensitive individual. It is an *in vivo* technique where a prescribed amount of antigen is placed into a nebulizer and it is applied to the mucous membranes. Subsequent reactions can be determined by the response. The amount of the secretion flow or increased airway resistance may be determined and quantified. This process is individually specific with a very high coefficient of reliability. It is also time consuming and technically demanding because it requires one agent to be tested at a time.

The *in vivo* techniques are employed by practitioners involved in therapeutic management by immunotherapy. These techniques frequently are performed by trained staff who are skilled in the application of the skin test and its interpretation. When performed properly the result should be reproducible. *In vitro* testing involves identification of antigen-specific IgE within blood. This can be performed by enzymatic or by radioactive absorbent testing. The *in vitro* test attempts to measure the specific IgE in a qualitative and quantitative manner. The test involves a sample of the patient's serum, which contains specific IgE. That serum is washed in a solution containing antigen-specific anti-IgE. The bound complex of the patient's IgE and the labeled antiserum is then measured. The higher the recording, the larger amount IgE within the patient. These tests can be performed in the office or an outside reference laboratory. For inhalant allergens there is a high coefficient of reliability, approximately 95%. The interpretation must always be correlated with the patient's condition and symptomatology to confirm the presence of allergy.

A reactive skin test or an elevated IgE obtained from an *in vitro* test simply correlates with the level of IgE within an individual. A positive test, by itself, does not mean that the antigen is biologically active in the patient. The correlation of elevated IgE to a specific antigen and the confirmation of symptoms during exposures to that agent are confirmatory of the allergic state.

MANAGEMENT OF THE ALLERGIC STATE

There are three methods by which allergy may be managed: avoidance, chemotherapy, and immunotherapy. Alone or in combination they will provide symptomatic relief for the affected individual. If there is a failed response to treatment, overlooked factors may be operative such as underlying infection or the failure to avoid salicylates in patients with the asthma–polyposis–aspirin triad.

Avoidance

If the allergic state is brought on by the interaction of an exogenous antigen which then triggers an inflam-

matory reaction, the avoidance of that offending agent will prevent the occurrence of symptoms. For avoidance to be effective, there must be an identification of the offending agents and it must be possible to avoid those agents. The nature of the offending agent usually can be obtained from the patient's history or through testing, as was mentioned previously. Avoidance is always the simplest method. The elimination of tobacco smoking from the house is an important method of avoidance especially for sensitized children. In the house-dust-sensitive patient, changing the filters on the furnace, cleaning the heat registers, removing dust-catching surfaces, and frequent cleaning may be of great benefit. The slight dampening of the lawn prior to mowing will cut down the amount of dust and diminish the density of mold spores that would be placed into the environment while mowing the lawn. The simple use of a mask can be effective.

During the summer months the air conditioning has been found to be an effective filtration of dust and pollen materials. This would reduce the allergic load. The allergic patient should be encouraged not to sleep with a window open.

To be effective in assisting the patient in avoiding possible offending agents, it is necessary for the practitioner to become aware of the environmental and occupational surroundings of the individual. A farmer will have different exposure from a secretary in an office building. By exploring the patient's life-style setting, many clues are obtained as to possible offending agents. Many may be untestable, such as chemicals in the environment. By alerting the patient to possible offending agents, insight may be reached as to those agents' impact on a given patient. An example would be a headache following the use of "White-out" by a secretary. The headache was induced from the chemicals in that product. Many times, avoidance is the only method of management, especially in the chemically sensitive patient.

Chemotherapeutic Agents

The primary purpose of this group of drugs is to block or modify the inflammatory response in such a way as to relieve symptoms. All these agents interact within one specific area: either the induction of the inflammatory response by the mast cell or the blockage of the chemical mediators released from the mast cell. Figure 3 shows a simplified version of the site of action of these chemotherapeutic agents (5).

Cromolyn Sodium

Cromolyn sodium inhibits the secretion of granules in mast cells and basophils. Cromolyn sodium does

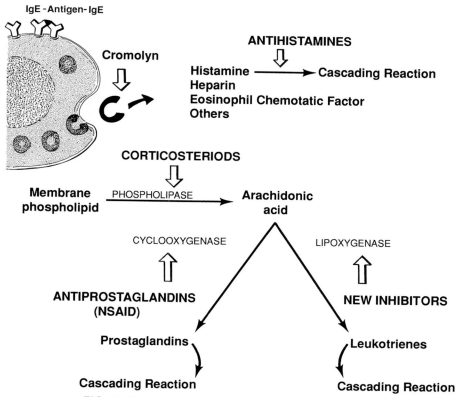

FIG. 3. Sites of action of chemotherapeutic agents.

not inhibit the binding of IgE and specific antigen. It suppresses the secretory response-degranulation of the mast cell and, in so doing, the subsequent allergic cascade does not occur. Cromolyn sodium is a prophylactic treatment of allergy. Cromolyn sodium is not effective after the inflammatory response has been initiated unless ongoing challenges are continuing to occur. It is a topical agent used in a nebulizer form that is distributed over the nasal mucosa. It also comes as an inhaler for tracheal and bronchial mucosa in prevention of asthma. Cromolyn sodium has been especially beneficial in the prevention of exertional asthma. The response to treatment is not always consistent, which could be a reflection of the timing of use and the fact that no delivery system can completely coat the nasal mucosa by simply spraying into the anterior nares. As with other prophylactic medications, it is difficult to educate patients on proper use of this agent. It frequently is used in conjunction with other agents such as antihistamines or topical corticosteroids. Some patients find it more effective in the dropper form, where the head is positioned to allow the liquid to more effectively coat the nasal and ostial mucosa.

Antihistamines

Clinically, there are six classes of H_1 blocking agents. These block the local effect of released hista-

mine from mast cells or basophils. By interfering with this phase, they attenuate the inflammatory response mediated by histamine. Other mediators, including the prostaglandins and leukotrienes, are not affected by these agents. Antihistamines, used in the prophylactic mode, are probably the mainstay of allergic management and the principal component in most over-the-counter preparations for allergy. The classes—ethanolamines, ethylenediamine, alkylamines, piperidine, astemizole, and terfenadine—have different biologic activity depending on the patient (Table 1). It is not that any one is more effective than another, but rather, one particular antihistamine may be more effective for a given patient. Sample packs of the different antihistamines are given to the patient. This allows the patient to select the drug that is pharmacologically the most effective in controlling his/her symptoms. At the same time, they are able to assess the one with the least side effects, the most common of which are drowsiness and dryness of the mouth.

It is important to realize that after symptoms have been initiated antihistamines cannot resolve the already existing inflammatory response. Use of antihistamine will not correct or relieve inflammatory changes already in existence. Administration of a cortisone preparation should relieve acute existing symptoms, allowing antihistamines to work in their prophylactic mode, thus allowing the trial to occur.

TABLE 1. *Antihistamine classes in clinical practice*

Class	Generic name	Trade name
Ethanolamine	Diphenhydramine	Benadryl (OTC)
	Clemastine	Tavist
Ethylenediamine	Methapyrilene	Histadyl
	Tripelennamine	PBZ
Alkylamine	Brompheniramine	Dimetane (OTC)
	Chlorpheniramine	Chlor-Trimeton (OTC)
	Dexchlorpheniramine	Polaramine
	Triprolidine	Actidil
Piperidine	Azatadine	Optimine
Astemizole	Astemizole	Hismanal
Terfenadine	Terfenadine	Seldane

Antihistamines have an effect on the contractility of smooth muscle. In some patients with cardiac arrhythmias, antihistamines may be contraindicated. Also, some older patients, both male and female, complain of urinary symptoms due to the enhancement of smooth muscle contractility of the bladder.

Antihistamines frequently are administered in combination with decongestants. Many side effects associated with these drugs, such as dryness of the mouth, insomnia, and hyperirritability, can be attributed to an associated sympathomimetic amine in the decongestant. Similarly, decongestants do have an effect on the muscular neck of the urinary bladder.

For this group of agents to be pharmacologically effective, they must be used in the prophylactic mode. The patient should be instructed on their proper usage, specifically, how and when. The patient who has difficulty after mowing the lawn should be instructed to use antihistamines prior to mowing. The most frequent reason for failure in the antihistamine group is their underuse. Frequently, numerous visits are required to educate the patient about the nature of his/her allergies and of the strategic timing for taking the medication. Antihistamines can be used in conjunction with other agents or as a supplement to immunotherapy.

Corticosteroids

The corticosteroids are effective both in topical and systemic forms in the management of allergic conditions. The primary mode of action is in the phase of

TABLE 2. *Nasal steroid sprays*

Steroid	Trade name
Beclomethasone	Vancenase
	Beconase
Flunisolide	Nasalide
Dexamethasone	Decadron

inhibition of the conversion of arachidonic acid to the leukotriene and prostaglandin pathways. These two groups of substances are probably the slow-reacting substance of anaphylaxis. The corticosteroids also have multiple other effects including vasoconstriction and antipyresis. They inhibit leukocyte mobilization and depress antibody formation. They are extremely effective in reversing the symptoms of acute allergy (6).

Topical application of corticosteroids by nebulizers or atomizers is effective in preventing and moderating symptoms. Some patients complain of local irritation from the vehicle in these products. The newer agents have forms of cortisone that are rapidly detoxified by the liver and are associated with minimal systemic side effects. Older products, using dexamethasone (Decadron), do have systemic effects if used chronically (Table 2). The newer agents have proved to be safe in children. The cortisone spray preparations are frequently used in conjunction with antihistamines.

As with other topical agents, there is a problem of distribution on the nasal mucous membranes that cannot always be achieved through the anterior nose.

Parenterally, cortisone is used frequently either orally or by injection. It often is used in conjunction with severe allergic symptoms during the peak of an allergy season or after an acute reaction due to some acute exposure.

Newer Agents

New pharmacologically active chemicals are being developed to intervene at the different phases of the allergic reaction. Early reports on agents that affect the 5-lipoxygenase enzyme are encouraging in their blockage of allergic symptoms (7,8). The antiprostaglandins (nonsteroidal anti-inflammatory agents) have not been universally effective in the management of allergy.

IMMUNOTHERAPY

Immunotherapy is a technique whereby the patient is tested, the offending antigens determined, and specific antigens are administered to the patient in a controlled fashion. The immunologic response is thus altered and controlled. Probably, it is the suppressor end of the immunologic process that is enhanced by immunotherapy (9). An analogy to this method of treatment is the everyday occurrence of acquiring a suntan. To protect against injurious effects of the sun, a fair-skinned individual absorbs an allocated amount of sunlight over time. In so doing, there is a modification in the epithelial cells of the skin to increase production of melanin. The injurious effects of the sun are modified. In a similar fashion, immunotherapy alters the immunologic environment of the patient and suppresses the allergic response.

Antigen selection in the testing format is determined by each practice location. The number and groups of antigens are dependent on the patient's exposure history and the type of flora available in a given location. A rural community will have different available antigens from an urban setting. The possible antigens that can pose clinical symptoms can be obtained from many sources. These include fellow colleagues who practice in the field of allergy, reference laboratories, and commercial manufacturers of antigen extracts. The number and groups of antigens change with time and experience within a given clinical practice. Therefore no table of minimum or maximum antigens can be provided.

The selection of antigens within the individual groups is determined by the patient's age and exposure history. Young children who have not had sufficient exposure time to be sensitized to the complete array of plant pollens do not need to be tested with these groups. House dust and dust mites are universal potential antigenic offenders. The danders to test should include those likely to be a problem: cat and dog dander for those who are exposed to these animals, and cattle, sheep, horses, and others based on the history of exposure. The molds to be tested include the ones encountered in the treatment location. These can be determined by culturing mold spore colonies from different locations within the treatment area. The area test must include inside and outside sites during the mold season. In selected mold-sensitive patients, sampling cultures from the patient's environment may be required. In agricultural areas, smut and rust usually are necessary testable antigens within the mold group.

Pollens in the tree, grass, and weed groups that should be tested are regionally determined by the available flora. Some downwind locations may need to include pollen from a distant source because of the targeted dispersion from the upwind area.

After determining the composition of antigens to be tested and potentially used in an immunologic treatment regime, the practitioner is ready to proceed. There are three methods currently in use to achieve this end. Two are *in vivo* tests, and one is an *in vitro* method. The individual methods have technique-specific requirements and training required for their successful application.

The first *in vivo* method uses prick–scratch testing with specific antigens followed by correlated immunotherapy. Pricks are made in the skin and concentrated specific antigen is applied to the scratched area. After 10 min the site is read. A wheal-flare reaction is used to determine qualitatively the presence of IgE-specific antigen. The reaction is recorded from 0 to 4+, with 0 being no reaction and 4+ being a large reaction with pseudopods. Based on these data, antigen mixtures are prepared in vials containing antigens in different concentrations from 1:1,000,000 to 1:100. Doses starting at 0.05 ml and progressing to 0.50 ml from each of the dilution vials are given on a weekly basis, starting with the weakest and progressing to the most concentrated dilution. The concentrated antigen dose is then given on a 3- to 4-week schedule to maintain the suppressive effect of the immunotherapy. There is individual variability on where to initiate the process and where to maintain the patient. At times, the patient cannot tolerate the higher antigen doses and is maintained on the highest tolerated dose. The patient is maintained on this dose for 2 to 3 years and a weaning from the therapy is then attempted. Many patients find sufficient alteration in the degree of reactivity to the antigen challenge in their lives that immunotherapy is discontinued. Some patients find that the control provided by immunotherapy is more satisfactory than being off shots and continue with this mode of treatment.

The second method of *in vivo* testing uses the serial dilution titration technique. Serial dilution titration is an intradermal method where by qualitative and quantitative information about the IgE-specific antigen is obtained. A 5-mm wheal (0.01 ml) of antigen is delivered intradermally using progressively more concentrated solutions (usually progressive 1:5 dilutions). When there is a reaction, a wheal of larger than 5 mm is observed. Progressively larger wheals—5 mm to 7 mm to 9 mm—demonstrate the end point of the titration. The 7-mm wheal marks the concentration of antigen where the patient biologically reacts to that antigen. This point then represents the concentration of antigen to start the desensitization process. This then allows a more rapid method of desensitization. The therapy progresses with weekly stronger concentrations of antigen extracts, until the maximum tolerated dose is achieved. Some practitioners use 25 to 50 times the dose of the end-point concentration, if clinical symptoms are controlled, as the maintenance dose. Therapy continues for 2 to 3 years and then a weaning process is initiated like the first method.

The controversy that exists between the two *in vivo* methods is the dose of antigen to maintain treatment. Ideally, the maximum dose should be that amount of antigen that can achieve IgE suppression, associated with an increase in antigen-specific immunoglobulin G (IgG). Tests for IgE and IgG levels are expensive and often unavailable. From a practical point of view, these objective points are rarely determined and the appropriateness of therapy is determined by the sense of well-being perceived by the patient.

In the hands of some practitioners, sublingual drops with the patient-reactive antigens are said to be effective. Subcutaneous injections remain the traditional mainstay of immunotherapy.

The third method is the *in vitro* technology using IgE levels from the serum to determine the offending antigen and the concentration to initiate treatment. These methods are referred as RAST, PRIST, or FAST tests depending on whether radioisotope, enzymatic spectrophotometric or enzymatic fluorometric technology is used. These methods determine the patient's IgE level by mixing the patient's serum with anti-IgE-labeled antibody. The resulting complex, IgE–anti-IgE, level is then read. The level or reading is used as a reference point to determine the presence or absence of antigen sensitivity in the patient. This information is then used to construct an antigen mix for immunotherapy with progressively stronger doses of antigen, similar to the method described in the *in vivo* techniques.

The three methods have proponents and opponents. By whichever method the outcome to the patient is satisfactory, the practitioner of that methodology is within the ethical bounds of medicine.

ALLERGY AND SURGERY

Allergies should be taken into account in the timing of any surgical procedure on the nose or its sinuses. If surgery is anticipated during a time of a maximal allergic challenge, that diathesis will cause a response that may be detrimental to the surgical outcome desired. If the surgery is elective, postponement to a nonreactive season may be desirable. If that is not feasible, then maximal allergic suppression should be instigated to ensure optimal surgical outcome. The use of cortisone may be indicated as well as the adjuvant use of antihistamines and topical cortisone sprays. It should be remembered that cortisone interferes with fibrous tissue formation and thus attenuates the healing process. The risk–reward balance must be assessed by the operating surgeon. If there is associated asthma, the surgical process may accentuate the asthmatic sensitivity because of packing of the nose and the synergistic response that surgical trauma induces.

ALLERGY AND INFECTION

The immunologically mediated allergic response and infection are both inflammatory responses that follow similar cascading biochemical reactions. One accentuates the other. Allergies cannot be managed if infection is present, nor can infection be controlled without allergy management. If the two coexist, which is frequently the case, they must be managed jointly. When allergy management is less than satisfactory, failure should alert the clinician that an underlying infectious process may be operative. This is especially true in obstructive ethmoid disease, where chronic infection can be difficult to find unless suspected. In any patient where there is a poor response to management and a history suggestive of possible osteomeatal obstruction of the sinuses, computed axial tomography (CAT) scans in the coronal projection frequently exhibit abnormalities, which reveal the coexistence of infection.

ALLERGIES AND OTHER CONDITIONS

Hypothyroidism accentuates and unmasks allergic symptomatology. The hypothyroid state makes any form of allergic management difficult at best. If there is a history of thyroid disorder within the family, positive physical findings, or other symptoms suggestive of a hypothyroid state, thyroid investigation should be initiated.

Rheumatoid arthritis and the associated sicca syndrome often confuse the diagnosis or give the impression of the allergic state. It should not be forgotten that allergy, affecting one in six in the population, can coexist with other conditions. The sicca syndrome, affecting the nose in the patient with allergies and rheumatoid arthritis, poses a difficult problem for the clinician. It demands an understanding on the part of the patient that not all the symptoms of dryness, congestion, and so on are the result of allergy alone, and failure of management of these symptoms is not a failure of management of the allergies.

Many patients receiving β-adrenergic and/or calcium channel blockers have symptoms that appear to be allergic. Furthermore, these drugs compound the difficulty in management of allergic patients. A careful history usually will show accentuation of symptoms associated with the onset of taking those medications. One should work in conjunction with the internist who has prescribed them, if it is felt that these medications are contributing to the nasal symptoms.

ALLERGIES AND CHEMICAL INHALANTS

Chemical and noxious fumes associated with sensitivity to the respiratory mucosa are an everyday event. There is, however, a significant group of patients who are difficult to diagnose who have a seemingly occult sensitivity. They are frequently patients who have been seen by multiple allergists, who have been told they do not have allergies because of very low skin reactivity and, yet, seem to have a typical allergic history. They will complain of sensitivity when around tobacco smoke. Frequently, there is absence of cosmetics and other adornments of chemically leeching materials. They will give a history of washing a new garment after purchasing it. They will have symptoms after purchasing a new car, rug, or piece of furniture. They frequently complain of nasal and periorbital congestion and pain. The pain is typically relieved by aspirin or other nonsteroidal anti-inflammatory agents. Similarly, it is not relieved by Tylenol or opiates in low doses. This class of patients favorably responds to information bringing awareness of probable chemical sensitivity as a triggering mechanism of their symptoms. These symptoms can frequently be controlled by avoidance of environmentally active agents such as room fresheners, toilet bowl fresheners, potpourri, perfumes, scented candles, rug fresheners, and other similarly scented products. House plants also give off a plant-specific odor, some of which may be bothersome to these individuals. These patients frequently respond to topical nasal steroids and the headache is diminished if they promptly use one of the nonsteroidal anti-inflammatory agents in the early stages of symptoms.

Many (greater than 80%) respond to immunotherapy with other inhalants for which they test positive. Positive response to therapy and diminution of symptomatology are related to the lowering of the allergic load by desensitization.

NASAL POLYPS

The management of nasal polyposis is one of the most frustrating to any otolaryngologist or allergist. Simple allergic reactions do not explain polyp formation. Their origin is multifactorial. Frequently, nasal polyps are exacerbated during mold seasons and less frequently during the peak of pollen seasons. One facet of nasal polyp formation may be salicylate sensitivity. The triad of asthma–nasal polyps–aspirin sensitivity has been described for many years. Salicylate may be a factor in polyp formation in some patients with or without the presence of asthma. Salicylates occur commercially as a dispersant of flavor and coloring in foods. They also occur naturally in many fruits (apples, oranges, grapes, and others) and in vegetables (toma-

TABLE 3. *Salicylate-free diet*

Beverages
Allowed: Coffee, grapefruit juice, milk, pear nectar, pineapple juice, postum, vodka
Avoid: Beer, birch beer, ciders, gin and all distilled drinks except vodka, juices of fruits to avoid (see below), Kool-aid and similar artificially flavored and colored beverages, soft drinks, diet drinks and supplements, tea, tomato juice and vegetable juice cocktail, wine

Breads and starches
Allowed: Any bread, English muffins, dinner rolls, frankfurter and hamburger buns, tortilla, rice, pastas, macaroni, spaghetti, popcorn, flour, biscuits, cornbread, muffins
Avoid: None, except those with artificial color and flavor

Cereals
Allowed: Shredded wheat, puffed cereals, cooked cereals, grits, cornmeal, and rice; any cereal without artificial flavor and coloring
Avoid: Any cereal with artificial flavor and colors

Desserts and snack foods
Allowed: Homemade cakes, cookies, doughnuts, ice cream, and pies; potato chips, corn chips, snack crackers with no artificial flavor and colors, nuts (except almonds)
Avoid: Commercial cakes and mixes, cookies, ice cream, sherbet, jello, pudding mixes, and almonds

Fats
Allowed: Avocado cream, cream cheese, vegetable oil, margarine with beta-carotene as coloring
Avoid: Commercial salad dressings, margarine with artificial flavor and color

Flavorings
Allowed: Cinnamon, honey, sugar, vanilla, most herbs and spices (except mint and cloves)
Avoid: Cloves, jams and jellies with artificial color and flavorings, oil of wintergreen

Fruits
Allowed: Bananas, dates, figs, grapefruit, melons, cantaloupe, honeydew, watermelon, pears, pineapple, tangerines
Avoid: Apples, apricots, blackberries, boysenberries, cherries, currents, dewberries, gooseberries, grapes (raisins), nectarines, oranges, peaches, plums (prunes), raspberries, strawberries

Meats or protein foods
Allowed: Beef, chicken, fish, pork, seafood (crab, lobster, shrimp), cheese (natural), dried beans and peas, eggs, peanut butter, tofu
Avoid: Any smoked meats, bacon, bologna, frankfurters, corned beef, ham, lunch meats, processed cheeses

Vegetables
Allowed: Asparagus, bean sprouts, beets, broccoli, brussel sprouts, cabbage, carrots, cauliflower, celery, eggplant, green beans, green pepper, greens (beet, mustard, spinach), lettuce, mushrooms, okra, onions, radishes, rhubarb, rutabaga, sauerkraut, summer squash, turnips, wax beans, zucchini, corn, lima beans, parsnips, peas, potatoes, pumpkins, winter squash, sweet potatoes, yams
Avoid: Cucumbers (pickles), tomatoes

toes and cucumbers). Avoidance of these foods, especially during the mold season, has proved to be effective in some patients with nasal polyps. A supplemental list of foods high in salicylates is given in Table 3).

Not all polyps are allergic. Some can be inflammatory. The management of the underlying infectious process must be undertaken.

This chapter was written with the intention that further excellent references would be sought for more in-depth discussion of these topics. Many of the concepts presented have practical clinical application and have worked in the author's clinical practice.

REFERENCES

1. Young P. *Asthma and allergies; an optimistic future*. Washington, DC: US Department of Health and Human Services, US Public Health Service, National Institutes of Health, CDIHD 80-3887, March 1980.
2. Durham SR, Kay AD. The laboratory investigation of mediators and inflammatory cells in asthma and rhinitis. *Clin Immunol Allergy* 1985;5(3):531–548.
3. Barnes PJ. Allergic inflammatory mediators and bronchial hyper-responsiveness. *Immunol Allergy Clin North Am* 1990;10(2):241–249.
4. Despot JE, Lemanske RF. Inflammatory mediators in allergic rhinitis. *Immunol Allergy Clin North Am* 1987;7(1):37–55.
5. Reed CE. Pharmacologic basis of the treatment of the allergic patient. *Immunol Allergy Clin North Am* 1991;11(1):1–15.
6. Claman HN. Anti-inflammatory effects of corticosteroids. *Clin Immunol Allergy* 1984;4(2):317–329.
7. Israel E, Dermarkarian R, Rosenberg M, et al. The effects of a 5-lipoxygenase inhibitor on asthma induced by cold, dry air. *N Engl J Med* 1990;323:1740–1744.
8. Knapp H. Reduced allergen-induced nasal congestion and leukotriene synthesis with an orally active 5-lipoxygenase inhibitor. *N Engl J Med* 1990;323:1745–1748.
9. DeWeck AL. New approaches to desensitization in IgE mediated allergy. *Clin Immunol Allergy* 1985;5(1):1–11.

CHAPTER 10

Food Allergies and Hypersensitivities

Richard J. Trevino

One area of clinical allergy and immunology requiring further study is hypersensitivity reactions induced by foods. This chapter presents current data demonstrating that the entire immune system is activated by foods to produce symptoms. Clinical testing and treatment modalities will be discussed and their immunologic bases elucidated.

In 1963, Coombs and Gell (1) classified the various immune mechanisms involved in the production of tissue damage into four basic types: I, anaphylactic; II, cytotoxic; III, antigen–antibody complexes; and IV, delayed hypersensitivity.

Type I, the anaphylactic reaction, is the classic allergic type of reaction mediated through immunoglobulin E (IgE), which attaches to the cell membrane of blood basophils or mast cells in the tissues. Following a reaction between antigen and the antibody IgE, certain vasoactive amines are released from these cells, producing symptoms that may be generalized or localized, depending on the mode and degree of administration of antigen. Generalized anaphylaxis may affect the respiratory tract (bronchial obstruction and laryngeal edema), the gastrointestinal tract (nausea and vomiting, cramping pain, diarrhea, bloating, and occasionally blood in the stool), the cardiovascular system (hypotension and shock), and the skin (hives). Allergic rhinitis and asthma are examples of localized respiratory reactions.

Cytotoxic reactions (type II) involve a combination of either immunoglobulin G (IgG) or immunoglobulin M (IgM) with antigenic determinants on the cell membrane. Alternatively, a free antigen or hapten may be absorbed into the tissue component of the cell membrane and antibodies subsequently combine with this absorbed antigen. Complement fixation may then occur, frequently leading to cell damage. A typical example of this type of reaction is the hemolytic reaction induced by a mismatched blood transfusion.

Type III reactions are caused by the formation of antigen–antibody complexes circulating in the blood also utilizing complement.

Initially, there is the formation of antigen–antibody complexes, generally in antigen excess, which fix complement. Release of complement components, which are chemotactic for leukocytes, occurs. There is also damage to the platelets, resulting in release of other vasoactive amines. Increased vascular permeability and precipitation of antigen–antibody complexes occur in capillary walls and tissues, resulting in inflammation and subsequent symptoms. Further fixation of complement and release of chemotactic factors with attraction of polymorphonuclear leukocytes may develop. Neutrophils ingest the immune complexes with release of lysosomal enzymes; this causes further tissue damage and deposition of fibrin. Finally, regression and healing of the lesion may occur if the exposure is a single dose of antigen, or chronic deposition and inflammation will result if there is continuing formation of immune complexes.

Cell-mediated immune reactions (type IV) occur as a result of the interaction between actively sensitized lymphocytes and specific antigens. Such reactions are mediated by the release of lymphokines, direct cytotoxicity, or both, occurring without the involvement of antibody or complement. The delayed skin reaction of poison oak—with its characteristic of mononuclear cell infiltrate developing over a period of 24 to 48 hr—is a typical type IV reaction.

The first requirement for any immunologic reaction to occur is the penetration of antigenic molecules through a tissue barrier of the body. It has been demonstrated that small, nutritionally insignificant amounts of antigenically intact food macromolecules are transmitted across the mature mammalian gut. For example, Danforth and Moore (2) noted that insulin injected into adult rat small intestine caused hypoglycemia, suggesting absorption in biologically active quantities. Bernstein and Ovary (3) demonstrated that haptens and larger antigens were absorbed from guinea pig small intestines in quantities that could produce passive cutaneous anaphylaxis. In human subjects, studies have shown that macromolecules, under normal physiologic conditions, can cross the mature mucosal barrier. Korenblatt et al. (4) showed that a considerable proportion, 15% to 30%, of normal adults develop milk precipitins after ingestion of milk protein. In earlier studies, Wilson and Walzer (5) reported uptake and transport of undigested protein, using a passive cutaneous anaphylactic technique to measure circulating food proteins, and demonstrated precipitins to these proteins in the serum of adults. Thus food antigens may be absorbed through the gastrointestinal mucosa into the body and stimulate immune responses.

Types of immunologic responses incriminated in the production of symptoms caused by food ingestion can be documented.

TYPE I (ANAPHYLACTIC) REACTION

The existence and mechanisms of reaginic IgE immediate-onset food sensitivities are well established. Signs and symptoms range from anaphylaxis to urticaria, asthma, rhinitis, vomiting, and diarrhea. The onset is usually within minutes after ingestion and lasts only a few hours. In 1974, Hoffman and Haddad (6) established that the radioallergosorbent test (RAST) could be used in the diagnosis of food sensitivities. They assembled patients with unequivocal histories of food allergies (i.e., ingestion of the food produced a reaction every time it was consumed and a reaction had occurred within the previous 6 months), often referred to as a fixed food allergy. A number of patients with non-life-threatening symptoms were placed on a strict elimination–challenge regimen to verify the clinical histories. Prick skin testing was performed, until two severe systemic reactions resulted in discontinuation of the test. The test group displayed reactions to 14 common foods. Age-matched control sera were

TABLE 2. *Correlation of RAST with symptoms from food ingestion in a group of patients with unequivocal histories*

Symptom	Number of patients	Percentage of RAST positive
Anaphylaxis	10	100
Bronchospasm	23	96
Angioedema	13	92
Atopic eczema	30	87
Urticaria	26	62
Diarrhea[a]	12	92
Acute gastrointestinal upset	6	33
Tension–fatigue syndrome	15	0

Adapted from ref. 6.
[a] Cases of disaccharidase deficiency, infection, and so on are not included.

tested by RAST and used to determine the normal range for each allergen (Table 1).

Allergen systems with adequate allergenic content—that is, more than a contaminant of the extract, such as codfish, peanut, and egg white—produced excellent correlation in patients with severe symptoms; correlation with less defined allergens, such as orange and chocolate, was not as significant. Positive RASTs correlate in patients with various symptoms and unequivocal histories (Table 2). Note the higher correlation for the more severe symptoms.

These investigators also studied children with severe respiratory allergy without a history of food allergy, finding that 12% were RAST positive to egg. Egg was removed from their diets with improvement of the allergic respiratory symptoms, suggesting that some patients previously presumed to have inhalant allergy alone might also have IgE-mediated food allergy. In 1978, May and Brock (7) reported a verification of the Hoffman–Haddad findings regarding the detection of specific IgE in food-sensitive patients. They found, in a large series, that those who exhibited high serum-specific food IgE levels were sensitive to those foods when challenged orally. There have now been a number of follow-up studies verifying that RAST can be used to diagnose IgE-mediated food sensitivities (8–17).

TABLE 1. *Number of patients with a positive RAST/number tested*

Foods	Anaphylaxis, angioedema, asthma	Eczema	Urticaria skin test	Other symptoms	Control
Codfish	11/11	5/5	6/7	0/2	0/15
Cow's milk	11/12	15/15	5/5	2/8	0/15
Peanut	3/3	8/8	3/3	0/1	0/15
Orange	5/7	7/9	2/5	0/1	0/15
Egg white	8/9	7/8	9/14	0/2	3/20
Chocolate	7/12	6/10	4/8	0/4	0/20
Walnut	5/5	3/3	6/9	0/1	0/15

Adapted from ref. 6.

TYPE II AND TYPE III REACTIONS

Type II or type III food sensitivity is much more difficult to diagnose than type I. These reactions are delayed rather than immediate, occurring from 4 hr up to several days after food ingestion. Patients commonly do not realize that their symptoms are secondary to food ingestion. Investigation of such delayed sensitivities was initiated with the study of complement. In 1936, Lippard et al. (18) used complement fixation to detect milk protein and the subsequent appearance of antibody in the sera of infants. By this technique, small quantities of milk proteins were found in the sera of infants in the first few months of life. The appearance of complement fixation antibodies was followed by the disappearance of antigens from the sera and the presence of precipitating antibodies.

In 1962, Heiner et al. (19) described multiple precipitins to cow's milk (see also ref. 20). In 1970, Mathews and Soothill (21) demonstrated a change in C3 complement level in a group of small children after oral challenge with a small amount of milk. Some had an immediate reaction and others had a delayed reaction when orally challenged. The group with immediate reactions showed no change in C3, whereas the group with delayed reaction did show activation of C3.

In 1977, Sandberg et al. (22) reported a study of children with nephrotic syndrome who had proteinuria after challenge with certain foods. When these foods were withheld from the diet, the nephrotic syndrome cleared and C3 dropped. Sandberg and co-workers also measured C3c, an early detected breakdown product of C3b, documenting an increase in C3c, indicating C3 had been activated. They then studied other children, challenging them with various foods, resulting in a number of delayed symptoms and an elevation of C3c. Sandberg and co-workers recommended that C3c levels be tested along with any oral challenge test performed. Although complement change may occur, it is important to remember that C3 can be activated not only by the immune system but also by the alternative system for complement activation.

In 1981, Trevino (23) demonstrated that the delayed food reaction was truly an immunologic reaction. The experimental group consisted of 55 patients, with 10 as a control group. One food showing a positive reaction on the leukocyte-cytotoxic test was chosen for each patient in the experimental group, and one food that reacted negatively was chosen for the control group. Each food was withdrawn from the patient's diet for 4 days. On the fifth day, the patients were instructed to ingest this food beginning with breakfast. Of the 55 patients in the experimental group, 53 reported some symptoms ranging from mild irritability, restlessness, and inability to sleep to severe migraine, nausea, vomiting, and angioedema. None of the controls reported symptoms. In those experiencing symptoms, C3 and C4 dropped significantly, with levels returning to normal the day following provocation. The control group evidenced no changes in C3 and C4. Since C4 activation occurs only by way of the classic pathway (IgG activation), delayed food hypersensitivity with complement activation is an immunologic phenomenon. Subsequent studies of delayed food sensitivities show that these early components of complement are activated by food antigens. Paganelli et al. (24) found circulating complement-fixing immune complexes bound to the specific food antigen to which their patients were clinically sensitive. Such immune complexes were seen in both normal and food-sensitive subjects, but the concentrations were considerably higher and clearance was slower in the food-sensitive patients.

The study of delayed food reactions has progressed from the investigations of complement, showing that complement is activated by way of the classic complement pathway stimulation, and on to the measurement of immune complexes. More recently, RASTs for specific food IgG have been developed, and studies continue to document what correlation, if any, exists among high IgG titers, complement use, and production of symptoms.

TYPE IV REACTIONS

Type IV (delayed hypersensitivity) reactions are the most difficult to demonstrate since the T-cell effect develops 24 to even 72 hr after the attachment of antigen to the target cell, and the attachment itself may not occur until several hours after ingestion. In 1971, Garcia et al. (25) described an in vitro procedure, the lymphocyte transformation test (LTT). When lymphocytes from the blood of sensitized patients are incubated with food antigens, certain foods increase the activity of the lymphocytes, transforming them to a more blastic form, whereas other foods produce no change. In 1972, May and Alberto (26,27) selected foods positive by the LTT and challenged patients with these foods. After harvesting the lymphocytes, they demonstrated these cells to be active and transformed even when not exposed to in vitro antigen. They postulated that ongoing in vivo proliferation of lymphocytes was induced by antigens absorbed in the challenge procedure. Transformation of lymphocytes, not subjected to food antigens in vitro, did not occur when the oral challenge was not performed. In 1976, Sheinmann et al. (28) repeated and confirmed these studies.

In 1980, Valverde et al. (29) studied 258 patients with idiopathic chronic urticaria and angioedema with the LTT for foods and additives. The LTT response index was positive in 238 patients: 44 positive to additives,

TABLE 3. *Number of patients registering a positive response index (RI) to additives, food extracts, or both*

Response	Number of patients (n = 238)
Positive RI to additives	44 (18.4%)
Positive RI to food extracts	83 (35.2%)
Positive RI to both	111 (46.6%)

From ref. 29, with permission.

83 to food extracts, and 111 to both foods and additives (Table 3). The implicated additives and foods demonstrating a possible LTT response were eliminated from the diets of patients, with complete remission of symptoms in 61.6%, partial remission in 22%, and no change in 16.2% (Table 4). These investigators concluded that the LTT was accurate in identification of foods responsible for patient's symptoms. Typically, patients with chronic idiopathic urticaria and angioedema have normal levels of total IgE. There is no evidence of IgG-mediated disease, biopsies of lesions demonstrating no vasculitis as observed in immune complex reactions, and no necrosis of the vessel walls or presence of nuclear dust. Neutrophils are not prominent in these biopsies, and immunofluorescent studies for the deposition of immunoglobulins and complement are negative. Thus there is no evidence of a type I IgE-mediated reaction or a type II or III IgG-mediated reaction. Nevertheless, the LTT is positive in these patients; that is, the lymphocytes are stimulated by foods, and the elimination of these foods improves the condition of the patients.

The immunologic reaction implicated in producing the urticaria is type IV delayed hypersensitivity. Valverde et al. (30) have performed similar experiments on patients with the allergic tension–fatigue syndrome, with total remission occurring in 86.3% of the patients. These studies are not direct evidence of T-cell activity but are deductive evidence. There is more direct evidence from studying enteropathy in patients with food-induced symptoms.

Ashkenazi et al. (31) studied cell-mediated immunity within the small intestinal mucosa in celiac disease utilizing a test for T-cell activation by measurement of

TABLE 4. *Response to special recommended diet on the basis of results obtained in vitro*

Response	Number of patients (n = 258)
Total remission	159 (61.6%)
Partial remission	57 (22.0%)
No change[a]	42 (16.2%)

From ref. 29, with permission.
[a] This group included 20 patients who did not show any response to foods or additives.

leukocyte inhibition factor (LIF), which decreases white cell migration. When the patient's T cells and the antigen are incubated together in an agar well, migration from the well (or lack of it) can be measured easily. This test obtained in a group of patients with celiac disease demonstrated that celiac disease symptoms resolved when specific foods producing a LIF-positive response were eliminated from the patients' diets. In 1980, Minor et al. (32) measured LIF responses to milk proteins in children with milk-induced enteropathy and verified a positive correlation in 75%. Withdrawal of the milk eliminated the enteropathy. Therefore T-cell type IV delayed-hypersensitivity reactions occur secondary to food antigenic stimulation and cause noxious effects. All four types of immunologic reactions may be stimulated simultaneously by food antigens, the one causing the most severe symptoms being the one that is recognized.

FOOD ALLERGY

Clinically, two types of food allergy occur—fixed and cyclic. The response to IgE type I anaphylactic fixed food allergy is usually prompt, seen within minutes to hours. The symptoms produced are the typical anaphylactic type of reactions, for example, urticaria, wheezing, bronchoconstriction, conjunctivitis, and angioedema. Sensitivity to the food usually persists for more than 2 years after the food is removed from the diet and may last indefinitely. This fixed food allergy accounts for about 5% of all immunologically induced adverse reactions to foods. Therefore treatment for IgE-mediated food sensitivity is elimination of the offending food.

The second type of food allergy is the cyclic form or the non-IgE-mediated delayed sensitivity, accounting for 60% to 80% of the food sensitivity problems seen in clinical practice. These are probably IgG-mediated, representing an immune complex disease. Identification of this type of sensitivity depends primarily on history taking. Verification may be accomplished with a measurement of specific IgG or immune complexes using RAST, but it must be noted that a high level of IgG or immune complexes does not necessarily mean that the person is clinically sensitive to this particular food. The immune response could just be protective in nature. Following the *in vitro* testing, the foods that show a high IgG level should be tested with an *in vivo* test.

Cyclic food allergy, unlike fixed food allergy, is exposure dependent. Increased frequency of ingestion leads to increased sensitivity; that is, the more frequently the food is eaten, the higher the concentration of specific IgG and immune complexes, and the greater the probability of symptom production. When exposure is present at nearly every meal, as occurs in such hidden foods as corn or milk, a condition of masked food allergy may occur in which a small amount of the food actually relieves symptoms for a short period of time. Treatment for this type of food sensitivity is elimination of the food. This elimination need not be indefinite, but rather for only 5 to 6 months. At that time, the food can be reintroduced into the diet, but not consumed every day. Foods should be rotated so that exposure to any food is no more frequent than every 4 to 5 days. Infrequent exposure commonly ensures that the specific IgG to these foods will not become elevated and symptom-producing levels will not be reached. The cyclic pattern of delayed food sensitivity may be explained through an IgG immune complex mechanism (Fig. 1).

Figure 1 demonstrates stage I masked sensitization. The food is eaten frequently, leading to immune complex disease with continuous chronic symptomatology. During this time, there is a phenomenon called masking in which a small amount of food is eaten and symptoms are relieved for a short period of time. This phenome-

non is explained through the effects of prostaglandin E.

Prostaglandins are intracellular components that function to fine-tune the metabolism of the cells. Their effect is on the cell itself. They might affect adjacent cells but have no effect on distant sites. They are rapidly inactivated in the circulation.

There are prostaglandins that have antagonistic actions to each other, but when prostaglandin E predominates, it has an effect on the cyclic nucleotides within the cell. Cyclic adenosine monophosphate (cAMP) is increased and cyclic guanosine monophosphate (cGMP) is decreased intracellularly. This has the effect of making the cell metabolically inactive and resistant to injury. This is the same mechanism utilized by epinephrine to eliminate the effects of anaphylaxis.

Small amounts of a noxious agent cause the cells to produce prostaglandin E. Thus when a small amount of food is eaten, prostaglandin E is produced and the symptomatology of the immune complex disease is alleviated. This effect is transitory, lasting a few hours, at which time, the effect of the prostaglandins comes

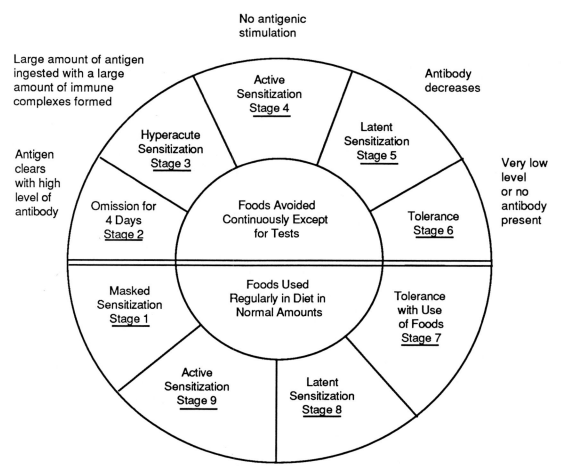

FIG. 1. Increased immune complex disease with increased antigen exposure. (From ref. 33, with permission.)

to an end, and the immune complex symptomatology reasserts itself.

Dependence on this masking action for continued well-being often results in food craving or addiction.

If the antigen or the food is omitted for a period of 4 or 5 days, the food antigen is cleared from the body; however, there is still a high level of IgG being produced. If a large amount of food is then consumed, large amounts of immune complexes form and an exacerbation of symptoms is incited. This is the basis of the oral challenge test in which a person acquires exaggerated symptoms after a 4- to 5-day fast from that food.

If the patient continues to omit the food in question from the diet, the level of IgG gradually falls until the tolerance phase (stage IV) is attained. At this point, there is a very low level of IgG, if any, to that food antigen. At this stage, if the food is reintroduced, there will be some elevation of IgG; but, with limitation of the exposure interval, the level of IgG with symptom production will not be reached. In this tolerance phase, the food or foods in question should be rotated to prevent symptom recurrence to a particular food. If the allergic individual again ingests the food frequently, the immune system will be stimulated to produce IgG, and eventually, the immune response will become elevated enough to produce symptoms once again.

Clinically, there are several ways to test for food sensitivities. For IgE-mediated allergic reactions, the RAST is diagnostic, but rarely necessary, since these food sensitivities are usually well known to the patient, producing immediate reactions. Two types of *in vivo* testing for the more delayed food sensitivities are available. The oral challenge test involves the elimination of a specific food for a period of 4 to 5 days followed by ingestion of that food in large amounts. If the patient has a delayed IgG type of sensitivity to this food, he/she will respond in an exaggerated symptomatic manner.

There are occasions, however, when certain foods cannot be eliminated or are very difficult to eliminate from the diet, for example, very common foods such as corn, soy, or wheat. Other common foods may be difficult to eliminate for a period of 4 to 5 months and to rotate in the diet, particularly for a person who travels frequently and is dependent on restaurants. In these cases, provocation with neutralization may be utilized.

NEUTRALIZATION

Three mechanisms (most likely working together) may explain the neutralization phenomenon. Two are immunologic, one is nonimmunologic, and more mechanisms may be involved that are still unknown.

In 1974, Jerne (34) proposed a hypothesis to explain the complex interactions that regulate antibody formation (Fig. 2), suggesting that the immune system is self-regulating and is composed of a network of idiotypes and anti-idiotypic antibodies. According to this hypothesis, an antigen elicits the production of an antibody (Ab_1) that creates a unique sequence of amino acids, the idiotype, in its antigen-binding region distinguishing it from other antibodies. The unique sequence displayed by idiotype 1 (Id_1) may also function as an immunogen in the same host, since this new array of amino acids is not recognized as self and stimulates the production of another antibody (Ab_2) that has anti-idiotypic specificity for Ab_1. At the same time it displays another unique idiotype, idiotype 2 (Id_2). Ab_2 suppresses the production of Ab_1. In a similar manner, Ab_2 will stimulate the production of Ab_3 and its own unique idiotype 3 (Id_3), displaying anti-anti-idiotypic antibody activity against Ab_2 and so on such that each idiotype that is expressed will stimulate the production of a corresponding anti-idiotypic antibody to suppress the production of the antibody (Ab) against which it was produced. It should be noted that the network can also involve T cells, whereby helper or suppressor T cells can suppress idiotypes identical to those displayed on antibody molecules. Perturbation of this network initiated by exposure to antigen evolves in interactions between idiotypes, anti-idiotypes, and anti-anti-idiotypes. They either turn on or turn off antibody formation to the activities of the various subsets of immunoregulatory T cells. With low doses of antigen exposure, this regulatory system is shifted toward shutting off Ab_1 to the original immunogen, and the person moves into the low-dose tolerance phase.

The second immunologic mechanism involved with low-dose therapy is the T-cell regulatory system. Figure 3 schematically represents proposed cellular interactions that might occur among the already recognized subsets of regulatory T cells. This mechanism involves the direct effect of antigen on T cells. Presentation of the immunogen to macrophages results in the activation of helper–effector T cells and helper–suppressor inducer cells, which cooperate with B cells to initiate antibody formation (pathway 1). At the same time, the helper–suppressor–inducer T-cell population is activated to stimulate the regulator T cells, which influence the suppressor–effector T cells to exert their regulatory suppressor effect (pathway 2).

It is currently believed that the suppressive effects initiated by the suppressor–effector T cells are manifest at the level of the helper–effector T cells rather than by direct action of B cells. In situations in which the immunogen appears to bypass interaction with macrophages (e.g., high antigen dose), suppressor–effector T cells can be activated directly by antigen (pathway 3). These cells also exert their suppressive effects at the level of the helper–effector T cell. This pathway

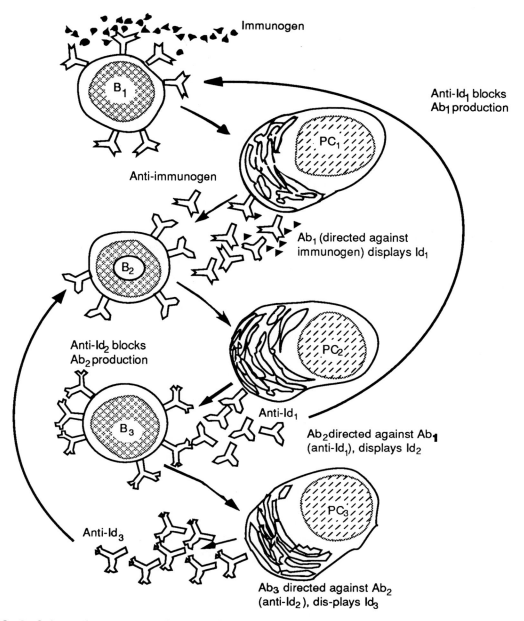

FIG. 2. Schematic representation of idiotype–anti-idiotype regulation of antibody formation. (Adapted from ref. 34.)

may explain the state of pseudotolerance that occurs in the presence of antigen excess.

The final pathway to consider, the contrasuppression circuit (pathway 4), is initiated by the activation of contrasuppressor–inducer T cells. It has a dual regulatory effect interfering with the suppressive activities of the suppressor–effector T cells as well as rendering the helper–effector T cells resistant to the activity of the suppressor–effector T cell.

With very high antigen stimulation, pathway 3 is dominant with suppression of antibody production, creating the pseudotolerance state. With less antigen

administration but still high dose, the level of optimal antibody production is reached and pathway 4 predominates. With less antigen administered or low antigen dose, the suppressive effect through pathway 2 predominates and this is the stage of low-dose tolerance. Thus with low-dose therapy the T-cell regulatory mechanism shifts more toward the suppression of antibody production. This eliminates immune complex disease.

The third mechanism that affords protection to cells when exposed to low-dose antigen exposure is not immunologic but rather involves prostaglandin produc-

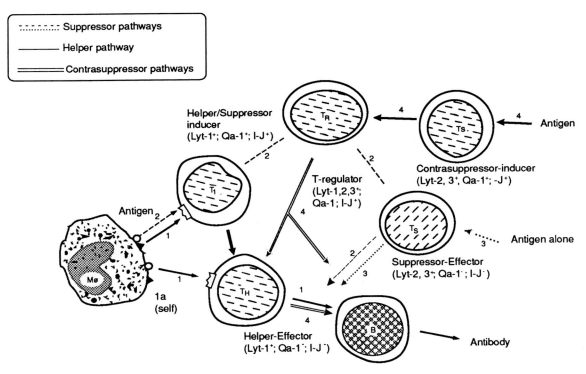

FIG. 3. Schematic representation of T-cell feedback regulatory circuits involved in the control of antibody formation.

tion. In 1979, Robert et al. (35,36) reported on cytoprotection by prostaglandin. These investigators gave rats oral administration of caustic substances (NaOH, HCl, H_2O_2), inducing extensive necrosis of the gastric mucosa. Pretreatment with exogenous prostaglandin either orally or subcutaneously prevented necrosis. They then produced endogenous prostaglandins by pretreating the rats orally with small amounts of the caustic material. This prevented the necrosis when the caustic concentration of the chemicals was given. They called this phenomenon the cytoprotective effect. Pretreatment of the rats with indomethacin completely ablated the cytoprotective effect of the low-dose oral feeding. Thus blocking endogenous prostaglandin production blocked the cytoprotective effect.

Based on these studies, Boris et al. (37) in 1983 studied this cytoprotective effect on antigen-induced asthma in humans. Bronchospasm was evaluated with pulmonary function testing in double-blind studies on 19 subjects with a history of wheezing to animal dander. The subjects were challenged with gradually increasing doses of inhaled animal dander until the dose that caused a 20% increase in forced expiratory volume in 1 sec (FEV_1) was achieved. Intradermal skin endpoint titration was then performed to ascertain the end point of the animal dander on each subject. The subjects were pretreated with subcutaneous injection of this end-point dose and the inhalation provocation was

repeated. There was significant prolongation of the FEV_1 up to 75% when an identical inhalation challenge dose was administered. The subjects were then pretreated with indomethacin, the end-point dose of antigen was administered by injection, and then rechallenge was performed by inhalation of the identical dose of animal dander as used previously. This pretreatment with indomethacin completely ablated the protection against bronchospasm that was produced by pretreatment with a low dose of injected antigen.

The studies of Sobotka et al. (38) and Mendoza and Kiminobu (39) document antigen-specific desensitization of basophils for high-dose histamine release by low-dose preincubation. This possible mechanism of neutralization is supported by Scadding and Brostoff (40) in their double-blind study of low-dose house dust mite treatment.

These phenomena have been applied clinically to patients with delayed food sensitivity. The process of provocation–neutralization for food sensitivities and treatment is still in its evolutionary phase and may change in the future. At the present time, the following methodology is being used.

The food antigen is first diluted using the standard fivefold dilution method. This is the same process used for preparing inhalant allergies for the serial end-point titration technique.

The dilutions are labeled in numerical order—1, 2,

3, 4, 5 and so on, with each successive dilution five times weaker than the dilution preceding it. Dilution #1 is five times weaker than the concentrate dilution in #2 is five times weaker than the first dilution and 25 times weaker than the concentrate, and so on.

A 0.05-cc dose of dilution #1 is applied intradermally and observed for a whealing response over a 10-min period. If there is a progression of swelling before 10 min, 0.05 cc of dilution #2 is applied and observed for 10 min. This process of applying successively weaker dilutions continues until a dilution is found that, when applied intradermally, will not provoke a whealing response. This is called the neutralizing dose and usually occurs with dilution #2 or #3.

This method of testing provides two important pieces of information:

1. It identifies the food to which the patient is reacting.
2. It identifies the concentration that will provoke prostaglandin E production and shut down all the reactive cells.

When possible, this particular food is eliminated from the diet. After 5 to 6 months of elimination, the food can be reintroduced on a rotation basis, every 4 to 5 days.

If the food cannot be eliminated from the diet, the dilution of antigen (determined by testing to be the neutralizing dose) is injected subcutaneously daily, prior to ingestion of the food. This therapy produces two results:

1. It protects the individual from the subsequent ingestion of that food because of the prostaglandin production.
2. After several days of subcutaneous injections of the food, antigen B cells are put into the low-dose tolerant phase. This is due to the B-cell feedback mechanism and the T-cell suppression mechanism and results in the cessation of IgG formation to that particular food and the subsequent immune complex disease.

Continuing antigen therapy over a period of several months results in the progressive diminution of the level of IgG until the patient loses the sensitivity to that food.

The theory and application of low-dose therapy for food sensitivities have been tested in a double-blind fashion by King et al. (41–43).

In conclusion, the field of food allergy and sensitivity is a diverse and stimulating field in which food proteins can cause a myriad of symptoms with different mechanisms. In efforts to give the food-sensitive patient the entire benefit of our knowledge, the clinician should be aware of all aspects of the immunological response to food sensitivities and be prepared to apply this knowledge in the relief of the patient's symptomatology.

The conclusion is that low-dose therapy gives protection to the shock organ, and this is accomplished through prostaglandins. The cells of the shock organ, when exposed to a small amount of a noxious substance, produce prostaglandins that cause an increase in cAMP and decrease in cGMP intracellularly, leading to a reduced metabolism and reactivity of the cell. This is the same effect that is produced by the antiasthmatic medication theophylline and the antianaphylactic medication epinephrine. Small doses of immunogen initially protect the cells from the noxious effects of larger doses of the same immunogen. That antigen dose that causes the shock organ to produce prostaglandins and thus increases cAMP and decreases cGMP, that causes the antibody feedback mechanism to shut off antibody production against that antigen, and that directly causes suppressor T-cell activity to shut off antibody production is called the neutralizing dose. Therefore small doses of immunogen protect the cells from the damaging effects of larger doses of the same immunogen.

REFERENCES

1. Coombs RR, Gell PG. *Classification of allergic reactions responsible for clinical hypersensitivity and disease: clinical aspects of immunology.* Oxford: Blackwell Scientific Publications, 1975;761.
2. Danforth E, Moore RD. Intestinal absorption of insulin in the rat. *Endocrinology* 1959;65:118.
3. Bernstein ID, Ovary Z. Absorption of antigens from the gastrointestinal tract. *Int Arch Allergy Appl Immunol* 1986;33:521.
4. Korenblatt RE, Rothberg RM, Minden P, et al. Immune response of human adults after oral and parenteral exposure to bovine serum albumin. *J Allergy* 1968;41:226.
5. Wilson SJ, Walzer M. Absorption of undigested protein in human beings. *Am J Dis Child* 1935;50:49.
6. Hoffman DR, Haddad ZH. Diagnosis of IgE mediated immediate hypersensitivity reaction to foods by radioimmunossay. *J Allergy Clin Immunol* 1974;54:165.
7. May CD, Brock SA. A modern clinical approach to food hypersensitivity. *Allergy* 1978;33:166.
8. Chua YY, Brenmer K, Lakdawalla N, et al. In vivo and in vitro correlates of food allergy. *J Allergy Clin Immunol* 1976;58:299.
9. Wraith DG, Merrett J, Roth A, et al. Recognition of food-allergic patients and their allergens by the RAST technique and clinical investigation clinic. *Allergy* 1979;9:25.
10. Merrett TG, Merrett J. The RAST principle and the use of mixed allergen: RAST as a screening test for IgE-mediated allergies. *Methods Enzymol* 1980;70:376.
11. Monro J, Brostoff J, Carini C, Zilki K. Food allergy in migraine: study of dietary inclusion and RAST. *Lancet* 1980;2:1.
12. Paganelli R, Levinsky RJ. Solid phase radioimmunoassay for detection of circulating food protein antigens in human serum. *J Immunol Methods* 1980;37:333.
13. Schwartz HR, Nerurkar LS, Spies JR, et al. Milk hypersensitivity: RAST studies using new antigens generated by pepsin hydrolysis of beta lacto globulin. *Ann Allergy* 1980;45:242.
14. Freed D. Laboratory diagnosis of food intolerance. *Clin Immunol Allergy* 1982;2:181.
15. Scudamore HH, Philips SF, Swedlund HA, Gleich GJ. Food allergy manifested by eosinophilia, elevated immunoglobin E

level, and protein-losing enteropathy: the syndromes of allergic gastroenteropathy. *J Allergy Clin Immunol* 1982;70:129.

16. Sampson HA, Alberto R. Comparison of results of skin test, RAST, and double-blind, placebo-controlled food challenges in children with atopic dermatitis. *J Allergy Clin Immunol* 1984;6:26.

17. Hattevig G, Kjellman B, Johansson SG, Bjorksten B. Clinical symptoms and IgE responses to common food proteins in atopic and healthy children. *Clin Allergy* 1984;14:551.

18. Lippard VS, Scloss OM, Johnson PA. Immune reactions induced in infants by intestinal absorption of incompletely digested cow's milk protein. *Am J Dis Child* 1936;51:562.

19. Heiner DD, Sears JW, Kniker WT. Multiple precipitins to cow's milk in chronic respiratory disease. *Am J Dis Child* 1962;103:634.

20. Holland HN, Hong R, Davis NC, West CD. Significance of precipitating antibodies to milk proteins in the serum of infants and children. *J Pediatr* 1962;61:181.

21. Mathews TS, Soothill JF. Complement activation after milk feeding in children with cow's milk allergy. *Lancet* 1970;2:893.

22. Sandberg DH, Bernstein CW, McIntosh RM, et al. Severe steroid responsive nephrosis associated with hypersensitivity. *Lancet* 1977;1:388.

23. Trevino RJ. Immunologic mechanisms in the production of food sensitivities. *Laryngoscope* 1981;91:1913.

24. Paganelli R, Levinsky RJ, Atherton DJ. Detection of specific antigen within immune complexes: validation of the assay and its application to food antigen–antibody complexes formed in healthy and food allergic subjects. *Clin Exp Immunol* 1981;46:44.

25. Garcia P, Rodriguez JC, Vinos J. A new rapid and more sensitive microcytotoxicity test. *J Immunol Methods* 1971;1:103.

26. May CD, Alberto R. In vitro responses of leukocytes to food proteins in allergic and normal children: lymphocytes stimulation and histamine release. *Clin Allergy* 1972;2:335.

27. May CD, Alberto R. In vivo stimulation of peripheral lymphocytes to proliferation after oral challenge of children allergic to foods. *Int Arch Allergy Appl Immunol* 1972;43:525.

28. Scheinmann P, Gendrel D, Charlas J, et al. Value of lymphoblast transformation test in cow's milk protein intestinal intolerance. *Clin Allergy* 1976;6:515.

29. Valverde E, Vich JM, Garcia-Colderon J, Garcia-Colderon PA. In vitro stimulation of lymphocytes in patients with chronic urticaria induced by additives and foods. *Clin Allergy* 1980;10:691.

30. Valverde E, Vich JM, Garcia-Colderon JV, Garcia-Colderon PA. In vitro response of lymphocytes in patients with allergic tension-fatigue syndrome. *Ann Allergy* 1980;454–185.

31. Ashkenazi A, Idar O, Handzel ZT, et al. An in vitro immunologic assay for diagnosis of coeliac disease. *Lancet* 1978;1:627.

32. Minor JD, Tolber SG, Frick OL. Leukocyte inhibition factors in delayed onset food allergy. *J Allergy Clin Immunol* 1980;66:319.

33. Rinkel HJ, Randolph TG, Zeller M. *Food allergy*. Springfield, IL: Charles C Thomas, 1951.

34. Jerne NK. Towards a network theory of the immune system. *Ann Immunol* 1974;125c:373.

35. Robert A, Nezamis JE, Lancaster C, Hanchar AJ. Cytoprotection by prostaglandins in rats: prevention of gastric necrosis produced by alcohol, HCl, NaOH, hypertonic NaCl and thermal injury. *Gastroenterology* 1979;77:761.

36. Robert A. Cytoprotection by prostaglandins. *Gastroenterology* 1979;77:761.

37. Boris M, Schiff M, Weindorf S. Injection of low dose antigen attenuates the response to subsequent bronchoprovocative challenge. *Otolaryngol Head Neck Surg* 1988;98:536.

38. Sobotka AK, Dembo M, Goldstein B, Lichtenstein LM. Antigen specific desensitization of human basophils. *Ann Immunol* 1979;122:511–517.

39. Mendoza GR, Kiminobu M. Subthreshold and suboptimal desensitization of human basophils. *Int Arch Allergy Appl Immunol* 1982;65:101–107.

40. Scadding GK, Brostoff J. Low dose sublingual therapy in patients with allergic rhinitis due to house dust mite. *Clin Allergy* 1986;483–491.

41. King W, Rubin W, Fadal R, Ward W, Trevino R, Pierce W, Stewart J, Boyles J Jr. Provocation–neutralization: a two-part study; Part I. The intracutaneous provocative food test: a multicenter comparison study. *Otolaryngol Head Neck Surg* 1988;99(3):263–271.

42. King W, Fadal R, Ward W, Trevino R, Pierce W, Stewart J, Boyles J Jr. Provocation–neutralization: a two-part study; Part II. Subcutaneous neutralization therapy: a multicenter study. *Otolaryngol Head Neck Surg* 1988;99(3):272–277.

43. King W, Rubin W, Fadal R, Ward W, Trevino R, Pierce W, Stewart J, Boyles J Jr. Efficacy of alternative tests for delayed-cyclic food hypersensitivity. *Otolaryngol Head Neck Surg* 1989;101(3):385–387.

CHAPTER 11

Background Considerations and Office Management of Food Allergy

Wellington G. Borges and Douglas C. Heiner

Adverse reactions to foods are an important clinical consideration for physicians including ear, nose, and throat specialists, particularly in dealing with infants, but also in the management of patients of any age. Reactions to food may be an occult cause of chronic disease or may cause acute symptoms that occasionally may be lethal. The diagnosis of food allergy is sometimes obvious, but it can be difficult and time consuming.

Unfavorable reactions to foods were recognized by Van Helmont, who in the 17th century described attacks of asthma precipitated by eating fish (1). Awareness of food-induced reactions has increased during the 20th century, stimulated by reports of severe reactions to foods (2–4). In recent years, a vast array of symptoms and disorders have been attributed to the ingestion of foods. The spectrum of clinical manifestations has broadened to include reactions that are delayed in onset and may involve the gastrointestinal tract, skin, respiratory system, or other parts of the body.

DEFINITION

The term "adverse food reaction" refers to any untoward reaction that results from the ingestion of a food or food additive. The term "food allergy" implies an abnormal or excessive immunologic response to one or more constituents of the food. "Food allergy" should not be used to describe all symptoms appearing after the ingestion of a food but only to describe those adverse reactions that are immunologically mediated. The term "food intolerance" is more appropriate to use for other adverse food reactions.

Definitions recommended by the Committee on Adverse Reactions to Food of the American Academy of Allergy and Immunology (5) are listed in abbreviated form in Table 1.

EPIDEMIOLOGY

The prevalence of allergy to specific foods may vary in different geographical areas and among different ethnic groups. Unfortunately, there are no universally accepted diagnostic criteria and no epidemiologic studies that permit an accurate estimate of the prevalence of the different types of food allergy and/or intolerance. There is little doubt that food allergy is perceived by the public to be a major health problem. Although its true prevalence is unknown, food allergy is probably less common than is generally perceived. Allergy to cow's milk has been reported to occur in 0.3% to 7.5% of the pediatric population (6,7), but some authors report a lower and some a higher incidence.

In a 3-year follow-up of 480 children, an adverse reaction to food was suspected in 28% of cases, but only 8% were confirmed by double-blind food challenges (DBFCs) (8). The prevalence of food allergy is probably increased among patients with immunoglobulin A (IgA) deficiency or preexisting intestinal disease (9). It may be as high as 33% in some patient groups, such as children with atopic dermatitis (10).

There is evidence that the incidence of food allergy changes with age (11). It is common knowledge among pediatricians that adverse reactions to cow's milk are much more common during the first 2 years of life than later in childhood. Based on history as well as on di-

TABLE 1. *Definitions of terms*

Adverse reaction (sensitivity) to a food: A general term applied to an abnormal response attributable to a food or food additive.

Food allergy (hypersensitivity): An adverse immunologic reaction resulting from ingestion of a food or food additive.

Food anaphylaxis: A severe, usually generalized adverse reaction to a food or additive in which IgE antibody and chemical mediator release are involved.

Food intolerance: A general term describing an abnormal physiologic response to an ingested food or food additive that is not proved to be immunologic in nature. It includes idiosyncratic, metabolic, pharmacologic, and toxic responses.

Food toxicity (poisoning): An adverse effect caused by the direct action of a food or an additive without the involvement of immune mechanisms; nonimmune release of chemical mediators may take place; toxins may be either from the food itself or from microorganisms.

Food idiosyncrasy: Quantitatively abnormal response to a food or food additive; response differs from its physiologic or pharmacologic effect and resembles a hypersensitivity reaction but does not involve recognized immune mechanisms.

Anaphylactoid reaction to a food: An anaphylaxis-like reaction presumed to result from nonimmune release of chemical mediators; mimics food allergy and is similar to idiosyncrasy.

Pharmacologic reaction: An adverse reaction caused by a food constituent that produces an effect similar to that of a drug.

Metabolic food reactions: Adverse reaction to a food or food additive as the result of effect of substance on metabolism of the host.

From ref. 5, with permission.

etary elimination and challenge, one group reported the prevalence of selected food allergies to increase between birth and 3 years of age, then to decline to approximately the adult prevalence by 6 years of age (12).

A history of food allergy or of other allergic disease in an immediate family member identifies a child to be at increased risk for food allergy. Food allergy was reported by Kjellman (13) to occur in 58% of children with bilateral parental family history of atopic disease as compared with 29% in children with one atopic parent, and 12% in children with no family history of atopic disease. Gerrard et al. (7) estimated that when a family has one child with milk allergy, a subsequently born sibling will have a 1:3 risk of having problems when fed cow's milk.

FOOD ALLERGENS

The foods that most frequently cause allergic reactions are those most commonly consumed and those with a relatively high protein content. Thus the preva-lence of specific reactivity to a food depends in part on the eating habits of a given population. Fortunately, the majority of patients with allergic food reactions react to a relatively small number of foods. Not all proteins found in foods are equally allergenic. Some foods with a high protein content, such as beef and chicken, are only rarely implicated in allergic disease. For most child populations, the proteins of milk, eggs, peanuts, soy, and wheat are the main food allergens. Adults have a higher proportion of reactions to fish, shellfish, and tree nuts. However, any food can cause an allergic reaction in a specifically sensitive individual at any age.

Most foods contain a large number of potentially allergenic proteins, among which there are one or more allergens to which the majority of allergic individuals react and many minor antigens to which a smaller group of people react (14). Most allergens are glycoproteins, with molecular weights between 17,000 and 40,000 daltons. It has been suggested that, in general, animal foods (shrimp, egg, fish) have more potent allergenic activity than fruits and vegetables, but there are exceptions such as the peanut, which is a potent allergen. Heat processing often weakens or abolishes the allergenicity of a protein (e.g., heat labile milk proteins, celery, potato, and banana allergens) (15). IgE-dependent reactions may also be caused by food additives (16).

PATHOPHYSIOLOGY

Food allergy develops as a result of the interaction between food allergens and sensitized cells in specific tissues or organs.

The gastrointestinal tract has immunoreactive cells that can cause local symptoms or systemic manifestations as a result of the release of chemical mediators from the gastrointestinal tract into the circulation. It also can act as a conduit for antigen uptake, which in turn can reach other organs, where it can react with sensitized cells and cause the release of mediators of inflammation. Absorbed antigens also can react with circulating sensitized basophils.

One function of the mature gastrointestinal tract is to reduce the absorption of immunoreactive food antigens. Infants gradually develop an extensive system of defense mechanisms within the intestinal tract. These features of the gastrointestinal tract ensure a nearly impermeable barrier to the uptake of antigens. Table 2 (17) lists some of the components of the mucosal barrier. These include enzymatic and mechanical mechanisms as well as antigen-specific dimeric IgA antibodies (Fig. 1), which retard the penetration of luminal antigens (18). The gastrointestinal tract also mini-

TABLE 2. *Components of the mucosal barrier to food antigens*

Nonimmunologic
  Gastric acidity, proteolysis
  Peristalsis
  Mucosal surface
    Mucus coat
    Epithelial membrane
    Microvillous enzymes
Immunologic
  Secretory IgA system
  Other immunoglobulins (IgM, IgG)
  Cellular immune system
Combination of immunologic and nonimmunologic
  Immune complex-mediated mucus release from goblet cells
  Immune complex-facilitated mucosal surface proteolysis
  Kupffer cell phagocytosis of immune complexes

Adapted from ref. 17.

TABLE 3. *Likely causes of excessive uptake of food antigens*

Immature gastrointestinal function (enzymes, mucosal barrier)
Malnutrition
Inflammation (inflammatory bowel disease, celiac disease, gastroenteritis)
Gastrointestinal anoxia
Transient or persistent IgA deficiency
Other immunodeficiencies

Adapted from ref. 17.

mizes systemic immune responses by favoring immune tolerance.

The usual result of a normal luminal immune response is an absence of adverse reactions to ingested foods. If the mucosal defense is disrupted (Table 3) (17), intraluminal food antigens may gain increased access to the immune system, leading to an increase in antigen-induced disease (Fig. 2).

The gastrointestinal tract normally is permeable to a small but immunogenic amount of the macromolecules that enter its lumen. This is particularly true during early infancy but is also true in adults (19), and the production of small to moderate amounts of IgG and IgA antibodies to most food proteins is a normal phenomenon. About 95% of normal babies develop antibodies to milk protein during the first 2 years of life (20). People with food allergy tend to have higher antibody titers of all immunoglobulin classes to specific food allergens than do healthy individuals.

Walzer (21) established that small amounts of immunoreactive food proteins may gain access to the circulation at various levels of the gastrointestinal tract, after which they are transported to distant target organs. Thus a variety of antigen–antibody complexes can occur not only in the gastrointestinal lumen but also within the systemic circulation, from which they may attach to the Fc fragment (crystallizable) of immunoglobulin and complement receptors in various tissues. It is likely that most food antigen–antibody complexes are harmless, but some, when in excess or of a particular composition, may participate in pathologic processes in the kidney or the skin and probably at other sites.

Paganelli and Levinsky (22) reported the presence of circulating food antigen–antibody complexes in a proportion of allergic individuals. It is possible that these complexes could activate the complement system and lead to mast cell/basophil degranulation. However, normal individuals also may have demonstrable circulating immune complexes, and no test is presently available to clinicians that will accurately determine which complexes are involved in symptom production.

Allergic reactions to foods can be classified into two

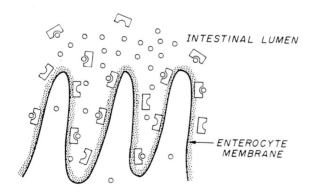

○ INTESTINAL ANTIGEN (Food, Bacteria)

▱ ANTIBODY

▱ IMMUNE COMPLEX

FIG. 1. Antibody acting as a barrier to antigen absorption at the mucosal surface of the gastrointestinal tract. Secretory antibodies in the intestinal lumen and on the mucosa surface inhibit absorption of most antigen molecules.

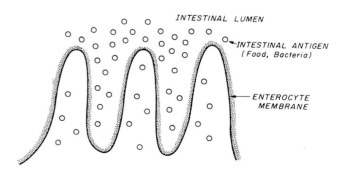

FIG. 2. Compromise of the antibody barrier at the surface of the gastrointestinal tract in subjects with IgA deficiency. The absence of secretory antibodies permits an increase in antigen uptake.

distinct categories. The first, which is most familiar, is usually precipitated by small amounts of food. This type is predominantly immunoglobulin E (IgE) mediated, the type I anaphylactic or immediate hypersensitivity mechanism of Coombs and Gell (23). IgE molecules, which are affixed to receptors on basophils or mast cells, react with food antigens and cause the release of chemical mediators including histamine, chemotactic factors, leukotrienes, and prostaglandins. These substances rapidly produce vasodilation and mucus secretion, increased muscle contraction, and stimulation of pain fibers. They also begin recruitment of inflammatory cells (24,25).

Local immune reactions may increase mucosal permeability and allow enhanced absorption of foreign antigens. In addition, it has been suggested that as foods traverse the intestinal tract and are digested, new antigens may be produced (26). It is possible that these neoantigens enter the circulation where they initiate mast cell degranulation at peripheral sites in the body. The clinical significance of new antigen generation in the gastrointestinal tract, however, is unknown.

The manifestations of IgE-mediated immediate hypersensitivity may begin seconds after the ingestion of an offending food, or they may occur only after 1 to 2 hr, the time required for maximal uptake of dietary allergens into the systemic circulation. They usually are associated with positive prick tests and radioallergosorbent tests (RASTs) to the offending food.

Activation of the complement cascade may also induce an immediate response resembling an IgE-mediated reaction. Indeed, C5a anaphylotoxin is a potent releaser of chemical mediators from mast cells (27).

In the second type of reaction, symptoms usually are precipitated by the ingestion of large amounts of a specific food. The symptoms usually are delayed, recurrent, or chronic and begin from a few hours to several weeks after the offending food is introduced into the diet. Such reactions may arise on the basis of type II (cytotoxic), type III (immune complex or Arthus reaction), or type IV (cell-mediated or delayed) hypersensitivity according to the Coombs–Gell classification (23). It is also possible that a patient with delayed-onset food sensitivity is reacting to a peptide breakdown fragment of a food protein and that symptoms do not occur until that fragment is produced and absorbed. There is some evidence that peptide fragments of food proteins formed in the gastrointestinal tract may interact with specific histocompatibility leukocyte antigen (HLA) molecules and initiate cellular immune responses (28).

In their series of nearly 120 children, Bock and May (29) found eight children who reacted to a food challenge more than 4 hr after antigen administration. One must be aware that delayed IgE-mediated responses may occur. These usually, but not always, follow several hours after an immediate-type reaction. Hill et al. (30) have reported eczematous skin eruptions only after 2 to 3 days of daily food antigen exposure. It is common knowledge that the clinical manifestations of celiac disease may not occur until days or weeks after wheat is introduced into the diet. A similar delayed-type response also may be seen in milk-induced gastroenteropathy (31,32). These conditions are in all likelihood immunologically mediated and are extreme examples of delayed clinical food hypersensitivity.

Moneret-Vautrin and Andre (33), studying 154 cases of food allergy, found that immediate type I (IgE-dependent) allergy is the most frequent (87% of cases), followed by type IV or delayed type (9% of the cases). Types II and III were thought to be exceedingly rare. However, one should remember that type I reactions are easiest to recognize, and more than one type of immune mechanism may contribute to any given adverse response.

CLINICAL FEATURES

Allergic reactions to foods take many forms. Manifestations vary in location and severity as well as time of onset. Signs and symptoms may be localized to the gastrointestinal tract or to distant organs including the skin, nose, lung, central nervous system, or circulatory system. Nasal manifestations may include rhinitis, sinusitis, and otitis media. The basis of preferential reactivity with one system over another is unknown. There could be a selective binding of certain IgE antibodies to the mast cells of a particular organ or tissue. Or there could be a heightened reactivity to chemical mediators of target cells in certain organs.

The clinical manifestations of food allergy range in severity from minimal skin manifestations or mild rhinitis to asthma, pulmonary infiltrates, and life-threatening anaphylaxis. Manifestations may be influenced by the age of the patient, the volume of food ingested, and the immunologic mechanisms at play. Some of the many possible signs and symptoms are listed in Table 4 (34).

A patient with type I hypersensitivity may have swollen lips within minutes of eating a food. The mouth and throat may tingle, and blebs of mucosal swelling may develop on the buccal surfaces. This is probably due to IgE antibodies. Such reactions are usually transient and may not be followed by other allergic manifestations. They are usually self-evident, and affected patients often solve the problem without medical help by avoiding the food that causes the symptoms.

Type II, III, or IV responses are more difficult to recognize. The manifestations are delayed rather than immediate, occurring from 2 hr to several days after the food ingestion. Patients commonly do not know

TABLE 4. *Food hypersensitivity reactions confirmed in blinded challenges*

Generalized reactions
  Anaphylaxis
Skin reactions
  Urticaria/angioedema
  Atopic dermatitis
  Dermatitis herpetiformis
Respiratory reactions
  Rhinoconjunctivitis
  Laryngeal edema
  Asthma
  Heiner's syndrome
Gastrointestinal reactions
  Vomiting and diarrhea
  Eosinophilic gastroenteritis
  Protein-losing enteropathy
  Gluten-sensitive enteropathy (celiac disease)
  Gastrointestinal blood loss
  Colic
Neurological reactions
  Migraine

Adapted from ref. 34.

that these symptoms are secondary to food ingestion. Reactions that are predominantly type IV may be the most difficult to recognize since the T cells involved may not cause a clinical effect for days after exposure.

ALLERGIC RHINITIS AND FOOD ALLERGY

Food-induced respiratory symptoms are often associated with other clinical manifestations of atopic diseases, for example, cutaneous or gastrointestinal (35). Sabbah et al. (36) found that in one-third of 261 cases, perennial rhinitis was related to food allergy, but food allergy without inhalant allergy was seen only in six patients.

The most common respiratory manifestation of food allergy in infants and young children is chronic rhinorrhea. Sneezing and a congested runny nose are the usual symptoms. Whenever rhinorrhea that persists for 6 weeks or longer is seen in a child under 1 year of age, the possibility must be considered that food allergy is at fault (37). Nasal symptoms have been noted in 13% to 31% of children with cow's milk allergy (38–41). Inhalant allergy is not common in children under 1 year of age.

The child may have breathing difficulty (mouth breathing), particularly during sleep. A lingering cough may be associated with a postnasal drip. The nasal mucosa usually appears edematous and pale. A nasal smear often reveals that more than 10% of the cells are eosinophils. Some children with frequent rubbing of the nose may have a transverse crease on the nasal bridge. Others may have a bluish discoloration and/or puffiness of the lower eyelid ("allergic shiners") as a

result of nasal allergy. Serous otitis media and thickening of the mucosal lining of the sinuses are common concomitants of nasal allergy. These set the stage for bacterial otitis media and/or sinusitis.

ALLERGIC RHINITIS AND SINUSITIS

Subjects with allergic rhinitis are especially prone to develop signs of sinusitis (42). Mucosal edema secondary to allergy can obstruct the sinus ostia, creating stasis (43), accumulation of mucus, and infection. Optimal treatment frequently must include measures to alleviate both the allergy and the infection.

There is a high prevalence of abnormal sinus radiographs in any group of children with chronic respiratory allergy. Thirty-seven subjects (or 53%) of one group demonstrated roentgenographic abnormalities and 15 (21%) had complete opacification of one or more sinus cavities (44).

Recently, Savolainen (45) studied 224 patients with *acute* maxillary sinusitis and allergy was documented in 56 (25%). Other studies confirm that *chronic* maxillary sinusitis and allergic rhinitis are closely linked (46,47). According to these workers, allergy may be an underlying factor in 38% to 67% of patients with chronic sinusitis.

Subjects with allergic rhinitis or asthma are likely to have more widespread involvement of the paranasal sinuses than patients without an allergic history.

The symptoms of sinusitis may be confused with those of allergic rhinitis, especially by patients (48). Chronic nasal congestion, puffiness and/or discoloration of eyelids, mouth breathing, rhinorrhea, fatigue, and irritability may be manifestations of either. In children, the most common symptoms associated with sinusitis have been reported to be chronic rhinorrhea (77% of cases), middle ear disease with eustachian tube obstruction (61%), and persistent cough (48%) (49). The presence of increased numbers of eosinophils on the nasal smear points toward allergic rhinitis, whereas numerous polymorphonuclear cells and the presence of large numbers of bacteria suggest infection. The presence of phagocytosed bacteria within neutrophils is particularly suggestive of infection.

In a study of the maxillary mucosa in nasal allergy associated with chronic sinusitis, Yamada (50) found that the number of mast cells in the nasal mucosa was similar to those in the maxillary mucosa, suggesting that type I allergic mechanisms can occur in the sinuses as well as in the nose. Ordinarily, there is a turnover of air in the maxillary sinuses about every 5 min (51).

Harlin et al. (52) showed that prominent eosinophilic infiltrates of the sinus mucosa were related to both chronic asthma and allergic rhinitis. In addition, they found strikingly similar histopathologic changes in the sinus and bronchial mucosae in allergic subjects including stromal edema, thickening of the basement membrane, hyperplasia of goblet cells, and mucus plugging. Charcot–Leyden crystals (from degenerated eosinophils) and Creola bodies (clumps of epithelial cells) can be found in both nasal and paranasal airways. They concluded that the major basic protein (MBP) contained in eosinophil granules may play a role in the physiopathology of allergic sinusitis by damaging paranasal respiratory epithelium in a manner similar to that described in chronic asthma (53,54).

DIAGNOSIS AND LABORATORY FINDINGS

The diagnosis of food allergy requires a thorough history and physical examination. As mentioned earlier, some food allergy is self-diagnosed. Self-diagnoses need not be wrong, but subjective impressions should not be the sole diagnostic criteria. The clinical history should include details of early postnatal life, the evolution of atopic manifestations in relation to the introduction of specific foods, and evidences of a repetitive association between a particular food and symptoms. The clinical history by itself is misleading about half the time (55).

If a convincing relationship between the ingestion of a food and symptoms is not forthcoming from the history, a diet diary may be helpful. Some of the advantages and disadvantages of diet diaries are indicated in Table 5 (56).

An important first step in diagnosis is the clinical demonstration that the patient's symptoms disappear while on an elimination diet. This involves either excluding a suspected food or using an arbitrary diet that excludes the most commonly suspected foods for 1 month. If symptoms clear before that time, foods may be reintroduced, one at a time, beginning a week after symptom amelioration. If symptoms persist during the

TABLE 5. *Diet diaries*

Advantages
Detailed records can be reviewed.
Consistent associations can be documented.
The cost is very low.
The patient and family will focus on the possibility of dietary contributions to symptomatology.
May be useful when there is no obvious connection between ingestion of a particular food and symptom production.
Disadvantages
Low yield, often of little help.
Patients may be confused by the findings unless assisted by an experienced physician.
Diet diaries may be suggestive but seldom are diagnostic of allergy.

Adapted from ref. 56.

month of elimination, the eliminated foods are individually reintroduced in goodly amounts at 3-day intervals to see if any induces an exacerbation. A disappearance or improvement in symptoms following an elimination diet must be followed by a recurrence after a specific food challenge before a presumptive diagnosis of specific food intolerance can be made.

The above probably is the most practical initial diagnostic approach to food allergy or food intolerance. Sometimes more objective evidence is needed. A separation of organic from psychologic factors is often possible by double-blind challenge testing. Even with a double-blind protocol there is a finite possibility that a patient will have a psychologic or placebo-induced reaction when the suspected food is given but not when placebo is given. Statistical considerations indicate that at least three challenges, one placebo and two food challenges, or vice versa, each double blind, are necessary to accurately separate allergic from placebo reactions. Subtle influences from medical personnel are difficult to avoid. Negative challenges offer good evidence that a particular food does not produce symptoms when administered in the amount given by double-blind challenge. However, one must remember that larger amounts of the food taken repetitively could cause or contribute to symptoms. With cooperation between the patient and an experienced physician, delayed-type reaction often can be sorted out.

From a practical point of view, appropriate challenge tests carried out nonblinded frequently will provide a satisfactory presumptive diagnosis. Symptoms while the patient is taking the food, disappearance of symptoms during an elimination diet, reappearance of symptoms when the specific food is reintroduced in amounts usually ingested, and clearing of symptoms once again on elimination of the food provide the presumption of food intolerance. Double-blind tests have shown many claims of an adverse food reaction to be unsubstantiated. Studies are needed to determine how often and under what circumstances double-blind challenge tests and long-term patient follow-up are superior to elimination–open challenge–repeat elimination plus long-term follow-up. Undoubtedly, the double-blind approach is more objective if sufficient challenges are undertaken using appropriate amounts of the food. One must remember that some allergies are triggered by proteins that are present only in trace amounts in a particular food. Because of this, type I reactions may occur only when rather large amounts of that food are ingested.

Well-planned double-blind challenges are seldom carried out in practice and may themselves be misleading. Nevertheless, they have a definite place in research investigations and in studying selected patients in the clinician's office.

Some medications suppress clinical as well as skin test responses to antigen challenge. The recommended times for avoiding selected medications prior to challenge are as follows: most β-agonists (12 hr), cromolyn (12 hr), theophyllin (12 hr), corticosteroids (48 hr), most antihistaminics (96 hr), hydroxyzine, terfenadine, and loratidine (1 week), and astemizole (4 weeks).

Patients of any age who have had a life-threatening reaction attributable to a food should not be subjected to challenge procedures. Instead, efforts should be made to identify immunological hypersensitivity by *in vitro* tests.

Presumptive identification of an immunologic basis for a non-life-threatening adverse reaction occurring within 2 hr of a food ingestion can be made by prick tests with an extract of the food and, if these are negative, by applying a freshly cut slice of the food directly to a newly made small scratch. A drop of milk or fresh fruit juice is equally satisfactory. A positive skin test is indicated by the development of a wheal that has a diameter 3 mm or more in excess of the diluent control, both measured 15 to 20 min after the prick or scratch is applied. One should also demonstrate that an identical prick or scratch test will not cause a nonspecific wheal in a nonallergic control subject. Prick tests with 1:10 or 1:20 wt/vol food extracts usually will detect IgE-mediated hypersensitivity. Remember that only about half the subjects with positive skin tests and a history suggesting allergy respond to double-blind challenge testing. A somewhat higher but as yet ill-defined number will respond to open challenge testing.

In one study, positive skin tests for milk were associated with positive double-blind challenges 47% of the time, for peanuts 55%, for eggs 63%, and for soybeans 33% of the time (57).

Some individuals may have positive skin tests with no clinical response to the food ingestion (58–60). Others may have bona fide food-induced symptoms in the absence of a positive prick test. However, immediate-type allergic reactions to foods seldom are associated with negative skin tests. Thus a negative skin prick test with an appropriate food antigen is a good indication that a given food will not cause an immediate-type hypersensitivity reaction. In general, the larger the skin test reaction, the more likely it is to be significant, but this is not always the case since some subjects with a 3- to 5-mm wheal have severe symptoms, whereas a few healthy controls have 5- to 10-mm wheals and can eat the food with impunity. Thus the value of skin testing with food antigens is largely limited to subjects in whom there is a suspicion of food allergy to one or more specific foods. Properly performed and interpreted skin prick tests are helpful in selecting those individuals for whom elimination diets and appropriate food challenges are indicated (61).

Intradermal testing only occasionally detects relevant food sensitivities that are missed by prick tests. In addition, intradermal tests result in a higher frequency of false-positive reactions (62) and involve a risk of anaphylaxis if not preceded by prick or scratch tests or if dilutions are improperly made. Patients with celiac disease, some with food-induced gastroenteropathy, and others with milk-induced occult intestinal bleeding typically have negative prick tests to the offending food. These diseases are probably due to non-IgE-mediated immune mechanisms (63).

RASTs and related *in vitro* tests for specific IgE antibodies to foods offer an alternative to skin tests. Positive RASTs to foods were found in 50% of patients who reported food intolerance (64), but the identification of circulating IgE antibodies generally offers little advantage over skin prick tests and the combined results of RASTs and skin prick tests seldom improve the diagnostic accuracy over the use of the individual test (65). *In vitro* tests are useful if skin disease precludes skin tests or if skin testing is judged to be unsafe (history of a severe anaphylactic reaction). In general, *in vitro* tests are both less efficient in identifying clinically relevant antigens (66) and more expensive than skin tests. Other disadvantages of *in vitro* tests include their availability for only a limited number of foods and the inherent delay in obtaining results. Individuals may be clinically symptomatic to only one or a few foods despite a large number of positive skin tests or positive RAST results.

A high level of IgG antibodies or immune complexes does not necessarily mean that the person is clinically sensitive to a particular food. Many immune responses undoubtedly are protective in nature. While it is true that high levels of IgG and IgA antibodies are seen more frequently in allergic than in nonallergic individuals, it is difficult to determine the role of these antibodies in the genesis of symptoms. Such antibodies simply may reflect an unusually vigorous immune response. Perhaps when certain IgG or IgA antibodies are involved in immune complexes or facilitate other mechanisms, they may contribute to symptom production.

Table 6 outlines an approach to the office evaluation of food hypersensitivity (67). Additional diagnostic aids can be used if challenge tests are inconclusive or unwarranted. These include studies of *in vitro* food antigen-induced lymphocyte proliferation or lymphokine production, basophil histamine release, and high titer precipitins to the food antigen. Responsible personnel must know the problems associated with each procedure, and both positive and negative controls must be included in each assay to ensure that the procedure is functioning properly.

PROGNOSIS

Fortunately, food allergy is not necessarily a life long affliction. This is particularly true for infants. One

TABLE 6. *Office evaluation of food hypersensitivity*

1. *History and physical exam*
2. *Prick skin tests with antigens suspected by history*
   Negative: Further work up for immediate-type hypersensitivity generally unnecessary.
   Positive: *Go to next step.*
3. *Strict allergen avoidance diet for 1 month*
   Unequivocal improvement and only one major[a] or one to two minor[a] foods involved: *Continue restricted diet.*
   Improvement equivocal or more than two foods involved: *Go to next step.*
4. *Single-blind challenge in office*
   If negative, discontinue restricted diet.
   If positive to one major food or less than four minor foods, institute appropriate restricted diet.
   If positive to more than one major food or more than four foods in total: *Go to next step.*
5. *Double-blind placebo-controlled challenge in hospital setting*

Adapted from ref. 67.
[a] Major foods: egg, cow's milk, soy, wheat; minor foods: any food other than "major."

study demonstrated the development of clinical tolerance in 42% of children after 1 to 2 years, varying somewhat according to the food antigen involved (60). Follow-up studies of children who were milk intolerant during early infancy showed that by the end of the first year of life 17% in one study (7) and 65% in another (38) were able to tolerate cow's milk in one form or another. The severity of symptoms did not appear to have a consistent influence on the prognosis (7). A recent report by Pastorello et al. (68) indicates that adults also may lose symptoms of food allergy after a period of elimination. We recommend a carefully planned repeat challenge about 6 months after the initial confirmation of food allergy. If this challenge remains positive, we challenge the patient under carefully controlled conditions at approximately yearly intervals thereafter to be certain the hypersensitivity persists.

It should be remembered that food allergy is dose related. In general, even small amounts of a food allergen cannot be tolerated when immediate-type hypersensitivity is the predominant immunopathological mechanism, but in other types of hypersensitivity (e.g., celiac disease, milk-induced gastroenteropathy), symptoms may occur only when much larger amounts of the food are ingested.

There may be a change in skin test reactivity following clinical remission. Ford and Taylor (69) found that skin test reactivity decreased when clinical sensitivity was lost, but Sampson and McCaskill (60) and Bock (70) reported that prick skin test and RAST results often remained positive in children who became clinically tolerant of the incriminated food.

TREATMENT

Once food allergy is diagnosed, the treatment of choice is avoidance of that specific food. There may be a problem, however, in obtaining complete patient compliance. It is impossible to discern at the onset how long the food must be avoided before it may be tolerated to some degree at a later time.

Since small amounts of allergically active proteins ingested by lactating women enter their breast milk (71,72), judicious elimination of suspected foods from the mother's diet may be all that is necessary to alleviate a breast-fed infant's symptoms (73). When such is the case, the infant is usually sensitive to very small quantities of the food and care must be taken when the child is first fed that food when weaned off the breast.

It is now known why the elimination of an offending food at times leads to the establishment of tolerance to that food. In the case of infants, it may be related to maturation of the gastrointestinal and immunologic systems. In older children and adults, intolerance to a food at one time and tolerance at another time may relate to the total allergen burden to which the subject is exposed at any given time. For example, it is not unusual to find adult patients who by history were intolerant of cow's milk during infancy yet at 2 to 3 years of age tolerated it without difficulty. However, when they became allergic to pollens later in childhood, or as adults, it became apparent that symptoms were much worse during the pollen season if milk was part of the diet than if milk was eliminated or its ingestion greatly reduced until the pollen season was past. A similar summation of effects from a second allergen also may occur in other situations; for example, when a person has mild or subclinical allergic responses to each of two different foods, there may be allergic symptoms only if both are in the diet. Similarly, exercise may cause symptoms only after the ingestion of a particular food and the food without exercise may not cause symptoms (food-related, exercise-induced anaphylaxis). The nature of the offending food may be an important factor relative to the disappearance of symptoms. For example, allergy produced by milk or egg may be more transient than those produced by peanuts or wheat (70).

Pharmacologic management of food hypersensitivity may be desirable in some situations in which compliance with a diet is extremely difficult. Oral cromolyn (Gastrocrom) is thought to help some subjects with multiple food sensitivities, although not all investigators agree on this point. Prophylactic administration of corticosteroids and/or antihistamines may permit a mild to moderately sensitive child to take small amounts of an offending food. This is not recommended as routine or something one would do with any frequency. We occasionally have suggested this when absolute avoidance appears to be psychologically crippling to a child. For example, a small serving of ice cream or cake at a friend's birthday party may be permitted if prior testing with premedication has shown the technique to be safe and effective. This obviously should not be attempted if the prior adverse reactions were severe or life-threatening in nature. Patients with severe anaphylactic reactions to a food should carry a device for self-administration of epinephrine for use in the event of accidental exposure to the food. Prednisone generally is ineffective for treatment or prophylaxis in patients with predominantly immediate-type reactions to a food.

Antihistamines, decongestants, nebulized cromolyn, and nasal corticosteroids are helpful in preventing, and sometimes in managing, sinusitis when it occurs in allergic subjects. Appropriate antibiotics should be given for 3 to 4 weeks to ensure the eradication of the sinus infections.

Pelikan (74) recently reported a double-blind placebo-controlled study that revealed a protective effect of oral cromolyn in 38 patients with perennial allergic rhinitis secondary to food ingestion.

There are several reports suggesting a beneficial role for hyposensitization (classic immunotherapy) in the treatment of food hypersensitivity (75,76). However, appropriately designed studies have not yet demonstrated the efficacy of immunotherapy with food antigens. At present, there is no indication to use food antigens in allergy "shots." There also is insufficient evidence in the literature to support sublingual or oral desensitization in the treatment of food allergy (77,78).

When sensitivity to common inhalant allergens such as house dust, molds, and mites have been excluded, or when their elimination and appropriate management have failed, a contribution of food allergy to the symptoms should always be considered in subjects with chronic rhinitis and/or sinusitis.

PREVENTION

Prevention is the best approach when it is feasible. Nevertheless, there is evidence that the risk of food allergy can be minimized by certain practices.

Exclusive breast-feeding is to be encouraged for the first 6 months of life. It may be protective in some infants against the development of atopic disease (79). If allergic symptomatology occurs in a breast-fed infant, attempts should be made to eliminate likely allergens from the maternal diet (73,80). Among high-risk infants (those with one or more allergic immediate family members) who are not breast fed, a casein hydrolysate formula is preferred. This may reduce the incidence of atopic disease in the child (81) and in some instances is more beneficial than breast-feeding without maternal dietary restrictions or the use of a soy-based formula (82). A partially hydrolyzed whey formula such as Good Start[R] may also be of value in prophylaxis but is not recommended for treating known milk allergies where the use of more completely hydrolyzed casein-based formulas is preferable.

One report suggested that the prevalence of allergic rhinitis, asthma, and inhalant sensitization was little affected by dietary manipulation (83). However, one of these investigators firmly believes in the possibility of minimizing allergy by dietary means as evidenced

TABLE 7. *Recommendations for the prevention of allergic disease in high risk infants*

Strategy	Method or measure
1. Identify at-risk infant prenatally or early post-natally	• Document atopy in one parent or sibling (35% risk); in both parents (65% risk). • Document elevated cord blood IgE (>1.0 IU/ml).
2. Avoid infant exposure to: 　a. Food allergens in breast milk	• Maternal lactation diet without egg, milk or peanut • Supplement maternal diet daily with 1500 mg elemental calcium.
b. Food allergens in infant diet	• Exclusive breastfeeding for 4–6 months if possible. • Supplement with protein hydrolysate formula if needed. • Delay solid foods until 6 months, then add strained fruits, vegetables, rice cereal, one new food every 4 days. Temporarily discontinue foods which appear to be associated with symptoms. • After 1 year, add at 2-week intervals if tolerated: milk, wheat, soy, corn, citrus, egg, fish, peanut-butter. Delay egg, peanut, fish until age 2 if child has shown any sign of allergy.
c. Inhalant allergens	• Minimize exposure to mites, molds, pets.
3. Avoid nonspecific environmental triggers	• No smoking in house during pregnancy or after birth. • Minimize household sprays (hair, deodorant, insecticide, etc.). Avoid accumulating magazines and newspapers. Fix leaky gas stoves. • Minimize infections (avoid early day care, visiting people with URI's).

Modified from ref. 84.

by his recommendations which are indicated in Table 7 (84).

Until it becomes possible to inactivate or replace the genes responsible for allergic disease, the optimal management of infants at risk for allergy will include breast-feeding with both maternal and infant diets designed to minimize food allergen exposure of the infant.

REFERENCES

1. *A history of medicine—Ralph H Major, MD,* Vol 1. Springfield, IL: Charles C Thomas, 1954;500–503,941–942.
2. Hutinel V. Intolerance pour le lait et anaphylaxie chez les nourrissons. *Clinique (Paris)* 1908;3:227–231.
3. Park EA. A case of hypersensitivity to cow's milk. *Am J Dis Child* 1920;19:46–54.
4. Smith HL. Buckwheat poisoning, with a report of a case in man. *Arch Intern Med* 1909;3:350–359.
5. *American Academy of Allergy and Immunology Committee on Adverse Reactions to Foods and National Institute of Allergy and Infectious Diseases: Adverse reactions to foods.* US Department of Health and Human Services Publ 84-2442. Bethesda, MD: National Institutes of Health, 1984.
6. Collins-Williams C. The incidence of milk allergy in pediatric practice. *J Pediatr* 1956;48:39–48.
7. Gerrard JW, McKenzie JWA, Goluboff N, et al. Cow's milk allergy: prevalence and manifestations in an unselected series of newborns. *Acta Paediatr Scand Suppl* 1973;234:1.
8. Bock SA. Prospective appraisal of complaints of adverse reactions to foods in children during the first 3 years of life. *Pediatrics* 1987;79:683–688.
9. Cunningham-Rundles C, Brandeis WE, Good RA, Day NK. Bovine antigens and the formation of circulating immune complexes in selective immunoglobulin A deficiency. *J Clin Invest* 1979;64:272–279.
10. Burks AW, Mallory SB, Williams LW, Shirrel MA. Atopic dermatitis: clinical relevance of food hypersensitivity reactions. *Pediatrics* 1988;113:447–451.
11. Buckley RH, Metcalfe D. Food allergy. *JAMA* 1982;248:2627–2631.
12. Kajosaari M. Food allergy in Finnish children aged 1 to 6 years. *Acta Pediatr Scand* 1982;71:815–819.
13. Kjellman N-IM. Development and prediction of atopic allergy in childhood. In: Bostrom H, Ljungstedt N, eds. *Theoretical and clinical aspects of allergic disease.* Skandia International Symposia, Oct 12–14, 1982. Stockholm: Almqvist & Wiksell, 1983;52–73.
14. King TP. Chemical and biological properties of some atopic allergens. In: Kunkel-Dixon F, ed. *Advances in immunology,* vol 23. San Francisco: Academic Press, 1976;76–105.
15. Bleumink E. Food allergy. The chemical nature of the substances eliciting symptoms. *World Rev Nutr Diet* 1970;12:505–570.
16. Wuthrich B, Huwyler T. Asthma due to disulfites. *J Suisse Med* 1989;119:1177–1184.
17. Walker WA. Pathophysiology of intestinal uptake and absorption of antigens in food allergy. *Ann Allergy* 1987;59:7–16.
18. Walker WA, Isselbacher KJ. Intestinal antibodies. *N Engl J Med* 1977;297:767–773.
19. Walker, WA, Isselbacher KJ. Uptake and transport of macromolecules by intestinal tract. *Prog Gastroenterol* 1974;67:531–550.
20. Gunther M, Aschaffenburgh R, Mathews RH, et al. The levels of antibody to the proteins of cow's milk in the serum of normal human infants. *Immunology* 1960;3:296–300.
21. Walzer M. Absorption of allergens. *J Allergy* 1942;13:554–562.
22. Paganelli R, Levinsky R. Solid phase radioimmunoassay for detection of circulating food protein antigens in human serum. *J Immunol Methods* 1980;37:333–341.
23. Coombs RRA, Gell PGH. Classification of allergic reactions responsible for clinical hypersensitivity and disease. In: Gell PGH, Coombs RRA, Lachman PJ, eds. *Clinical aspects of immunology.* London: Blackwell, 1975;761.
24. Lemanske RF Jr, Atkins FM, Metcalfe DD. Gastrointestinal mast cells in health and disease. I. *J Pediatr* 1983;103:177–184.
25. Lemanske RF Jr, Atkins FM, Metcalfe DD. Gastrointestinal mast cells in health and disease. II. *J Pediatr* 1983;103:343–351.
26. Haddad ZH, Kubra V, Verma S. IgE antibodies to peptic and peptic tryptic digests of betalactoglobulin: significance in food hypersensitivity. *Ann Allergy* 1979;42:368–372.
27. Frank MM. Complement & kinin. In: Stites DP, Terr AI, eds. *Basic and clinical immunology.* Norwalk, CT: Appleton & Lange, 1991;161–174.
28. Johnsen G, Elsayed S. Antigenic and allergenic determinants of ovalbumin-III. MHC Ia-binding peptide (OA 323–339) interacts with human and rabbit specific antibodies. *Mol Immunol* 1990;27:821–827.
29. Bock SA, May CD. Adverse reactions to food caused by sensitivity. In: Middleton E, Reed CE, Ellis EF, eds. *Allergy: Principles and practice.* St Louis: CV Mosby, 1983;1415–1427.
30. Hill DJ, Ford RPK, Shelton MJ, Hosking CS. A study of 100 infants and young children with cow's milk allergy. *Clin Rev Allergy* 1984;2:125–142.
31. Heiner DC. Allergy to cow's milk. *NESA Proc* 1981;2:192–197.
32. Visakorpi JK, Immonen P. Intolerance to cow's milk and wheat gluten in the primary malabsorption syndrome in infancy. *Acta Paediatr Scand* 1967;56:49–56.
33. Moneret-Vautrin DA, Andre CI. *Immunopathologie de l'allergie alimentaire et fausses allergies alimentaries.* Paris: Masson, 1983.
34. Sampson HA. Differential diagnosis in adverse reactions to foods. *J Allergy Clin Immunol* 1986;78:213.
35. Novembre E, de Martino M, Vierucci A. Foods and respiratory allergy. *J Allergy Clin Immunol* 1988;81:1059–1065.
36. Sabbah A, Drouet M, Millet B, Biset T. Perennial rhinitis from food allergy. *Allerg Immunol (Leipz)* 1990;22:51–55.
37. Wraith DG. Asthma and rhinitis. *Clin Immunol Allergy* 1982;2:101.
38. Clein NW. Cow's milk allergy in infants. *Pediatr Clin North Am* 1954;4:949–962.
39. Lebenthal E. Cow's milk protein allergy. *Pediatr Clin North Am* 1975;22:827–833.
40. Clein NW. Cow's milk allergy in infants and children. *Int Arch Allergy* 1958;13:245–256.
41. Bachman KD, Dees SC. Milk allergy. II. Observations on incidence and symptoms of allergy to milk in allergic infants. *Pediatrics* 1957;20:400–407.
42. Shapiro GG. Role of allergy in sinusitis. *Pediatr Infect Dis* 1985;4:S55–S58.
43. Slavin RG. Sinusitis. *J Allergy Clin Immunol* 1984;73:712–716.
44. Rachelefsky GS, Katz RM, Siegel SC. Diseases of paranasal sinuses in children. In: Gluck L, ed. *Current problems in pediatrics,* vol 12, no 5. Chicago: Year Book, 1982.
45. Savolainen S. Allergy in patients with acute maxillary sinusitis. *Allergy* 1989;44:116–122.
46. Kogutt MS, Swischuck, LE. Diagnosis of sinusitis in infants and children. *Pediatrics* 1973;52:121–124.
47. van Dishoeck HAE. Allergy and infections of paranasal sinuses. *Adv Otorhinolaryngol* 1961;10:1–29.
48. Shapiro GG. The sinuses: sinusitis in children. *J Allergy Clin Immunol* 1988;81:1025–1027.
49. Shaprio GG. The role of nasal airway obstruction in sinus disease and facial development. *J Allergy Clin Immunol* 1988;82:935–940.
50. Yamada H. A study of infiltrated cells in the maxillary mucosa in nasal allergy and chronic sinusitis. *Nippon Jibiinkoka Gakkai Kaiho [J Otorhinolaryngol Soc Jpn]* 1990;93:1999–2008.
51. Aust R. Measurements of the ostial size and O_2 tension in the maxilary sinus. *Rhinology* 1976;14:43–46.
52. Harlin SL, Ansel DG, Lane SR, Myers J, Kephart GM, Gleich GJ. A clinical and pathologic study of chronic sinusitis: the role of the eosinophil. *J Allergy Clin Immunol* 1988;81:867–875.
53. Hogg JC. The pathology of asthma. *Clin Chest Med* 1984;5:567.

54. Salvato G. Some histological changes in chronic bronchitis and asthma. *Thorax* 1968;23:168.
55. May CD. Objective clinical and laboratory studies of immediate hypersensitivity reactions to foods in children. *J Allergy Clin Immunol* 1976;58:500.
56. Metcalfe DD. A current practical approach to the diagnosis of suspected adverse reactions to foods. *NER Allergy Proc* 1987; 8:22–26.
57. Bock SA, Lee W-Y, Remigio LK, May CD. Studies of hypersensitivity reactions to foods in infants and children. *J Allergy Clin Immunol* 1978;62:327–334.
58. Atkins FM, Steinberg SS, Metcalfe DD. Evaluation of immediate adverse reactions to foods in adult patients. I. Correlation of demographic, laboratory, and prick skin test data with response to controlled oral food challenge. *J Allergy Clin Immunol* 1985;75:348–335.
59. Atkins FM, Steinberg SS, Metcalf DD. Evaluation of immediate adverse reactions to foods in adult patients. II. A detailed analysis of reaction patterns during oral food challenge. *J Allergy Clin Immunol* 1985;75:356.
60. Sampson HA, McCaskill CM. Food hypersensitivity and atopic dermatitis: evaluation of 113 patients. *J Pediatr* 1985;107: 669–675.
61. Bock SA, Buckley J, Holst A, May CD. Proper use of skin tests with food extracts in diagnosis of hypersensitivity to food in children. *Clin Allergy* 1978;7:375–383.
62. Bock SA, Lee WY, Remigio L, Holst A, May CD. Appraisal of skin tests with food extracts for diagnosis of food hypersensitivity. *Clin Allergy* 1978;8:559–564.
63. Kuitunen P, Visakorpi JK, Savilahti E, Pelkonen P. Malabsorption syndrome with cow's milk intolerance. *Arch Dis Child* 1975; 50:351–356.
64. Hoffman, DR, Haddad ZH. Diagnosis of IgE mediated hypersensitivity reactions to food antigens by radioimmunoassay. *J Allergy Clin Immunol* 1974;54:165–173.
65. Sampson HA, Albergo R. Comparison of result of skin tests, RAST and double-blind, placebo-controlled food challenges in children with atopic dermatitis. *J Allergy Clin Immunol* 1984; 74:26.
66. Chua YY, Bremner K, Lakdawalla N, Llobet JL, Kokuba H, Orange RP, Collins-Williams C. "In vivo" and "in vitro" correlates of food allergy. *J Allergy Clin Immunol* 1976;58:299–307.
67. Sampson HA. Immunologically mediated food allergy: The importance of food challenge procedures. *Ann Allergy* 1988;60: 262–269.
68. Pastorello EA, Stocchi L, Pravettoni V, et al. Role of the elimination diet in adults with food allergy. *J Allergy Clin Immunol* 1989;84:475–483.
69. Ford RPK, Taylor B. Natural history of egg hypersensitivity. *Arch Dis Child* 1982;57:649.
70. Bock SA. The natural history of food sensitivity. *J Allergy Clin Immunol* 1981;69:173–177.
71. Kaplan M, Solli N. Immunoglobulin E to cow's milk protein in breast-fed atopic children. *J Allergy Clin Immunol* 1979;64: 122–126.
72. Host A, Husby S, Hansen LG, Osterballe O. Bovine β-lactoglobulin in human milk from atopic and non-atopic mothers. Relationship to maternal intake of homogenized and unhomogenized milk. *Clin Exp Allergy* 1990;20:383–387.
73. Gerrard JW. Cow's milk and breast milk. In: Brostoff J, Challacombe ST, eds. *Food allergy and intolerance.* Philadelphia: Bailliere Tindal, 1987;344–355.
74. Pelikan Z. Effects of oral cromolyn on the nasal response due to foods. *Arch Otolaryngol Head Neck Surg* 1989;115:1238–1243.
75. Miller JB. A double-blind study of food extract injection therapy; a preliminary report. *Ann Allergy* 1977;38:185–191.
76. McEwen LM. Enzyme potentiated hyposensitization. Five case reports of patients with acute food allergy. *Ann Allergy* 1975; 35:98–103.
77. Golbert TM. A review of controversial diagnostic and therapeutic techniques employed in allergy. *J Allergy Clin Immunol* 1975; 56:170–190.
78. Morris DL. Use of sublingual antigen in diagnosis and treatment of food allergy. *Ann Allergy* 1969;27:289–294.
79. Juto P, Moller C, Engberg S, Bjorksten B. Influence of type of feeding on lymphocyte function and development of infantile allergy. *Clin Allergy* 1982;12:409–416.
80. Jakobson I, Lindberg T. Cow's milk as a cause of infantile colic in breast-fed infants. *Lancet* 1978;2(8097):437–439.
81. Chandra RK, Puri S, Hamed A. Influence of maternal diet during lactation and use of formula feeds on development of atopic eczema in high risk infants. *BMJ* 1989;299:228–230.
82. Chandra RK, Singh G, Shridhara B. Effect of feeding whey hydrolysate, soy and conventional cow milk formulas on incidence of atopic disease in high risk infants. *Ann Allergy* 1989;63: 102–106.
83. Zeiger RS, Heller S, Mellon MH, Forsythe AB, O'Connor RD, Hamburger RN, Schatz M. Effect of combined maternal and infant food-allergen avoidance on development of atopy in early infancy: a randomized study. *J Allergy Clin Immunol* 1989;84: 72–89.
84. Zeiger RS. Prevention of food allergy in infancy. *Ann Allergy* 1990;65:430–441.

CHAPTER 12

Nonallergic Rhinitis

Jack L. Gluckman

DEFINITION

Chronic rhinitis is an inflammation of the nasal tissue, which results in a symptom complex consisting of nasal obstruction due to mucosal swelling secondary to blood vessel engorgement; rhinorrhea secondary to glandular hypersecretion and tissue transudate; sneezing due to neural reflexes; and pruritis secondary to histamine release from mast cells and basophils (1–3). This represents a limited response of a target organ to allergy or a wide range of nonspecific external and internal stimuli. This chapter reviews and categorizes the various causes of nonallergic rhinitis, emphasizing the approach to diagnosis and treatment.

INCIDENCE

Nonallergic rhinitis represents 40% to 70% of all chronic rhinitides, afflicting 30 to 40 million Americans with a prevalence of 20% (4–6). Although not a life-threatening condition, rhinitis may cause significant discomfort and altered feelings of well-being due to congestion, pruritis, sneezing, anosmia, disturbed sleep, fatigue and irritability, dry mouth, bothersome rhinorrhea, and/or postnasal drainage (7). This leads to untoward social ostracism, and when summated, significant economic impact. It is estimated that between $250,000 and $500,000 per year is spent on doctors' fees and drug costs, with between 10 million and 28 million lost work or school days and restricted days per year, and up to 6 million bedridden days per year (5,6). When thus measured, the significant individual and social impacts of this simple condition become obvious.

NASAL ANATOMY AND HISTOLOGY

Essentially, the nasal fossae are paired, tubular structures separated by the septum with variegated, redundant lateral walls affording a large surface area of erectile tissue with humoral and neurologic control subtending the primary nasal functions (8). The lateral nasal walls are closely related to the paranasal sinus ostia, eustachian tube orifices, and the nasolacrimal system; hence any diseases affecting the mucosa may have secondary effects on the functions of these structures.

The vasculature of the mucosa includes arteries and arterioles, which are resistance vessels under α-adrenergic control regulating regional flow. The capillaries are fenestrated, porous vessels contributing to fluid extravasation under certain pathologic conditions. The venules and sinusoids within the nasal mucosa are capacitance vessels under parasympathetic control, possessing erectile properties (1,8).

The autonomic nerve supply to the nasal mucosa derives from both sympathetic and parasympathetic fibers. The sympathetic fibers exert primary control over the nasal vasculature, while the parasympathetic fibers supply the mucosal glands with only secondary effects on the vasculature. Preganglionic parasympathetic nerve fibers have their cell bodies in the superior salivatory nucleus, leave the brain stem via the nervus intermedius, travel with the facial nerve through the geniculate ganglion, form the greater superficial petrosal nerve, synapse in the pterygopalatine ganglion, and give off postganglionic parasympathetic fibers that innervate the glands and capacitance vessels of the nasal mucosa. The preganglionic sympathetic nerve fibers originate in the upper thoracic intermediolateral gray column, travel in the cervical trunk, and pass through the pterygopalatine ganglion via the deep petrosal nerve to innervate the vasculature of the nasal mucosa (2,8).

The nasal mucosa consists of stratified squamous epithelium in the anterior one-third and pseudostratified, ciliated columnar epithelium in the posterior two-thirds of the nose. Goblet cells within the mucosa secrete mucus, which, with the cilia, forms a mucociliary blanket (8,9). The nasal epithelium overlies a well-defined basement membrane, deep to which is the lamina propria overlying the bony and cartilaginous framework of the nose (9). The lamina propria contains seromucous glands, blood vessels, nerves, ground substance and connective tissue, and cellular elements.

The ground substance is an amorphous colloid containing cells and other components including acid mucopolysaccharides of hyaluronic acid and chondroitin sulfate. This ground substance exists in a gel/sol state controlled by hyaluronidase. The connective tissue consists of fibers of collagen, reticulin, elastin, and oxytalan, and various cells including fibroblasts, macrophages, mast cells, and plasma cells. The fibroblasts produce the fibers, as well as the acid mucopolysaccharides, while the mast cells and plasma cells are responsible for histamine release (10). The mast cells may play some role in the regulation of nasal physiology, with control of local blood flow via release of histamine and heparin (8,11).

The mucous blanket overlying the nasal mucosa has protective and humidifying functions. It consists of an exudate synthesized by goblet cells, serous and seromucous glands, and a tissue transudate via the fenestrated capillaries (1,9). The various nasal secretions are under parasympathetic cholinergic, as well as histamine and vasoactive intestinal polypeptide (VIP), control. Nasal secretions are comprised of mucus-like proteins, immunoglobulins, secretory component, lactoferrin, lysozyme, kallikrein, antiprotease, tissue transudate, and various cells (3).

PHYSIOLOGY

As already stated, the microvasculature supplying the nasal mucosa is controlled by the vasomotor system. The α-adrenergic, sympathetic control of resistance vessels (arteries and arterioles) controls regional blood flow; however, parasympathetic control of capacitance vessels (venules and sinusoids) controls engorgement of tissues. The mediator of parasympathetic stimulation leading to vasodilatation and decreased nasal patency is at present unclear (12). This stimulus is not blocked by atropine; hence it is not felt to be cholinergic mediated. Likewise, there is no evidence that parasympathetic stimulation is mediated via prostaglandins. Possible mediators, however, do include kinins and vasoactive intestinal polypeptide (2,3).

There is a constant, baseline, low-output level α-adrenergic sympathetic tone, which by controlling the capacitance vessels governs the blood content of the nasal mucosa (13). High-output α-adrenergic stimulation, on the other hand, decreases blood flow to nasal

mucosa and is abolished by α-adrenergic blockers. β-Adrenergic stimulation causes no change in regional blood flow.

The normal physiologic nasal cycle, with a periodicity of approximately every 30 min, results from a constant, baseline balance between sympathetic and parasympathetic vasomotor control (2). This results in cyclic congestion and decongestion of the turbinates alternating from one side to the other.

Nasal glandular secretion is under parasympathetic cholinergic control (3,12). In addition to acetylcholine, it is felt that vasoactive intestinal polypeptide and histamine also control nasal secretions, with histamine probably enhancing the effects of acetylcholine (11). There is also a baseline parasympathetic output with a constant secretory output (12). Parasympathetic, acetylcholine-mediated stimulation causes a profuse watery secretion blocked by atropine. In addition, the parasympathetic nervous system innervates the contractile and secretory elements of the nasal glands. Nasal secretion is also under indirect α-adrenergic sympathetic control of the nasal vasculature (9). Loss of sympathetic stimulation with parasympathetic vasodilatation causes vessel engorgement and increased tissue transudate, which contributes to nasal secretion.

The mucociliary system consists of a sol layer (serous component of plasma transudate) and a gel layer (mucous component). This system is pH and temperature dependent, trapping and clearing particles between 5 and 10 μm. The immunologic component of filtration includes secretory immunoglobulin A (IgA) (1,3,6,9).

There are four major functions of the nose. These are airway protection, air conditioning, olfaction, and resonance. Alteration in the mucosal physiology may affect these functions to some degree.

PATHOLOGIC MECHANISM OF RHINITIS

A number of intrinsic and extrinsic pathologic mechanisms alter normal nasal function and cause the symptoms of rhinitis.

The extrinsic factors include allergens, irritants, cold air, odors, infectious agents, pharmacologic agents, and exercise. The intrinsic factors include food metabolites, hormonal and endocrine substrates, infiltrating cells, vasoactive mediators, and the autonomic nervous system.

The autonomic nervous system can mediate the various intrinsic and extrinsic factors causing rhinitis or can cause rhinitis directly via an imbalance with hyperactive parasympathetic activity. For example, antihypertensive agents may cause unchecked parasympathetic activity with decreased sympathetic activity. Irritants, temperature changes, and alcohol also increase parasympathetic activity and vasomotor instability. Estrogens and hypothyroidism potentiate parasympathetic cholinergic stimulation while hyperthyroidism is a sympathomimetic (2,8,9,14).

These extrinsic and intrinsic causes of rhinitis also may be mediated by non-IgE-activated vasoactive substances, including histamine, kinins, and vasoactive intestinal polypeptide (7,15).

In summary, a wide variety of both extrinsic and intrinsic factors have a significant effect on nasal function. The symptoms of rhinitis, caused by these factors, can be explained on the basis of autonomic nervous system imbalances, non-IgE- activated vasoactive mediators, and changes in the composition of ground substance with interstitial edema. These ground substance changes may be a direct result of the insulting agent or may be mediated via histamine or kinins (10,16,17).

CLASSIFICATION OF RHINITIS

Rhinitis can be due to multiple causes, but this chapter will deal only with nonallergic, noninfectious causes of rhinitis (Table 1). Obviously, in many patients the etiology is multifactorial and will defy categorization.

SPECIFIC CAUSES OF NONALLERGIC RHINITIS

Structural Abnormalities

Structural abnormalities such as nasal valve collapse or nasal septal deformity, adenoid hypertrophy, and

even choanal atresia may result in secondary mucosal abnormalities. Neoplastic conditions, both benign (papilloma, angiofibroma) and malignant, as well as granulomatous processes also may evoke classic symptoms of rhinitis by virtue or their mass effect and nasal obstruction. In the elderly patient, loss of cartilage support may cause the anterior nares to collapse with each inspiratory effort, which may cause or aggravate the nasal obstruction. A deviated septum frequently is associated with turbinate hypertrophy in the concavity of the septum, which will have to be addressed if adequate relief of the nasal obstruction is to be obtained by nasal surgery.

Rhinitis Medicamentosa

Rhinitis medicamentosa is a drug-induced rhinitis representing 5% of all chronic rhinitis syndromes and characterized by rebound nasal congestion with edematous, red, engorged, friable nasal mucosa (6). It is the end result of prolonged, sustained use of topical vasoconstrictors (α-adrenergic stimulators) or systemic drugs, particularly antihypertensive agents (8) (Table 2).

Frequent and prolonged use of topical vasoconstrictors results in a rebound vasodilatation (rebound rhinitis), which may become permanent because of vascular atony. For this reason, topical vasoconstrictors should not be used for longer than five consecutive days;

TABLE 1. Classification of nonallergic, noninfectious rhinitis

Structural abnormalities
  Deviated nasal septum
  Obstructing masses
    Intranasal
    Paranasal
    Nasopharyngeal
  Foreign body
Rhinitis medicamentosa
Endocrine
  Pregnancy
  Hypothyroidism
  Diabetes
  Menstrual cycle
Irritative
Idiopathic
  Vasomotor rhinitis
  Eosinophilic nonallergy rhinitis
  Mixed cellular rhinitis
  Nasal mastocytosis
Miscellaneous
  Postlaryngectomy rhinitis
  Tracheostomy rhinitis
  Recumbency rhinitis

TABLE 2. Drugs causing rhinitis medicamentosa

Systemic
  Antihypertensive agents
    Methyldopa
    Guanethidine
    Reserpine
    Hydralazine
    Prazosin
  Beta-blockers
    Propanolol
    Nadolol
  Antidepressants and tranquilizers
    Thioridazine
    Chlordiazepoxide–amitriptyline
    Perphenazine
    Alprazolam
  Oral contraceptives and estrogen therapy
  Aspirin and nonsteroidal anti-inflammatory agents
  Ergot alkaloids
  Antithyroid drugs
  Iodides
  Alcohol
  Tobacco
  Hashish
  Marijuana
Topical
  Vasoconstrictors
  Cocaine

otherwise the patient will become a "nose-drop addict."

Oral medications may include reserpine, hydralazine, guanethidine, methyldopa, propanolol, thioridazine, and perphenazine (1). These medications all cause depletion of norepinephrine stores in one way or another; for example, reserpine inhibits norepinephrine transport to storage pools, and guanethidine causes active release of norepinephrine from these pools. Reserpine is the drug most likely to cause problems. In addition, aspirin, alcohol, tobacco, iodides, hashish, and marijuana also may cause rhinitis medicamentosa. Aspirin alters prostaglandin metabolism, causes degranulation of mast cells, and lowers the threshold of the nasal mucosa to histamine (9). Oral contraceptives also may cause the symptoms and signs of rhinitis.

In treating rhinitis medicamentosa due to topical decongestants, the physician must attempt to identify the underlying cause for the nasal obstruction that initiated the use of the topical medication in the first place. The patient must stop using the topical decongestant and topical or systemic steroids (5), together with saline nose sprays or systemic decongestants (14) substituted to alleviate the symptoms during the withdrawal period. If permanent changes have occurred with resultant chronic hypertrophic turbinates, some form of turbinectomy may become necessary. If the rhinitis is due to systemic drug administration, this will need to be replaced with an alternate drug if feasible.

While cocaine has been described as a potential cause of rhinitis medicamentosa, this is an unlikely scenario as most abusers do not use the drugs frequently enough and also most cocaine sold illicitly is usually "cut" and therefore is unlikely to cause problems. On the other hand, the irritation from its use together with the vasoconstrictive effect may cause crusting, ulceration, septal necrosis, and even collapse (18).

Nasal Polyposis, the Aspirin Triad, and Nonallergic Rhinitis

A small percentage of patients with asthma and rhinitis (4%) or just rhinitis (2%) have associated nasal polyposis. Of those patients with nasal polyposis, approximately 14% to 31% have associated aspirin sensitivity characterized by bronchospasm (70%), urticaria (13%), rhinitis (10%), or a combination of symptoms (7%). Of all the patients with aspirin intolerance, about 45% have associated polyps. There is an increased incidence in individuals older than 30 years. Of those patients with nasal polyposis, a greater percentage have negative rather than positive skin tests to common allergens. When patients with known aspirin intolerance are challenged with aspirin, they develop bronchospas-

tic and/or naso-ocular symptoms, which are unaltered by pretreatment with steroids or aminophyllin. About 30% of these patients have been found to have a different end organ response on rechallenge, and 10% are found to have no response on rechallenge with aspirin (19–21).

The various nonallergic rhinitides, as well as other conditions, have been associated with the subsequent development of nasal polyposis and/or the aspirin triad. One such predictor is rhinitis associated with eosinophilia (5,6,22); however, the specific nonallergic, eosinophilic rhinitis has no associated or subsequent development of polyposis, a negative aspirin challenge test, and no evidence of hyperactive airway disease (7). Other predictors of polyposis and aspirin intolerance include perennial, nonallergic rhinitis (1); cystic fibrosis (25% of children with cystic fibrosis have associated nasal polyps, and 40% of children with nasal polyps are found to have cystic fibrosis) (1); atopic, nonallergic perennial rhinitis demonstrating a strong hereditary pattern (23); and patients with a neutrophilic nasal transudate (9).

The pathologic mechanisms of aspirin intolerance and formation of nasal polyps include prostaglandin synthesis abnormalities and connective tissue alterations. Aspirin and other nonsteroidal anti-inflammatory agents inhibit prostaglandin pathways with the buildup of metabolites, hydroxyeicosatetraenoic acid (HETE), and slow-reacting substance of anaphylaxis (SRS-A), which are chemotactic for eosinophils and neutrophils and may cause degranulation of mast cells and a lower threshold for the histamine response. Aspirin also alters the ratio of prostaglandin E_2, a bronchodilator, and prostaglandin F_2, a bronchoconstrictor. Aspirin also may cause IgE-mediated angioedema and urticaria. It also may affect the composition of connective tissue and ground substance with subsequent polyp formation (9,10,19,20).

Polyps contain active fibroblasts, collagen, and abundant ground substance composed of acid mucopolysaccharides (10), eosinophils, plasma cells, and neutrophils (9). Nasal polyps also have been shown to release histamine, SRS-A, eosinophilic chemotactic factor of anaphylaxis (ECF-A), and serotonin (19).

The management of nasal polyposis includes surgery and systemic or topical steroids (5,21). Systemic steroids and/or surgery may be necessary to reduce the bulk of the nasal polyps before topical steroids may be effective. Since nasal polyposis generally is not associated with antigen-specific allergy, desensitization is usually ineffective (21).

Endocrine and Hormonal Causes of Rhinitis

While rhinitis medicamentosa affects the autonomic nervous system and microvasculature of the nasal mucosa, the hormonal causes of rhinitis affect the matrix and ground substance of the submucosa. These causes of rhinitis include pregnancy, menstruation, oral contraceptives, hypothyroidism, and diabetes mellitus.

The rhinitis of pregnancy is an estrogen-induced rhinitis (5). Estrogens increase the hyaluronic acid component of ground substance, causing increased tissue hydration and tissue edema (10,17). During the second trimester there is an increase in estrogens and an increase in mucous glands, a decrease in ground substance, and the development of large cavernous areas with an atrophic basement membrane in the nasal mucosa. In addition, the estrogen effects on the nasal mucosa include squamous metaplasia, intraepithelial edema due to tissue hydration, increase in collagen fibers and fibroblasts, congested capillaries, loss of cilia, and hyperplastic mucous glands with increased secretory activity (17).

The rhinitis of pregnancy is characterized by nasal congestion without sneezing, pruritis, or rhinorrhea. It occurs during the second and third trimesters. Although the treating physician should always consult with the patient's obstetrician, judicious corticosteroid use, particularly topical steroids with minimal absorption, would appear a relatively safe method of treatment (24–26). Systemic decongestants and antihistamines, too, can probably be used safely, but in the final analysis, the obstetrician and patient should participate in the decision whether to treat the patient at all.

Hypothyroidism induces thyrotropic hormone release, which stimulates acid mucopolysaccharide production with increased turgidity and edema of the turbinates, congestion of subcutaneous tissues, and mucous gland hypertrophy (8,10). The premenstrual "cold" also may be due to hormonal changes.

It has been shown, in some patients, that wide swings in blood levels of glucose, as occur in uncontrolled diabetes mellitus, result in altered molecular configurations of ground substance acid mucopolysaccharides with more short-chain hydrophilic polysaccharides, increased osmotic pressure, edema, collagen and elastic tissue deposition, and the eventual formation of fibromyxomatous nasal polyps. Meticulous control of blood sugar levels is necessary to control this rare cause of rhinitis (16).

Irritative Causes of Rhinitis

Persistent irritation of the nasal mucosa may cause chronic rhinosinusitis. The most common irritants are occupational (dust, fumes, chemicals), but environmental factors such as pollution may play a role. Control of pollution is becoming a serious problem for the future.

Idiopathic Causes of Nonallergic Rhinitis

Vasomotor Rhinitis

Vasomotor rhinitis (1,2,4–7,27) is a diagnosis made only after excluding all other causes of rhinitis previously described. Hence true vasomotor rhinitis represents only a small percentage of the perennial, nonallergic, noninfectious rhinitides. It is characterized by nonspecific airway obstruction with postnasal drainage and profuse rhinorrhea. There is no associated pruritis or sneezing. The family history is negative for allergy. The skin tests are also negative. The serum IgE is normal, and the nasal smears show few, if any, eosinophils. There may, however, be other associated autonomic abnormalities such as irritable bowel syndrome.

Vasomotor rhinitis is felt to be the result of an unstable autonomic nervous system with a hyperresponsive parasympathetic outflow and a hyperresponsive mucosa. Nonspecific irritants such as fumes, tobacco smoke, odors, changes in temperature, and weather changes may trigger this already hyperresponsive, unstable autonomic nervous system with the nasal mucosa as the end organ. Likewise, anxiety, hostility, guilt, depression, and constant frustration all can affect the autonomic nervous system with resultant vasomotor rhinitis.

Eosinophilic Nonallergic Rhinitis

Eosinophilic nonallergic rhinitis is a specific entity affecting a defined patient population (7). This perennial condition, with no geographic variation, presents with paroxyms of sneezing, watery rhinorrhea, and pruritis. There is an absence of hyperactive airway and negative methacholine and aspirin challenge tests (23), a normal serum IgE, negative skin tests, and prominent nasal eosinophilia. Nonspecific irritants such as strong odors, dust, smoke, and weather changes are noted to evoke change in 15% to 30% of afflicted patients. This condition is noted in patients older than 20 to 30 years of age, presents in paroxyms, and is worse in the morning and better later in the day.

Within these parameters, eosinophilic nonallergic rhinitis is a specific subgroup of all the rhinitides associated with eosinophilia. These include allergic rhinitis, nasal polyposis, nonallergic asthma with rhinitis, and aspirin sensitivity. As noted, eosinophilic nonallergic rhinitis, whatever the cause, is intermittent, characterized by rhinorrhea and induced by nonspecific irritants with negative skin tests. On the other hand, eosinophilic rhinitis associated with allergy is continuous or seasonal and is induced by specific antigens with positive skin testing. Approximately 25% of patients with eosinophilic rhinitis have associated nasal polyps.

Despite the cause, eosinophilic rhinitis is characterized histologically by a thickened submucosa; a mixed infiltrate of plasma cells, lymphocytes, eosinophils, and neutrophils; an intense local IgE staining; and a damaged basement membrane.

Presumptive mechanisms for eosinophilic rhinitis include altered prostaglandin synthesis or metabolism, aberrant eosinophil chemotactic factors, a persistent reaction to bacterial or viral infection, vasomotor instability, nonspecific irritants, and undiagnosed specific allergies (1,6).

Eosinophilic rhinitis is treated by removal of the offending irritants, surgical removal of the polyps, avoidance of aspirin, and the use of antihistamines (4,5,28) and topical steroids. Asthma, if present, should be treated with the appropriate bronchodilating agents.

Mixed Cellular Rhinitis

Mixed cellular rhinitis represents up to 50% of the chronic rhinitides (4). This condition is characterized by rhinorrhea, congestion, and a red, inflamed mucosa. The nasal smears contain mixed lymphocytes, plasma cells, and eosinophils. There is a normal serum IgE and negative skin tests.

Nasal Mastocytosis

Nasal mastocytosis (6,8,9,29) is a rare condition, found mostly in adults and characterized by rhinorrhea and congestion without pruritis. There is an idiopathic increase in mucosal mast cell content from a normal of 200 to 400 cells/mm^3 to 2000 cells/mm^3. There are few eosinophils, skin tests are negative, and serum IgE is normal. This condition may have its onset with associated upper respiratory tract infection. Approximately 15% of patients afflicted with nasal mastocytosis have a past medical history of cluster headaches, and another 15% have associated rhinitis with alcohol ingestion. The mast cell infiltrate is due to unknown, nonspecific stimuli, which attract mast cells and cause release of mediators, which account for the symptoms of rhinorrhea and congestion.

Miscellaneous

Recumbency rhinitis is a nonspecific vasomotor congestion characterized by the dependent side of the nose becoming congested while sleeping on one's side. In patients with a laryngectomy or tracheostomy, where the nose is excluded from the airflow, a vasomotor reaction occurs with the mucosa becoming congested and boggy.

PATIENT EVALUATION

History

As in the evaluation of any other medical complaint, the workup for rhinitis begins with a detailed history. The chief complaint will be one of nasal obstruction, anterior and/or posterior nasal drainage, nasal irritation, sneezing, or a combination of all these symptoms. Symptoms of nasal itching and sneezing may be indicative of an allergy or eosinophilic nonallergic rhinitis. Intermittent nasal congestion and blockage may be due to the normal nasal cycle or to any of the conditions previously described. If the nasal congestion is constant, an anatomic obstruction such as nasal polyps or chronic end-stage hyperplastic rhinitis should be considered. If the obstruction is recent in onset and the patient has not undergone an operation to the nose or sustained an injury, the problem probably is due to mucosal disease.

The history should include the onset, frequency, duration, character, and severity of the symptoms. Any precipitating factors, as well as response to any previous treatment, should be documented.

The onset of the symptoms may be in childhood, as an adult, after trauma or an upper respiratory tract infection, or following a move from one geographic location to another. The onset of symptoms early in life may indicate an allergic etiology, while symptoms beginning in adulthood are more likely to be due to nonallergic rhinitis.

The symptoms may be seasonal or perennial, constant or episodic and paroxysmal, acute (less than 10 days duration) or chronic. The character of the nasal drainage, whether watery, mucoid, or purulent, may help distinguish between allergic, nonallergic, or infectious rhinitis.

The severity of the symptoms, disability, and the social and economic impacts should be noted and quantified if possible.

Any precipitating factors such as allergens, irritants, weather changes, and medications should be identified. These factors may be deduced by questioning the patient as to whether the symptoms occur indoors or outdoors, at home or at work, during a particular season, or in a specific geographic location. Obviously, a detailed drug history to include prescription medications, over-the-counter preparations, alcohol, tobacco, and illicit drugs is necessary. Patients sensitive to aspirin may also experience similar symptoms with other nonsteroidal anti-inflammatory agents, as well as dyes and preservatives such as tartrazine, sodium benzoate, and sulfur dioxide.

Associated symptoms also should be noted. This would include hyposmia or anosmia, disturbed sleep, mouth breathing with associated dry mouth, snoring, fatigue, and irritability.

The efficacy or failure of previous treatment modalities, whether medical or surgical, should be documented and considered in establishing the diagnosis and planning any further treatment.

The past medical history should include specific inquiry as to hypertension, diabetes, thyroid dysfunction, pregnancy, estrogen therapy and other endocrine abnormalities, and other conditions associated with autonomic nervous system abnormalities.

A detailed family history of asthma, rhinitis, hayfever, and atopic dermatitis should be noted.

The Physical Examination

A patient presenting with rhinitis requires a complete otolaryngologic–head and neck examination as well as at least a cursory evaluation of the lower respiratory tract. The conjunctiva should be inspected for injection or edema, the chest auscultated for wheezing, and the skin inspected for urticaria. The patient should be evaluated for the stigmata of hypothyroidism.

Before routine rhinoscopy, the external nose and caudal septum should be inspected for gross, obstructing deformity. Gentle upward traction on the lower lateral cartilages may relieve symptoms of obstruction due to nasal valve collapse.

Rhinoscopy should be undertaken with a nasal speculum and brilliant illumination, both before and after vasoconstriction. Any secretions, particularly if directly visualized in the middle meatus, are evaluated as to their character, and any obvious masses either benign or malignant are documented. The contour of the nasal septum and the relevance of the nasal valve are assessed for possible contribution to symptoms of obstruction. The characteristics of the mucosa are noted. Pale, boggy, gray mucosa is seen in a nonallergic rhinitis and hypothyroidism, while engorged reddened mucosa may be seen in rhinitis medicamentosa. Thin, crusted mucosa is characteristic of atrophic rhinitis and may be associated with a foul odor (ozena). These changes may or may not be useful in diagnosing the etiology. The size of the turbinates is evaluated both before and after vasoconstriction with 4% cocaine solution or any other topical vasoconstrictor. Turbinate hypertrophy, significant enough to cause nasal obstruction unresponsive to vasoconstrictive agents, may require surgical therapy. Do not forget that sarcoidosis may mimic chronic hyperplastic rhinitis.

Probably all patients with chronic rhinitis should undergo *paranasal sinus radiographs*. Twenty percent of patients with perennial rhinitis have mild mucosal changes, while another 20% have dense clouding of the paranasal sinuses on x-ray evaluation. Ethmoid cloud-

ing is a frequent finding. The mechanisms of paranasal mucosal changes include ostial blockage due to middle meatal mucosal edema, secondary sinus infection, or a similar reaction of the sinus mucosa to the cause of the nonallergic rhinitis. Obvious conditions primarily affecting the sinuses may cause secondary nasal mucosal changes.

The nasopharynx should be evaluated carefully to exclude the presence of obstructing masses, which may cause secondary rhinitis. In an adult, this can be accomplished by indirect mirror examination or fiberoptic nasopharyngoscopy. In a child, a lateral radiograph of the nasopharynx may suffice.

The Laboratory Evaluation

The laboratory evaluation of a patient presenting with rhinitis is dependent on the history and physical findings. Nasal smears may be evaluated for eosinophils, mast cells, or neutrophils. A nasal mucosal biopsy and electron microscopy will be necessary for the diagnosis of immotile cilia syndrome or sarcoidosis.

When indicated, blood work for serum IgE, total eosinophil count, thyroid hormone levels, estrogen levels, blood glucose levels, and drug levels should be obtained. A sedimentation rate may be useful if occult infection is suspected as the underlying cause of the patient's symptoms.

Skin testing may be helpful if the history and physical findings are suggestive of an allergic etiology.

TREATMENT OF NONALLERGIC RHINITIS

The treatment of nonallergic, noninfectious rhinitis may be either medical or surgical. As causes of rhinitis fall on a continuum between antigen-specific rhinitis and nonspecific, idiopathic, perennial vasomotor rhinitis, the treatment of rhinitis may be specific and directed to the etiologic agent or directed solely toward symptomatic control. Specific treatment modalities are best used in true allergic rhinitis and include avoidance of the offending antigen, measures to cleanse the air, and immunotherapy. Likewise, nonallergic rhinitis also may be treated by avoidance of offending irritants, hormones, and medications that may induce the symptoms. Symptomatic treatment includes use of antihistamines, oral vasoconstrictors, anticholinergics, corticosteroid nasal sprays, and cromolyn sodium (30,31). It has been suggested by some that sleeping with the head of the bed elevated and regular exercise help minimize the symptoms.

Antihistamines

Antihistamines selectively block H_1 receptors and suppress those symptoms mediated by histamine. The response of nonallergic rhinitis to antihistamines is variable and depends on the contribution of histamine to the symptoms, as well as the chemical structure of the particular histamine. Antihistamines also exert an anticholinergic-like effect on rhinorrhea; however, non-histamine-mediated symptoms such as nasal stuffiness are not affected.

The side effects of antihistamines include drowsiness, dry mouth, irritability, and dizziness. In larger doses, delirium, hallucinations, ataxia, muscle twitching, fevers, convulsions, and death have been reported. Little is known about the teratogenicity of antihistamines; however, brompheniramine (24) and diphenhydramine (25) have been associated with congenital malformations. Antihistamines interact with medications producing drowsiness, as well as anticholinergics such as the tricyclic antidepressants.

There is little correlation between the wheal suppression and the half-life of antihistamines; hence dosing of antihistamines remains empiric (30,31).

Sympathomimetic Agents

Sympathomimetic agents stimulate α-adrenergic receptors, constrict vessels, decongest mucous membranes, and provide an overall decrease in nasal airway resistance. They are also felt to increase cyclic adenosine monophosphate (cAMP) and inhibit release of mediators.

Sympathomimetics such as pseudoephedrine and phenylpropanolamine are given orally and are the first-line drugs used for symptoms of nasal congestion. Side effects of oral sympathomimetics include nervousness, insomnia, irritability, and difficulty urinating in elderly males. No effect on blood pressure is noted in normotensive individuals; however, an increase in diastolic blood pressure in patients with labile or overt hypertension or individuals taking monoamine oxidase (MAO) inhibitors may be noted.

For control of the multiple symptoms of rhinitis including obstruction, rhinorrhea, sneezing, and pruritis, combination antihistamine–sympathomimetic preparations are available. The strengths of these preparations are fixed; therefore the physician may need to alter the dosage schedule to obtain optimal benefit (30–32).

The topical sympathomimetics are phenylephrine and oxymetazoline. These agents have a marked short-term effect followed by rebound congestion and rhinitis medicamentosa after prolonged use. Therefore these agents should be used only sparingly and for short periods of acute situations requiring rapid mucosal decongestion (i.e., acute sinusitis).

Anticholinergic Agents

Anticholinergics such as propantheline and belladonna may be effective in reducing the rhinorrhea of vasomotor rhinitis. These drugs have not found widespread clinical use in the treatment of rhinitis and, at any rate, should be avoided in patients with tachyarrhythmias, obstructive uropathy, and narrow-angle glaucoma. Studies comparing glucocorticoids to anticholinergics in the treatment of nonallergic perennial rhinitis, however, have found no significant decrease in severity of symptoms for the anticholinergics. As noted, secretions are controlled by other mediators in addition to acetylcholine; hence anticholinergics should not be expected to be as effective in control of the symptoms of rhinitis (30,33).

Topical Steroids

Topical steroids suppress the local inflammatory response caused by the release of vasoactive mediators. Steroids also reduce the sensitivity of irritant receptors, thus diminishing the sneeze response, reduce the reactivity of acetylcholine receptors with some decrease in rhinorrhea, and decrease the total basophil and eosinophil counts. There is also experimental evidence to show *in vitro* inhibition of mediator release, a phenomenon previously not attributed to topical steroids (31,34,35).

The topical steroid preparations in common use are beclomethasone dipropionate and flunisolide. Both medications are delivered in a propylene glycol carrier via a mechanical pump, thus avoiding use of fluorocarbon aerosol (Freon) propelled sprays. Neither flunisolide or beclomethasone inhibit the hypothalamic–pituitary–adrenal axis at recommended doses (30,34,36). However, reports of adrenal suppression at increased doses of flunisolide have been noted (31).

Both beclomethasone and flunisolide are shown to cause a significant improvement in the symptoms of rhinitis when compared to placebo. The symptoms of congestion are particularly affected both subjectively and objectively with documented decrease in nasal airway resistance. Nasal steroids are effective in allergic as well as nonallergic rhinitis, including vasomotor rhinitis and nasal polyposis. When used for vasomotor rhinitis, the primary benefit is relief of nasal obstruction rather than rhinorrhea and postnasal drainage. In particularly severe cases of nasal obstruction or polyposis, a short course of oral steroids may be necessary to provide initial decongestion or shrinkage of the polyps, which can then be maintained with subsequent use of the topical steroids.

Side effects of topical steroids include mucosal edema, mild erythema, burning, drying, epistaxis, and occasionally a stinging sensation upon application. Development of subsequent candidiasis with prolonged use of nasal steroids has not been a problem (30,31, 34,36). A relatively new topical steroid, fluocortin butyl, has been evaluated recently in a multicenter double-blind placebo-controlled study for both allergic and nonallergic rhinitis. This medication is breath activated and delivered as an odorless, tasteless powder in a lactose carrier. There is a significant reduction in symptoms and use of concomitant medication versus placebo, with relatively few side effects (37).

Cromolyn Sodium

Cromolyn sodium prevents mast cell degranulation and inhibits the release of histamine. This medication may be of some benefit in IgE-mediated allergic rhinitis; however, no benefit over oral antihistamines alone has been shown for the nonallergic rhinitides. A recent evaluation of 4% cromolyn sodium in eosinophilic nonallergic rhinitis revealed no significant difference between the cromolyn sodium and placebo in the control of symptoms (30,38).

Surgical Management of Nonallergic Rhinitis

The surgical management of nonallergic rhinitis involves the correction of any anatomic abnormalities including the removal of tumors or polyps and the surgical debulking of chronic turbinate hypertrophy. Often, a combination of abnormalities necessitates a combination of procedures to afford relief.

Anatomic abnormalities usually include bony and cartilaginous deformities of the septum, external nose, and nasal valve area. Various septorhinoplastic techniques have been popularized to restore a normal nasal airway. Do remember that not every deviated septum requires surgical correction; only if it is felt to be contributing to the nasal obstruction should this be performed. As noted, a wide variety of benign, malignant, and granulomatous processes also may affect the nasal cavity and mimic the symptoms of rhinitis. Therapy for these lesions ranges from simple biopsy for diagnosis to radical ablative surgery for removal of malignant neoplasms.

Nasal polyps, if small, may be managed successfully using topical steroids. Those refractory to this management or large multiple polyps should be removed surgically intranasally or via the sinuses, if necessary or if they should recur after intranasal extraction. The use of topical steroid therapy after surgical removal should prevent their recurrence.

Vasomotor rhinitis refractory to conservative therapy even if the mucosa has not undergone chronic hyperplastic change may be managed by cryosurgery or submucous diathermy to the turbinates or even vidian neurectomy. Cryosurgery to the turbinates has been described as effective in treating vasomotor rhinitis with nasal obstruction but less effective for excessive rhinorrhea (39,40). Vidian neurectomy only provides short-term relief for rhinorrhea and sneezing of vasomotor rhinitis and was not very useful for the nasal obstruction. It is not commonly performed any longer.

Chronic turbinate hypertrophy that is unresponsive to medical management is a late sequela of rhinitis, of whatever cause. Diagnosis of this condition is characterized by a failure of the turbinates to shrink after application of topical vasoconstrictors. This end-stage, chronic hypertrophic rhinitis may be managed by a number of surgical techniques including intraturbinate steroid injection, turbinate outfracture, cauterization, cryosurgery, laser vaporization, submucous resection of the conchal bone, partial inferior turbinate resection, and total inferior turbinectomy (41). Surgery is considered only after failure of an adequate trial of medical management, as already discussed. The middle turbinates are not usually the cause of airway obstruction but, if felt to be the problem, can easily be outfractured or, if particularly prominent, crushed. Middle turbinectomy in our experience is complicated frequently by prolonged postoperative crusting until the area heals. In general, it is the inferior turbinates that warrant the surgical attention.

Intraturbinate steroid injection using triamcinolone acetonide is accomplished by injecting 0.5 cc submucosally into the anterior tip of the inferior turbinate gently to minimize the described rare complication of blindness due to retinal vasospasm or embolization (42). While many patients are delighted with the results, others do not obtain long-term relief of symptoms.

Turbinate outfracture is usually not very successful, as at best a "greenstick fracture" is created and the turbinate gradually drifts back into its original position. Surface cautery using silver nitrate or an electric current usually only affects the mucosa, sparing the submucosa, and therefore is likewise not very effective for true hyperplastic rhinitis. Surface cryosurgery, on the other hand, will cause not only mucosal but submucosal necrosis. This is quite successful, but there is significant prolonged postoperative nasal congestion and the eschar takes a long time to separate. Damage to the adjacent nasal septum may be difficult to avoid.

Submucous resection of the inferior turbinate has been proposed by many authors as the most ideal method of debulking the inferior turbinate (43–45). However, this is technically quite difficult, frequently results in significant bleeding, and results in a floppy residual inferior turbinate that does not give the desired result in relieving airway obstruction.

Submucosal diathermy along the length of the turbinate may be very successful provided the obstruction is not due predominantly to bony enlargement. It also avoids the crusting seen with surface cautery. Necrosis of the underlying bone has been described as a complication.

Rhinomanometric data have implicated the anterior end of the inferior turbinate as the major site of obstruction owing to its proximity to the nasal valve and excellent improvement has been reported following removal of just the anterior half of the turbinate (46). It has been our experience, however, that frequently the obstruction is due to a hyperplastic posterior segment obstructing posterior choanae, which would fail to be resolved by this technique. A subtotal turbinectomy, which essentially consists of removal of the entire length of the inferior turbinate, has, in our hands, proved an excellent method of achieving relief of nasal congestion due to turbinate hypertrophy. It is technically simple with excellent results being reported by many authors (47,48). Complications include significant hemorrhage and crusting, particularly when performed in dry climates. In general, rhinitis sicca and atrophic rhinitis have not proved to be a problem even after many years.

The technique consists of initially in-fracturing the turbinates and applying a straight hemostat (Kelly clamp) along the length of the turbinate, just medial to its attachment to the lateral wall. After waiting approximately 1 min, the clamp is removed and the turbinectomy performed by cutting along the crushed tissue caused by the clamp. A suction-cautery is then used to cauterize the stump of tissue remaining for hemostasis as indicated. The packing is removed the following day and the eschar usually spontaneously becomes dislodged at approximately 10 days.

REFERENCES

1. Simons FER. Chronic rhinitis. *Pediatr Clin North Am* 1984; 31(4):801.
2. Kimmelman CP, Ali GHA. Vasomotor rhinitis. *Otolaryngol Clin North Am* 1986;19:65.
3. Druce HM. Nasal physiology. *Ear Nose Throat J* 1986;65:201.
4. Ballow M. Allergic rhinitis and conjunctivitis. Help for the weeping nose and eyes. *Postgrad Med* 1984;76:197.
5. Buss WW. Chronic rhinitis. A systematic approach to diagnosis and treatment. *Postgrad Med* 1983;73:325.
6. Meltzer EO, Zeiger RS, Schatz M, Jalowayski AA. Chronic rhinitis in infants and children: etiologic, diagnostic and therapeutic considerations. *Pediatr Clin North Am* 1983;30:847.
7. Jacobs RL, Freedman PM, Boswell RN. Nonallergic rhinitis with eosinophilia (NARES syndrome). Clinical and immunologic presentation. *J Allergy Clin Immunol* 1981;61:253.
8. Connell JT. Nasal disease: mechanisms and classification. *Ann Allergy* 1983;50:227.
9. Zeiger RS, Schatz M. Chronic rhinitis: a practical approach to diagnosis and treatment. Part I: Diagnosis. *Immunol Allergy Prac* 1982;4:63.
10. Weisskopf A. Connective tissue: a synthesis of modern thought and its impact on the understanding of nasal disease. *Laryngoscope* 1960;70:1029.
11. Rucci L, Cirri-Borghi B, Pantaleo T, Cagnoli A. Effects of vidian nerve stimulation on the nasal and maxillary sinus mucosa. A light and electron microscopic study. *J Laryngol Otol* 1984;98:597.
12. Anggard A. The effects of parasympathetic nerve stimulation on the microcirculation and secretion in the nasal mucosa of the cat. *Acta Otolaryngol (Stockh)* 1974;78:98.
13. Anggard A, Edwall L. The effects of sympathetic nerve stimulation on the tracer disappearance rate and local blood content in the nasal mucosa of the cat. *Acta Otolaryngol (Stockh)* 1974; 77:131.
14. May M, West JW. The "stuffy" nose. *Otolaryngol Clin North Am* 1973;6:655.
15. Silber G, Naclerio R, Eggleston P, et al. *In vivo* release of histamine by hyperosmolar stimuli. *J Allergy Clin Immunol* 1985;75:176.
16. Smith MP. Dysfunction of carbohydrate metabolism as an element in the set of factors resulting in the polysaccharide nose and nasal polyps (the polysaccharide nose). *Laryngoscope* 1971; 81:636.
17. Topposada H, Topposada M, El-Ghazzawi I, Elwany S. The human respiratory nasal mucosa in females using contraceptive pills. *J Laryngol Otol* 1984;98:43.
18. Parker GS, Mehlum DL, Bacher-Wetmore B. Ciliary dyskinesis: the immotile cilia syndrome. *Laryngoscope* 1983;93:573.
19. Mygind N, Thomsen J, Balslev (Jorgensen) M. Ultrastructure of the epithelium in atrophic rhinitis—transmission electron microscopic studies. *Acta Otolaryngol (Stockh)* 1974;78:106.
20. Greenberger P, Patterson R. Safety of therapy for allergic symptoms during pregnancy. *Ann Intern Med* 1978;89:234.
21. Hill RM, Tennyson LM. The effect of maternal allergy medications on the fetus. *Immunol Allergy Prac* 1985;7:80.
22. Mabry RL. The management of nasal obstruction during pregnancy. *Ear Nose Throat J* 1983;62:16.
23. Nelson HS. What is atopy? Sidestepping semantics. *Postgrad Med* 1984;76:118.
24. Siegel CJ, Dockhorn RJ. An evaluation of childhood rhinorrhea. *Ann Allergy* 1982;47:9.
25. Connell JT. Nasal mastocytosis. *J Allergy* 1969;43:182.
26. Settipane GA, Chafee FH. Nasal polyps in asthma and rhinitis. A review of 6,037 patients. *J Allergy Clin Immunol* 1977;59:17.
27. Pleskow WW, Stevenson DD, Mathison DA, Simon RA, Schatz M, Zeiger RS. Aspirin-sensitive rhinosinusitis/asthma: spectrum of adverse reactions to aspirin. *J Allergy Clin Immunol* 1983;71:574.
28. Webb DR. Clinical characteristics and therapy of nasal polyps. *J Allergy Clin Immunol* 1978;61:185.
29. Mullarkey MF, Hill JS, Webb DR. Allergic and non-allergic rhinitis: their characterization with attention to the meaning of nasal eosinophilia. *J Allergy Clin Immunol* 1980;65:122.
30. Rupp GH, Friedman RA. Eosinophilic non-allergic rhinitis in children. *Pediatrics* 1982;70:437.
31. Hendeles L, Weinberger M, Wong L. Medical management of noninfectious rhinitis. *Am J Hosp Pharm* 1980;37:1496.
32. Norman PS. Review of nasal therapy: update. The John Sheldon Memorial Lecture. *J Allergy Clin Immunol* 1983;72:421.
33. Broms P, Malm L. Oral vasoconstrictors in perennial nonallergic rhinitis. *Allergy* 1982;37:67.
34. Bende M, Rundcrantz H. Treatment of perennial secretory rhinitis. *J Otorhinolaryngol Relat Spec* 1985;47:303.
35. Knight A, Kilin A. Long-term efficacy and safety of beclomethasone dipropionate aerosol in perennial rhinitis. *Ann Allergy* 1983; 50:81.
36. Wihl JO. Topical corticosteroids and nasal reactivity. *Eur J Respir Dis Suppl* 1982;122:205.
37. Patow CA, Kaliner M. Corticosteroid treatment of rhinologic disease. *Ear Nose Throat J* 1983;62:14.
38. Arbesman C, Bernstein IL, Bierman CW, Bocles JS, Katz R, Lieberman PL, Mattuci K, Meltzer EO, Middleton E, Noyes J, Pearlman DS, Pence HL, Slavin RG, Spector SL. Multicenter, double-blind, placebo-controlled trial of fluocortin butyl in perennial rhinitis. *J Allergy Clin Immunol* 1983;71:597.
39. Nelson BL, Jacobs RL. Response of the non-allergic rhinitis with eosinophilia (NARES) syndrome to 4% cromolyn sodium nasal solution. *J Allergy Clin Immunol* 1982;70:125.

40. Bumsted RM. Cryotherapy for chronic vasomotor rhinitis: technique and patient selection for improved results. *Laryngoscope* 1984;94:539.

41. Moore JRM, Bicknell PG. A comparison of cryosurgery and submucous diathermy in vasomotor rhinitis. *J Laryngol Otol* 1980;94:1411.

42. Kirtane MV, Prabhu VS, Karnik PP. Transnasal preganglionic vidian nerve section. *J Laryngol Otol* 1984;98:481.

43. William JD. Laser vidian neurectomy. *Ann Otol Rhinol Laryngol* 1983;92:281.

44. Mabry RL. Surgery of the inferior turbinates: How much and when? *Otolaryngol Head Neck Surg* 1984;92(5):571.

45. Fanous N. Anterior turbinectomy. A new surgical approach to turbinate hypertrophy: a review of 220 cases. *Arch Otolaryngol Head Neck Surg* 1986;112:850.

46. Ophir D, Shapira A, Marshak G. Total inferior turbinectomy for nasal airway obstruction. *Arch Otolaryngol* 1985;111(2):93–95.

47. Martinez SA, Nissen AJ, Stock CR, Tesmer T. Nasal turbinate resection for relief of nasal obstruction. *Laryngoscope* 1983;93:871–875.

48. Moore GF, Freeman TJ, Ogren FP, Yonkers AY. Extended follow-up of total inferior turbinate resection for relief of chronic nasal obstruction. *Laryngoscope* 1985;95:1095.

CHAPTER 13

Barotrauma

Jack L. Gluckman

In this day and age of routine air travel and the rising popularity of scuba diving as a recreational sport plus the increasing use of hyperbaric oxygen chambers, barotrauma affecting the air-filled cavities of the head has become a common presenting complaint to the practicing otolaryngologist irrespective of geographic location. While barotrauma to the middle ear is by far the most common injury, the paranasal sinuses are the second most common site affected (1), particularly the frontal sinus (2). Barosinusitis (aerosinusitis) was first described by Marchoux and Nepper in 1919 after experiments in a decompression chamber (3) and was subsequently elaborated on by Campbell (4–6) after extensive experience obtained with aviators involved in high-altitude flying during World War II.

All commercial aircraft have pressurized cabins, thereby protecting the passengers and crew from barotrauma. If, however, the patient has a congested upper respiratory tract that prevents pressure equalization in the sinuses, barosinusitis will result. This condition is more likely to occur in military aircraft where the crew is subject to repeated abrupt changes in pressure or in small private aircraft that do not have pressurized cabins.

The development of the Self-Contained Underwater Breathing Apparatus (SCUBA) in 1943 by Jacque-Ives Cousteau and Emile Gagnon resulted in an explosion of interest in the sport of scuba diving with more than a quarter of a million recreational divers being trained annually in the United States alone. Unfortunately, but predictably, this has led to a concomitant dramatic increase in the number of patients presenting to the otolaryngologist with barotrauma.

In recent years, the use of hyperbaric oxygen has increased in popularity for the treatment of chronic nonhealing infections and injuries, as well as a myriad of other conditions. Such chambers are now found in many medical centers and patients treated by this means are extremely vulnerable to barotrauma.

PHYSICS AND PHYSIOLOGY

Barotrauma refers to tissue damage sustained from changes in the volume of gas (air) in a self-contained space secondary to alteration in the ambient pressure. In barosinusitis, this affects the lining mucosa in one or more sinuses.

Pressure is expressed in atmospheres (atm), pounds per square inch (psi), and millimeters of mercury. Atmospheric pressure is the amount of force exerted by the earth's atmosphere on the body surface and varies with elevation. At sea level it is 1 atm, that is, 14.7 psi, and is ideal for human life. As one descends below the surface of sea water, the pressure increases by 1 atm for every 33 ft. On the other hand, for every 18,000 ft one ascends into the atmosphere, the pressure decreases by 0.5 atm.

The behavior of air, like other gases, is affected by temperature, pressure, and volume with the relationship being defined by Boyle's law. This states that at a constant temperature, the volume of gas varies inversely with the pressure to which it is subjected ($P = K/V$), where K is a constant. Therefore if the pressure of a gas is doubled, it must be compressed to half its volume with obviously significant effect on the air-filled spaces of the ear and paranasal sinuses (Fig. 1).

Three mechanisms of barotrauma have been described: squeeze, reverse squeeze, and mixed squeeze (7).

Squeeze

As the scuba diver descends into the depths of the ocean or a plane descends from high altitudes, the ambient pressure increases and the volume of gas in the body air spaces halves, necessitating constant equalization of the pressure to prevent barotrauma.

The paranasal sinuses are particularly vulnerable to

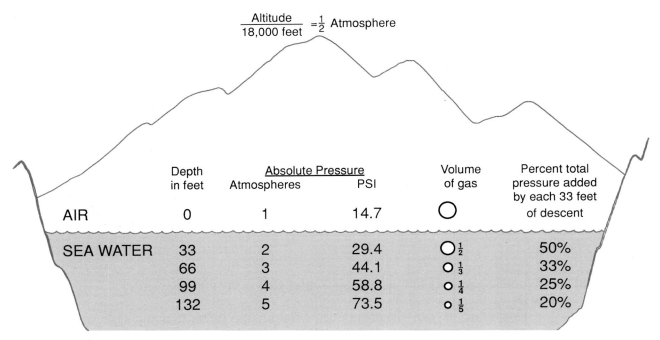

FIG. 1. Effect on volume of gas by changes in pressure.

barotrauma because of their narrow ostia and the fact that the rigid walls of the cavities do not permit change in the size of the air-filled space as the pressure changes. If the air in the sinuses cannot equilibrate, a negative vacuum effect results in engorgement of the blood vessels, mucosal edema, mucosal and submucosal hemorrhage, and ultimately bleeding into the involved sinus, which will partially equalize the pressure (2,8). Any pathology that narrows the ostia may predispose to this barotrauma. This may be as subtle as a mucus plug or minimal mucosal thickening confined to the middle meatus or more overt such as a deviated nasal septum, polyps, tumor, or bacterial rhinosinusitis.

Reverse Squeeze

This phenomenon occurs during ascent when, due to a ball-valve action at the sinus ostia because of mucosal edema, air is allowed to enter during descent but is prevented from escaping from the sinus into the nose during ascent. This trapped air expands and may cause significant trauma to the mucosa and even bone of the sinus.

Mixed Squeeze

This is a combination of squeeze and reverse squeeze, which may occur during the same dive or aircraft flight.

CLINICAL FEATURES

The most common symptom of barotrauma is pressure and/or sharp *pain* over the affected sinus, which may last minutes to hours, often leaving the patient with a residual ache that may persist for days (1). This pain most commonly manifests over the frontal sinuses but also may be present over the maxillary sinus and between or behind the eyes. If the sphenoid is involved, the pain may be referred to the occipital area. This pain usually increases as the aircraft approaches lower altitudes or as the diver descends deeper. *Epistaxis,* if it occurs, is usually mild and intermittent, although it may persist for some days after the acute event.

If the patient should experience reverse sinus squeeze during ascent, the pain may be even more intense because of the air trapped in the sinuses expanding. Rarely, it may produce anesthesia or paraesthesia in the distribution of the infraorbital nerve if the maxillary sinus is involved (9,10), and even more rarely fracture of the overlying bone may occur (7), which may result in subcutaneous emphysema (11). Most commonly, however, the air forces secretions consisting of blood and mucus through the ostia, resulting in a serosanguinous discharge.

The findings on examination depend on how long after the acute event the patient is seen. The sinuses may be mildly tender to palpation and examination of the nose may reveal no abnormality other than evidence of the underlying causative problem, for example, polyp or deviated septum.

Radiographic Findings

These findings also will depend on the stage at which the patient is initially seen. In 80% of patients, there are abnormal findings varying from mucosal thickening to an air–fluid level or a completely opaque sinus filled with blood (9). These findings may take weeks to resolve, persisting long after the patient is asymptomatic.

A clinical grading according to degree of severity of the sinus barotrauma has been proposed (2) but probably is of very little practical value.

Grade 1: Mild, transient sinus discomfort without radiographic changes.
Grade 2: Localized pain over the affected sinus persisting for 6 to 24 hr. Radiographic evidence of sinus mucosal thickening.
Grade 3: Pain lasting for days. Sinus radiographs may reveal a polypoid mass due to a submucosal hematoma or an air–fluid level.

Differential Diagnosis

The diagnosis of acute barotrauma to the sinuses is usually self-evident; however, the condition may need to be differentiated from other conditions.

Barodontalgia (Aerodontalgia)

Pain may result from air trapped in air pockets in carious teeth, periodontal abscess, or under fillings in patients who recently have undergone dental restoration where the gas is caught underneath inadequate packing or filling. This is particularly a problem if the dental pulp has been damaged. While this classically causes symptoms during ascent when the air expands, it may occur during descent as well. The pain from this condition, which usually is confined to the affected tooth, may radiate into the maxilla and be confused with maxillary sinus barotrauma. Pain from maxillary sinus barotrauma, on the other hand, may cause discomfort in a number of teeth, but the teeth are normal to inspection and palpation.

Other causes of headache and facial pain and even acute suppurating sinusitis should always be considered when evaluating the patient on the initial examination. One of the more difficult problems is to differentiate between blood and pus in a completely opaque antrum after barotrauma. Magnetic resonance imaging using a combination of T1 and T2 weighted images may distinguish hemorrhage from mucosal reaction and sinus effusion (12), and certainly if any doubt persists, an antral lavage should be performed in the case of the maxillary sinus or the frontal sinus trephined.

TREATMENT

Prevention

Patients, particularly those with a prior history of barotrauma, should be advised to avoid flying, entering a hyperbaric oxygen chamber, or scuba diving in the presence of a significant upper respiratory tract infection. If this activity is essential, the use of topical nasal decongestants immediately preceding the event may obviate the development of barotrauma. In the case of flying, this should be sprayed a half-hour prior to both ascent and descent.

Treatment of Acute Barotrauma

If acute barotrauma should develop, the scuba diver is instructed to ascend and then commence descent at a slower rate, or if the diver is ascending, he/she should descend and then ascend slower. Likewise, if a pilot experiences severe barotrauma, it is advisable to regain an altitude where the symptom is not as severe and then change altitude more slowly.

If the patient is seen by the physician shortly after the acute event, the following steps should be taken and are dependent on the severity of the condition.

If mild barotrauma is present, simple reassurance that the discomfort will disappear within a short period of time, together with administration of topical decongestants and analgesics, is all that is necessary. In moderately severe cases, topical decongestants and the appropriate analgesics are indicated, as well as prophylactic antibiotics if the possibility of a secondary infection is suspected. In severe barotrauma, hospitalization to permit adequate decongestion and analgesia may be necessary. Drainage either by antral lavage or frontal sinus trephination may become necessary.

Aviators who have experienced severe barotrauma are required to be tested in an altitude testing chamber after resolution of their symptoms and the reestablishment of normal radiographs, to ensure that return to flight status is safe.

Treatment of Recurrent Barotrauma

Recurrent barotrauma is a syndrome that is to be differentiated from a solitary acute episode, which usually occurs while flying or diving with an upper respiratory tract infection. Recurrent barotrauma represents a significant problem, particularly for career pilots, who fly high-performance aircraft where they are subject to wide fluctuations in barometric pressure, as well as professional scuba divers. These patients should be evaluated carefully to rule out any anatomic abnormality that may predispose to impaired ventilation or drainage of the sinus. This evaluation may include allergy assessment and treatment, and therapy should be directed to sinus drainage procedures, nasal polypectomy, or correction of a deviated nasal septum (12,13). If the nose and sinuses appear normal clinically and radiographically, a computed tomography scan may be necessary to exclude subtle middle meatal abnormalities. Standard sinus drainage procedures may occasionally not be helpful, and in the appropriate case, functional endoscopic sinus surgery directed to the osteomeatal complex may be the treatment of choice (14,15).

REFERENCES

1. Fagan P, McKenzie B, Edmonds C. Sinus barotrauma in divers. *Ann Otol Rhinol Laryngol* 1976;85:61–64.
2. Weisman B, Green RS, Roberts P. Frontal sinus barotrauma. *Laryngoscope* 1972;82:2160–2168.
3. Singletary E, Reilly J. Acute frontal sinus barotrauma. *Am J Emerg Med* 1990;8:329–331.
4. Campbell PA. Aerosinusitis. *Arch Otolaryngol* 1942;35:107–114.
5. Campbell PA. Aerosinusitis—its cause and treatment. *Ann Otol Rhinol Laryngol* 1944;53:291–301.
6. Campbell PA. Aerosinusitis—a resume. *Ann Otol Rhinol Laryngol* 1945;54:69–83.
7. Garges LM. Maxillary sinus barotrauma case report and review. *Aviat Space Environ Med* 1985;56:796–802.
8. Stucker FJ, Echols WR. Otolaryngologic problems of underwater exploration. *Milit Med* 1971;136:896–899.
9. Dickey LS. Diving injuries. *J Emerg Med* 1984;249–262.
10. Neuman T, Settle H, Beaver G. Maxillary sinus barotrauma with cranial nerve involvement—case report. *Aviat Space Environ Med* 1975;46:314–315.
11. Leitch DR. Unusual case of emphysema. *Br Med J* 1969;1:383.
12. Simmerman RA, Bilaniuk L, Harkney D. Paranasal sinus hemorrhage. Evaluation with MR imaging. *Radiology* 1987;162:499–503.
13. Barrs DM, Shagets FW. Surgical treatment of recurrent frontal sinus barotrauma. *Aviat Space Environ Med* 1982;53:69–71.
14. Yarrington CT. Surgical treatment of recurrent frontal sinus barotrauma. *Aviat Space Environ Med* 1982;53:72.
15. Bolger WE, Parsons DS, Matson RE. Functional endoscopic sinus surgery in aviators with recurrent sinus barotrauma. *Aviat Space Environ Med* 1990;61:148–156.

CHAPTER 14

Sinusitis

Jack L. Gluckman, Paul D. Righi, and Dale H. Rice

Sinusitis is a common health problem in the United States affecting approximately 30 million people and accounting for nearly 16 million physician visits in 1989 (1). Given the magnitude of the problem, it is somewhat surprising that a standard definition and clear-cut nomenclature for sinusitis have never been widely adopted. In general terms, sinusitis can be defined as inflammation of the paranasal sinuses (2), the etiology of which includes both infectious agents and allergic mechanisms. The most significant risk factor for the development of sinusitis is a prior viral upper respiratory tract infection (URI); it is estimated that 0.5% of cases of URI are complicated by sinusitis (3). The reason that the exact incidence is difficult to determine is that clinically the early symptoms of sinusitis are indistinguishable from a simple URI. However, recent advances in radiologic imaging and new endoscopic techniques have improved both diagnostic and therapeutic capabilities. While sinusitis can be categorized in many ways, the most common description is by the duration of symptoms. Therefore, in this discussion, *acute* sinusitis will refer to symptoms lasting less than 4 weeks; *subacute* sinusitis 4 weeks to 3 months; and *chronic* sinusitis longer than 3 months (4,5).

PATHOGENESIS

Bacterial Sinusitis

The pathogenesis of sinusitis is multifactorial and involves a complex interaction between host defense mechanisms and the infecting organism. In order to understand the pathologic events that result in clinical sinusitis, it is necessary to review the normal physiology of the paranasal sinuses.

The key to normal sinus function is the mucociliary transport system. The nose and paranasal sinuses are lined by ciliated pseudostratified columnar epithelium (6). Epithelial goblet cells and submucosal seromucous glands produce a secretory blanket that has two components—a surface mucous layer and a deeper aqueous layer (7,8). Ciliary action moves the mucus layer toward the natural sinus ostia and then to the nasopharynx. Replenishment of the mucous layer is an ongoing process. Mucociliary transport functions as a barrier to infection by removing bacteria and inhaled particulate matter from the nose and sinuses. Moreover, the aqueous layer beneath the mucus contains immunoglobulins such as secretory IgA, IgG, IgM, and other molecules that contribute to host defense (8). Alteration in sinus ostia patency, ciliary function, or quality of secretions causes disruption of the system and leads to sinusitis (9).

The most important factor in the pathogenesis of sinusitis is the patency of the sinus ostia (10). The normal size of the ostium varies for the different sinuses but may be as small as 1 to 2 mm, which is the usual diameter of the ostia of the ethmoid sinus. Ostium size may decrease further under normal activities such as recumbency and perhaps during nasal cycle because of mucosal congestion (2). It is generally felt that the most common cause of sinus ostial obstruction, and thus secondary acute sinusitis, is viral upper respiratory tract infection (11,12) with more than half of individuals with viral upper respiratory tract infections demonstrating thickening of the sinus mucosa on radiographic imaging (13–15). Because of their unique anatomic structure with narrow ostia, the ethmoid sinuses are probably the most susceptible to ostial obstruction and infection. While usually the whole complex is affected, occasionally just a group of cells will be diseased. While obstruction of the sinus ostia in acute sinusitis is most often due to mucosal edema, in chronic sinusitis, an anatomic abnormality that interferes with drainage through the ostia is frequently present.

Obstruction of the sinus ostia, partial or complete,

results in stagnation of secretions, decreased pH (16), and lowered oxygen tension within the sinus (17,18). These changes create an environment that favors bacterial growth (16). Stagnant secretions and bacterial infection in turn cause mucosal inflammation. Subsequent damage to the mucosal epithelium and the cilia is, in large part, due to proteolytic enzymes released by leukocytes. True bacterial mucosal invasion is uncommon. With the additional swelling of the mucosa, the sinus ostia obstruct completely and the "sinusitis cycle" described by Reilly (16) is perpetuated. Oxygen tension within an obstructed sinus may drop to virtually zero, promoting growth of anaerobic and facultative bacteria (17,18), which has important implications in chronic sinusitis. Host defense mechanisms are impaired by conditions of low oxygen tension with the generation of oxygen free radicals by leukocytes being depressed, which impairs bacterial killing (2). Leukocyte function is further impaired by the low concentration of IgA, IgG, and IgM found in purulent sinus secretions (19).

Disruption of mucociliary transport in the paranasal sinuses is another key factor in the pathogenesis of sinusitis. Normal ciliary beat frequency is greater than 700 beats per minute; however, during sinusitis, the ciliary beat frequency decreases to less than 300 beats per minute. In addition, the inflammation stimulates the conversion of ciliated cells to mucus-secreting goblet cells and eventually irreversible change of the respiratory epithelium occurs (6).

In addition, the quality and character of sinus secretions change during sinusitis. Inspissated mucus, which cannot be cleared effectively from the sinuses, becomes a source of inflammation and a culture medium for bacterial growth. In addition, thickened secretions block the sinus ostia and stimulate the sinusitis cycle. This is a particular problem in patients with cystic fibrosis with failure of exocrine gland function, which results in thickened sinus secretions with the majority of patients developing sinusitis (20).

Of note is the relatively recent discovery that normal paranasal sinuses are not sterile and, in fact, harbor the same bacteria that cause acute sinusitis, confirming the important role of obstruction of the ostia. Brook demonstrated that 12 out of 12 normal patients grew anaerobic organisms, from their maxillary sinuses, with seven also growing aerobic organisms (21). The anaerobes isolated in this study were predominantly *Bacteroides* species, anaerobic gram-positive cocci, and *Fusobacterium*. Predominant aerobes were β- and α-hemolytic *Streptococci*, *Streptococcus pneumoniae*, *Hemophilus influenzae*, and *Staphylococcus aureus*. Likewise, Su and colleagues (22) found aerobic and facultative bacteria in the sinuses of seven normal patients.

Fungal Sinusitis

Fungal infection of the sinuses involves a spectrum of disease ranging from a fungus ball in the sinus to invasive fungal sinusitis. Fungal sinusitis most commonly afflicts immunosuppressed patients or those with chronic debilitating diseases such as diabetes (23). Fungal sinusitis can be categorized into noninvasive, invasive, and allergic fungal sinusitis.

Noninvasive fungal sinusitis occurs in immunocompetent hosts as a localized process. It usually involves the maxillary sinus and runs an indolent course (23). Occasionally, it may occur in an apparently normal host. Sinus ostial obstruction is the most likely precipitating event in this type of sinusitis as hypoxic conditions favor fungal growth (23). Inoculation of the sinus with a massive fungal load is another possible pathogenic mechanism (24). The nidus of fungal infection slowly increases in size within the sinus (fungus ball) without true invasion of tissue, although erosion of bone due to pressure is possible, but most unusual.

Invasive fungal sinusitis occurs predominantly as an opportunistic infection in an immunocompromised host. Patients with lymphoproliferative neoplasms such as acute leukemia are at highest risk (25). In this disease, invasion of blood vessels by fungi leads to thrombosis of the vessels and ultimately tissue necrosis. Destruction of surrounding bone is common and the risk of disseminated disease is significant.

Allergic fungal sinusitis was recognized as a separate clinical entity in 1983 by Katzenstein et al. (26), who described seven cases of allergic *Aspergillus* sinusitis in normal hosts. Histopathologically, allergic *Aspergillus* sinusitis is indistinguishable from allergic bronchopulmonary aspergillosis with mucinous material containing eosinophils, Charcot–Leyden crystals, and fungal hyphae found in both conditions. The pathogenesis of allergic fungal sinusitis probably involves a combination of types I and III Gell and Coombs hypersensitivity reactions (24). Eosinophils and fungus-specific IgE play a central role in the local tissue response. Mucosal inflammation and thickened, inspissated mucus (allergic mucin) contribute to ostial obstruction and local tissue hypoxia, which promotes fungal growth (27). Histopathologically, only a small amount of fungi are detected in allergic mucin and there is no evidence of tissue invasion. Bone erosion can occur in longstanding cases (26).

ETIOLOGY

Predisposing Factors

There are several well-recognized predisposing factors for bacterial sinusitis. As already stated, the most common of these is recurrent viral upper respiratory tract infections (11). In normal hosts, a viral URI increases the amount and decreases the viscosity of the mucus. Ciliated cells can be damaged severely by the viral infection and may take may months to recover normal function. Other predisposing factors for acute bacterial sinusitis include allergy, dental procedures, presence of a foreign body (e.g., nasotracheal tube, nasogastric tube, or nasal packing), and barotrauma. Iatrogenic causes of sinusitis are obviously becoming increasingly prevalent. Kaplan and Hoyt (28) studied adult patients hospitalized in a trauma unit and found that sinusitis accounted for 5% of all nosocomial infections observed over a 2-year period. Nosocomial sinusitis occurred in 100% of patients on mechanical ventilation, 81% of patients with nasogastric tubes, 34% of patients with facial or cranial fractures, 19% of patients with nasotracheal tubes, and 6% of patients with nasal packing. In a separate study of 111 head trauma patients by Grindlinger et al. (29), sinusitis developed in 19 patients, 16 of whom had nasotracheal intubation as opposed to oral tracheal intubation.

Factors that predisposed to chronic sinusitis include allergic rhinitis, aspirin sensitivity with hypertrophic rhinitis, nasal polyposis, various immunodeficiency disease syndromes, anatomical disorders such as septal deviation, cystic fibrosis, and immotile cilia syndromes.

Risk factors for fungal sinusitis are related to the patient's immune competency. While unusual in a normal host, fungal sinusitis occurs as a result of either hypersensitivity to the fungus (26) or as a result of changes in the local tissue milieu within the sinus, which favor fungal growth (27). Immunocompromised hosts are at risk for opportunistic fungal infections that may be life-threatening. Diabetics who develop fulminant mucormycosis infection are an example. The most significant immune deficiencies predisposing to invasive fungal sinusitis involve T-cell deficits and severe neutropenia (24).

Bacteriology

Acute Bacterial Sinusitis

The bacterial pathogens responsible for acute sinusitis in adults have been identified in studies by performing maxillary sinus aspiration on previous untreated patients. These studies show that nonencapsulated *Hemophilus influenzae* and *Streptococcus pneumoniae* account for the majority of community-acquired sinusitis (30,31). Anaerobic organisms such as *Bacteroides, Peptostreptococcus,* and *Fusobacterium* account for only 6% to 10% of acute sinus infections and are usually associated with dental infections (30). The prevalence of β-lactam-producing strains of *Hemophilus influenzae* and *Streptococcus pneumoniae* has increased in recent years. In one study, 52% of *H. influenzae* strains were β-lactam producers (31).

In children, the bacteria responsible for acute sinusitis are nearly the same as that for adults, with *H. influenzae* and *S. pneumoniae* playing a major role. However, *Moraxella catarrhalis* is responsible for approximately 20% of acute sinusitis in children. Both *H. influenzae* and *M. catarrhalis* may be β-lactamase producing, making them resistant to amoxicillin (9,32,33). The prevalence of resistant strains varies with geographic location. Recently, 75% of *M. catarrhalis* and 30% of *H. influenzae* were found to be β-lactam positive in the Pittsburgh area (33).

In nosocomial sinusitis, gram-negative bacteria predominate. In Kaplan and Hoyt's study (28), *Pseudomonas aeruginosa* was the most common organism isolated, followed by *Klebsiella pneumoniae, Enterobacter* species, *Proteus mirabilis,* and *Escherichia coli.* In the Grindlinger et al. (29) study of head-injured patients, the most common gram-negative bacilli were *Pseudomonas aeruginosa* and *Escherichia coli.* Occasionally, nosocomial sinusitis can be caused by *Actinomyces* or *Nocardia.*

Chronic Bacterial Sinusitis

Anerobes play a significant role in chronic sinusitis in adults (22,34). In a recent study, Brook (35) found that anaerobes were present in 88% of culture-positive specimens from adults with chronically inflamed maxillary sinuses. Predominant anaerobes were anaerobic cocci and *Bacteroides* species. In 21 cases (32% of aspirates), a mixture of aerobes and anaerobes was isolated. *Streptococcus* species and *Staphylococcus aureus* were the predominant aerobes. Brook (35) theorized that β-lactam-producing anaerobes liberate the enzyme into the sinus cavity, thereby protecting penicillin-susceptible bacteria, which may account for the presence of a mixed flora.

The microbiology of chronic sinusitis in children is more controversial than in adults in terms of the prevalence of anaerobic organisms. Brook (36) isolated anaerobes such as anaerobic cocci, *Bacteroides,* or *Fusobacterium* in 37 out of 40 patients with chronic sinusitis. *Staphylococcus aureus* was the most common aerobic organism found. Muntz and Lusk (37), however, isolated anaerobes in only 6% of cases of children with chronic sinusitis. Review of the methodology and patient population in these studies has led Wald (32) to conclude that in children with longstanding symptoms or symptoms severe enough to require surgery, anaerobic organisms and *Staphylococci* should be suspected.

Fungal Sinusitis

Noninvasive fungal sinusitis is most commonly caused by *Aspergillus* species (24), but other organisms have been reported including *Pseudallescheria boydii, Schizophyllum commune,* and *Alternaria* species (3). *Aspergillus* species is also the most common organism responsible for invasive fungal sinusitis in immunocompromised patients. In a recent study, *Candida* was a distant second to *Aspergillus* as an etiologic agent in sinusitis afflicting immunocompromised children (25). *Mucor* species and *Pseudallescheria boydii* have also been reported (3). While *Aspergillus* was the initial pathogen identified in allergic fungal sinusitis, many other fungal species have been implicated. *Bipolaris specifera* (38), *Alternaria* species, and *Curvularia lunata* have all been implicated in allergic fungal sinusitis (27).

CLINICAL EVALUATION

In general, sinusitis complicating a viral upper respiratory tract infection diffusely involves all the paranasal sinuses to some degree (pansinusitis). If the acute infection involves one sinus, an underlying cause should be sought (e.g., dental infection or local anatomic abnormality).

Bacterial Sinusitis

The clinical features of acute bacterial sinusitis in adults are difficult to distinguish from the common cold or even allergic rhinitis in the early phase of illness. Purulent nasal discharge and facial pain are the most common clinical findings in acute sinus infection (2). The location of the facial pain is related to the particular sinus involved. Typically, maxillary sinusitis causes pain in the cheek while ethmoid sinusitis is felt most in the area of the medial canthus. Frontal sinusitis typically gives pain in the region of the forehead and medial orbit, while sphenoid sinusitis produces retro-orbital or occipital pain. Other less frequent signs and symptoms include vague headache, halitosis, anosmia, and postnasal drip with cough. Fever is present in 50% of adult patients with acute sinusitis (4).

Physical examination often reveals a mucopurulent discharge in the region of the middle meatus, which can be secondary to maxillary, ethmoid, or frontal sinusitis. Pus in the region of the superior meatus implicates the posterior ethmoid or sphenoid sinuses. In addition, the mucosa is diffusely congested. The paranasal sinuses may be tender to palpation. In the case of dental infection secondarily involving the maxillary sinus, the offending tooth is usually tender to percussion.

The symptoms of chronic bacterial sinusitis in adults are similar to those of acute sinusitis except that the nasal congestion and purulent nasal discharge are protracted (2). Evidence of purulence emanating from the sinuses is usually present on physical examination. An underlying cause for the chronicity is usually apparent; for example, an anatomic obstruction of the sinus ostia is often found. Nasal polyps, deviated nasal septum, and persistent mucosal edema from recurrent infection or allergy are just a few of the possible etiologies of chronicity.

The symptoms of acute bacterial sinusitis in children are less specific than in adults. Children are less likely to complain of headache and facial pain. Rather, symptoms of a URI such as nasal congestion and day-time cough that persist beyond 7 days are suspicious for sinusitis (9). In addition, children with a high fever (greater than 39°C) and purulent nasal discharge associated with an upper respiratory infection probably have sinusitis, especially if there is associated mild periorbital edema (39). Physical examination is less informative in children than in adults in terms of the diagnosis of sinusitis. One may detect mild facial swelling over the involved sinus or occasionally periorbital swelling. Tenderness over the maxillary sinus is often present (39). Intranasal examination is limited to anterior rhinoscopy except in older children. Evidence of frank pus in the nose and the presence of a deviated nasal septum can often be detected by this method. Flexible or rigid endoscopy improves visualization of the sinus drainage areas and can be used on occasion in older children (40).

Subacute and chronic sinusitis in the pediatric age group usually manifests as purulent rhinorrhea with or without postnasal drip. Cough and occasionally episodes of wheezing can be present as well (41). Of note, 50% of children with chronic sinusitis demonstrate associated chronic otitis or recurrent otitis media (6) and chronic sinusitis is frequently diagnosed in children with asthma or allergic rhinitis (39). As in adults, the child suspected of having chronic sinusitis must be evaluated for a mechanical obstruction of the sinus ostia.

Fungal Sinusitis

Noninvasive fungal sinusitis is an indolent disease process that usually affects only one sinus. Characteristic symptoms include nasal congestion and facial pain (2), but it may be asymptomatic. Symptomatology and findings on physical examination usually do not distinguish this condition from chronic bacterial infection. It can, however, present with a mass effect, distorting the orbit and for practical purposes resembling a neoplasm.

Patients with *allergic fungal sinusitis* are typically healthy young adults with nasal polyposis, a history of asthma, and chronic sinusitis refractory to medical therapy. In addition, many patients have had some form of sinus surgery without relief of symptoms. It is difficult to distinguish allergic fungal sinusitis from chronic bacterial sinusitis on clinical grounds. For this reason, immunologic parameters (eosinophil count, antigen-specific IgE levels, skin sensitivity tests) and radiologic criteria are helpful to make the diagnosis preoperatively (27).

Invasive fungal sinusitis is a fulminant disease that occurs most often in immunocompromised patients. Facial pain and fever were the most common clinical findings noted in a series of pediatric patients with neoplasms who developed invasive fungal sinusitis (25). However, adults patients may be desperately ill with fungal invasion of blood vessels causing tissue ischemia and necrosis. This initially presents as black mucosal patches in the nose and palate (e.g., mucormycosis in diabetics). Progression of disease is rapid and may include intracranial extension and death (24). For this reason, a high index of suspicion should compel the clinician to constantly examine the nose for early signs of necrosis.

SPECIAL INVESTIGATIONS

A variety of diagnostic maneuvers and procedures are available to aid the clinician in establishing the diagnosis of sinusitis. The simplest of these maneuvers is *transillumination* of the maxillary and frontal sinuses, which, although still practiced by some clinicians, has been pretty much abandoned because of concern as to its clinical significance. In patients with a dull maxillary sinus on transillumination, only one-third were found to have culture-positive sinus aspirates (30), leading some authors to suggest that this technique should be discarded (42). More sensitive diagnostic modalities such as the computed tomography (CT) scan and the use of fiberoptic endoscopy have also discouraged the use of transillumination. Despite these objections, transillumination is useful in following patients for resolution of an opacified maxillary sinus initially demonstrated by sinus radiography, thereby avoiding multiple radiation exposures, particularly in patients who are pregnant (43). Wald (9) argues that in children over 10 years of age, transillumination of the sinuses is useful if it is interpreted as being completely normal.

Nasal culture for the purpose of identifying pathogenic organisms in sinusitis is not advised. Poor correlation between nasal culture results and sinus aspiration results has been well documented with contamination by *Staphylococcus aureus* being the major confounding problem (44).

Nasal cytology has been described as a means of differentiating acute sinus infection (polymorphonuclear cells) from allergic rhinitis (eosinophils). While this method is sensitive (45), it is not, in our opinion, of any real value and certainly not a substitute for sinus radiography (46).

Nasal endoscopy using the newer rigid endoscopes has greatly improved the ability to diagnose and evaluate the results of therapy for sinusitis. Visualization of the accessible components of the osteomeatal complex and a thorough evaluation of nasal anatomy are certainly possible (47) and easily performed as an office procedure under topical anesthesia. Nasal endoscopy is most suitable for adult and adolescent patients, who can cooperate as needed, but is less suitable for young children (39).

Aspiration of the maxillary sinus secretions for microscopy, culture, and sensitivity has been suggested as a diagnostic technique in those cases of sinusitis refractory to medical therapy, or in patients who are at increased risk, such as immunocompromised patients (9). Puncture is performed transnasally via the inferior meatus under local anesthesia. This can be performed quite easily in most adults and older children.

While a complete blood count and sedimentation rate have little clinical value in the evaluation of patients with symptoms of sinusitis, an absolute eosinophil count, fungus-specific IgE levels, and immediate skin test to fungal antigens are important in the diagnostic workup for fungal sinusitis (24,38).

IMAGING

The radiologic evaluation of patients with sinusitis can involve a wide range of techniques that differ in their sensitivity, specificity, indications, costs, and risks to the patient. The four modalities in current use include sinus plain films, ultrasound, CT scan, and MRI scan.

Sinus Radiographs

Plain films of the sinus are the traditional imaging technique used in evaluating patients with symptoms of sinusitis. A routine sinus series includes anteroposterior, lateral, and occipitofrontal projections (48). While plain films provide a rapid and noninvasive evaluation of the maxillary, frontal, sphenoid, and posterior ethmoid sinuses and the lower one-third of the nasal cavity, the critical area of the osteomeatal complex and the anterior ethmoid sinuses are poorly visualized (49). The specificity and sensitivity of sinus films have been examined in several studies, which compared the results of radiographs with the results of maxillary sinus puncture. From these studies, it is clear that a significant number of patients with radiographic sinus abnormalities do not have sinusitis (50). The most reliable and specific signs of sinusitis on radiographs include sinus opacification, mucosal thickening greater than 3 mm, and air–fluid levels. While very specific, these findings yield a sensitivity of approximately 50% (50). Problems with interpretation of plain films of the sinuses are magnified in children. In one study, 50% of children with no clinical evidence of sinusitis had opacified sinuses on radiograph (51). In contrast, Kovatch et al. (48) found that in children older than 1 year without signs or symptoms of upper respiratory infection, abnormal maxillary sinus radiographs were infrequent. They questioned whether adequate screening of the control group for evidence of URI had been done in previous studies.

Despite conflicting data, several points regarding the usefulness of sinus plain films can be made. A clear sinus radiograph makes significant sinus pathology unlikely. The presence of an air–fluid level in the sinus is significant in all age groups, whereas mucosal thickening remains nonspecific especially in young children. Unilateral complete opacification of a sinus is clearly abnormal and correlates well with sinusitis (50).

In summary, the usefulness of sinus radiographs in the evaluation of both children and adults with sinusitis has been diminished by the emergence of more sensitive and specific techniques such as nasal endoscopy and CT scan. However, the expense of newer modalities and the need for sedation of pediatric patients mean that sinus radiographs will likely continue to play a role in the evaluation of patients with sinusitis (52).

Computed Tomography

Computed tomography (CT) is now recognized as the single best imaging technique for paranasal sinus disease. Optimal demonstration of the ethmoid sinuses and the osteomeatal complex is achieved with thin coronal sections. Axial sections are most helpful in the evaluation of orbital complications of sinusitis. Contrast injection is rarely necessary for a benign process but may be of value if there is concern that malignant disease may coexist with bone destruction or extension outside the sinus (52). CT scan of the paranasal sinuses is indicated in the evaluation of chronic refractory sinusitis, sinusitis with complications, or possible underlying malignancy. It is also used for preoperative evaluation before endoscopic and conventional sinus surgery.

Magnetic Resonance Imaging

Magnetic resonance imaging (MRI) is emerging as a valuable tool for the evaluation of specific conditions and diseases of the paranasal sinuses. MRI has superior soft-tissue resolution compared with CT and is better at distinguishing fungal sinusitis, sinus neoplasia, and intracranial extension of sinus disease (50). Another important feature is the avoidance of ionizing radiation, which is particularly significant for children. There are several limitations of MRI, however. Resolution of bony landmarks is poor, and therefore MRI has limited value in planning endoscopic sinus surgery. Other limitations include the high cost, the small size of the machine portal (claustrophobia), and the need for sedation of most young children due to the long imaging times (52).

Ultrasonography

The role of ultrasound (US) in the evaluation of sinusitis remains unclear despite a growing experience with this technique. A-mode ultrasound, the most commonly used modality for sinusitis, emits sound waves along the axis of the transducer and produces a one-dimensional scan that is displayed on an oscilloscope (53). The transducer is placed directly over either the maxillary or frontal sinus during testing. The locations of the ethmoid and sphenoid sinuses prohibit evaluation with ultrasound. The sound waves produced are transmitted by fluid but reflected at tissue interfaces such as bone and fluid or bone and air (50). Use of this technique to diagnose sinusitis has met with varying success (50,53,54). Ultrasound appears to detect accurately fluid in the maxillary sinus, but its capacity for diagnosing mucosal thickening is limited. In one study, the low sensitivity of ultrasound led the authors to advise that a negative scan should be followed by radiographs if clinical suspicion were high (53). Currently, ultrasound is not widely used for evaluating sinusitis in the United States but is common in Europe. However, continued evaluation of this modality is probably warranted as it is a noninvasvie technique, is inexpensive, does not expose the patient to ionizing radiation, and requires minimal patient cooperation.

MEDICAL MANAGEMENT

Acute Sinusitis—Adults

The primary treatment of acute sinusitis in adults involves antibiotic therapy and decongestants (4,55,56). Use of mucolytic agents, nasal irrigation, antral lavage, and either topical or systemic steroids is usually decided on a case-by-case basis.

Antibiotic therapy is the primary treatment of acute bacterial sinusitis despite 40% of cases spontaneously resolving (9). Antibiotics are felt to facilitate recovery from the acute episode, to prevent complications of sinusitis, and to prevent progressive mucosal changes that could result in chronic sinusitis. The efficacy of antibiotics in the treatment of sinusitis has been well documented (3). Evans et al. (57) found antibiotics useful if the organism was sensitive to the agent being used. Carenfelt and Lundberg (58) showed that bacteriocidal and bacteriostatic antibiotics are equally effective, provided the concentration reached in the sinus secretions exceeds the minimum inhibitory concentration for the bacteria isolated.

Antibiotic selection in acute adult sinusitis is most often empiric as nasal cultures are unreliable and maxillary sinus aspiration is unnecessary and not performed in most uncomplicated cases. The likely pathogens are as noted above and elsewhere in this book. Duration of therapy should be at least 7 to 10 days, but a minimum of 14 days and even longer if clinically indicated has been advocated. In adults, amoxicillin, ampicillin, Ceclor, cefuroxime axetil, trimethoprim-sulfamethoxazole, and clarithromycin (58a, 58b) have all proved clinically effective (2). The choice of a particular agent depends on several factors including history of drug allergies, cost, prior tolerance to the drug, and the incidence of β-lactam-producing organisms in a particular geographic area (31). In particular, β-lactam-producing strains of *Hemophilus influenzae* and *Branhamella catarrhalis* can be problematic if ampicillin or amoxicillin are employed. However both ampicillin and clavulanate appear to be effective in irradicating most B lactainase producing *H. influenzae* (58b).

The antibiotic chosen should be given in sufficient dose to reach the minimum inhibitory concentration of likely pathogens within the sinus secretions. Eneroth and Lundberg (59) studied antibiotic levels achieved in the sinus mucosa and secretions with ordinary clinical doses of penicillin and tetracycline. They found adequate levels in only 45% of patients treated with penicillin, whereas 93% of patients treated with tetracycline achieved adequate levels. They noted that an adequate level in the secretions ensured an adequate mucosal level. These findings were confirmed by Carenfelt et al. (60) while studying penicillin, azidocillin, tetracycline, and doxycycline. They found that when antibiotic levels failed to reach the minimum inhibitory concentration for the bacteria isolated, bacterial growth was present in almost all samples aspirated 2 to 3 days after initiation of therapy. When the levels exceeded the minimum inhibitory concentration, eradication of bacteria occurred in 50% of cases. A similar study performed by Reynolds, Catlin and Cluff (61) found that 86% of patients responded within 14 days if treated with a correct antibiotic as compared to 65% treated with an incorrect or no antibiotic.

In most cases of sinusitis, *decongestants* play an important ancillary role in therapy. Decongestants are α-adrenergic drugs that produce vasoconstriction and

may be administered topically or systemically. Use of topical decongestants should be limited to 5 days or less to minimize the risk of rebound rhinitis (rhinitis medicamentosa). Beyond 5 days, decongestant therapy should consist of a systemic preparation. There are two commonly available systemic decongestants—pseudoephedrine and phenylpropanolamine. While effective in reducing nasal congestion, these medications may produce undesirable stimulation of the central nervous system and cardiovascular system. Blood pressure elevation in patients with labile hypertension can occur with use of these drugs although the risk of inducing hypertension in otherwise normal subjects is minimal (62). Because of their potential stimulatory effect, it is prudent to administer the evening dose of a decongestant several hours before bedtime or reduce the evening dose to avoid insomnia. Use of *antihistamines* in the treatment of acute purulent sinusitis is not advised as thickening of mucous secretions may further inhibit sinus drainage and ventilation.

It may be helpful to include a *mucolytic agent* in the treatment program to decrease the tenacity of the mucus. Numerous preparations have been promoted for this purpose ranging from chicken soup and horseradish to a variety of medications. Iodide preparations increase ciliary action, split mucoproteins, and possibly stimulate fibrin breakdown. However, documentation of the value of a saturated solution of potassium iodine (SSKI) is essentially anecdotal. Organic iodine, however, has been shown to be an effective mucolytic and expectorant in patients with bronchitis, although its role in treating sinusitis is less well established. Guanefesin, another mucolytic agent, is frequently used in the management of sinusitis (63). Unfortunately, guanefesin acts as an emetic in large doses and has a low therapeutic ratio. Therefore patients may experience gastrointestinal side effects from this preparation when used in appropriate dosages.

In many patients with sinusitis, great benefit is derived from regular saline *nasal irrigations* delivered with a bulb syringe or nasal irrigator (64). Saline irrigations help to move thickened secretions through the nasal cavity. To be effective, the irrigations must be thorough and must be performed several times per day.

It may, on occasion, become necessary to use a *nasal steroid aerosol* to achieve maximum reduction of edema in the area of the osteomeatal complex, especially when allergy is a precipitating factor (4). In theory, one should initiate antibiotic therapy well before adding topical steroids because steroids may inhibit the natural defense mechanisms of the sinuses. Furthermore, nasal aerosol steroids are only effective if they reach the area of sinus drainage. Obstacles to the accurate placement of nasal steroid preparations include anterior nasal edema, polypoid disease in the nose, or septal deviation with hypertrophy of the inferior turbinates. Moreover, several days of treatment with topical nasal steroids are required before a clinical effect is noted and the maximum benefit is achieved only after 1 to 2 weeks of treatment. For these reasons, the benefit of nasal aerosol steroids in sinusitis should be questioned and in our opinion is contraindicated. However, if nasal steroids are to be used, there are several preparations available to select from including beclomethasone (65), flunisolide, and triamcinolone (66).

It has been suggested that, occasionally, the treatment of bacterial sinusitis will necessitate the use of systemic steroids to improve the clinical response to therapy, particularly if the condition is proving refractory to conventional therapy. It is our belief that this should very rarely be considered and it may be frankly contraindicated in the presence of fulminant infection.

Antral lavage is indicated for patients with acute sinusitis who have proved refractory to 3 to 5 days of antibiotics with increasing discomfort and in those patients who are at risk for opportunistic infection where the rapid identification of a specific pathogen and its pattern of drug susceptibility is crucial to a favorable outcome. Details of the technique for antral lavage are discussed by Gluckman in Conventional Surgery for Infection of the Maxillary Sinus.

Acute Sinusitis—Children

Treatment of acute sinusitis in the pediatric population consists of antimicrobial therapy, decongestants, and, rarely, simple maxillary sinus puncture and irrigation (9,40). A variety of antimicrobials are available, which provide adequate coverage of the likely pathogens of acute sinusitis, and include amoxicillin, erythromycin, sulfisoxazole, trimethoprim, sulfamethoxazole, Ceclor, and Augmentin. In choosing an antibiotic, one must again consider the patient's history of drug allergies, potential side effects, previous antibiotic treatment, and the increased prevalence of β-lactamase-producing strains of *H. influenzae* and *M. catarrhalis*, which are resistent to amoxicillin and ampicillin. While *M. catarrhalis* is rarely pathogenic in adults, it is responsible for approximately 20% of acute bacterial sinusitis in young children (9).

In an uncomplicated case of maxillary sinusitis, initial therapy with amoxicillin for 10 to 14 days is reasonable. Failure to demonstrate clinical improvement over 48 to 72 hr should prompt selection of an alternative antibiotic that covers β-lactam-positive organisms. Improvement, but not resolution, of symptoms after 10 to 14 days of therapy requires continuation of the antibiotic until all symptoms have resolved (9).

While decongestants or antihistamines are often employed as adjuvant therapy in children with sinusitis, the effectiveness of these preparations has not been adequately studied (9). As discussed previously, antihistamines may have a deleterious effect by increasing the tenacity of secretions and are not recommended.

While maxillary sinus irrigation and drainage can dramatically improve symptoms in acute sinusitis, it is not used routinely in pediatric patients as antimicrobial therapy is usually adequate for acute sinusitis and sinus puncture often requires either intravenous sedation or a general anesthetic in the pediatric population, especially in young children (9). Antral lavage, however, plays a role in symptomatic children who fail to respond to medical therapy or who have a threatened complication of sinusitis. Much like the adult, immunocompromised children may require early sampling of maxillary sinus contents to determine a specific pathogen because they are at increased risk.

Chronic Sinusitis—Adults

Compared to acute sinusitis, the role of medical therapy in the treatment of chronic sinusitis is of limited value. Chronic sinus infection is a sequelae of persistent sinus obstruction, the underlying cause of which must be addressed (67). Prolonged antibiotic therapy, decongestants and topical nasal steroids, and even immunotherapy (if allergy is felt to be a causative factor) constitute the basic medical regimen used in chronic sinusitis. The microbiology of chronic sinusitis in adults differs from the acute process in that anaerobes or a mixture of aerobes and anaerobes are recovered frequently in chronic infection (2,35). Antibiotics that cover anaerobes, such as penicillin VK or clindamycin, are the appropriate choice for the treatment of chronic sinusitis. However, a recent study of chronic sinusitis in adults revealed that 44% of anaerobic isolates were β-lactamase positive (68). In these cases, penicillin would be ineffective and Augmentin or clindamycin is preferable. Minimum duration of antibiotic therapy in chronic sinusitis is 4 weeks. Decongestants, as already described, may be of some value.

Topical nasal steroids such as beclomethasone may be beneficial in chronic sinusitis especially if allergy is a predisposing factor. Unfortunately, the role of nasal steroids has not been well defined for chronic sinusitis.

Immunologic therapy is appropriate for a patient with chronic sinusitis with underlying allergy. It is an adjunctive treatment and not a substitute for either medical or surgical management. While safe and effective, immunotherapy routinely requires 6 months of treatment before a clinical benefit is noted (69).

Chronic Sinusitis—Children

The medical management of subacute and chronic sinusitis in children is, in general, similar to treatment in adults. A prolonged course of antibiotic therapy and systemic or topical decongestants as well as topical nasal steroids and appropriate immunotherapy form the cornerstones of treatment of chronic pediatric sinusitis. Selection of an appropriate antibiotic must be done carefully for several reasons. While the microbiology of subacute pediatric sinusitis is similar to acute sinusitis (5), anaerobic bacteria are commonly found in chronic sinusitis (36). In addition, most children with chronic sinusitis have failed previous antibiotic regimens and one can anticipate a high rate of β-lactamase-producing pathogens in this setting (5). Tinkelman and Silk (41) advocate maxillary sinus puncture early in the workup of children with chronic sinusitis to ensure the effectiveness of the antibiotic chosen.

As with adults, decongestants are commonly used in pediatric chronic sinusitis to decrease nasal congestion and promote sinus ventilation. In addition, topical nasal steroids play a role in the treatment of allergy-based nasal congestion because of their anti-inflammatory effects.

In children with immunodeficiency syndromes, immunotherapy in the form of immunoglobulin replacement therapy may be helpful in controlling refractory sinusitis (70).

SURGICAL TREATMENT OF CHRONIC SINUSITIS

The surgical treatment of adults with chronic sinusitis has been described comprehensively in other chapters. However, it is worthwhile to reiterate several key points. The pathogenesis of chronic sinusitis involves ostial obstruction of the sinuses with secondary bacterial infection. As such, the role of surgery in chronic sinusitis is to reestablish sinus ventilation and drainage and allow for gradual resolution of mucosal disease (47). Patients who fail comprehensive medical therapy, with demonstrated abnormalities of the osteomeatal complex on endoscopy and CT scan are candidates for surgical intervention (43,47). In addition, patients with intracranial or intraorbital complications of sinusitis will require drainage of the involved sinuses together with the surgical treatment of the complication.

The surgical management of chronic sinus disease in children is controversial. Multiple surgical approaches have been advocated including endoscopic sinus surgery, adenotonsillectomy, and inferior meatal antrostomy. The value of each of these approaches is a matter of debate. While an association exists between adenoid and tonsil disease and sinusitis, the precise relationship remains unclear. Specific indications for adenotonsillectomy in the management of chronic sinusitis, unfortunately, do not exist (71), but it stands to reason that if these are grossly enlarged or repeatedly infected,

surgical removal is appropriate. The role of endoscopic sinus surgery in the pediatric population is controversial but appears appropriate for a small minority of patients. Specific indications for surgery include true chronic sinusitis refractory to comprehensive medical therapy, suppurative complications of sinusitis, and serious underlying disease aggravated by recurrent sinusitis (72).

TREATMENT OF FUNGAL SINUSITIS

A chapter is dedicated to this condition elsewhere in this book; however a few general points can be made.

The management of both noninvasive and invasive fungal sinusitis is primarily surgical and involves debridement of diseased tissues and drainage of the involved sinuses. Noninvasive fungal sinusitis most commonly involves the maxillary sinus and is treated by surgical debridement using either a standard Caldwell–Luc approach (24) or newer endoscopic techniques (73). In these cases the fungal ball is curetted out and no bone need be removed. Usually, antifungal chemotherapy is not indicated. Invasive fungal sinusitis can be life-threatening and requires both aggressive surgical debridement and immediate antifungal chemotherapy (23,24). In fact, in high-risk patients such as immunosuppressed patients, facial pain associated with abnormal sinus radiographs may even prompt empiric antifungal and antibacterial therapy (25). Allergic fungal sinusitis is treated by surgical drainage of the involved sinus and systemic antifungal medications do not appear to be necessary (27). However, use of either intranasal steroids (74) or systemic steroids (27) seems to prevent recurrence of this condition. Duration of systemic steroid therapy is empiric currently but usually entails a tapering dose over several months (27).

SUMMARY

Sinusitis is a common health problem in both children and adults. While a minority of patients have unusual diseases that predispose them to sinusitis, most cases of sinusitis develop as a complication of viral upper respiratory tract infections. The central role of sinus ostial obstruction in the pathogenesis of acute and chronic sinusitis is only now being appreciated. Medical therapy alone is sufficient in the vast majority of cases of acute sinusitis while surgical intervention plays a major role in the treatment of refractory or chronic sinusitis. Fungal sinusitis is uncommon in immunocompetent patients, but an increasing number and variety of cases are being reported in immunocompromised patients, in part due to improvements in diagnostic and imaging techniques. Complications of sinusitis can be severe if diagnosis is delayed; urgent medical and surgical therapies are required. As our knowledge of the pathogenesis and pathophysiology of sinusitis increases, we are better able to prevent the development of chronic sinus disease and better able to treat such problems should they occur.

REFERENCES

1. Kennedy D. Overview. *Otolaryngol Head Neck Surg* 1990; 103(5):847–855.
2. Malow JB, Creticos CM. Nonsurgical treatment of sinusitis. *Otol Clin North Am* 1989;22(4):809–818.
3. Bamberger DM. Antimicrobial treatment of sinusitis. *Semin Respir Infect* 1991;6(2):77–84.
4. Stafford CT. The clinician's view of sinusitis. *Otolaryngol Head Neck Surg* 1990;103(5):870–875.
5. Wald ER, Byers C, et al. Subacute sinusitis in children. *J Pediatr* 1989;115(1):28–32.
6. Yonkers AJ. Sinusitis—inspecting the causes and treatment. *Ear Nose Throat J* 1992;71(6):258–262.
7. Wagenmann M, Naclerio RM. Anatomic and physiologic considerations in sinusitis. *J Allergy Clin Immunol* 1992;90(3):419–423.
8. Kaliner MA. Human nasal host defense and sinusitis. *J Allergy Clin Immunol* 1992;90(3):424–430.
9. Wald ER. Sinusitis in infants and children. *Ann Otol Rhinol Laryngol* 1992;101:37–41.
10. Slavin RG. Sinusitis in adults. *J Allergy Clin Immunol* 1988;81: 1028.
11. Gwaltney JM. Sinusitis. In: Benett MD, ed. *Principles and practice of infectious disease.* New York: Wiley, 1979;458.
12. Turner BW, Cail WS, Hendley JO, et al. Physiologic abnormalities in the paranasal sinuses during experimental rhinovirus colds. *J Allergy Clin Immunol* 1992;90(3):474–478.
13. Rachelefsky GS, Kate RM, Siegel SC. Chronic sinus disease with associated reactive airway disease in children. *Pediatrics* 1984;73:526–529.
14. Naclerio RM. Allergic rhinitis. *New Engl J Med* 1991;325: 860–869.
15. Slavin RG. Sinusitis—present state of the art. *Allergy Proc* 1991; 12:163–165.
16. Reilly JS. The sinusitis cycle. *Otolaryngol Head Neck Surg* 1990;103(5):856–862.
17. Carenfelt C, Lundberg C. Purulent and non-purulent maxillary sinus secretions with respect to Po_2, Pco_2 and pH. *Acta Otolaryngol* 1977;85:116.
18. Drettner B, Aust R. Pathophysiology of the paranasal sinuses. *Acta Otolaryngol* 1977;83:16.
19. Daley CL, Sande M. The runny nose: infection of the paranasal sinuses. *Infect Dis Clin North Am* 1988;2:131.
20. Ramsey B, Richardson MA. Impact of sinusitis in cystic fibrosis. *J Allergy Clin Immunol* 1992;90(3):547–551.
21. Brook I. Aerobic and anaerobic bacterial flora of normal maxillary sinuses. *Laryngoscope* 1971;92:372.
22. Su W, Liu C, Hung SY, Tsai WF. Bacteriological study in chronic maxillary sinusitis. *Laryngoscope* 1983;93:931.
23. Parnes LS, Brown DH, Garcia B, et al. Mycotic sinusitis: a management protocol. *J Otolaryngol* 1989;18(4):176–180.
24. Corey JP, Romberger CF, et al. Fungal diseases of the sinuses. *Otolaryngol Head Neck Surg* 1990;103(6):1012–1015.
25. Kavanagh KT, Hughes WT, Parham DM, et al. Fungal sinusitis in immunocompromised children with neoplasms. *Ann Otol Rhinol Laryngol* 1991;100:331–336.
26. Katzenstein AA, Sale SR, Greenberger PA. Allergic *Aspergillus* sinusitis: a newly recognized form of sinusitis. *J Allergy Clin Immunol* 1983;72(1):89–93.
27. Corey JP. Allergic fungal sinusitis. *Otolaryngol Clin North Am* 1992;25(1):225–230.
28. Kaplan ES, Hoyt NJ. Nosocomial sinusitis. *JAMA* 1982;247: 839.
29. Grindlinger GA, Niehoff J, Hughes L, et al. Acute paranasal sinusitis related to nasotracheal intubation of head injured patients. *Crit Care Med* 1987;15:214.
30. Winther B, Gwaltney JM. Therapeutic approach to sinusitis: anti-infectious therapy as the baseline of management. *Otolaryngol Head Neck Surg* 1990;103(5):876–879.
31. Gwaltney JM, Scheld WM, Sande DM, et al. The microbial etiology and antimicrobial therapy of adults with acute community-acquired sinusitis: a fifteen-year experience at the University of Virginia and review of other selected studies. *J Allergy Clin Immunol* 1992;90(3):457–461.
32. Wald ER. Microbiology of acute and chronic sinusitis in children. *J Allergy Clin Immunol* 1992;90(3):452–456.
33. Wald ER. Antimicrobial therapy of pediatric patients with sinusitis. *J Allergy Clin Immunol* 1992;90(3):469–473.
34. Frederick J, Braude AL. Anaerobic infection of the paranasal sinuses. *N Engl J Med* 1974;290:135.
35. Brook I. Bacteriology of chronic maxillary sinusitis in adults. *Ann Otol Rhinol Laryngol* 1989;98:426–428.
36. Brook I. Bacteriologic features of chronic sinusitis in children. *JAMA* 1981;246:967–969.
37. Muntz HR, Lusk RP. Bacteriology of the ethmoid bulla in children with chronic sinusitis. *Arch Otolaryngol Head Neck Surg* 1991;117:179–181.
38. Gourley DS, Whisman BA, Jorgensen NL, et al. Allergic *Bipolaris* sinusitis: clinical and immunopathologic characteristics. *J Allergy Clin Immunol* 1990;85:583–591.
39. Fireman P. Diagnosis of sinusitis in children: emphasis on the history and physical examination. *J Allergy Clin Immunol* 1992; 90(3):433–436.
40. Lusk RP, Lazar RH, et al. The diagnosis and treatment of recurrent and chronic sinusitis in children. *Pediatr Clin North Am* 1989;36(6):1411–1421.
41. Tinkelman DG, Silk HJ. Clinical and bacteriologic features of chronic sinusitis in children. *Am J Dis Child* 1989;143:938–941.
42. Druce HM. Diagnosis of sinusitis in adults: history, physical examination, nasal cytology, echo, and rhinoscope. *J Allergy Clin Immunol* 1992;90(3):436–441.
43. Richtsmeier WJ. Medical and surgical management of sinusitis in adults. *Ann Otol Rhinol Laryngol* 1992;101:46–50.
44. Gwaltney JM, Sydnor A, et al. Etiology and antimicrobial treatment of acute sinusitis. *Ann Otol Rhinol Laryngol Suppl* 1981; 90:68–71.
45. Wilson NW, Jalowayski AA, et al. A comparison of nasal cytology with sinus X-rays for the diagnosis of sinusitis. *Am J Rhinol* 1988;2:55–59.
46. Gill FF, Neiburger JB. The role of nasal cytology in the diagnosis of chronic sinusitis. *Am J Rhinol* 1989;3(1):13–15.
47. Kennedy DW. Surgical update. *Otolaryngol Head Neck Surg* 1990;103(5):884–886.
48. Kovatch AL, Wald ER, et al. Maxillary sinus radiographs in children with nonrespiratory complaints. *Pediatrics* 1984;73(3): 306–308.
49. Zinreich SJ. Imaging of chronic sinusitis in adults. X-ray, computed tomography, and magnetic resonance imaging. *J Allergy Clin Immunol* 1992;90(3):445–451.
50. Kuhn JP. Imaging of the paranasal sinuses: current status. *J Allergy Clin Immunol* 1986;77(1):6–8.
51. Maresh MM, Washburn AH. Paranasal sinuses from birth to late adolescence: clinical and roentgenographic evidence of infection. *Am J Dis Child* 1940;60:841.
52. Diament MJ. The diagnosis of sinusitis in infants and children: X-ray, computed tomography, and magnetic resonance imaging. *J Allergy Clin Immunol* 1992;90(3):442–444.
53. Rohr AS, Spector SL, Siegel SC, et al. Correlation between A-mode ultrasound and radiography in the diagnosis of maxillary sinusitis. *J Allergy Clin Immunol* 1986;78(1):58–61.
54. Landman MD. Ultrasound screening for sinus disease. *Otolaryngol Head Neck Surg* 1986;94(2):157–164.
55. Aust R, Drettner B. Oxygen tension in the human maxillary sinus under normal and pathological conditions. *Acta Otolaryngol* 1974;78:264.
56. Axelsson A, Chidekel N. Symptomatology and bacteriology correlated to radiologic findings in acute maxillary sinusitis. *Acta Otolaryngol* 1972;74:118.

57. Evans FO Jr, Syndor JB, Moore WE, et al. Sinusitis of the maxillary atrum. *N Engl J Med* 1975;293:735.
58. Carenfelt C, Lundberg C. Aspects of the treatment of maxillary sinusitis. *Scand J Infect Dis Suppl* 1976;9:78.
58a. Dubois J, Saint-Pierre C, Tremblay C. Efficacy of clarithromycin vs. amoxicillin/clavulanate in the treatment of acute maxillary sinusitis. *ENT Journal* 1993;72(12):804–810.
58b. Karma P, Pukander J, Penttila M, et al. The comparative efficacy and safety of clarithromycin and amoxycillan in the treatment of outpatients with acute maxillary sinusitis. *J Antimicrob Chemother* 1991;27(Suppl A):83–90.
59. Eneroth CM, Lundberg C. The antibacterial effects of antibiotics in the treatment of maxillary sinusitis. *Acta Otolaryngol* 1976; 81:475.
60. Carenfelt C, Eneroth CM, Lundberg C, Wretland B. Evaluation of the antibiotic effect of treatment of maxillary sinusitis. *Scand J Infect Dis* 1975;7:259.
61. Reynolds RC, Catlin RI, Cluff LE. Bacteriology and antibiotic treatment of acute maxillary sinusitis. *Bull Johns Hopkins Hosp* 1964;114:269.
62. Mabry RL. Pharmacotherapy with immunotherapy for the treatment of otolaryngolic allergy. *Ear Nose Throat J* 1990;69:63–71.
63. Ziment I. Help for an overtaxed mucociliary system: managing abnormal mucus. *J Respir Dis* 1991;12:21–33.
64. Druce HM. Adjuncts to medical management of sinusitis. *Otolaryngol Head Neck Surg* 1990;103(5):880–883.
65. Mabry RL. Use and misuse of cromolyn and corticosteroids. *Am J Rhinol* 1991;5:121–124.
66. Storms WW. Clinical experiences with triamcinolone in rhinitis. *J Respir Dis Suppl* 1991;12:S34–S39.
67. Lanza DC, Kennedy DW. Current concepts in the surgical management of chronic and recurrent acute sinusitis. *J Allergy Clin Immunol* 1992;90(3):505–510.
68. Brook I. Diagnosis and management of anaerobic infections of the head and neck. *Ann Otol Rhinol Laryngol* 1992;101:9–13.
69. Evans R III. Environmental control and immunotherapy for allergic disease. *J Allergy Clin Immunol* 1992;90(3):462–468.
70. Polmar SH. The role of the immunologist in sinus disease. *J Allergy Clin Immunol* 1992;90(3):511–514.
71. Lusk RP. Surgical modalities other than ethmoidectomy. *J Allergy Clin Immunol* 1992;90(3):538–542.
72. Manning SC. Surgical management of sinus disease in children. *Ann Otol Rhinol Laryngol* 1992;101:42–45.
73. Stammberger H. Endoscopic surgery for mycotic and chronic recuring sinusitis. *Ann Otol Rhinol Laryngol Suppl* 1985;119: 1–11.
74. Allphin AL, Strauss M, et al. Allergic fungal sinusitis: problems in diagnosis and treatment. *Laryngoscope* 1991;101:815–820.

CHAPTER 15

Orbital Complications of Sinusitis

Paul J. Donald

Because of the proximity of the paranasal sinuses to the eyes, orbital complications can arise from acute to chronic infection in any of the sinus cavities (Fig. 1). Moreover, most of the walls common to the orbit and the sinuses are exceptionally thin and occasionally dehiscent. In Lang's series (1) of 117 adult specimens, 14% of the time, the course of the infraorbital nerve is dehiscent in the roof of the maxillary sinus. He also found a 35% incidence of rarefication and 11.7% incidence of dehiscence between the orbit and the anterior ethmoidal cells. Furthermore, between the posterior cells and the orbit, rarefication is seen in 26% and dehiscence in 14% of cases. Between anterior cells and the orbit, rarefications were found by Ohnishi (2) in 38% of specimens and 14% showed actual defects. These areas of thinning and rarefaction were principally found along the courses of the anterior and posterior ethmoidal nerves. The barriers to the spread of infection in those natural dehiscences or those that are the result of bone erosion by infection are limited to the submucosa of the sinus and the periorbita lining the orbit.

The floor of the orbit is shared in common with the roof of the maxillary sinus. The medial orbital wall, the lamina papyracea, is in common with the medial wall of the ethmoids. The roof of the orbit anteriorly is variably comprised of the floor of the orbital ethmoid cells and the floor of the frontal sinus. The sphenoid sinus is related superiorly to the optic nerve, the canal of which is often very thin, even less than 1 mm thick in some patients, but is rarely ever dehiscent. In Lang's series, no dehiscences at all were found in the sphenoid sinus. A more anteriorly extending sphenoidal sinus will be related to the posteromedial aspect of the globe's apex. The nerve is usually found in the superolateral aspect of the sinus and often projects into the sinus lumen. The optic canal wall thickens as a more posterior progression is made and the chiasm is approached.

The other vital neurovascular area at the orbital apex, other than the optic canal, is the superior orbital fissure (Fig. 2). The fissure has a club-like appearance with the handle directed superiorly and the expanded end inferiorly. Exiting from the anterior aspect of the middle cranial fossa, the contents of this fissure are responsible for the motility and sensation of the globe. In addition, the sensory supply to the periorbital tissues is subserved as well. The superior and inferior orbital fissures are confluent and form a boomerang-like configuration with the apex pointed medially. Near their point of juncture, but more into the inferior fissure, is located the foramen rotundum. The optic canal lies independently and sits just medial but slightly superior to the angle of the boomerang. The contents of the compartment are divided by the annulus of Zinn (Fig. 3). This fibrous structure is the origin of the rectus muscles of the eye. The ring is attached posteriorly to dura and laterally to the lesser wing of the sphenoid medially and the greater wing laterally. The lateral attachment in part is through a spine of the greater wing (the spine of Merkel) (3). The superior oblique and levator palpebral superioris arise from the lesser wing just posterior and medial to the annulus. The optic nerve goes through the central portion of the annulus and a leash of nerves and vessels through its lateral part. It has been dubbed the oculomotor foramen (4) (Fig. 4). This lateral part spans the inferior portion of the superior orbital fissure dividing the fissure's contents into two parts (Fig. 3). Within the oculomotor foramen emanates the superior and inferior divisions of the oculomotor nerves laterally. Medially, the nasal branch of the ophthalmic division of the trigeminal nerve exits superiorly and the abducens nerve inferiorly. Outside the annulus, superiorly in the fissure, lies the lacrimal nerve superiorly and the frontal nerve inferolaterally—both branches of the first division of the fifth cranial nerve. Inferomedially in this compartment,

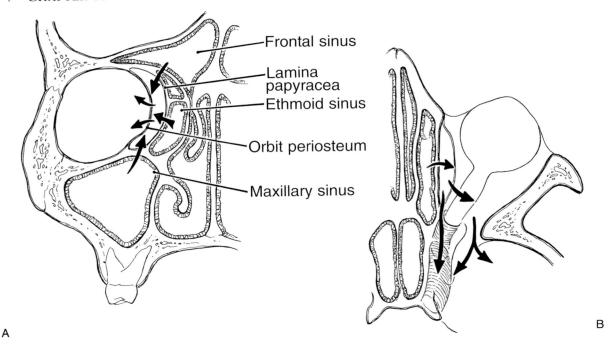

FIG. 1. Routes of spread of paranasal sinus infection to the orbit. **A:** Spread from ethmoid and maxillary sinuses. **B:** Spread from posterior ethmoid and sphenoid sinuses.

lying in a small separate fibrous sheath, is the trochlear nerve. The superior ophthalmic vein runs through the supra-annular compartment and the inferior ophthalmic vein through the infra-annular part. These veins lead directly into the cavernous sinus.

Inflammatory conditions of the sphenoid sinus can profoundly influence the orbital contents because of the immediate proximity of the lateral sinus wall to the medial aspect of the cavernous sinus (Fig. 5). Indeed, the intracranial sphenoid periosteum at this site provides the medial wall of the cavernous sinus. The internal carotid artery with the abducent nerve plastered against its lateral wall is so intimately related to the lateral wall of the sphenoid sinus that it commonly produces an easily recognizable ridge (Fig. 6).

The anterior extension of the cavernous sinus is the

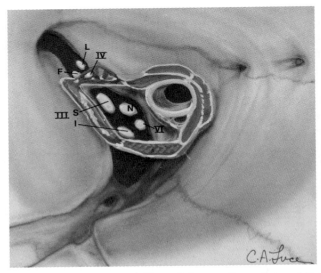

FIG. 2. Relationship of the superior orbital fissure, optic foramen, and inferior orbital fissure. Note position of the foramen rotundum near the junction of the superior and inferior orbital fissure. SOF, superior orbital fissure; FR, foramen rotundum; IOF, inferior orbital fissure. (From ref. 4, with permission.)

FIG. 3. The annulus of Zinn. It forms the origin of the rectus muscles of the eye (see text). L, lacrimal nerve; F, frontal nerve; S, superior branch of the oculomotor nerve; I, inferior orbital nerve; N, nasal nerve.

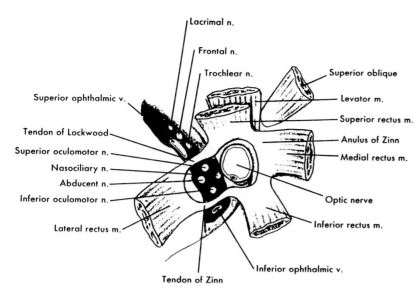

FIG. 4. The contents of the oculomotor foramen. Note that the superior oblique and the levator muscles take origin from the lesser wing of the sphenoid just outside the annulus of Zinn. (From ref. 3, with permission.)

coalescence of the inferior and superior ophthalmic veins. This is an important consideration in cavernous sinus thrombosis. The cavernous sinus is the site of confluence of a number of intracranial sinuses and extracranial veins (Fig. 7). The inferior and superior petrosal sinuses provide the most significant contribution in terms of sinuses, but a smaller connection called the circular sinus serves to join the cavernous sinus across the midline. This sinus travels in the dural reflections of the diaphragma sellae around the pituitary stalk. This connection is the reason why afflictions such as cav-

ernous sinus thrombosis are so commonly bilateral. Another link between these sinuses is provided by the basilar venous plexus. This midline structure is found on the cranial surface of the clivus and is an interconnecting lacework of venous channels. The inferior petrosal sinuses connect with the plexus both superiorly and inferiorly and are also directly connected superiorly to the cavernous sinus. The plexus has its connections to the cavernous sinus via the corticocavernous branches (6).

The extracranial connections of the cavernous sinus permit access for microbes from superficial facial and oral cavity infections to enter into the intracranial cavity. The inferior and superior orbital veins coalesce in the orbital apex as a single vessel that then drains into the anterior aspect of the cavernous sinus. The connec-

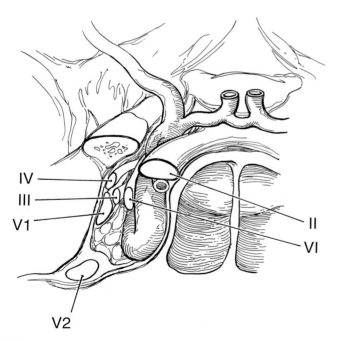

FIG. 5. Coronal section of the sphenoid sinus showing the immediate relationship of the cavernous sinus.

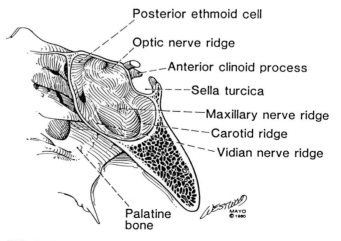

FIG. 6. Lateral wall of the sphenoidal sinus showing the ridges produced by structures contained within the cavernous sinus. (From ref. 5, with permission.)

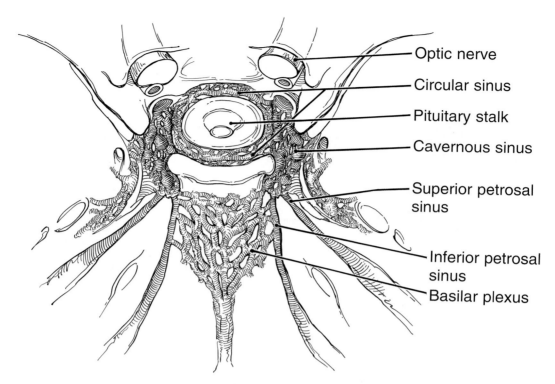

FIG. 7. Cavernous sinus and its connections.

tion of the angular vein in the anterior midface, traversing the nasal jugal area, to the inferior ophthalmic vein provides a route of spread of infection to the sinus. The pterygoid plexus within the medial and lateral pterygoid muscles close to their origins from the pterygoid plates constitute a robust venous network that connects to the sinus inferiorly through the so-called unnamed foramen of Vesalius. This plexus provides access for infection from the upper teeth and the maxillary and ethmoid sinuses.

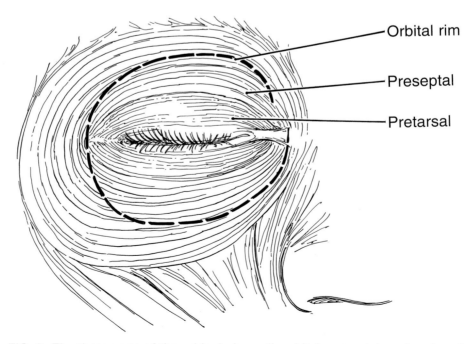

FIG. 8. The three parts of the orbicularis oculi: orbital, preseptal, and pretarsal.

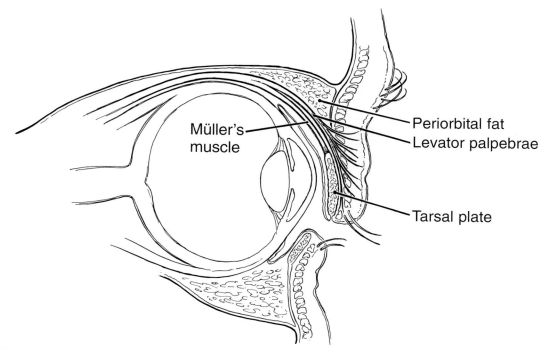

FIG. 9. Anatomy of the upper eyelid. Note orbital septum dividing lid into preseptal and postseptal parts.

Finger-like projections of the sinus often protude along the maxillary and especially the mandibular branches of the trigeminal nerve. The sinus commonly invests part or all of the gasserian ganglion as it sits in Meckel's cave. Venous channels coursing with the inferior alveolar nerve provide direct access from the mandibular teeth to the cavernous sinus.

An understanding of the compartmentalization of the periorbital soft tissues allows for a clearer comprehension of the pathophysiology of orbital infection. The loose skin of the eyelids lies directly over the orbicularis oculi with only scant subcutaneous fat between. The orbicularis has three parts: orbital, preseptal, and pretarsal (Fig. 8). Deep to the muscle lies the tarsal plate inferiorly and between the superior limbus of the tarsus and the orbital rim lies the septum orbitale. The septum orbitale is the continuation of orbital periosteum that connects the rim with the tarsal plate (Fig. 9). In the upper lid, the levator palpebrae superioris and the underlying Müller's palpebral muscle traverse the roof of the orbit and descend in the upper lid. Posterior to the orbital septum, the levator becomes aponeurotic, blends with the septum orbitale, and inserts on the tarsal plate. Some fibers of the levator are inserted into the skin at the upper level of the tarsal plate, but the main insertion is to the lower two-thirds of the anterior aspect of the plate itself. Müller's muscle inserts directly on the superior limbus of the tarsal plate.

In the lower lid, no analogue to the levator exists but a muscle similar to the Müller's muscle—Horner's muscle—acts as a sympathetically innervated retractor. The major retractor, although weak compared to the levator complex of the upper lid, is the capsulopalpebral part of the inferior rectus muscle. The periorbital fat is present behind the septum orbitale and with age bulges forward as the septum thins, constituting pseudoherniations at these sites.

An important consideration in the compartmentalization of the eye is the presence of lateral and medial extensions of the levator aponeurosis to the orbital rim margins. These extensions are strong and thick laterally and divide the lacrimal gland into two portions. However, they are much thinner and more flimsy medially as they encircle the superior oblique tendon and insert on the medial canthal tendon (7).

The eye is further divided by the presence of the muscular cone. The intraconal compartment exists within the extraocular muscles as they traverse the orbit from the annulus to their insertion on the globe. The extraconal space is within the periorbita but outside the ocular muscles.

PATHOGENESIS AND PATHOPHYSIOLOGY

Approximately 75% of all orbital infections in patients are directly related to sinusitis. In most cases, this arises as a result of ethmoid disease (8,9). The spread to the orbit may occur in several ways: direct

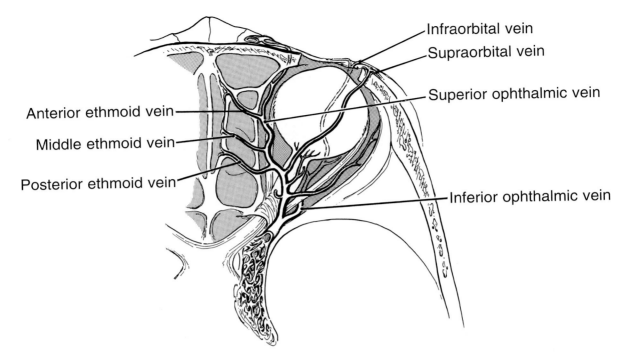

FIG. 10. The ethmoid veins and the venous drainage of the orbit.

penetration through bony dehiscences, osteitis of bone, and retrograde thrombophlebitis. The spread along the penetration of vessels through vascular foramina and via the veins within these natural eventrations in bone is a common route. The manifold connections between the ethmoid veins and those of the orbit are illustrated in Fig. 10. The fact that these veins are valveless probably facilitates the spread of infection along their course.

Orbital complications of sinusitis are more commonly seen in children. The site of origin is related at least in part to the stages of sinus development. Thus maxillary sinus infection is a common predisposing infection in infants and very young children, ethmoiditis in school-age children, and ethmoid and frontal sinusitis in adolescents and adults (10). Fearon et al. (11) believe that the increased frequency of orbital complications in children is related directly to their frequency of upper respiratory tract infection, increased diploic bone in sinus walls, and the greater degree of bony vascularity. The relative thinness of the individual bones and the openness of suture lines are other contributing factors. In addition, the relatively small sinus ostia are predisposed to obstruction from inflammation more quickly than in the adult.

In young children, the commonest organism cultured in these infections is *Hemophilus influenzae pneumoniae;* other streptococci and *Staphylococcus aureus* are less commonly seen. In the Rabinstein and Handler (12) series, 74% of all *H. influenzae* cultured were from children under the age of three. In the Schramm et al (9)

series of 303 orbital complications following sinusitis, positive blood cultures were seen in 33% of children under 4 years old, 16% in those aged 4 to 8, an 5% in older children and adults. They found that *H. influenzae* was commonest in young children. Blood cultures in adults were of little value. On the other hand, cultures from periorbital abscesses and purulent nasal secretions are much more revealing (7,13). *Staphylococcus* and *Streptococcus pneumoniae* are most common. Mixed cultures and those containing penicillin-sensitive *Bacteroides* are also seen (13). Approximately 33% to 50% of cultures grow no organisms, presumably due to pretreatment with antibiotics prior to obtaining the swab.

Cultures of abscess contents, purulent nasal secretions, nasopharyngeal drainage, and eye secretions should always be done in an attempt to establish the etiologic agent. Although controversial, Rabinstein and Handler (12) as well as Borkin et al. (14) have data to support the utility of culture of conjunctival aspirates.

Mucormycosis, a particularly virulent variety of sinusitis, usually presents with orbital complications. A detailed discussion of this disease entity is presented in the chapter, Fungal Infections, by Donald.

Orbital complications may occur as inflammatory sequelae initiated by disease processes other than acute and chronic sinusitis. The presence of foreign bodies can initiate inflammation directly or cause sinusitis by obstruction of natural ostia. Both benign and malignant tumors produce inflammation also from sinus obstruc-

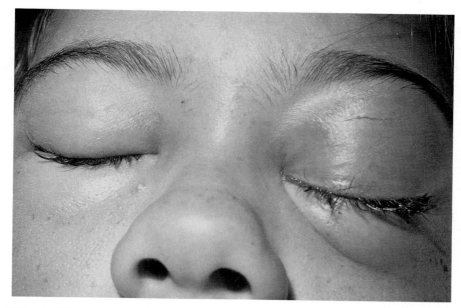

FIG. 11. Patient with cavernous sinus thrombophlebitis secondary to swimming in dirty water.

tion and from tumor necrosis, as well as blockage of venous and lymphatic pathways. Maxillofacial trauma can set the stage for infection by mucosal disruption, sinus obstruction, and hematoma formation. Wegener's granulomatosis may present with orbital inflammatory manifestations. Orbital cellulitis may be a manifestation of a number of systemic diseases such as leukemia, immunodepressive disorders, sickle cell anemia, rheumatoid arthritis, or diabetes (10).

Certain predisposing factors such as swimming in dirty water (Fig. 11), barosinusitis induced from rapid ascent or descent in a pressurized environment, and excessive nose blowing (15) in the presence of sinusitis can set the stage for an orbital complication.

CLINICAL PRESENTATION

Chandler et al. (16) in 1970 introduced a schematic of inflammatory orbital complications of gradually increasing severity. This was based on a commonly encountered scenario in an era when effective antibiotics were not as available as they are presently for the management of severe acute sinusitis. There appeared to be a natural progression of worsening of the condition with time. This model of a series of relatively distinct diagnoses as a spectrum of disease is clinically very useful, although each entity can exist without those of lesser severity preceding it in time. These five groups or stages of disease (Fig. 12) were originally proposed by Hubert (17) in 1937. These stages are listed in Table 1.

The first and most benign stage is that of *periorbital cellulitis*. This is most commonly seen in children; and

in the modern era with rapid access to health care and the early use of antibiotics, orbital inflammatory disease rarely progresses beyond this point. In the series by Fearon et al. (11) 133 of 159 cases of orbital complications from sinusitis were periorbital cellulitis. The group of 303 patients with orbital involvement followed by Schramm et al. (9) contained 82% with periorbital cellulitis. In maxillary sinusitis the lower lid is most commonly involved, while in the ethmoids it is usually the upper eyelid. The limitation of spread of edema and erythema is imposed by the septum orbitale. The septum presents a significant barrier to the spread of infection into the orbit proper. Periorbital cellulitis has been described by some as "preseptal cellulitis" (18). In the series by Goodwin et al. (8), 97% of orbital complications were located anteriorly to the septum. This comes about by the presence of venous obstruction and the local inflammatory response.

Although the lids may be swollen shut (Fig. 13), there is no chemosis, loss of visual acuity, interference with ocular motion, or proptosis. The eye is painful and tender. Funduscopic exam is normal.

When infection breaks through the septum or penetrates directly from the ethmoid sinuses through the lamina papyracea, there is an acute inflammatory response throughout the soft tissues that encircle the globe. This is called orbital cellulitis. Edema, inflammatory cells, and distended vessels cause proptosis. The inflammatory process can be postseptal and extraconal or intraconal in location or can occupy all or parts of these spaces (19). Obstruction to conjunctival lymphatics results in conjunctival edema and is called chemosis (Fig. 14). Swelling of the conjunctival tissues

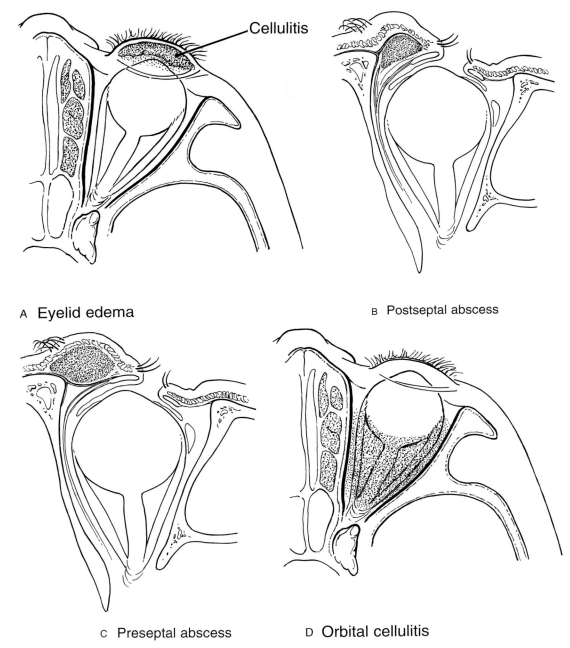

FIG. 12. Various forms and stages of orbital inflammatory disease progressing from less severe periorbital cellulitis to cavernous sinus thrombophlebitis.

may progress to such a degree that they may protrude between the lids. Ulceration may ensue that can lead to a panophthalmitis and loss of the eye. In *H. influenzae* infections, the coloration of the swollen lids as well as the congested nasal mucosa is said to be purplish in color.

As inflammation of the muscles proceeds with immediate extraconal and intraconal involvement, reduction of ocular motility ensues. Movement of the eye is painful as well as impeded. With intraconal involvement,

inflammation of the fat and connective tissues around the optic nerve leads to diminished visual acuity.

A *subperiosteal abscess* results from the accumulation of pus under the periosteum lining the orbit. These subperiorbital abscesses evolve from extensions from any of the sinuses adjacent to the orbital walls. By far, the commonest source of these abscesses is from infection of the ethmoid labyrinth. The next commonest is the frontal sinus and the least common is the maxillary. The frontal sinus source is usually from a

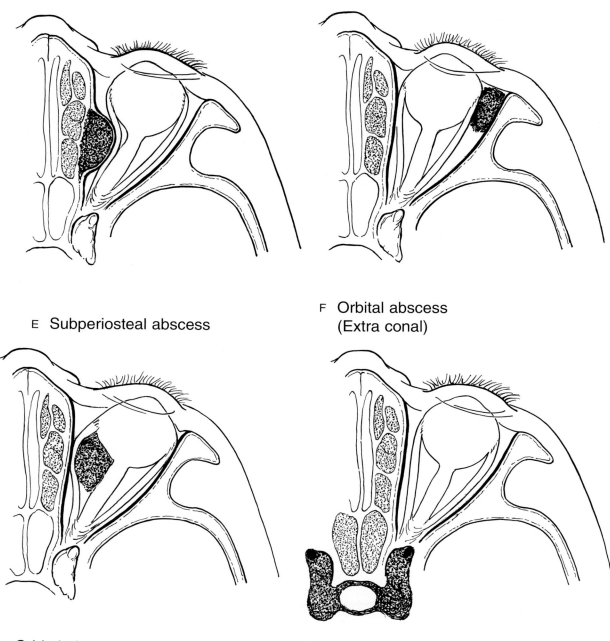

E Subperiosteal abscess

F Orbital abscess
(Extra conal)

G Orbital abscess
(Intra conal)

H Cavernous sinus
thrombosis

FIG. 12. *Continued.*

TABLE 1. *Stages of disease*

1. Periorbital cellulitis
2. Orbital cellulitis
3. Inflammatory orbital hematoma (20)
4. Subperiosteal abscess
5. Orbital abscess
6. Cavernous sinus thrombosis

mucopyocele. The purulent accumulation displaces the globe (Fig. 15) away from the collection. Proptosis and displacement in an outer and downward direction are the most usual (13).

In rare instances, a subperiosteal abscess may be preceded by a *subperiosteal hematoma*. This hematoma is not traumatic in origin but results from sudden enlargement of the veins from secondary inflammation in the area with subsequent rupture. Necrosis of these

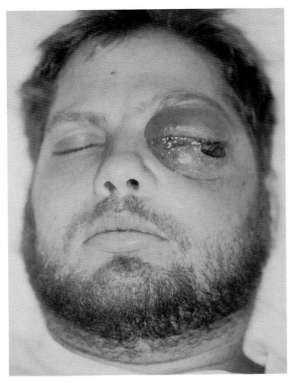

FIG. 13. Patient with periorbital cellulitis secondary to ethmoid sinusitis.

vessels by the infection may also be responsible for this hematoma. This was first associated with acute ethmoiditis by Choi et al. (20) in 1988 but was probably first described by Wheeler (21) in 1937 associated with a frontal sinusitis. Harris et al. (22) in 1978 and Calcaterra and Trapp (23) in 1988 also described a similar

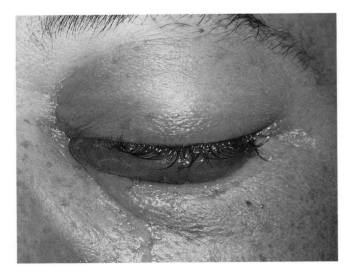

FIG. 14. Chemosis of conjunctiva.

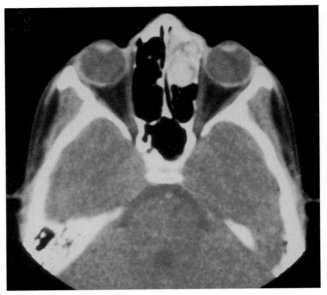

FIG. 15. CAT scan of subperiosteal abscess of the orbit showing lateral displacement of the globe.

scenario, the former from a frontal sinusitis and the latter from an ethmoid sinusitis. Severe sudden painful proptosis is a common presenting symptom.

Orbital abscess is a most serious complication of sinus infection. Infection has broken through a preseptal abscess or cellulitis or subperiosteal abscess. Direct erosion through the periorbita by a rapidly progressing sinusitis or the coalescence of an orbital cellulitis can produce an orbital abscess.

The pus loculates often medially adjacent to the infected ethmoid sinus. Multiple abscesses may occur throughout the various compartments of the orbit. Gas-producing organisms will produce gas bubbles within the purulent collection and are pathognomonic of abscess. The pus bathes the periorbital muscles and the optic nerve (Fig. 16). Intraconal abscesses rapidly produce a fixed globe and blindness. Severe proptosis, displacement in the direction opposite to the location of the abscess, complete ophthalmoplegia, chemosis, optic neuritis, vascular ischemia, and blindness rapidly ensue. Irreversible optic nerve head degeneration and retinal damage occur with vascular occlusion longer than 90 minutes (24).

The most catastrophic and feared complication of sinus infection and orbital involvement is *cavernous sinus thrombosis*. It was originally described by Bright in 1831 and since then over 1000 cases have been described in the literature (25–30). It is in reality a cavernous sinus thrombophlebitis. Retrograde thrombophlebitis from the supraorbital or infraorbital veins extends into this vascular space. Any infection with venous drainage into this central watershed can result in cav-

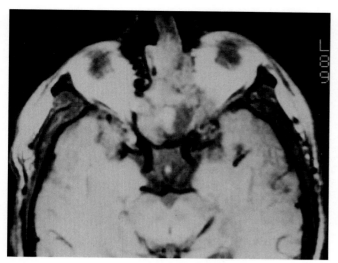

FIG. 16. CAT scan of orbital abscess showing pus in area of optic nerve and ocular muscles.

ernous sinus thrombosis. Infections from such disparate sites as the nasal tip, molar tooth, or ear and mastoid can spread to this area. The commonest source, however, is from an orbital complication of sinusitis, usually an orbital abscess. In the author's experience this is a very rare complication and is usually seen most often as the result of mucormycocis. In the Schramm (9) and Fearon (11) series only 1% of patients with orbital complications developed cavernous sinus thrombosis.

This condition is usually bilateral and only very occasionally it is unilateral. Although beginning unilaterally, bilaterality often evolves within a few hours. Severe headache, symptoms of meningitis, eye pain, and rapidly diminishing vision are visual symptoms. The temperature that accompanies the other complications becomes high and swinging in cavernous involvement. This is likely due to the periodic intravascular shedding of septic emboli from the infected venous spaces. Patients are profoundly ill, often in coma. Bilateral proptosis, total ophthalmoplegia by involvement of all the nerves of the superior orbital fissure, chemosis, and rapidly progressive bilateral blindness comprise the usual scenario. Historically, the prognosis was dismal with a 1961 literature review of 874 cases indicating an 80% mortality rate (25). Early diagnosis and swift intervention can be life-saving.

Ophthalmologic examination is mandatory in all orbital complications. A continuous vigilance for failing visual acuity with frequent vision checks and motility examination are essential. Retinoscopy must also be done repeatedly especially in the face of a threat of cavernous sinus thrombosis. As the retina becomes ischemic, it acquires a pallor secondary to edema and then as it begins to infarct turns gray. Disk pallor secondary to nerve head edema is seen. Venous engorgement is an ominous sign of increasing venous pressure from early involvement of the cavernous sinus. As complete vascular obstruction ensues, layering of the blood in the vessels is seen. Damage is usually irreversible at this point. Unfortunately, these early changes may be absent in cavernous sinus thrombosis and were seen in only two cases in the four patients of Price et al. (29).

Tests of ocular motility in the cardinal directions of gaze help to evaluate the severity of the ocular involvement and early on sometimes help in the localization of orbital abscesses. Observation for ptosis indicating superior division of oculomotor dysfunction and pupillary reaction especially to contralateral stimulation (in the face of intact vision) may aid in detecting inferior division third cranial nerve dysfunction. Complete lid immobility indicates compromise of the sympathetic supply to Müller's muscle as well. Involvement of the trigeminal nerve is primarily of the ophthalmic division with forehead, eyelid, and cornea anesthesia. The second division may also be involved but involvement of the mandibular branch is rare.

Orbital apex syndrome can occur independently of the classic scenario of progression of orbital complications from orbital cellulitis through the spectrum of disease to cavernous sinus thrombophlebitis. The sphenoid and posterior ethmoid sinuses are situated in direct proximity to the orbital apex. Direct spread of inflammation from these sinuses across the medial orbital wall at its posterior extremity can result in inflammatory changes in the optic nerve as well as the nerve emanating from the orbital apex. This is unaccompanied by periorbital edema or inflammation or proptosis (Fig. 17). The entity was first described by Rochon Du Vigneaud in 1896 and ascribed to syphilis (26). In 1945, Kjoer (27) clearly delineated the syndrome and established it as a complication of posterior ethmosphenoiditis. The patient presents with ophthalmoplegia and failing vision due to inflammatory changes in the oculomotor nerves of the orbital apex and optic nerve. It is fortunately very rare probably because of the thick, tightly bound periosteum of the posterior orbit compared to the thinner more loosely applied tissue of the anterior part. In addition, there are no vascular foramina at the apex with the occasional exception of a more posteriorly placed posterior ethmoid foramen. Finally, the bone is much thicker in the medial wall of the posterior orbit than in the lamina papyracea (28).

The inflammation causes swelling and compression in the narrow unforgiving confines of the posterior orbit. This results in necrosis of the neural structures (27) and the rapid onset of blindness, which is the unfortunate result in the majority of cases. Rapid, early

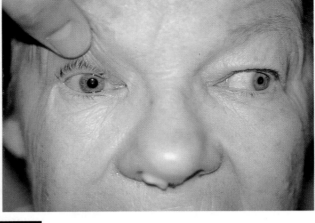

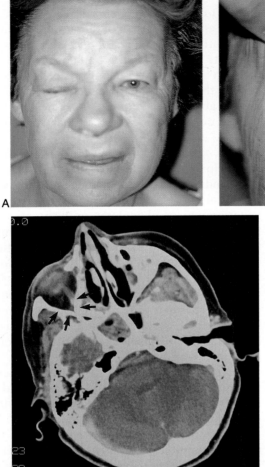

FIG. 17. **A:** Superior orbital fissure syndrome. Note ptosis without inflammation. **B:** Complete ophthalmoplegia. **C:** Axial CAT scan showing pus at orbital apex and swelling of optic nerve *(dark arrows).*

intervention with ethmosphenoidectomy and orbital decompression may be vision-sparing.

DIAGNOSIS

The computer-assisted tomography (CAT) scan and magnetic resonance imaging (MRI) evaluation of orbital involvement are critical in aiding in the establishment of localization and severity of orbital involvement from sinusitis. In most instances, computed tomography (CT) will most clearly delineate the extent of sinus disease. As indicated in the chapter, Radiology, by Rice, marked thickening of the sinus mucosa is readily seen. In the ethmoid sinuses, the thin bone of the labyrinth may lose definition, become hazy and indistinct, or be completely effaced by the opacification due to infection. The walls become obscured by a process of decalcification, most probably secondary to the hyperemia induced by the inflammatory reaction (31). Frank bone erosion is less common, especially in acute dis-

ease. Contrarily, bone erosion in the presence of a mucocele or mucopyocele of the frontal sinus (Fig. 18) and more uncommonly occurring in the ethmoid sinus (Fig. 19) is usually the rule. Mucoceles are often mistaken by the untutored eye as a tumor. Their appearance as a mass in the orbit with global displacement appears quite ominous (Fig. 20). Erosions from maxillary and sphenoid sinusitis are quite rare.

Soft tissue swelling of the preseptal area, although discernible on CT scan, is much clearer with MRI. Localization of preseptal abscesses as distinct from edema and swelling is more readily differentiated with MRI, which will show up as a bright signal in the case of abscess, rather than the more mild increase seen in cellulitis.

Orbital cellulitis is characterized by a diffuse clouding of the periorbital fat. Some minor diffuse enlargement of the ocular muscles may be seen as well (Fig. 21).

Subperiosteal abscess is well displayed on MRI, but its relationship to the lamina papyracea is much clearer

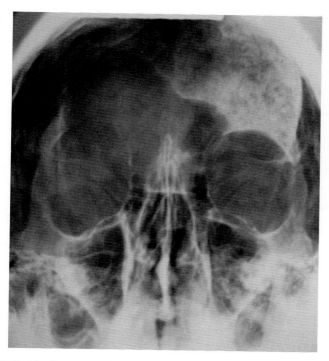

FIG. 18. Bone erosion of superior orbital wall secondary to frontal sinus mucocele.

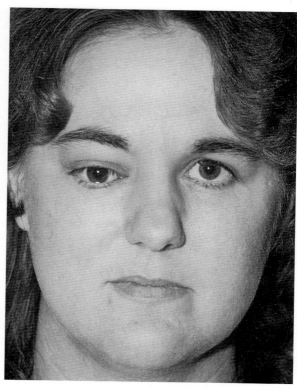

FIG. 20. Mucocele of frontal sinus displacing globe.

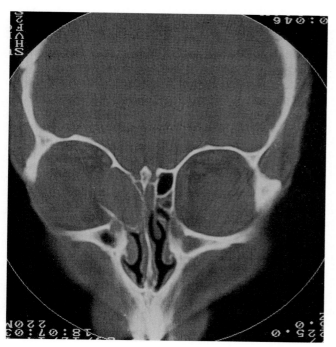

FIG. 19. Bone erosion of medial orbital wall secondary to ethmoid mucocele.

on CT scan (Fig. 15). Although some adjacent cloudiness and mild increase in density in the extraconal space are detected, they are clearly different from the diffuse changes of orbital cellulitis. The adjacent medial rectus muscle is usually swollen. The presence of gas bubbles make an abscess uniquely distinct from

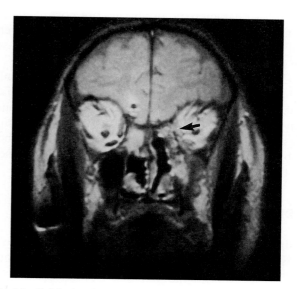

FIG. 21. Orbital cellulitis showing swelling of muscles (black arrow).

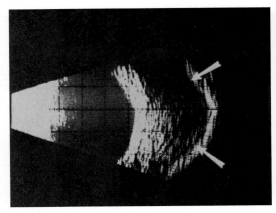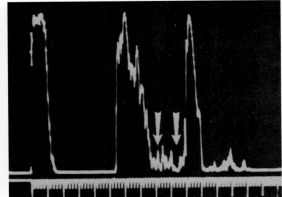

FIG. 22. The two types of orbital ultrasonic scan: A scan on left and B scan on right. The characteristic pattern of reflectivity of abscess formation is delineated by the *arrows*. (From ref. 8, with permission.)

cellulitis. Orbital abscess may be single or multiple and intraconal, extraconal, or both. Both CAT scanning and MRI are helpful in localizing the site of abscess (Fig. 16). This is essential for precisely directing the surgeon to the sites for drainage. A fluid density and surrounding edema indicate the purulent collection. The globe is displaced in the direction opposite to the abscess. Adjacent ocular muscles are swollen and increased in size. In intraconal abscess, the optic nerve is seen to be swollen as well.

Ultrasonic localization of abscesses was the method of choice up until the popularization of CT scans and MRI (Fig. 22). The method is office-based, inexpensive, and quick. However, it does take considerable skill on the part of the operator. The display of sound reflection emitted from a hand-held probe is portrayed in two modes. The A mode produces a visual two-dimensional tracing, where areas of low sound wave reflectivity characteristic of abscess are portrayed. The B mode demonstrates an oscilloscope tracing of vertical departure from baseline in which an abscess will be portrayed as an area of low short spikes.

Cavernous sinus thrombosis is usually accompanied by a severe pansinusitis of all sinuses on the initially infected side; however, bilateral involvement is generally the rule. Opacification of all paranasal sinus cavities is accompanied by diffuse increase in signal in both orbits and in both cavernous sinuses. This is best seen in the coronal and axial projections.

TREATMENT

In children with a reactive preseptal periorbital cellulitis, the quick institution of appropriate antibiotics usually given intravenously will stop the progression to a more serious complication. Periorbital cellulitis in this group is a common accompaniment to acute sinus-

itis and the administration of antibiotics usually results in rapid resolution. Because *H. influenzae* is so common in this age group, drugs not neutralized by β-lactamase must be used.

The problem of the appropriate antibiotic treatment choice is under constant evolution and change because of the periodic emergence of antibiotic-resistant organisms and the development of new antimicrobials. Any advice indicating the most effective antibiotic to treat these serious infections must be taken with this rapidly changing situation in mind. Presently, the non-β-lactamase producing *H. influenzae* is generally highly susceptible to ampicillin and amoxicillin. Ampicillin is administered in doses of 100 mg/kg/day orally in four divided doses and amoxicillin in three doses totaling 40 mg/kg/day. The incidence of β-lactamase production is highly variable, both on a geographic basis and on a community versus tertiary care hospital-based population. The addition of clavulinic acid to amoxicillin in the drug Augmentin overcomes the resistance produced by β-lactamase. The potassium clavulinate binds the β-lactamase, thus restoring the original potency and effectiveness of the amoxicillin component (32).

If the condition is more advanced, the ampicillin can be given intravenously, but at a higher dose in the range of 200 mg/kg/day, often combined with chloramphenicol, 100 mg/kg/day. An alternative is cefuroxime of 150 to 200 mg/day. For older children and adults, when staphylococci and streptococci are much more prevalent, penicillin is usually very effective. Penicillinase-producing organisms are treated with nafcillin at 150 mg/kg/day. Other organisms appearing in culture are treated with the antibiotics that show specific sensitivity. Supportive measures such as decongestants and antihistamines are given to reduce mucosal edema.

In teenagers and adults, periorbital cellulitis is a little

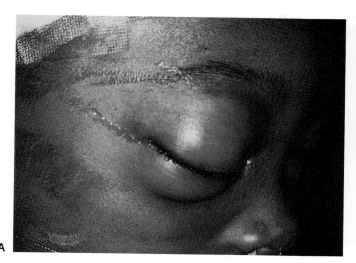
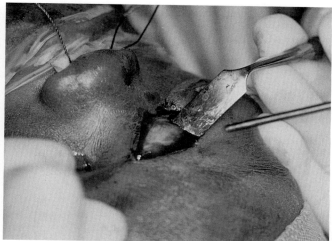

FIG. 23. Child with orbital abscess. **A:** Preoperative photograph. **B:** Intraoperative photograph with pus welling into the wound.

more ominous than in young children. It may be the forerunner of a more serious complication and indeed such an event may actually be in progress. Hospitalization and intravenous antibiotics, usually beginning with high-dose penicillin or nafcillin, are given until a culture and sensitivity indicates the specific drug to be given. In most instances, this combined with a strong intranasal astringent such as Afrin and a decongestant will be sufficient to produce amelioration of the condition. Pain relief may require the use of narcotic medication as the discomfort from sinusitis, especially with any orbital complication, is often intense. Nasal polyps may need to be removed acutely. A fluid level or persistent opacification of the maxillary sinuses in the face of antibiotic therapy will require antral lavage. Preseptal and postseptal abscesses require incision and drainage.

In orbital cellulitis, a more aggressive surgical approach is seldom necessary. Surgical treatment of a predisposing chronic sinusitis should be delayed if the acute episode is successfully treated conservatively until all evidence of the acute process has abated. If there is no resolution within 48 to 72 hr or especially if progression of the disease is evident, then surgical intervention should be invoked. One must continually be on guard for central complications. Any suggestion of meningitis would force early surgical intervention. Endoscopic surgery may be all that is required to manage the problem. This is as long as there is not extensive development of the supraorbital ethmoid cells precluding adequate exposure and drainage of this area. If any doubt exists concerning the ability to completely clear the disease via the endoscopic route, then an external ethmoidectomy should be performed. Acute periorbital cellulitis or pretarsal abscess secondary to a frontal sinus mucocele or mucopyocele cannot be well

handled by endoscopic surgery. External trephination and drainage are more successful, especially when followed by definitive management of the mucocele soon after the acute process has become quiescent (see the chapter, Surgical Management of Frontal Sinus Infections, by Donald).

Orbital cellulitis has to be treated expectantly with frequent observation of the clinical status including repeated tests of visual acuity and ocular motility, spread of periorbital erythema, checks of temperature and general physical condition, and progress of pain. Radiographs to assess the severity of sinus disease and rule out the presence of abscess may need to be repeated at 6- to 12-hr intervals. High-dose intravenous antibiotics, guided in part by Gram stains of intranasal pus or conjunctival secretions, are instituted immediately. Small cocaine packs in the middle meatus are repeated on a 4-hr basis to enhance sinus drainage. If chemosis is present, meticulous care of any herniated conjunctiva is essential to prevent ulceration and a secondary ophthalmitis. Liberal application of an antibiotic ointment, in addition to wet saline dressings, will maintain moisture and help prevent infection.

If rapid resolution does not ensue or if there is any evidence of progression of disease, immediate surgical intervention is necessary. External ethmoidectomy, wide sphenoidotomy, and opening of the natural maxillary sinus ostia are done to provide wide surgical drainage and decompress the orbit. The use of steroids is controversial, but their employment in the face of serious infection, I think, is a dubious practice.

Subperiosteal and orbital abscesses are absolute indications for surgery (Fig. 23). The initial establishment of an adequate blood level of antibiotics over a 4-hr period, at which time radiographic studies for localization are done, should be followed by appropriate

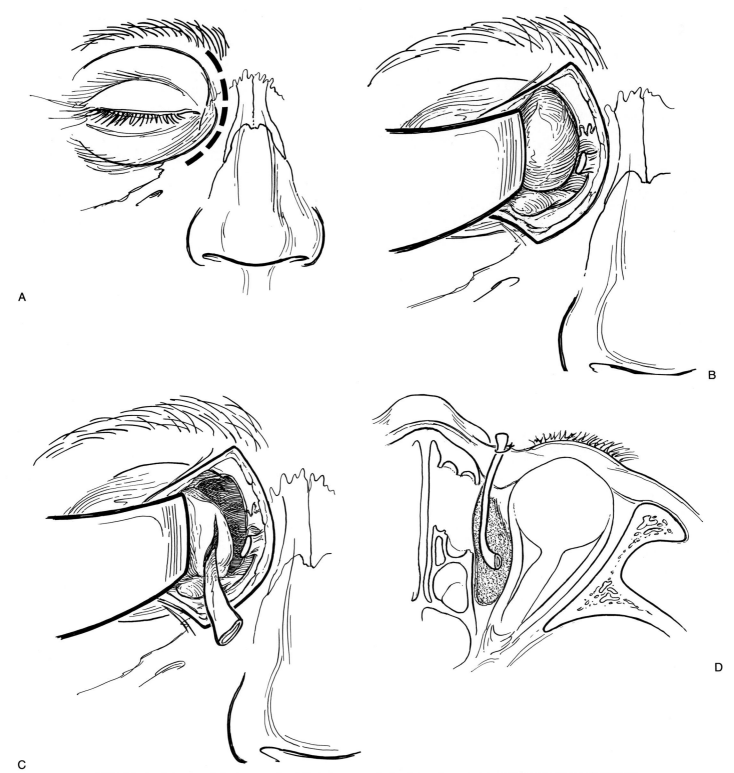

FIG. 24. Incision and drainage of orbital abscess. **A:** Incision in nasal-jugal area midway between inner canthus of the eye and the midline of the nose. **B:** Periorbita exposed. **C:** Penrose drain projecting through periorbita from the intraconal space done through an external ethmoidectomy approach. **D:** Horizontal section showing drain position.

sinus surgery, done by the external route, and incision and drainage of each abscess cavity. Once the purulent collections have been identified within the orbit, Penrose drains are inserted for irrigation and drainage (Fig. 24). In the subperiosteal space, although the lamina papyracea must be resected, it is unnecessary to penetrate surgically beyond the periorbita. Indeed, one must take care not to go beyond this layer for fear of introducing organisms into the soft tissues around the globe.

Cavernous sinus thrombosis is a rare, but extremely severe, complication of sinusitis. Earlier quotes of an 80% mortality rate have been transformed to a 70% to 80% survival rate. Lumbar puncture and repeated CT scans are done to rule out intracranial complications that occur as high as 75%. At the first inkling of cavernous sinus thrombosis, high doses of broad-spectrum antibiotics are administered intravenously. Heparinization is advised by some in doses of 5000 to 10,000 units. In Yarrington's (24) review, he felt that anticoagulation should not be done. Fibrinolysins may be used to cause dissolution of the clot. Corticosteroids may also be used, but usually only to counteract the effects of pituitary inflammation and subsequent suppression of the pituitary–adrenal axis.

Early surgical intervention may be ocular-saving and even life-saving. Ethmosphenoidectomy, maxillary drainage, and frontal trephine may be required. Blindness occurs in 15% and ocular palsies in 30% of patients (25,33).

High-dose antibiotics, sophisticated supportive care, early surgical intervention of sinus disease, and early detection and management of central complications are probably the key elements in the improved survival rates of modern times.

REFERENCES

1. Lang J. *Clinical anatomy of the nose, nasal cavity and paranasal sinuses.* New York: Thieme Medical Publishers, 1989;72–82.
2. Ohnishi T. Bony defects and dehiscences of the roof of the ethmoid cells. *Rhinology* 1981;19:195–202.
3. Lemke BN. Anatomy of the ocular adnexa and orbit. In: Smith BC, Rocca RCD, Nesi FA, Lisman RD, eds. *Ophthalmic plastic & reconstructive surgery,* vol 1, St Louis: CV Mosby, 1987;52.
4. Zide BM, Jelks GW. *Surgical anatomy of the orbit.* New York: Raven Press, 1985;8.
5. Pearson B, Laws ER. Anatomical aspects of the transsphenoidal approach to the pituitary. In: Laws ER, Randall RV, Kern EB, Alboud CF, eds. *Management of pituitary adenomas and related lesions with emphasis on transsphenoidal surgery.* New York: Appleton-Century-Crofts, 1982;4–7.
6. Lang J. *Clinical anatomy of the posterior cranial fossa and its foramina.* New York: Thieme Medical Publishers, 1991;7–8.
7. Anderson RL, Beard C. The levator aponeurosis attachments and their clinical significance. *Arch Ophthalmol* 1977;95:1437.
8. Goodwin WJ, Winshall M, Chandler JR. The role of high resolution computerized tomography and standard ultrasound in the evaluation of orbital cellulitis. *Laryngoscope* 1982;92:728–731.
9. Schramm VL, Curtin HD, Kennerdell JS. Evaluation of orbital cellulitis and results of treatment. *Laryngoscope* 1982;92:732–738.
10. Lawson W. Orbital complications of sinusitis. In: Blitzer A, Larson W, Friedman WH, eds. *Surgery of the paranasal sinuses,* 2nd ed. Philadelphia: Saunders, 1991;457–469.
11. Fearon B, Edmonds B, Bird R. Orbital-facial complications of sinusitis in children. *Laryngoscopy* 1979;89:947.
12. Rabinstein JB, Handler SD. Orbital and periorbital cellulitis in children. *Head Neck Surg* 1982;5:15.
13. Goodwin JW. Orbital complications of ethmoiditis. *Otolaryngol Clin North Am* 1985;18:139–147.
14. Borkin RM, Todd JK, Amer J. Periorbital cellulitis in children. *Pediatrics* 1978;62:390.
15. Wald ER. Rhinitis and acute and chronic sinusitis. In: Bluestone CD, Stool SE, Scheetz MD, eds. *Pediatric otolaryngology,* 2nd ed. Philadelphia: Saunders, 1980;729–744.
16. Chandler JR, Langenbrunner DJ, Stevens ER: The pathogenesis of orbital complications in acute sinusitis. *Laryngoscope* 1970;9:1414–1428.
17. Hubert L. Orbital infections due to sinusitis. A study of 114 cases. *NY J Med* 1937;37:1559.
18. Smith TF, O'Day D, Wright PF. Clinical implications of preseptal (periorbital) cellulitis in childhood. *Pediatrics* 1978;62:1006.
19. Mauriello JA, Flanagan JC. Orbital inflammatory disease. In: Mauriello JA, Flanagan JC, eds. *Management of orbital and ocular adnexal tumors and inflammations.* New York: Springer-Verlag, 1990;19–46.
20. Choi S, Lawson W, Urken ML. Subperiosteal orbital hematoma: an unusual complication of sinusitis. *Arch Otolaryngol* 1988;14:1164.
21. Wheeler JM. Orbital cyst without epithelial lining. *Arch Ophthalmol* 1937;18:356.
22. Harris GJ, Kay MC, Niles JJ. Orbital hematoma secondary to frontal sinusitis. *Ophthalmology* 1978;85:1229.
23. Calcaterra TC, Trapp TK: Unilateral proptosis. *Otolaryngol Clin North Am* 1988;21:53.
24. Maniglia AJ, Mintz DH, Novak S. Cephalic phycomycosis: a report of 8 cases. *Laryngoscope* 1982;92:755–760.
25. Yarrington CT. The prognosis and treatment of cavernous sinus thrombosis. *Ann Otol* 1961;70:263–267.
26. Kronschnabel EF. Orbital apex syndrome due to sinus infection. *Laryngoscope* 1974;84:353–371.
27. Kjoer I. A case of orbital apex syndrome in collateral pansinusitis. *Acta Ophthalmol* 1945;23:357–366.
28. Tarazi AE, Shikani AH. Irreversible unilateral visual loss due to acute sinusitis. *Arch Otolaryngol* 1991;117:1400–1401.
29. Price CD, Hameroff SB, Richards RD. Cavernous sinus thrombosis and orbital cellulitis. *South Med J* 1971;64:1243.
30. Fairbanks DNF, Vanderween TS, Boardley JE. Intracranial complications of sinusitis. In: English GM, ed. *Otolaryngology.* Philadelphia: Lippincott, 1991;18–19.
31. Dodd GD, Jing BS. Radiology of the nose, paranasal sinuses and nasopharynx. In: *Golden's diagnostic radiology, section 2.* Baltimore: Williams & Wilkins, 1977;113.
32. Wald ER, Pang D. Diagnosis and treatment of sinusitis and its complications. In: Johnson JT, ed. *Antibiotic therapy in head and neck surgery.* New York, Marcel Dekker, 1987;125–150.
33. DiNubile MJ. Septic thrombosis of the cavernous sinuses. *Arch Neurol* 1988;45:567.

CHAPTER 16

Intracranial Complications of Sinusitis

Jack L. Gluckman and James E. Freije

INCIDENCE

In the preantibiotic era, intracranial infection was a frequent and dreaded complication of sinusitis and the literature was replete with large series dealing with this problem (1). Following the introduction of antibiotics in the 1940s, the frequency of intracranial complications dramatically declined, but when they did occur, they were associated with a high mortality rate usually due to late presentation. In the more recent era, early detection by high-resolution computed tomography (CT) scan and magnetic resonance imaging (MRI) together with aggressive medical and surgical intervention has further decreased the morbidity and mortality rates, but unfortunately late diagnosis remains the rule because of a low index of suspicion and masking of the classic symptoms and signs by inadequate antibiotic therapy (2).

Intracranial complications secondary to sinusitis remain comparatively rare with an incidence varying from 3.7% to 10% (3). However, sinusitis has surpassed middle ear and mastoid disease as the most common source of infection in patients with brain abscesses (2,4,5).

The frontal sinus is the most common sinus associated with intracranial infection followed by the ethmoid, sphenoid, and maxillary sinus (6,7). Intracranial complications occur most commonly in adolescent or young adult males, which may be related to a peak in the vascularity of the diploic system and growth of the frontal sinus between the ages of 7 and 20 years (8–10). In many patients an underlying immunosuppression may be present.

Of the intracranial complications of paranasal sinusitis encountered, frontal lobe abscess and meningitis are the most common, depending on the series and the era reported on. Not infrequently, there may be more than one type of intracranial infection in a single pa-

tient. Although osteomyelitis of the cranial bone is not an intracranial complication per se, it is usually listed as such as it is a frequent cause of, or associated with, these complications.

PATHOGENESIS

Intracranial complications usually result from either acute or subacute exacerbations of chronic sinusitis, which in turn may be secondary to any process that alters normal sinus anatomy or physiology (e.g., allergy, trauma, barotrauma). Rarely, it may follow a solitary episode of acute sinusitis.

The mechanism of spread of infection from the sinuses intracranially may be *hematogenous* via thrombophlebitis along valveless diploic veins or *direct* extension through congenital dehiscences (e.g., sphenoid, frontal); normal anatomic pathways (e.g., craniopharyngeal canal, perineural sheaths); areas of avascular osteonecrosis secondary to osteomyelitis, pressure caused by neoplasm, mucocele, or infection; or finally, through fracture sites either accidental or iatrogenic (e.g., nasal or sinus surgery) in origin. Occasionally, underlying immunosuppression or a particularly aggressive organism (e.g., mucormycosis) may be causative.

Of these, the most significant route is thrombophlebitis. There exists a direct connection between the mucosa of the frontal sinus and the dural veins, via small valveless diploic veins (veins of Breschet), which permit blood and hence the infection to flow easily in either direction. Other sites for thrombophlebitic spread are via the small veins that accompany the olfactory nerves through the cribriform plate or via the ethmoid veins that drain into the cavernous sinus via the ophthalmic veins. Likewise, veins in the maxillary and sphenoid sinuses all directly or indirectly communicate with the cavernous sinus (1). A rare roundabout route of spread is to the superior longitudinal sinus via the parietal emissary veins secondary to a scalp infection following frontal sinusitis (1).

BACTERIOLOGY

Non-β-hemolytic *Streptococcus* is the organism most commonly encountered in intracranial complications (11) and these may frequently be anaerobic (5). *Staphylococcus* has been described in subdural empyema (8,12,13) and brain abscess (4,14,15), cavernous sinus thrombophlebitis (16,17), and osteomyelitis (6,7,18). Hemolytic *Streptococcus,* followed by *Pneumococcus* and *Hemophilus influenzae,* was found most commonly in meningitis of upper respiratory tract etiology (7). Anaerobes may account for 50% of nontraumatic brain abscesses (6). Negative cultures for anaerobes and aerobes occur in 21% of patients (14,19), almost certainly reflecting previous antibiotic therapy. *Pneumococcus, Proteus,* and *Bacteroides* also may be etiologic factors (12). Frequently, multiple pathogens may be encountered.

In general, the causative organism usually reflects the era in which the series was written and whether the patient was on previous antibiotics.

PRINCIPLES OF DIAGNOSIS AND TREATMENT

In general, the clinician should have a high index of suspicion for the development of intracranial complications in patients with acute and chronic sinusitis, particularly where the course is prolonged and the symptomatology is disproportionately severe. Headaches, persistent fever, lethargy, meningism, impaired consciousness, and altered personality are suggestive, while seizures and focal neurologic deficits are late developments and ominous predictive signs of subsequent morbidity and mortality.

Today, the high-resolution CT scan is the diagnostic aid of choice in diagnosing intracranial sepsis, although MRI is assuming an increasing role (Fig. 1). This imaging technique should be performed at the onset of the illness and then repeatedly as long as the index of suspicion persists. This is important not only for diagnosis of the intracranial problem but also to delineate the extent of disease in the paranasal sinuses. Both horizontal and coronal images with contrast may be needed for precise diagnosis. It is particularly useful in determining bone erosion. Magnetic resonance imaging has proved most useful for diagnosis of subtle intracerebral inflammation (5). Because of the potential catastrophic complications of intracranial sepsis, particularly if diagnosed late, it is not unreasonable to suggest that all patients with severe sinusitis, particularly frontal sinusitis requiring drainage, should routinely have a head CT scan before discharge from the hospital even if the patients are asymptomatic (5).

Lumbar puncture is really only useful in diagnosing meningitis, particularly to obtain cultures, but adds little to the diagnosis of the other intracranial complications. Because of the risk of uncal herniation in patients with intracranial abscess, this test should never be performed without initially obtaining a CT scan to rule out the presence of an intracranial abscess. Angiography, while quite useful for evaluating the presence of intracranial pus, may miss more subtle collections and has been superseded by the CT scan as the definitive diagnostic test. A technetium-99m mandibular dysostosis and peromelia (MDP) bone scan and a gallium-67 citrate scan are useful in establishing the diagnosis and progression of osteomyelitis (20).

The management of these critically ill patients should be multidisciplinary with an infectious disease specialist, ophthalmologist, neurosurgeon, and neurologist all being consulted as appropriate.

The initial treatment, irrespective of the intracranial complication suspected, consists of commencing intravenous systemic antibiotics with adequate gram-positive aerobic and anaerobic coverage. An empiric regimen may include aqueous penicillin, a penicillinase-resistant penicillin, and chloramphenicol (5,15), although third-generation cephalosporins together with metronidazole may be adequate (14,18). As soon as culture and sensitivity results have been obtained from either the sinus or intracranial abscess, these medications should be altered accordingly. In general, 2 weeks of intravenous therapy followed by a further 4 weeks of oral therapy should be administered. A sedimentation rate is a good technique for monitoring resolution of the intracranial process.

Anticonvulsant therapy should be commenced prophylactically in cases of severe intracranial complications, as the incidence of seizures may be as high as 80% (15).

Steroids have been advocated in order to decrease cerebral edema and they seem quite useful for this role. It has been suggested that steroids may minimize the inflammatory response and decrease the incidence of cerebral abscess formation but this seems unlikely. There is really no evidence that steroids have any effect on mortality rates, abscess formation, or intensity of inflammatory response (21).

Surgical treatment consists of drainage of the intracranial sepsis together with drainage of the sinus. Drainage of the sinus may consist of frontal sinus trephination, repeated antral lavage, nasoantral window, ethmoidectomy, or sphenoidotomy. If there is evidence of chronic sinus disease, a more definitive procedure may be performed at the same time as the neurosurgical procedure or at a later stage. Osteomyelitis will require adequate debridement.

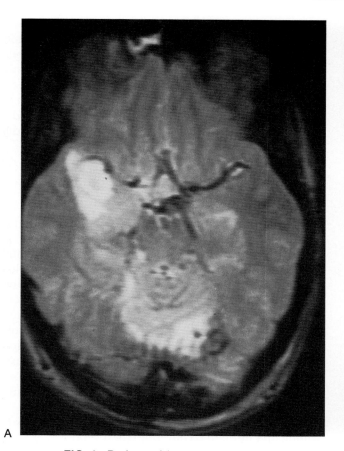
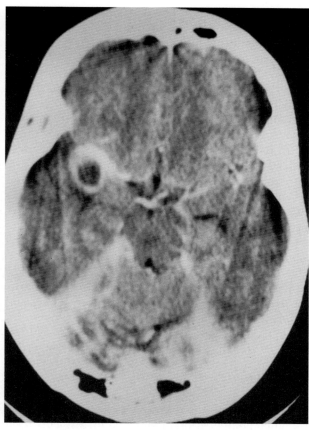

A   B

FIG. 1. Patient with severe sphenoid sinusitis and clinical evidence of cavernous sinus thrombo-phlebitis. **A:** T2 weighted axial MR image revealing ring-like increased signal in the right temporal lobe (abscess). There is irregular increased signal along the tentorium (subdural empyema). **B:** Postcontrast CT scan showing right temporal ring enhancement (abscess) and diffuse thickened enhancement along the tentorium bilaterally.

OSTEOMYELITIS

Although osteomyelitis of the cranial bones is not a true intracranial complication of sinusitis, it is often a precursor to or associated with intracranial sepsis. It involves most frequently the frontal bone and is most commonly seen in adolescents and young adults, possibly because the diploic system is more extensive (6,7). *Staphylococcus* is the most common organism isolated in frontal osteomyelitis followed by aerobic and anaerobic streptococci (6,7,13,18). Infection in the sinus results in thrombophlebitis of the diploic veins with secondary impairment of the arterial supply to the bone with resultant avascular necrosis, sequestra formation, further spread of infection, subperiosteal abscess, and further compromise of the blood supply. There are really two clinical forms of osteomyelitis—a localized, well-circumscribed variety and a more diffuse, spreading type due to progressive thrombophlebitis, which can achieve significant size if left untreated.

Involvement of the anterior table of the frontal sinus with subperiosteal abscess results in a doughy swelling of the forehead (''Pott's puffy tumor''). Involvement of the posterior table of the frontal sinus commonly results in an extradural abscess or the other intracranial complications. The tenderness associated with osteomyelitis may be difficult to differentiate from the tenderness of empyema of the frontal sinus.

Radiographic confirmation of the diagnosis of osteomyelitis may be difficult to establish especially early in the course of the infection. Plain radiographs are notoriously normal early and even a CT scan, which usually is obtained to rule out other intracranial complications, may only show evidence of bony erosion 7 to 10 days after the onset of the infection. The characteristic radiographic picture is the ''moth-eaten'' pattern due to decalcification and sequestra. A technetium bone scan and gallium scan may provide additional information in equivocal cases (20). Positive technetium and gallium scans, especially if the findings extend beyond the limits of the sinus, indicate acute osteomyelitis. Osteomyelitis is most unlikely in the presence of a negative technetium scan. A negative gallium scan indicates resolution of the osteomyelitis and may be useful in monitoring long-term therapy.

Treatment of osteomyelitis requires wide debridement of necrotic bone followed by prolonged antibiotic therapy. At least a 1-cm margin of healthy bone should be obtained at surgery (7). Antibiotics should be continued for at least 6 weeks but on their own are ineffective because of the avascular nature of the disease process. In the well-circumscribed cases, debridement is technically relatively easy. On the other hand, in the more extensive cases, this is more complicated and may require massive resection of cranial bone. No matter what the resultant cosmetic defect, aggressive debridement is necessary. Reconstruction of bony defects should be delayed for up to 1 year following resolution of the infection (18).

The prognosis of osteomyelitis is generally very good with a mortality rate of less than 5% (7,17); however, the problem may recur many years later, and therefore the patient should be subject to long-term follow-up.

MENINGITIS

Meningitis usually is regarded as the most common intracranial complication of sinusitis (6,16). This term refers to leptomeningitis, that is, inflammation of the pia mater, as opposed to pachymeningitis, which refers to inflammation of the dura mater. Th sphenoid and ethmoid sinuses followed by the frontal are the most common sinus sources of infection (7,13,16). While meningitis may be an immediate consequence of sinusitis, it may develop many years after a sinus fracture or may simply follow an episode of diving, with the infection being forced intracranially via olfactory perineural spaces.

The classical presentation of meningitis includes headache, fever, nuchal rigidity, and irritability followed by somnolence and delirium, although these may be masked in patients inadequately treated with antibiotics (16). There may be focal neurologic deficits due to involvement of the cranial nerves at the skull base or secondary to inflammation over the hemispheres.

When the diagnosis of meningitis is suspected, a CT scan should always be obtained prior to lumbar puncture to rule out a space-occupying lesion that potentially could result in brain herniation from the lumbar puncture. In meningitis, the CT scan will be normal or demonstrate mild ventricular or cistern enlargement. The findings on lumbar puncture are increased pressure, increased cerebrospinal fluid (CSF) protein, decreased glucose, leukocytosis, and identification of the offending organism by Gram stain (16).

Treatment of meningitis consists of intravenous antibiotics and, as soon as the patient is well enough, drainage of the affected sinus. Steroids for cerebral edema and anticonvulsants, if indicated, should be administered. Despite prompt surgical and medical intervention, significant neurological sequelae may occur in up to 30% of patients (6,18), including chronic seizure disorders, focal motor deficits, and mental retardation due to hydrocephalus and subdural effusion.

EPIDURAL (EXTRADURAL) ABSCESS

An epidural abscess by definition is a collection of pus between the bony calvarium and dura. It may be secondary to acute or chronic sinusitis with associated osteomyelitis or due to thrombophlebitis of the diploic veins with the bone being intact. The loose attachment of the dura to the inner table of the frontal sinus facilitates the collection of pus in this area (6). In less severe cases, the infection may consist of a granulomatous exudate over the dura without overt abscess formation. Obstruction of blood flow in the major dural sinuses by the epidural abscess may cause secondary increased intracranial pressure. Rarely, the abscess may rupture through the dura into the subdural space.

The signs and symptoms of epidural abscess may be subtle and difficult to differentiate from those of acute frontal sinusitis. Neurologic symptoms may be minimal or absent. It certainly should be considered in all patients with persistent headache and spiking fever. A large collection of pus may lead to focal motor or sensory deficits, seizures, and an altered level of consciousness.

A CT scan is the diagnostic study of choice. The classical radiographic picture is a collection in the extradural space with underlying cerebral edema and occasionally a defect in the posterior table of the frontal sinus. A lumbar puncture, if performed, may reveal normal or raised pressure and a normal chemical and cellular picture.

Treatment of an epidural abscess consists of intravenous broad-spectrum antibiotics and surgical drainage of the epidural space. The surgical approach depends on the extent of the epidural infection and the site of the collection. If the abscess extends above the frontal sinus, a bifrontal craniotomy may be necessary. If the collection is limited to the area behind the posterior wall of the frontal sinus, an osteoplastic flap approach to the sinus and drainage of the abscess through the sinus with cranialization of the sinus should be performed. Simple trephination of the frontal sinus is probably inadequate to accomplish drainage of the epidural abscess (14). All granulation tissue should be cleaned from the dura and it is our experience that the dura should not be violated, as it is an excellent barrier to infection. Some, however, advocate that the subdural space should be explored because of the difficulty in determining the presence of an associated subdural abscess (15). Prompt recognition and treatment of an epidural abscess will result in a favorable prognosis.

SUBDURAL ABSCESS

Subdural abscess by definition is pus in the space between the dura and pia mater. Sinusitis-induced subdural empyema is a disease of predominantly adolescents and young adult men (8). It is a rare complication of sinusitis, representing less than 10% of the intracranial complications (14), which is most fortunate as it is associated with a high morbidity and mortality rate. It usually develops secondary to retrograde thrombophlebitis from acute frontal sinusitis but may be secondary to direct rupture of an extradural abscess into the subdural space.

The most common organisms encountered in subdural empyema are aerobic and anaerobic streptococci as well as *Staphylococcus aureus* (8,12,19), although there may be a mixture of organisms and occasionally no pathogens are identified. Initially, the empyema may be located over the frontal lobes, often in the parafalcine space, but it may occasionally be present over the occipital cortex, possibly due to gravity in the supine patient (15), or may spread diffusely over the surface of the cerebral hemispheres. Secondary cortical thrombophlebitis may result in multicentric abscesses or cerebral venous infarction. The mass effect of the subdural empyema is usually of no clinical consequence.

Subdural empyema usually has a fulminant course and should be considered a neurosurgical emergency. Early symptoms include intense headache, meningism, and fever. As the process continues, an altered level of consciousness, hemiparesis, and seizures may develop.

The diagnosis is confirmed by CT scan or MRI, which demonstrates a thin enhancing collection over the cerebral convexity and/or fissures (12) (Fig. 2). Bilateral or multiple collections are not uncommon. A false-negative CT scan is possible (8). A lumbar puncture will reveal mildly increased pressure, increased protein, and white cells and therefore is not diagnostic. These findings together with the danger of herniation render this a superfluous and even dangerous test.

Medical treatment consists of broad-spectrum antibiotics and anticonvulsants, which probably should be administered prophylactically. Steroids may be helpful in decreasing the underlying cerebral edema.

The ideal technique for adequate surgical drainage of a subdural empyema is somewhat controversial and may be performed via multiple burr holes or craniot-

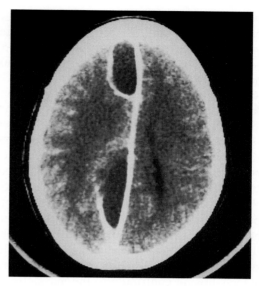

FIG. 2. Postcontrast CT scan showing diffuse thickening of the falx with two pockets of subdural empyema.

omy. Patients drained by burr holes appear to have a significantly higher mortality rate and higher recurrence rate than those treated by craniotomy (12,19). This is felt to be due to difficulty in draining multiple loculations and the thick pus adequately because of the limited exposure. On the other hand, more accurate modern imaging studies may localize the pus more precisely and allow better drainage by burr holes (8), but the overall sentiment is that craniotomy offers the most effective approach (12,19).

The affected sinus (usually the frontal sinus) should be drained at the time of the neurosurgical procedure. If the posterior wall is osteomyelitic and eroded, cranialization of the sinus should be performed. If trephination alone is performed, the sinus will require obliteration at a later stage.

Despite advances in diagnostic techniques, the mortality rate of subdural empyema remains high and long-term morbidity (e.g., focal neurologic deficits and chronic seizure disorders) is common (5,8,12). If the patient is obtunded on admission, the prognosis is particularly grim (19). Therefore the key to successful outcome remains early diagnosis.

CEREBRAL ABSCESS

Cerebral abscess, along with meningitis, is regarded as the most common intracranial complication of sinusitis. Sinusitis accounts for 13% to 40% of all brain abscesses that develop (4,13,14,22). Brain abscesses of sinogenic origin develop most commonly in the frontal lobe and are usually secondary to infection in the frontal or ethmoid sinuses, either as isolated infections or part of pansinusitis. Temporal lobe abscess, while usually otitic in origin, may be secondary to sphenoid sinusitis. Aerobic and anaerobic streptococci and *Staphylococcus aureus* are the most common causative organisms (4,14,15).

The pathogenesis of cerebral abscess formation is usually the result of retrograde thrombophlebitis with access to the cerebral parenchyma via the afferent venous system. It also may be secondary to subdural empyema with spread of infection diffusely over the cerebral hemispheres with resultant multiple foci of cortical thrombophlebitis. The intraparenchymal infection commences as a cerebritis and if necrosis and liquification occur, abscess formation results with surrounding cerebral edema. Encapsulation usually develops in 10 to 14 days. Thickening of the abscess wall, liquification of the cavity contents, cerebral edema, and surrounding encephalitis all contribute to the mass effect (6).

The clinical features depend on the various phases of abscess formation. The initial stage of cerebritis results in mild symptoms from parenchymal edema and may last for 1 to 2 weeks. These include fever, lethargy, and agitation with persistent headache being an important symptom. As the inflammatory process progresses, central liquification and necrosis occur without expansion. This represents the "quiescent" period with few, if any, new clinical symptoms or signs. With organization and expansion of the abscess, signs of increased intracranial pressure and mass effect occur (i.e., seizures and focal neurologic signs). It should be remembered that the frontal lobes are notorious "silent" areas and small abscesses may be asymptomatic other than subtle mood changes (11). If the condition progresses without treatment, death due to either uncal herniation or abscess rupture into the ventricular system may result.

The confirmatory diagnosis of cerebral abscess is made with high-resolution CT scans, which usually also demonstrate the offending paranasal sinus (Figs. 3 and 4). Sophisticated and sensitive radiology techniques are now able to diagnose the abscess at the stage of cerebritis. Lumbar puncture rarely is used because of the danger of cerebral herniation (16).

In patients suspected of having a brain abscess, high-dose broad-spectrum antibiotics should be commenced immediately with the definitive therapy dependent on the culture results. Steroids and/or mannitol may be useful in reducing intracranial pressure and prophylactic anticonvulsants should be administered. Anticonvulsants should be administered for at least 2 years following treatment. It has been claimed that in some cases, where the diagnosis is made at the stage of cerebritis, early and aggressive medical therapy may prevent progression of the infection and surgery may be avoided (5,23,24); however, this is rarely successful

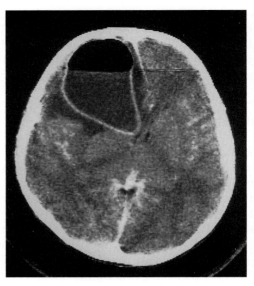

FIG. 3. Postcontrast CT scan showing thin-walled right frontal abscess with air–fluid level.

and most abscesses treated medically eventually require surgical treatment (14,22).

Total excision of a well-encapsulated abscess that does not involve a primary cortical area is the preferred surgical treatment and may be performed *ab initio* or following drainage. In severely ill patients, drainage through a burr hole with subsequent irrigation through a catheter is the treatment of choice.

Mortality rates from sinogenic brain abscesses until recently remained high in spite of intensive antibiotic therapy because of late diagnosis (4,9,14,25,26). However, since the advent of the CT scan and because of

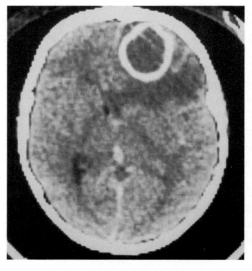

FIG. 4. Postcontrast CT scan showing the enhancing wall of a left frontal abscess. There is moderate surrounding edema and mass effect.

more aggressive surgical therapy, the mortality rate has dropped to 5% to 10% (27), although mortality rates as high as 25% have been reported (4). Significant long-term morbidity (e.g., chronic seizure disorders and occasionally hemiplegia) still occur in one-third to one-half of patients (4,7,14). Early identification and treatment are therefore the key to minimizing the morbidity and mortality in these patients.

VENOUS SINUS THROMBOPHLEBITIS

Venous sinus thrombophlebitis as a complication of sinusitis involves the cavernous sinus and the superior longitudinal sinus.

Sinogenic *cavernous sinus thrombophlebitis* is seen most frequently as a result of sphenoid or ethmoid sinusitis but can follow infection in any of the sinuses (6,7). Septic thrombi may gain direct access to the cavernous sinus via the ophthalmic veins. The cavernous sinus traps the bacteria and the resultant inflammation and stasis eventually lead to thrombosis. The most common organism isolated in cases of cavernous sinus thrombosis is coagulase-positive *Staphylococcus aureus* (16,17).

The classical orbital findings of cavernous sinus thrombophlebitis are chemosis and periorbital edema, which develop early, followed by proptosis with limitation of ocular movement initially due to edema then III, IV, and VI nerve palsies. A late development is decreased visual acuity and retinal edema and anesthesia in the distribution of VI. The pupil may be fixed and dilated but occasionally is pinpoint (28). The process may spread to involve the contralateral cavernous sinus with the development of contralateral eye signs. Epistaxis from venous obstruction may occur and edema over the mastoid process may develop. A "picket fence" fever with temperature spikes corresponding to showers of septic emboli is characteristic. As the infection and inflammation progress, widespread cortical thrombophlebitis and meningitis may result in seizures and a depressed level of consciousness. Jugular vein thrombophlebitis with multiple systemic septic emboli may occur.

The diagnosis is usually clinical and, of course, needs to be differentiated from purely orbital infection. In general, focal intraorbital and periorbital abscesses will have more local orbital features and less evidence of venous stasis. Likewise, ophthalmoplegia and deteriorating vision will make one more suspicious of cavernous sinus involvement. A high index of suspicion always should be present for the development of cavernous sinus thrombophlebitis in the presence of orbital infection. CT scan will demonstrate lack of contrast enhancement in the cavernous sinus (16), although MRI is more accurate (Fig. 1). Angiography,

while helpful, is dangerous in an extremely ill patient (7) and may accelerate the formation of thrombi (24). Invariably, a positive blood culture can be obtained.

Treatment consists of intravenous antibiotics with close monitoring for the development of any other associated intracranial complication. Anticoagulation for cavernous sinus thrombosis remains controversial. In theory, anticoagulation is useful in preventing propagation of the thrombus and facilitating recanalization (28) and is recommended by most clinicians. Others, however, believe that the clot may help contain the infection and anticoagulation may be detrimental (29). The affected sinus should be drained as soon as the patient is well enough to withstand the procedure.

Although the mortality rate has decreased dramatically to almost 20% (17), long-term morbidity, particularly permanent cranial nerve palsies and blindness, may occur in up to 50% of cases (28,29). A rare chronic slowly progressive variant of cavernous sinus thrombophlebitis has been described (28).

Superior longitudinal sinus thrombophlebitis usually is associated with an epidural or subdural empyema. Its pathogenesis is identical to cavernous sinus thrombophlebitis. Occlusion of cortical tributaries of the sinus results in focal neurologic deficits and seizures. Cortical vein obstruction in this area may affect the motor supply to the legs, usually unilaterally. Progression of the thrombosis may lead to stupor and coma, due to increased intracranial pressure in severe cases. Diagnosis is difficult but a CT scan with contrast may demonstrate an edematous lucency rostral to the point of obstruction. Treatment is similar to cavernous sinus thrombophlebitis, consisting of antibiotics with or without anticoagulants. The prognosis is generally poor, and in survivors neurologic sequelae are common (6,7).

INTRACRANIAL MUCOCELES

A mucocele of the sinus develops after prolonged obstruction of the natural ostium. This may be secondary to chronic infection, allergy, benign neoplasms, or trauma. This results in an expanding mass, which may erode intracranially. Sinuses that are commonly affected include the posterior ethmoid, sphenoid, and frontal sinuses. Superimposed infection of the mucocele (mucopyocele) will facilitate the expansion and extension of these lesions.

Clinical features include increasing headache and other symptoms and signs depending on the site of origin and extent of the intracranial component of the mucocele; for example, sphenoid mucoceles may erode the optic nerves, internal carotid artery, and pituitary, while a frontal mucocele may cause significant orbital signs before extending intracranially (30).

The diagnosis is confirmed by CT scan, which also will define the site of origin and exact extent of the lesion.

Treatment consists of broad-spectrum antibiotics if infection is suspected and surgical extirpation. Several approaches to the surgical drainage, marsupialization, and removal of mucoceles have been described with varying degrees of success (30–35). An excellent technique for frontal sinus mucoceles is exposure via an osteoplastic flap approach, removal of the mucocele in its entirety, and obliteration of the sinus. If there is extensive intracranial extension or complete removal of the lining mucosa is not possible, marsupialization of the mucocele into the nose via an external frontoethmoidectomy is indicated. Some authors have reported successful marsupialization using endoscopic nasal techniques (35). If the intracranial extension is significant, a craniotomy may be necessary to attain adequate removal (33).

INTRACRANIAL POLYPOSIS

Rare cases of aggressive sinonasal polyposis from chronic sinus disease with intracranial extension have been reported (18,36,37). The sequence of events with sinus obstruction, expansion, and destruction that occurs with extensive polyposis is similar to sinus mucoceles. The possibility of a malignant neoplasm or a concomitant infectious process also must be considered. CT scan and biopsy demonstrating benign polyps confirm the diagnosis. Treatment consists of surgical removal of the polypoid disease by whatever technique appears appropriate and reestablishment of proper sinus drainage, with the approach being the same as for the sinus mucoceles.

MISCELLANEOUS DISORDERS

Isolated cases of more unusual intracranial disorders associated with sinusitis also have been reported. Two cases of extradural hematoma complicating frontal sinusitis have been described (38). The bleeding most likely results from the diploic vessels and may be difficult to diagnose preoperatively. A case of pontocerebellar infarction with cavernous sinus thrombosis following sphenoethmoid sinusitis has been described (39). Various isolated cranial nerve palsies can occur in isolation secondary to sinusitis (e.g., VI nerve palsy), but usually they are seen as part of a cavernous sinus thrombophlebitis or as a consequence of other intracranial complications (40). Internal carotid artery spasm secondary to sinusitis has been described (41).

CONCLUSION

Although the incidence of morbidity and mortality associated with intracranial complications of sinusitis have decreased substantially over the past 50 years, a significant number of young, otherwise healthy, patients are still afflicted by these complications, which carry a high morbidity. While high-resolution CT scan has become a very sensitive technique for early recognition of intracranial complications, a low threshold for obtaining this study should be present in all patients in whom an intracranial complication is even remotely considered. This is particularly true today when the frequent use of over-the-counter sinus medications and the liberal use of antibiotics may mask the clinical features that herald the onset of these intracranial complications.

REFERENCES

1. Courville CB, Rosenvold LK. Intracranial complications of infections of the nasal cavities and accessory sinuses. *Arch Otolaryngol* 1938;27:692–731.
2. Chalstrey S, Pfleiderer AG, Moffat DA. Persisting incidence and mortality of sinogenic cerebral abscess: a continuing reflection of late clinical diagnosis. *J R Soc Med* 1991;84:193–195.
3. Bluestone C, Steiner R. Intracranial complications of acute frontal sinusitis. *South Med J* 1965;58:1–10.
4. Bradley PJ, Manning KP, Shaw MD. Brain abscesses secondary to paranasal sinusitis. *J Laryngol Otol* 1984;98:719–725.
5. Maniglia AJ, Goodwin WJ, Arnold JE, et al. Intracranial abscesses secondary to nasal, sinus, and orbital infections in adults and children. *Arch Otolaryngol Head Neck Surg* 1989;115:1424–1429.
6. Blitzer A, Carmel P. Intracranial complications of disease of the paranasal sinuses. In: Bliter A, Lawson W, Friedman WH, eds. *Surgery of the paranasal sinuses*. Philadelphia: Saunders, 1985;328–337.
7. Fairbanks D, Vanderveen T, Bordley J. Intracranial complications of sinusitis. In: English G, ed. *Otolaryngology*, vol II, chap 38. New York: Harper & Row, 1983;1–28.
8. Kaufman DM, Litman N, Miller MH. Sinusitis-induced subdural empyema. *Neurology* 1983;33:123–132.
9. Wenig BL, Goldstein MN, Abramson AL. Frontal sinusitis and its intracranial complications. *Int J Pediatr Otolaryngol* 1983;5(3):285–302.
10. Kaplan R. Neurological complications of infections of the head and neck. *Otolaryngol Clin North Am* 1976;9:729–737.
11. Daya S. A "silent" intracranial complication of frontal sinusitis. *J Laryngol Otol* 1990;104:645–647.
12. Wackym PA, Canalis RF, Feuerman T. Subdural empyema of otorhinological origin. *J Laryngol Otol* 1990;104:118–122.
13. Rice DH, Fishman SM, Barton RT, et al. Cranial complications of frontal sinusitis. *Am Fam Physician* 1980;22(5):145–149.
14. Clayman GL, Adams GL, Paugh DR, et al. Intracranial complications of paranasal sinusitis: a combined institutional review. *Laryngoscope* 1991;101:234–239.
15. Wald ER, Pang D, Milmore GJ, et al. Sinusitis and its complications in the pediatric patient. *Pediatr Clin North Am* 1981;28(4):777–796.
16. Rood SR, Schramm VL, Masciotra JN, et al. *Complications of acute and chronic sinus disease*. SIPAC American Academy of Otolaryngology–Head and Neck Surgery Foundation, 1982.
17. Kaplan R. Neurological complications of infections of the head and neck. *Otolaryngol Clin North Am* 1976;9(3):729–749.
18. Parker GS, Tami TA, Wilson JF, et al. Intracranial complications of sinusitis. *South Med J* 1989;82(5):563–568.
19. Bannister G, Williams B, Smith S. Treatment of subdural empyema. *J Neurosurg* 1981;55:82–88.
20. Gardiner LJ. Complications of frontal sinusitis: evaluation and management. *Otolaryngol Head Neck Surg* 1986;95:333–343.
21. Schroeder KA, McKeever PE, Schoberg DR. Effect of dexa-

methasone on experimental brain abscess. *J Neurosurg* 1987; 66:264–269.

22. Johnson DL, Markie BM, Weiderman BL, et al. Treatment of intracranial abscesses associated with sinusitis in children and adolescents. *J Pediatr* 1988;113(1):15–23.

23. Kamin M, Biddle D. Conservative management of focal intracerebral infection. *Neurology* 1981;31:103–106.

24. Rosenblum M, Hoff J, Norman D. Non-operative treatment of brain abscesses in selected high risk patients. *J Neurosurg* 1980; 52:217–225.

25. Garfield J. Management of supratentorial intracranial abscess: a review of 200 cases. *Br Med J* 1969;2:7–11.

26. Wright RL, Ballantine H. Management of brain abscesses in children and adolescents. *Am J Dis Child* 1967;114:113–122.

27. Rosenblum M, Hoff JJ, Norman D. Decreased mortality from brain abscesses since advent of computerized tomography. *J Neurosurg* 1978;49:658–688.

28. Karlin RJ, Robinson WA. Septic cavernous sinus thrombosis. *Ann Emerg Med* 1984;13:449–455.

29. Yarington CT. The prognosis and treatment of cavernous sinus thrombosis. *Ann Otol Rhinol Laryngol* 1961;70:263–267.

30. Schaeffer SA, Anderson Rg, Carder HM. Epidural mucopyocele: diagnosis and management. *Otolaryngol Head Neck Surg* 1981;89:523–529.

31. Hardy JM, Montgomery WW. Osteoplastic frontal sinusotomy: an analysis of 250 operations. *Ann Otol Rhinol Laryngol* 1976; 85:523–532.

32. Evans C. Aetiology and treatment of frontal–ethmoidal mucocele. *J Laryngol Otol* 1981;95:361–375.

33. Stiernberg CM, Baily BJ, Calhoun KH, et al. Management of invasive frontoethmoidal sinus mucoceles. *Arch Otolaryngol Head Neck Surg* 1986;112:1060–1063.

34. Neel HB, McDonald TJ, Facer GW. Modified Lynch procedures for chronic frontal sinus diseases: rationale, technique, and long-term results. *Laryngoscope* 1987;97:1274–1279.

35. Kennedy DW, Josephson JS, Zinreich SJ, et al. Endoscopic sinus surgery for mucoceles: a viable alternative. *Laryngoscope* 1989;99:885–895.

36. Winestock DP, Bartlett PC, Soundheimer FK. Benign nasal polyps causing bone destruction in the nasal cavity and paranasal sinuses. *Laryngoscope* 1978;88:675–679.

37. Parker GS, Tami TA, Wilson JF. Aggressive sinonasal polyposis. *Am J Rhinol* 1988;2(1):1–5.

38. Rajput AJ, Rozdilsky B. Extradural hematoma following frontal sinusitis. *Arch Otolaryngol* 1971;94:83–86.

39. Macdonald RL, Findlay JM, Tator CH. Sphenoethmoidal sinusitis complicated by cavernous sinus thrombosis and pontocerebellar infarction. *Can J Neurol Sci* 1988;15:310–313.

40. Weisberger EC, Dedo HH. Cranial neuropathies in sinus disease. *Laryngoscope* 1977;87:357–364.

41. Whitehead E, Desouza FM. Acute sphenoid sinusitis causing spasm of the internal carotid artery. *Can J Otolaryngol* 1974; 32:216–218.

CHAPTER 17

Surgical Management of Frontal Sinus Infections

Paul J. Donald

Since the advent of antibiotics in the management of sinusitis, this disease process has received much less attention in otolaryngologic training programs. In the preantibiotic era, the treatment of acute and chronic sinusitis was a large part of the otolaryngologist's practice. The frontal sinus was a particularly dangerous site to sustain an infection because of its potential for life-threatening complications. The problems of meningitis, subdural abscess, brain abscess, and cranial osteomyelitis were continuous threats, especially in a particularly virulent infection or in a compromised host.

In the 1880s, the usual treatment for an unresolved frontal sinusitis was external trephination (1). This procedure, with some modification, is still the operation of choice in refractory acute sinusitis today. In 1884, Ogston described drainage of the frontal sinus not only through the anterior wall, but intranasally as well (2). However, the first surgeon to describe an intranasal drainage procedure for infection was Jurasz (3) of Berlin; but the first actual operative incursion into the frontal sinus, at which time some form of obliteration was done, was by Runge in 1750 (4).

The interest in establishing intranasal drainage engendered by Jurasz and Ogston stimulated Schaeffer (5) in 1890 to design a puncture procedure done intranasally to hopefully reach the interior of the frontal sinus through its floor in the region of the frontonasal duct. The site of puncture was placed just anterior to the leading tip of the middle turbinate. Numerous complications ensued and the procedure fell into disrepute. One of the fatalities was reported by Mermod (6) who, at autopsy, found that the patient had no frontal sinuses and discovered two puncture wounds through the cribriform plate.

In 1893, Luc (7), one of the cofounders of the Caldwell–Luc operation on the maxillary sinus, described a procedure similar to Ogston's. This was a frontal trephination combined with an enlarging of the frontonasal ducts through the anterior ethmoids. The Ogston–Luc operation or some modification was the standard form of surgical procedure done for many years to come.

The first surgeon to describe actually removing the anterior wall for the management of inflammatory disease was Kuhnt (8) in 1895. He attempted to collapse this skin against the posterior wall of the sinus, but, unfortunately, in addition to not successfully obliterating the sinus cavity in some patients, the procedure also produced a marked deformity. In 1902, Jansen (9) described a method of frontal sinus obliteration in which the anterior sinus wall and periosteum were collapsed against the posterior wall once all intervening diseased mucosa was excised. This unfortunately also produced a cosmetic deformity and had its share of complications.

In 1889, Riedel (10,11) described the most radical of frontal sinus operations, which under certain circumstances is still done today. This operation entails the removal of the anterior and inferior walls of the sinus. The forehead skin is collapsed against the posterior wall but often leaves a hideous deformity (Fig. 1). Killian (12), in 1903, described his variation of the Riedel operation. He recommended leaving a 1-cm high bar of bone in the supraorbital area to diminish the amount of deformity. He also attempted to reconstruct the nasofrontal duct area with a mucoperiosteal flap. The results of this procedure were unsatisfactory as nasal mucosa grew back into the cavity and mucocele formation ensued (1,13).

Because of the unsightly deformity that results from the excision of the anterior wall, the basic principle of establishing frontonasal drainage by Ogston and Luc

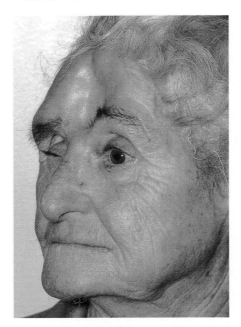

FIG. 1. Riedel ablation showing marked deformity.

was pursued by surgeons using a transorbital approach. In 1908, Knapp (14) first described an approach through the medial orbital wall, performing an extensive ethmoidectomy, leaving the anterior frontal sinus wall intact but removing diseased mucosa and enlarging the frontonasal duct. In 1914, Lothrop (15) designed an operation that attempted to maximize the concept of enlarging the frontonasal ducts because of the problems of re-stenosis and closures encountered with the various duct-enlarging procedures of the time—problems that still plague these procedures. He resected a large portion of the frontal sinus floor adjacent to the ducts and the intersinus septum but in addition removed the upper aspect of the nasal septum and that which adjoins the nasal bone. Dental burs were used to excise bone but not all sinus mucosa was removed. This procedure unfortunately did not meet with uniform success (13). Lynch (16), in 1921, proposed an operation that was based on the prior procedure of Jansen and Ritin and, like Knapp's, approached the sinus through the orbit. His operation entailed removing part of the frontal sinus floor and as much of the sinus mucosa as possible and inserting a stent into the orifice thus created to maintain patency. In the next year, Howarth (17) published a series of patients and helped popularize the operation. This operation has been cursed over the decades by repeated failures (13,18) and has been abandoned by many surgeons since the development of the osteoplastic flap procedure. In 1952, Boyden (19) described a mucoperiosteal flap that was later refined in 1973 by Baron et al. (20) that improved the success rate of the Lynch operation. The most popular frontal sinus procedure done

today, the osteoplastic flap with fat obliteration, had its beginnings in the construction of an anterior osteo-periosteal flap by Schonborn (21) in 1894 and Brieger (22) in 1895. This procedure was described in various modifications near the turn of the century by many investigators, mostly Europeans (23–26). It was Beugara and Itoiz (27,28) and Tato et al. (29) from South America who were the first to describe the osteoplastic operation using fat as an obliterating agent. They based their operation on the basis of cat experiments in which an inferiorly based anterior wall osteoplastic flap was created and frontal sinus mucosa was completely excised, then the cavity obliterated with abdominal fat. They found that autograft fat persisted as such and prevented osteoneogenesis and especially the ingrowth of mucosa from the nose. Further research on this method was done by Goodale and Montgomery (30–32), who found that the grafts in cats undergo minimal absorption of up to 15% of their volume with the remainder of the cavity being obliterated by fibrous tissue and osteoneogenesis. McBeth and Bosley (33,34) have contested that fat obliteration is unnecessary and that the cavity will fill in by osteoneogenesis. They advocate drilling of the mucosa only, without the implantation of an obliterating agent.

A summary of the various operations according to walls excised is seen in Fig. 2. Table 1 summarizes the chronology of the development of frontal sinus surgery.

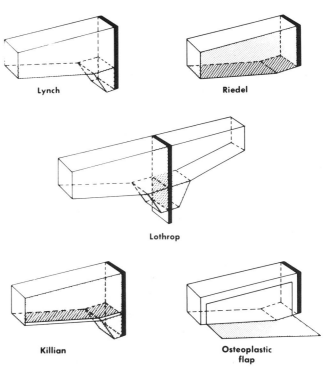

FIG. 2. Diagram of various types of frontal sinus procedures. (From ref. 13, with permission.)

TABLE 1. *Outline of the history of external surgery on the frontal sinus*

Trephine	Ogston (1884)	Trephine of anterior wall.
	Luc (1896)	
Collapse	Kuhnt (1891)	Removal of anterior wall.
	Riedel (1898)	Removal of anterior and inferior walls.
	Killian (1903)	Removal of anterior and inferior walls with preservation of supraorbital ridge.
Transorbital	Jansen (1902)	Removal of inferior wall, collapse of anterior wall.
	Ritter (1911)	Removal of inferior wall, ethmoidectomy.
	Knapp (1908)	
Osteoplastic flap	Schonborn (1894)	Osteoperiosteal flap of anterior wall.
	Brieger (1895)	
Septoplasty	Lothrop (1912)	Removal of intersinus septum.
Obliteration	Marx (1910), Tato et al. (1954), Bergara and Itoiz (1955), Good and Montgomery (1956), MacBeth (1954), Adson and Hempstead (1937), Malecki (1959)	Adipose tissue. Natural. Cranialization.

(From ref. 35)

The indications for frontal sinus surgery for infection are detailed in the chapter, Radiology, by Rice. The usual indication for surgery is lack of responsiveness to conservative medical therapy or irreversible chronic disease.

Adequate preoperative radiographic evaluation is mandatory. With the exception of the occasional case of trephination, most frontal sinus operations are done under general anesthesia. The anesthesia is augmented by cocainization of the nose in order to reduce bleeding, especially in the intranasal phases of the procedures. Since the eyes will be exposed during the procedure, either Frost stitches or corneal shields are used for corneal protection. Usually, a full facial prep is done with Betadine or other germicidal soap. The drapes are usually sutured in place to maintain sterility.

A local anesthetic with 1/100,000 epinephrine is injected as an aid in hemostasis to any facial or scalp incision. The agent should be injected 5 to 15 min prior to the creation of a skin incision to be maximally effective.

TREPHINATION

The trephination operation is among the oldest of the operative procedures and has stood the test of time in one form or another as an effective means of draining pus from the frontal sinus. It is most commonly used for an active frontal sinusitis, when the sinus remains completely opacified radiologically and there is no improvement of symptoms after intensive, appropriate antibiotic therapy (see the chapter, Radiology, by Rice).

The operation can be done under local or general anesthetic. A general anesthetic is preferred. An incision is marked 12 to 15 mm in length in the medial one-fourth of the eyebrow just through the inferior hairs

(Fig. 3). The incision line is injected with 1% xylocaine and 1/100,000 epinephrine. As the incision is made, the knife blade is slanted in the direction of the follicles of the brows. The incision is carried down through subcutaneous tissue and orbital orbicularis oculi to periosteum, and the underlying periosteum incised, then dissected along the upper medial wall and roof of the orbit using a periosteal elevator such as a Cottle or Joseph. It is important to remember that the trochlea is located approximately 15 mm from the orbital rim at this location. On some occasions, the trochlea may be dissected from its fossa. Fortunately, it almost always returns to its fossa and with usually no resultant disturbance of function.

A 6-mm dental cutting bur is then taken and a hole made in the anterior aspect of the frontal sinus floor (Fig. 4). The cavity of the frontal sinus is entered and specimens are taken for aerobic and anaerobic culture. The opening is enlarged to a diameter of about 8 mm to allow the passage of one or two drainage tubes. This sinus cavity is gently irrigated with warm saline. Mixing a nasal astringent such as epinephrine or cocaine into the irrigant may assist in opening the frontonasal

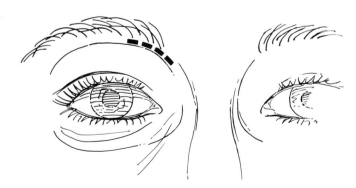

FIG. 3. Trephination incision.

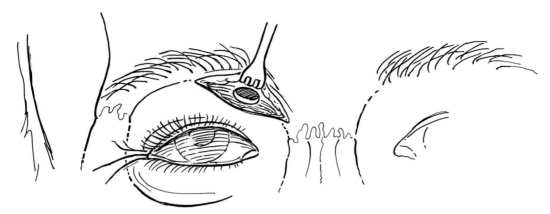

FIG. 4. Dental bur creating fenestration in floor of frontal sinus.

duct. If the opposing frontal sinus cavity is opacified, a large hole in the intersinus septum may promote drainage of both sinus cavities through the single trephination hole. The bur is inserted through the 8- to 10-mm trephination hole and the intersinus septum is removed. An attempt should be made to make this connection as low on the septum as possible to prevent localization of pus in the opposite sinus (Fig. 5).

I prefer the instillation of a large single drainage tube of plastic. The tube is sutured securely to the edge of the cutaneous incision with a nonabsorbable suture (Fig. 6). Irrigations with an antibiotic-containing solution are done on a daily basis until no further pus emanates from the tube and antibiotic-containing liquid drains into the nose. Once this has been accomplished, the tube is withdrawn and the soft tissue wound is lightly packed with medicated gauze for 24 to 48 hr; then the pack is removed and the wound is dressed with antibiotic ointment. During this time, the drain is in, and for 10 to 14 days after its removal, the patient is treated with the appropriate systemic antibiotic and a nasal astringent such as Afrin.

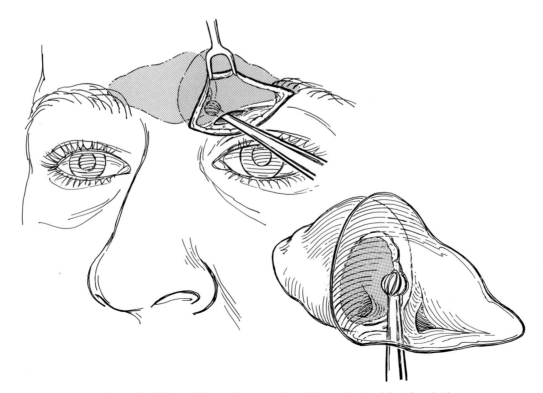

FIG. 5. Excision of intersinus septum through trephination hole.

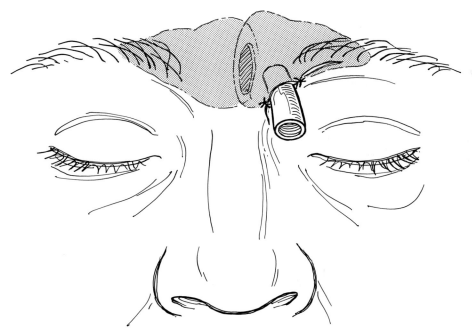

FIG. 6. Large-bore plastic tube is inserted into sinus and sutured to the cutaneous edge.

Very commonly, an individual who requires a trephination usually requires further exenterative surgery of the frontal as well as the ethmoid sinuses at a later time when the disease has become quiescent.

FRONTAL SINUS ABLATION

In patients who have severe irreversible frontal sinus disease, especially with a concomitant acute infectious process, a more radical procedure is required. The radical exenterative procedure proposed by Riedel (10,11) is still probably the safest and most reliable frontal sinus operation for infection in existence today. The only unsafe aspect is that it leaves the patient more vulnerable to brain injury if subsequent trauma is suffered to the frontal area. With the frontal sinus intact, the stout curved arch-shaped anterior wall serves as an excellent buffer against injury. However, when only the thin posterior wall is present, especially if it is dehiscent, the individual is more susceptible to major injury.

The operation may be done through a coronal incision or a brow incision. Since the second stage of this operation is a cranioplasty, done usually 12 months later, a coronal incision is preferred in order to avoid an incision that overlies the site of the proposed graft.

The brow incision is carried through the inferior hairs of the eyebrow for the medial two-thirds of each brow, then joined in a crease-line in the region of the nasion (Fig. 7). Each brow incision is carried in a curvilinear fashion down to a point midway between the caruncle of the eye and the midline of the nasal dorsum before being joined to its fellow on the opposing side. The blade, while in the brow, is inclined in an inferior direction parallel to the attitude of the follicles. Subcutaneous tissue and orbicularis oculi are incised down to periosteum. Periosteum is incised, as are usually the supraorbital and supratrochlear neurovascular bundles. Functional return of these nerves is unfortunately highly unpredictable. The periosteum is dissected up over the anterior table of the frontal sinus. In most instances in which this operation is employed, there is partial destruction of the anterior frontal sinus wall by osteomyelitis. This may follow the rare case of a failed osteoplastic flap with recurrent infection, a frontal sinus mucocele, but more especially a mucopyocele, or osteomyelitis from severe chronic frontal sinusitis. Usually, a prior trephination has been done so that any such eventrated area can serve as a start for the excision of bone. A Kerrison rongeur or other bone-biting instrument is used to remove the anterior wall of the sinus in its entirety (Fig. 8). A periosteal elevator is used to separate the periorbita from the floor of the frontal sinus. There may be an intervening ethmoid cell, which will require exenteration as well. As excision proceeds, great care is taken to also excise all necrotic bone found on the posterior wall. A periosteal elevator or dural elevator such as a Love–Adson is used to carefully separate dura from the necrotic bone (Fig. 9). This is especially important in the elderly whose dura is very brittle and easily torn. Any cerebrospinal fluid (CSF) leaks are noted and carefully sutured

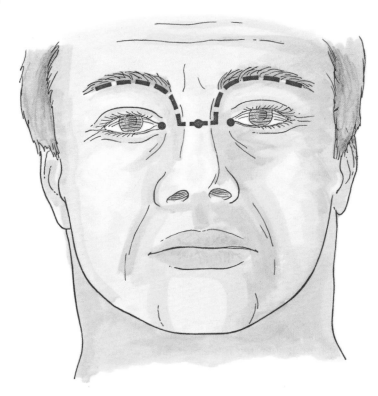

FIG. 7. Brow incision.

or patched as they form an easy pathway for infection with resultant meningitis.

The edges of the bony excision are trimmed up with the cutting bur. Once the bone of the sinus is completely removed, preserving as much of the posterior wall as possible, the soft tissue of the forehead is collapsed into the defect. The wound is sutured and dressed. The soft tissues are kept in position by the pressure exerted by fluffed gauze and a pressure dressing. It is difficult to maintain pressure just over the supraorbital area and an extensive all-over dressing like that for a facelift is most effective.

The dressing is removed at about 72 hr, and the sutures are removed in 5 days. It is common for considerable edema to exist in the flap in the first few weeks following the surgery. The defect does not look quite so bad initially as it does when the edema recedes. A delay of 10 to 12 months usually ensues prior to cranioplastic reconstruction. During this time, the aesthetic defect in the forehead is extremely noticeable,

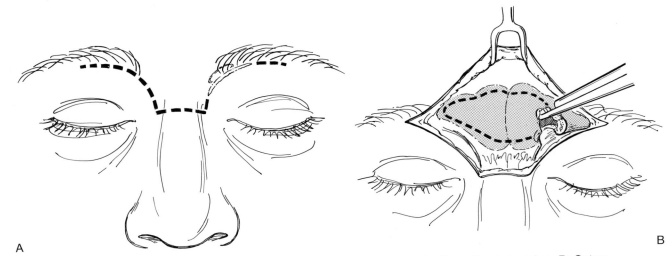

A   B

FIG. 8. Excision of anterior frontal sinus wall beginning in trephination site. **A:** Incision. **B:** Osteomyelitic bone removed from anterior wall.

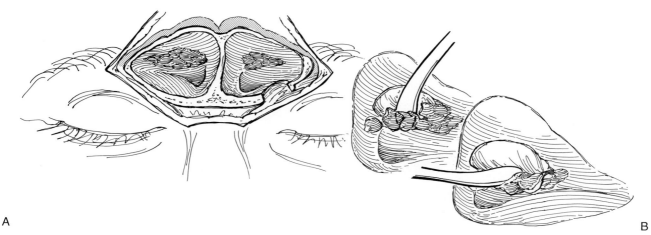

FIG. 9. A: Anterior wall completely removed. **B:** Separation of dura from osteomyelitic bone of posterior wall.

but amazingly well tolerated by patients, some of whom decline reconstructive surgery.

Case 1

Patient is a 58-year-old man who presented with a markedly erythematous swelling near the medial aspect of the eyebrow. The upper eyelid was swollen and sites of previous drainage were obvious (Fig. 10). He had a long history of purulent nasal drainage and obstruction. Every spring and fall, he suffered from seasonal allergic rhinitis. He had a history of over six instances of periorbital abscess treated by antibiotic

therapy with incision and drainage. A computer-assisted tomography (CAT) scan showed total opacification of the ethmoid and frontal sinuses. On plane films, there was a suggestion of bone erosion in the frontal sinus floor. The bony outline of the sinus was fuzzy and indistinct (Fig. 11).

Inspired with enthusiasm by the recent introduction of endoscopic sinus surgery into our therapeutic arma-

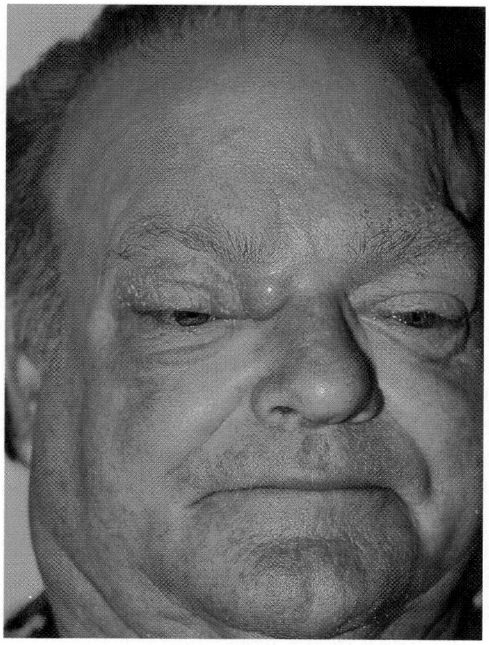

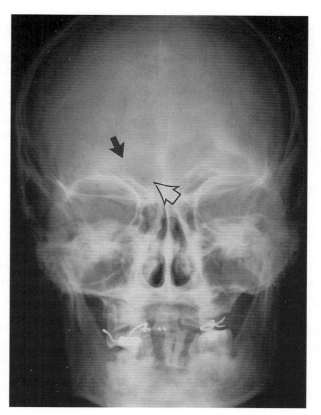

FIG. 11. Plane film of Case 1 showing erosion of floor and indistinct margin of frontal sinus *(closed arrow)*.

FIG. 10. Patient with periorbital abscess.

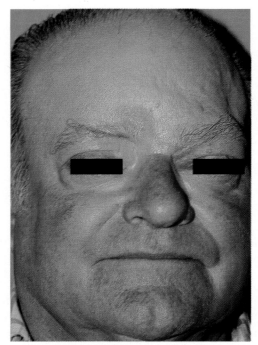

FIG. 12. Patient at 1 year following Riedel ablation.

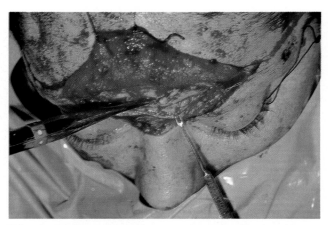

FIG. 13. Patient with mucopyocele extending into the anterior cranial fossa.

mentarium and its promise as a possible panacea for sinus disease, an attempt to cure the disease was made endoscopically. A complete ethmoidectomy and opening of the frontoethmoid cells revealed a large ethmoidal mucocele that was removed. This was followed by an asymptomatic period of 6 months.

A recurrent periorbital abscess was incised and drained and a frontal sinus trephination done. Once the infection became quiescent, a Riedel type frontoethmoidectomy was performed. The patient has been asymptomatic for 18 months and despite his marked deformity has declined reconstructive frontal cranioplasty (Fig. 12).

Case 2

Patient is a 23-year-old man who, in the year prior to his presentation, while in another state, was shot through the head with a small-caliber, low-velocity handgun. The bullet entered the right side of the anterior calvarium and crossed to the opposite side where it was lodged against the inner table of the skull (see Fig. 2A from the chapter, Frontal Sinus Fractures, by Donald). Three months prior to presentation, he suffered a near fatal case of meningitis. He was asymptomatic when first seen. A CT scan showed an opacification of the frontal sinuses and a defect in the posterior wall (see Fig. 26 from the chapter, Frontal Sinus Fractures, by Donald).

A diagnosis of frontal sinus mucopyocele was made and a Riedel procedure planned. A coronal scalp flap

was turned and the frontal sinus entered. A large mucopyocele was seen extending through the posterior sinus wall into the anterior cranial fossa (Fig. 13). The entire lining of the mucopyocele and all residual mucosa were removed from the frontal sinus. Portions of necrotic posterior sinus wall and all of the anterior wall and floor of the frontal sinus were removed.

The patient was left with a marked frontal sinus defect, which was obliterated at 1 year by a frontal cranioplasty using acrylic (Fig. 14).

LYNCH FRONTOETHMOIDECTOMY

The Lynch frontoethmoidectomy was a revolutionary operation in its time because it was such a marked departure from the more radical operations then popular. As Lawson (35) so correctly points out, Jansen (9) and Ritter (36) were the real founders of the procedure; and the currently used version was originally described by Knapp (14). The great advantage of saving the patient from a hideous deformity attracted many advocates of this procedure. Neither Lynch (16) nor Howarth (17) performed the frontoethmoidectomy that bears their names today. Lynch removed only a part of the frontal sinus floor and curetted all mucosa. Howarth in a review of greater than 200 cases resected the entire frontal sinus floor but did not remove the mucosa from the rest of the sinus cavity.

The facial preparation and use of corneal shields are the same as that seen for the Riedel operation. The nose is cocainized. The patient is positioned in a 30-degree head-up position to make perforation of the cribriform area more difficult. Once the fovea is exposed, the head position may be changed. The incision is not unlike a trephination incision. It begins in the medial one-third of the lower hairs of the eyebrow and extends in a curvilinear fashion through a point midway

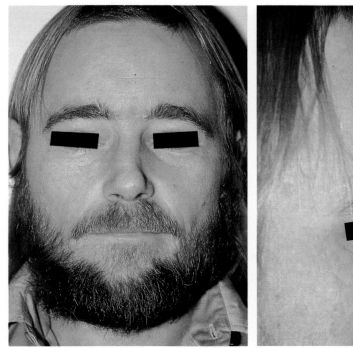
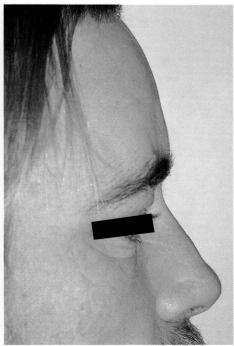

FIG. 14. Patient showing forehead profile 6 months after frontal cranioplasty. **A:** Frontal view. **B:** Lateral view.

between the medial canthus of the eye and the midline of the adjacent nasal dorsum (Fig. 15). A small angular flap may be introduced midway along the nasal orbital portion of the incision, the so-called Chiari modification (37). This helps to avoid scar contracture that sometimes occurs with the regular curvilinear incision (Fig. 16). The angular vein lies directly underneath the incision and troublesome bleeding can be avoided by careful dissection in the deeper soft tissues once the skin incision has been made. The vessel is tied with absorbable suture or cauterized. The periosteum over the nasal process of the frontal bone and frontal process of the maxilla is incised with a blade. Further incision of the periosteum of the orbital roof, which is common with either the floor of the frontal sinus or that of an orbital ethmoid cell, is done. The medial canthal tendon is dissected away from the frontal process of the maxilla and the anterior lacrimal crest with a Cottle or Freer elevator (Fig. 17). Small skin hooks are used for retraction. The medial skin margin is now retracted by the placement of two silk sutures in the skin that are suspended onto the opposite side of the face.

The anterior lacrimal crest is exposed and great care is taken as the lacrimal sac is dissected out of its fossa. The last remnants of the medial canthal tendon and Horner's muscle are dissected from the posterior lacrimal crest. Dissection superiorly prizes the fibrocartilaginous pulley, the trochlea, from its fossa. Displaced along with the trochlea will be the superior oblique

tendon that will be dislocated in an out and downward fashion as the periorbita is retracted to expose the frontal sinus floor (Fig. 18).

The skin hook that has been used for medial retraction is now replaced by a broad curved ribbon retractor. The best retractor adapted to this maneuver is the Sewell retractor. The assistant must constantly be reminded, however, to release the pressure the retractor exerts on the globe every 30 to 45 seconds to ensure no compromise of ocular circulation.

The next step in the procedure is to identify the anterior and posterior and, when present, the middle ethmoidal arteries, which are usually found in the frontoethmoidal suture line. The frontoethmoidal suture line also marks the level of the cribriform plate in many individuals, as does the interpupillary line. An understanding of the variability of the location of the ethmoidal arteries is a key point in maintaining a relatively bloodless field during the ethmoidectomy part of the operation. In the original procedures described by Jansen, Ritter, Knapp, and Lynch, no attempt was made to secure these vessels. It was not until 1926 that Sewall (38) described how to obtain hemostasis by ligating the ethmoidal arteries. It is noteworthy to mention that he did the procedure under local anesthesia.

Lang (39) in his meticulous dissections has illustrated the course, declination, and widths of the vascular canals of the ethmoidal arteries (Figs. 19 and 20). The paths of the anterior, posterior, and middle arteries

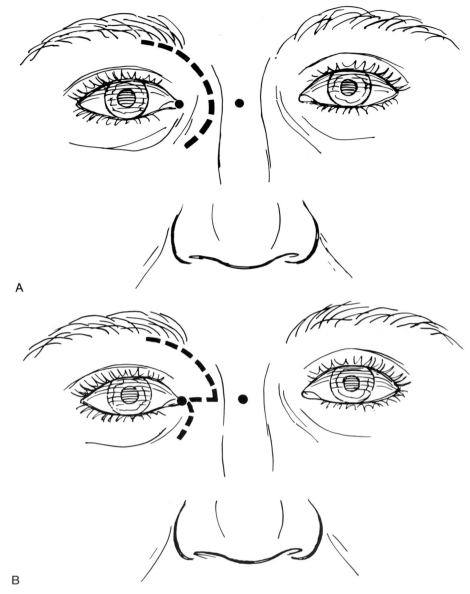

FIG. 15. Brow incision for frontoethmoidectomy. **A:** Standard Lynch incision. **B:** Chiari modification.

are observed to go either above or below the cribriform plate. Critical to the well-controlled frontoethmoidectomy is an understanding of the entry of the ethmoidal vessels from the orbit into the labyrinth (Fig. 21). Kirchner et al. (40) studied 150 orbits and found the anterior ethmoidal artery within the frontoethmoidal suture line in 68% of cases and within 1 to 4 mm above it in 32%. The distance from the anterior lacrimal crest to the anterior ethmoidal foramen was 14 to 18 mm in 64% of the specimens studied, but the distance between the anterior and posterior ethmoidal foramina was 10 to 11 mm. The posterior canal was in the frontoethmoidal suture line in 87% of cases and just above this site in the rest. The posterior foramen was absent in 22 of the

70 orbits dissected. They found the distance between the posterior ethmoidal foramen and the optic canal to be 4 to 7 mm in 84% of the specimens studied. Lang (39) states that the posterior ethmoidal artery was never closer than 2 mm to the optic canal in any of his dissections. Lawson (35) makes the excellent point that the optic nerve on its course to the optic canal will pass to within 2 mm of the posterior ethmoidal artery. Tertiary vessels (of the middle ethmoidal artery) were not mentioned in the Kirchner et al. (40) article but were found in 33 of Lang's specimens. The diameters of the tertiary vessels are about one-half the diameter of the anterior ethmoidal artery. The latter in turn is almost always larger than the posterior artery.

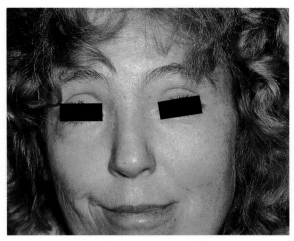

FIG. 16. Scar contracture after standard frontoethmoid incision.

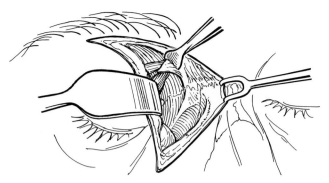

FIG. 18. The lacrimal sac is dissected out and the trochlea is displaced from its fossa.

Hemostasis is secured by the placing of a ligature or hemostatic clip or the use of the bipolar cautery. The cautery should not be used in the posterior ethmoidal artery. The posterior artery is only ligated if it is large and located relatively anteriorly. The cutting of the anterior, tertiary, and posterior ethmoidal arteries allows the freeing up of the periorbita over the medial and superior orbital wall.

The bony resection begins by either working through an already dehiscent area in the lamina papyracea with a bone-biting forceps such as the Blakesley or by resecting the posterior lacrimal crest with the Kerrison rongeur. During the removal of the posterior crest, cau-

tion is taken to carefully retract and guard the lacrimal sac. The ethmoid cells are judiciously excised with the bone-biting forceps and the lamina papyracea is methodically removed. The operator initially stays within the confines of the medial wall of the middle turbinate and its attachment to the lateral nasal wall, thus avoiding damage to the cribriform plate. Also, at the initial steps of the procedure, the lamina papyracea resection is limited to that area below the frontoethmoidal suture line. Resection is carried through the lacrimal fossa and for a short distance into the frontal process of the maxilla with a Kerrison rongeur. With this exposure, the agger nasi cells can be removed using both the external and intranasal approaches. Posterior excision continues back to the posterior ethmoidal artery. The thin cell walls, thickened mucosa, and polypoid material are all carefully removed with the resection for-

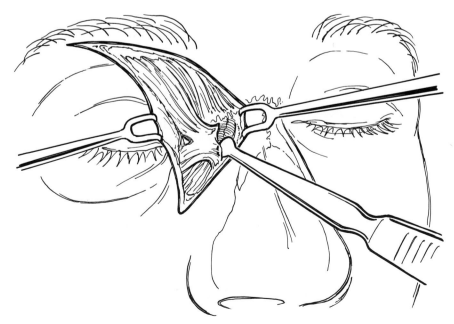

FIG. 17. Retraction of wound edges with skin hooks. Dissection of periosteum of orbital roof and medial orbital wall. Insertion of medial canthal tendon dissected away.

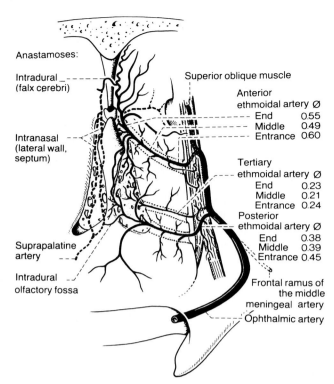

FIG. 19. The ethmoidal arteries and the diameter of their bony canals. (From ref. 39, with permission.)

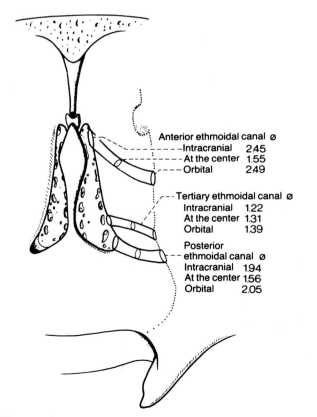

Anterior ethmoidal canal ø
Intracranial 2.45
At the center 1.55
Orbital 2.49

Tertiary ethmoidal canal ø
Intracranial 1.22
At the center 1.31
Orbital 1.39

Posterior ethmoidal canal ø
Intracranial 1.94
At the center 1.56
Orbital 2.05

FIG. 20. Course declination and diameter of ethmoidal arterial canals. (From ref. 39, with permission.)

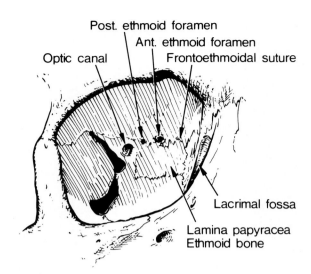

FIG. 21. The medial wall of the orbit. (From ref. 35, with permission.)

ceps. Bleeding is occasionally a problem, and this is controlled with a pack of ½- or ¾-in. wide ribbon gauze soaked in a solution of xylocaine and 1/100,000 epinephrine. After the pack is left in place for 5 min, hemostasis usually results.

At this point in the resection, a fairly capacious cavity has been created and the extent of orbital cells, if any, can be appraised (Fig. 22) (see also the chapter, Conventional Surgery for Ethmoid and Sphenoid Sinusitis, by Donald). A Kerrison rongeur is now used to bite away the remaining medial orbital wall above the level of the frontoethmoidal suture to expose the fovea ethmoidalis and the floor of the frontal sinus. With the orbital cells open, the ethmoidectomy proceeds posteriorly where the remaining posterior cells are removed to the level of the anterior wall of the sphenoid. Care is taken to go no further posteriorly with resection than the level of the equator of the globe because of risk to the optic canal. The anterior sphenoid face is removed and sphenoid mucosa removed. Attention is now turned anteriorly. If a former trephination has been done, then this provides a signpost to the frontal sinus. In its absence, entrance to the frontal sinus is made by punching through the anteromedial aspect of the orbital roof. This can be done with a small osteotome or cutting bur but is most often accomplished with the edge of the bone-biting forceps (Fig. 23).

The entire frontal sinus floor is removed up to the intersinus septum. If bilateral disease is present, then the intersinus septum is removed. The opposite frontal sinus floor in such cases will then have to be removed by a frontoethmoidectomy on the opposite side (Fig. 24).

One of the difficulties in this operation is complete

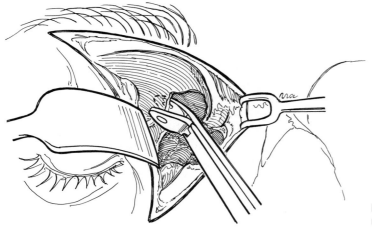

FIG. 22. Resection of anterior ethmoid cells beginning resection of orbital ethmoid cells.

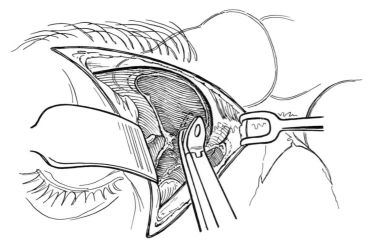

FIG. 23. Orbital ethmoid cells are removed and frontal sinus cavity is entered through the sinus floor.

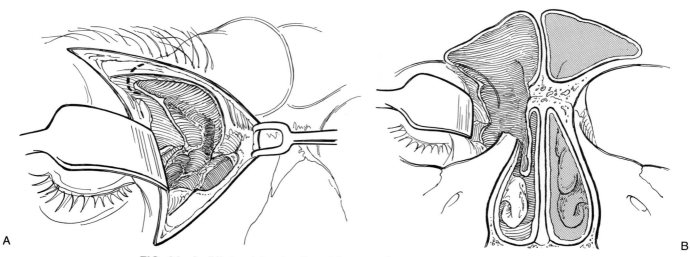

A   B

FIG. 24. A: Bilateral frontoethmoidectomy is complete. **B:** Coronal view.

removal of the entire frontal sinus mucosa. It has been shown by Lotta and Schell (41), Schenk (42), Ettin (43), and Donald (44) that damaged frontal sinus mucosa regrows in an abnormal fashion. However, many early proponents of the operation (16,17) emphasized neither complete mucosal removal nor removal of the entire sinus floor. An emphasis on the total removal of frontal sinus mucosa using a dental drill was made in 1962 by Williams and Holman (45). They also pointed out the danger of an intersinus cell that may be contained within the intersinus septum as a potential cause of failure if not exenterated. They reported 50 cases of success using this technique.

The next problem is maintaining patency of the frontonasal connection. It would seem an easy chore seeing that the entire floor of the sinus is being removed. Unhappily, stenosis of the frontonasal duct following frontoethmoidectomy is its commonest complication. Many workers throughout this century have advocated tubes of various materials and various sizes left in place for varying amounts of time. Table 2 outlines some of the materials used for stenting. The commonest early material used was rubber tubing. This met with a high degree of failure. Prolonged implantation was tried to see if the success rate could be improved, but McNally and Stuart (47) showed closure of the duct merely weeks after a 6-month placement of the tube. Barton (55) reported 100% success in 34 patients who had a permanent indwelling Dacron tube. However, in a later report, two cases had surgery using an osteoplastic flap because of recurrent purulent discharge around the tube and periorbital cellulitis (57). The use of Silastic sheeting has been advocated by Neel et al. (56). Originally, Silastic tubing was used but was accompanied by a high incidence of recurrence of disease and required reoperation. There was only one failure in the group in which Silastic sheeting was used. Most of the patients (12/14) were followed for at least 2 years. Mucosa

in the region of the newly created duct was left and, as was seen in dog experiments, mucosal regrowth into the sinus was not uncommon. Unfortunately, on the whole, the track record in those patients who have serious irreversible mucosal disease when frontal sinus mucosa regrows is not good.

The most successful method of maintaining duct patency is with mucosal flaps. Mucosal free grafts were first tried in 1928 by Mihoefer (58). Negus (59) and Smith (60) tried split-thickness skin grafts, all with limited success.

Sewall (38) was the first to devise the creation of a mucosal flap to swing into the defect created by a Lynch frontoethmoidectomy to reline the duct area. He proposed a large flap based on the nasal septum and extending over the lateral nasal wall. The operation was refined by contributions from Smith (61) and Simpson (62). In 1936, McNaught (63) reported a variation of Sewall's operation in which the flap was pedicled laterally and contained the tough mucoperiosteum of the septum. Sewall taught the operation to Kistner (20) who, then at the University of Oregon, introduced it to Boyden (64,65), who in turn popularized it in the 1950s. The definitive description of this flap in modern times was by Baron et al. (20) in 1973.

In Baron's modification of Sewall's technique (20), he removes a substantial portion of the lateral nasal wall with a cutting bur (Fig. 25). As the mucosa is approached, he switches over to a diamond bur so as not to damage the mucosa. Only 2 to 3 mm of bone are left on the lateral nasal wall near the dorsum. Care is taken to preserve the attachment of the upper lateral cartilage to the bone by leaving an additional 2- to 3-mm bony strip inferiorly. The mucoperiosteum is carefully dissected down to the tips of the middle and superior turbinates (Fig. 26). The frontoethmoidectomy is done posteriorly to the flap with great care taken to avoid damage to the flap. The inferior end of the flap is cut 90 degrees to the plane of the nasal dorsum and is made as long as possible, usually 1 to 3 cm. The inferior end of the flap is now developed through the nose. Parallel incisions at the extremity of this rostral cut are extended by the lateral nasal wall over the dome to the septum. The flap is packed out of harms way until the rest of the frontosphenoid–ethmoidectomy is done. After the frontal sinus floor and intersinus septum have been removed, care is taken to meticulously remove all vestiges of frontal sinus mucosa with the elevator and then polish the cavity with a bur.

At the completion of the sinus exenteration, the flap is turned into the cavity. The ethmoid cavity is packed with medicated gauze and a Poretex or Silastic tube is placed as a stent for 7 to 10 days. The packing should not contact the flap. No postoperative irrigation is used and only nasal spray with saline and the removal of crusts are done in the early postoperative period.

TABLE 2. *Materials used to maintain nasofrontal duct patency*

Surgeon	Material
Lynch[16]	Rubber
Howarth[17]	Rubber
Scharfe[46]	Tantalum foil
McNally & Stewart[47]	Tantalum foil
Goodale[48]	Tantalum foil
Harris[49]	Tantalum foil
Erich & New[50]	Acrylic
Woolflority & Solomon[51]	Protex
Ingals[52]	Gold
Anthony[53]	Gold
Lyman[54]	Gold
Barton[55]	Dacron
Neel et al[56]	Silicone

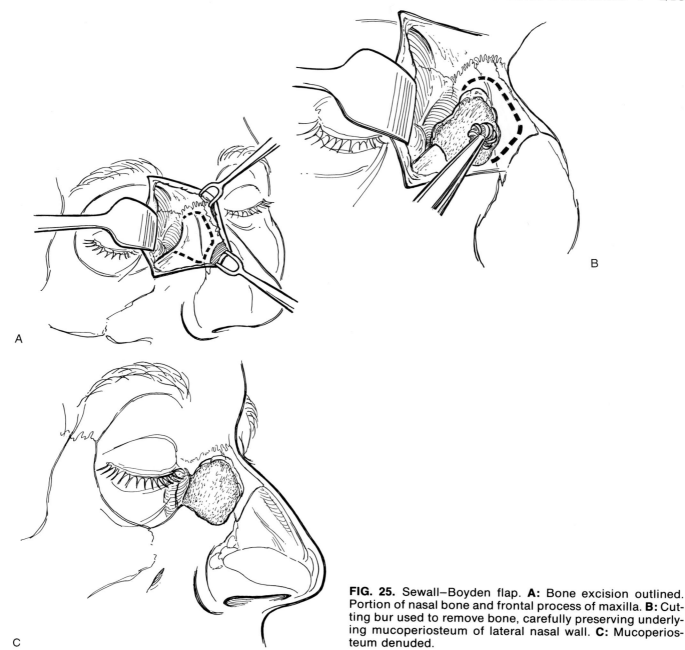

FIG. 25. Sewall–Boyden flap. **A:** Bone excision outlined. Portion of nasal bone and frontal process of maxilla. **B:** Cutting bur used to remove bone, carefully preserving underlying mucoperiosteum of lateral nasal wall. **C:** Mucoperiosteum denuded.

The laterally based flap requires more bone removal from the nasal dorsum. The flap is pedicled on the mucoperiosteum of the lateral nasal wall and the end of the flap is on the septum near the maxillary crest. Mucoperichondrium and mucoperiosteum are elevated off the quadrilateral cartilage and the perpendicular plate of the ethmoid. A flap 1 to 3 cm wide is created by two parallel incisions made from the extremities of the horizontal incision initially created above the maxillary crest (Fig. 27). The flap is elevated over the nasal dome and then turned into the frontal sinus defect. The flap is best used in those cases in which extensive surgery

had been done to the frontal sinus or in those that require a wide field resection. A much longer and wider flap is then required.

According to Baron et al. (20), Boyden reported 97 cases of this operation using these flaps without a failure; and furthermore that he himself and Dedo had never experienced a failure. McNally and Stuart (66) reported one failure in seven cases, and Ogura et al. (67) one failure out of 21. Dokianakis et al. (68) reported two failures in 22 patients with inflammatory disease of the frontal sinus. Their flap is a modification of the McNaught flap but uses the mucoperiosteum of

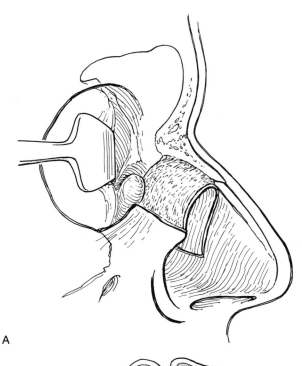

A

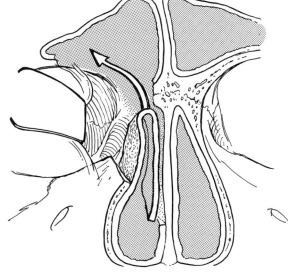

B

FIG. 26. Sewall–Boyden flap. **A:** The flap is pedicled on the lateral nasal wall and runs over the nasal dorsum, then onto the septum. **B:** Coronal view showing flap placed into the sinus.

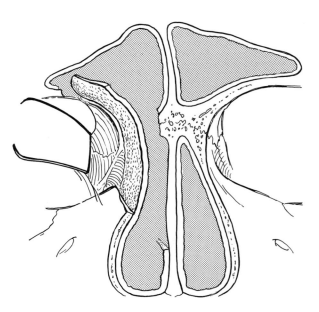

the middle turbinate as part of the flap. The average follow-up period was only 28 months.

These results are a vast improvement over those of early workers who report a 20% of 33% failure in their cases of a Lynch–Howarth type of frontoethmoidectomy (45,49,69).

OSTEOPLASTIC FLAP

One of the most popular and most effective methods of treating chronic frontal sinusitis, either with or with-

out a mucocele, is with the osteoplastic flap and fat obliteration operation. The fashioning of an osteoplastic cranial flap for the exenteration of chronic frontal sinus infection was first reported in 1894 by Schonborn (21) and in 1895 by Brieger (22) in the German literature. In the next 10 years, a number of others reported on modifications of this procedure (24–26) and introduced the notion of having a preoperative radiograph in these cases (23,70).

The osteoplastic flap procedure was introduced in the western hemisphere by Beugara and Itoiz (27,28,71) and Tato (29,72) from Argentina. Beugara

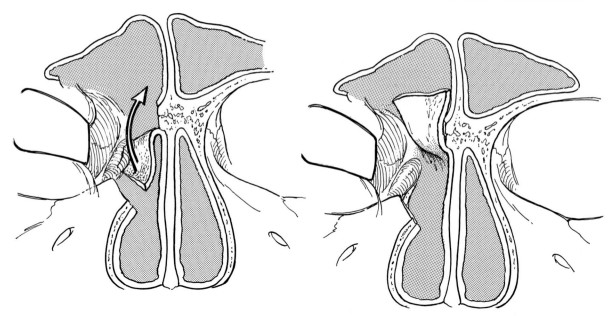

FIG. 27. The McNaught modification of the Sewall flap. The flap is pedicled on the nasal septum and run onto the lateral nasal wall.

actually began this operation as early as 1934. These investigators showed initially in dog experiments the transformation of part of the adipose tissue to fibrous tissue and in others a zone of osteogenesis on the inside of the sinus (73). It is curious that Marx (74) first suggested using fat as an obliterating agent in 1910. The earlier work by Beugara and Itoiz (71) showed that fat traumatized by boiling resorbed and was replaced by fibrosis whereas undamaged fat remained unchanged.

Montgomery and Pierce (75) showed in cat experiments that fat grafts usually remained at about 85% of their initial volume when the mucosa was meticulously removed. Donald (44) demonstrated the reverse in a series of cat experiments similar to those of Montgomery and Pierce (75) but in which the mucosa was simply stripped from the sinus cavity. None of the inner cortical lining was cut away with a bur. An attempt was made to ablate the cavity with fat in some and collagen in others. Epithelium regrew in 70% of the sinus cavities and there was evidence of infection in 67% (44). It became quite clear from this evidence that all vestiges of mucosa must be removed in order for the sinus to be successfully obliterated. Subsequent investigations have shown that the frontal sinus mucosal lining invaginates into the foramina of Breschet. Some of these imbrications may be amputated during stripping of the mucosa. Only a final polishing with a cutting bur will eliminate these vestiges (44). Montgomery and Ormon (76) showed that the fat graft inhibits osteoneogenesis and picks up a blood supply from the burred surface of the sinus cavity bone within a few days (77). This has been confirmed by the author both

clinically and in the laboratory. McNeil (78) showed fat survival in the cat frontal sinus but emphasized the problems of fat necrosis and infection if the graft was traumatized or active infection remains. In one group of controls, he noted that if no implant was used and the membrane is simply stripped, few changes occurred in the sinus wall. However, in those in whom the inner table was burred, osteoneogenesis ensued. He also showed that fat grafts in the maxillary sinus were successful in humans in alleviating symptoms of sinusitis. No radiographic follow-up was done.

The issues of whether an obliterating agent should be used and, if so, what type and, furthermore, whether alloplasts will work as well as tissue are controversial. Fat is the most commonly used obliterating agent, but McBeth (79) recommended that no obliterating agent at all need be implanted. He observed in his patients the tendency of the cavity to obliterate by the growth of osteoneogenesis. This confirmed the findings in animals by Samolineko, who in 1913 showed that bone filled in the sinus after stripping away the mucosa (80). This experimental finding was confirmed by Hilding (81) and Walsh (82), both of whom found that the denuded sinus filled in with both bone and fibrous tissue. Walsh, however, showed that the mucosa regenerated if removed only from the sinus cavity and that mucosa must also be removed from the frontonasal duct to achieve complete obliteration. Similar findings were also observed more lately by Abramson and Eason (83). However, they used only four dogs and one later formed a mucus-lined cyst and incomplete obliteration.

These were all animal experiments and McBeth (79) was the first to confirm these findings in humans.

Bosely (34) reviewed McBeth's experience in doing this operation in 100 consecutive patients who all had a minimum follow-up of 6 months. The review included six cases of trauma, 13 patients with osteoma, and 81 patients treated for frontal sinusitis, 25 of whom had prior frontal sinus surgery and 56 who did not. None of the trauma patients were new patients. All had complications secondary to trauma such as CSF leakage or mucopyocele. Over half the osteoma patients had chronic frontal sinusitis. On follow-up, persistent headache was a complaint in 15% of all the operated on cases, of which a total of seven cases were not completely obliterated. In the trauma patients, one-fifth had incomplete obliteration and six of the 56 patients with infection did not completely obliterate with bone. Since Bosley's landmark report, a number of patients operated on using the McBeth technique have required reoperation because of failure (84).

Most individuals doing the osteoplastic flap procedure obliterate the cavity with some type of material; fat being the most common. However, many investigators have tried a host of materials, some in experimental animals and some in patients.

Sessions et al. (85) described an experiment in cats in which they duplicated the usual clinical experience; that is, they produced an active infection in the frontal sinus and plugged the nasofrontal duct. Once the sinus formed an abscess, they then obliterated it with either fat, blood clot, synthetic collagen, or Silastic medical grade elastomer. Although they state that the animals did well and there was no infection, there were no details concerning the number of animals in each group or the duration of observation or technique of analysis. They reviewed 72 patients treated by osteoplastic flap and fat obliteration. Unfortunately, only a few patients were able to be observed for longer than 1 year. The results on the short term were excellent with only one patient having a relapse of chronic infection. A technical point they stress is the importance of obliterating the nasofrontal duct with fascia.

Abramson et al. (86) attempted cavity obliteration with cancellous bone chips from the iliac crest in dogs. The most successful results were in those animals in which the sinus cavity was completely packed with the chips. Despite this, in some instances, there was regrowth of mucosa in the form of cysts. In the long term (6 to 26 weeks), nine out of 24 animals had mucous cysts. It is difficult whether to indict the obliteration technique or criticize the thoroughness of mucosal excision as the authors admit they did not use a drill for mucosal removal.

The notion of autogenous bone obliteration of the frontal sinus is not new. Lierle and Huffman (87) described the procedure over 40 years ago. It was reinforced by Knouff (88) in 1963 and described again more recently by Wolfe and Johnson (89). They believe the method is superior to fat obliteration but, as Luce (90) points out, given there were no long-term results on a significant number of patients, it is difficult to conceive of the results as conclusive. One could also argue the morbidity of procuring a hip graft against the taking of a subcutaneous fat graft.

Naumann (91) has reported filling the sinus with plasma, fibrin, and Gelfoam. Siirala (92) reported the successful obliteration in four patients using deproteinized bovine bone. Beeson (93) implanted six dogs with plaster of Paris in the frontal sinus and successfully obliterated all sinuses at up to 24 weeks follow-up. There was much fibrovascular reaction, many chronic inflammatory cells, and some evidence of osteoneogenesis. Cotzee (94) used plaster of Paris in three patients as an obliterating agent after large mucopyoceles had been exenterated from the frontal sinus. The duration of follow-up on these patients is uncertain; but there were no complications mentioned in either these or the 117 others that had plaster of Paris obliteration for a host of head and neck defects, the majority of which resulted from mastoidectomy. In our own small series of cat frontal sinus obliteration with plaster of Paris, none were successful (P. J. Donald and M. Ettin, *unpublished data*).

A variety of alloplastic materials have been implanted in experimental animals and patients. Dickson and Hohmann (95) implanted, among other materials, closed pore Silastic, Teflon paste, and paraffin. The follow-up was only 8 weeks in their animals. The closed pore Silastic had fibrosis and osteoneogenesis up to the implant. There was no fibrosis or osteoneogenesis in either the paraffin-filled or Teflon-injected sinuses. Whereas there was no evidence of fibrous ingrowth in the Teflon-paste-obliterated animals of Dickson and Hohmann, Janeke et al. (96) discovered the ingrowth of osteoid material into Proplast inserted into the frontal sinus. Proplast is a Teflon fluorocarbon that is combined with vitreous carbon and is very porous. Schenk et al. (97) confirmed this finding in animal studies, whose sinuses remained obliterated for a year. Barton (57) treated eight patients with Proplast obliteration and they remained without complication or recurrent disease 1 to 8 years following surgery.

Failla (98) describes his rationale for using methylmethacrylate to obliterate the frontal sinus after fracture. He does not describe its use in infection. He alludes to the fact that a host of alloplasts have been used to reconstruct facial and cranial defects. Included in the list of materials are aluminum plates, Vitallium, gold, zirconium, tantalum plates and mesh, polyvinyl sponge, stainless steel, glass wool, celluloid, and preformed acrylic plates. In fracture patients, he eliminates the anterior wall, excises all the frontal sinus

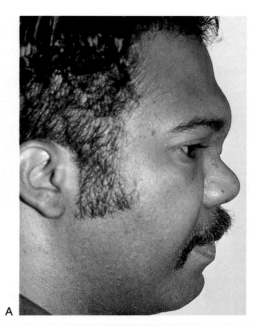

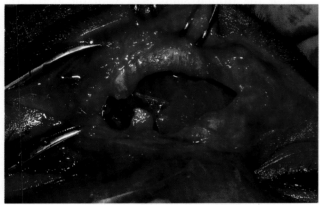

FIG. 28. Infected acrylic in frontal sinus. **A:** Patient preoperatively. Note Pott's puffy tumor. **B:** Intraoperatively, purulent material exuding around infected acrylic graft.

mucosa, and pours in the acrylic mixed at the operating table. In 18 patients followed for 2 to 73 months, there have been no complications and no mucoceles.

Unfortunately, in the author's experience, acrylic poured into a freshly exenterated sinus is frequently fraught with complications (Fig. 28). I strongly advise against the use of alloplastic materials in the frontal sinus, especially when treating infection and agree with Montgomery's statement (99) that alloplasts such as bone wax and acrylic are "frontal sinus poisons."

OSTEOPLASTIC FLAP AND FAT OBLITERATION

Despite the manifold surgical options claiming the best management of chronic frontal sinus disease, probably the most prevalent method in use today is

the osteoplastic flap and fat obliteration. The report by Hardy and Montgomery (100) describing their 250 cases with only a 6% failure rate on long-term follow-up attests to the efficacy and safety of this procedure.

The incisions used can be either the coronal or "butterfly" incisions through the brows (Fig. 29). The coronal gives the best access and is usually done in women or in men who have a full head of hair in which to hide the scar. It is also necessary in patients with tall frontal sinuses. The brow incision is used in male pattern baldness patients and those with short frontal sinuses. Prior to either incision, the area is injected with xylocaine and epinephrine. A preoperative culture is taken from the nasal cavity.

The eyelids are sutured together with a 5-0 nonabsorbable suture, or the eyes are protected by corneal shields. The brow incision is carried almost the length of the brow, depending on how much retraction is needed. It is carried through the most inferior hairs of the brow with the blade slanted in the direction of the hair follicles. The incision dips down through a crease line in the nasion to the opposite brow and is made symmetrically. Some criticism of the incision within the brows is the problem of the resultant scar, producing a "split brow" appearance. This has not been a problem in our experience. The frontalis muscle is cut through at just above the level of the brows. A submuscular, but extraperiosteal, dissection is carried to a point above the level of the frontal sinus.

The coronal incision is placed approximately 2 cm

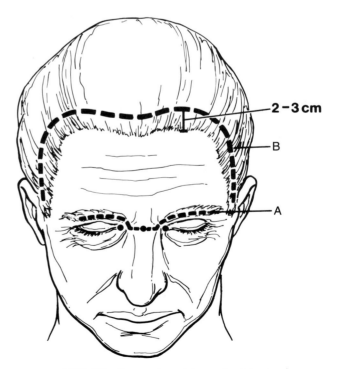

FIG. 29. Coronal and brow incisions.

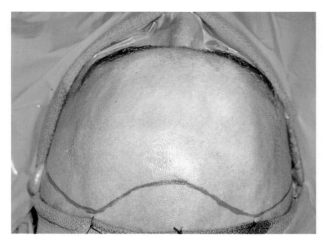

FIG. 30. Coronal incision marked out.

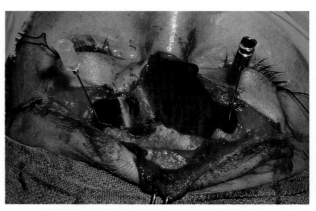

FIG. 32. Radiographic template is hammered into the bone with needles.

behind the hair line and carried over the vertex into the area anterior to, but just above, the pinna (Fig. 30). The incision is through the gala aponeurotica and not through the pericranium. Care is taken laterally to protect the temporalis fascia and therefore the frontal branch of VII. Hemostasis is obtained first by pressure and then with Rainey clips (Fig. 31). The flap is dis-

sected with a combination of sharp and blunt dissection down to the brows in the subgaleal plane. Lateral elevation is done to the extent that will just permit exposure of the frontal sinus area with the flap turned forward.

The area of the frontal sinus is determined by taking a 5- or 6-foot Caldwell view radiograph and cutting out the shape of the sinus. Some surgeons recommend that

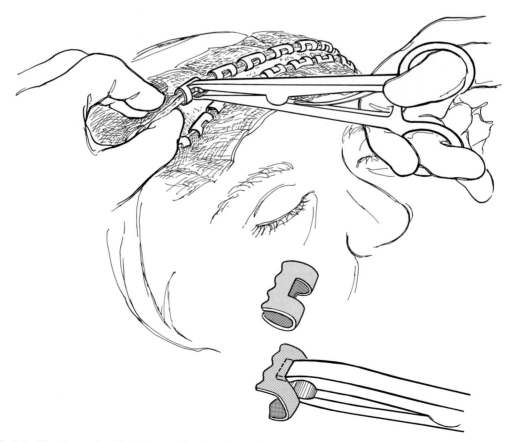

FIG. 31. Flap turned with Rainey clips in place. Folded over 4 × 4 and application of clips. **Inset** shows clip and clip applier.

one tape on a metal wire in the form of a cross over the frontal sinus area skin, take the radiography, and then maintain the wire until the patient is asleep. The template can be matched up with the crossed wire, and the sinus can then be marked out with methylene blue through the skin to bone. At the time of operation, once the cutaneous galeal flap is elevated, the template is fixed to the calvarium with either towel clips at the brows or hypodermic needles hammered into the outer calvarium (Fig. 32). The frontal sinus is outlined by passing a nonsiliconized needle soaked in methylene

blue through the pericranium, conforming to the outline of the template and twisted, thereby marking the underlying calvarium (Fig. 33). The periosteum is incised approximately 1 cm behind these marks in the outline of the sinus as taken from the template. A periosteal elevator is used to dissect the periosteum up to and just beyond the blue marks in the calvarium.

A penetrating drill is used to make multiple holes from the marks into the lumen of the sinus (Fig. 34). The drill is angled at about 60 to 45 degrees in order to create a beveled edge. This serves two purposes:

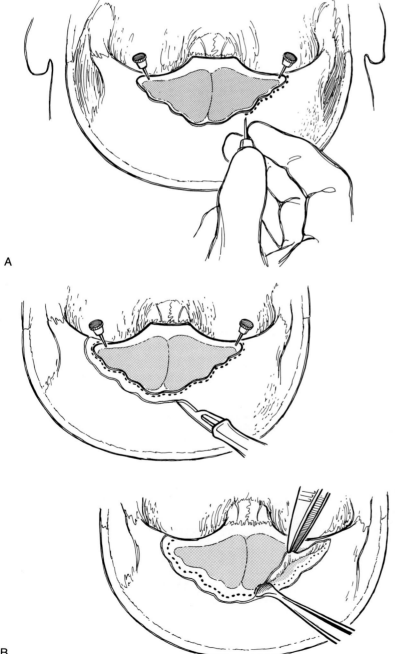

A

B

FIG. 33. A: The frontal sinus template is outlined with methylene blue and a nonsiliconized needle. **B:** Cuff of pericranium is incised outside proposed site of drill holes.

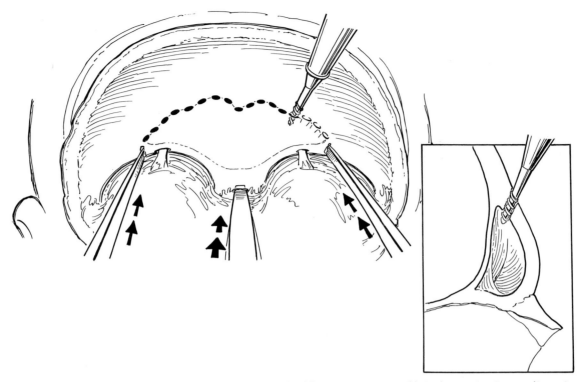

FIG. 34. Penetrating drill holes are connected with an osteotome. Note key osteotomy sites at nasion and brows. **Inset** shows obliquity of penetrating drill.

first, to avoid entering into the intracranial cavity if the size of the template turns out to be too large; and second, to prevent prolapse of the osteoplastic flap into the frontal sinus cavity postoperatively.

Once all the drill holes are made, they are connected with either a small osteotome or an angled round ended saw (Fig. 35). The outline of the frontal sinus is conformed to as closely as possible. The oblique cut toward the sinus lumen made with the drill is continued with the larger cutting tools. Since the flap will be

greenstick fractured across each anterior roof of the orbits, it is essential to cut through the brows and just below the glabella (Figs. 34 and 36) with the saw or osteotome. A small osteotome is insinuated between the anterior and posterior table of the sinus along the intersinus septum and driven to the sinus floor. The flap is gently pried forward with a broad osteotome, creating the greenstick fracture (Figs. 37 and 38). With the flap forward, the pathology becomes obvious. The commonest findings are mucoceles, mucopyoceles,

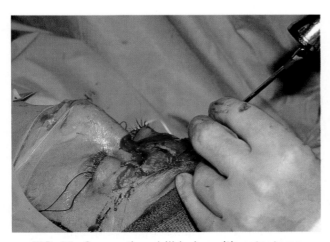

FIG. 35. Connecting drill holes with osteotome.

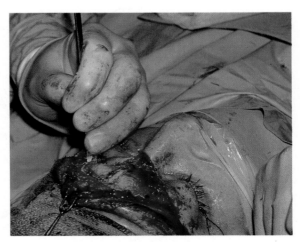

FIG. 36. Osteotome cut at brows.

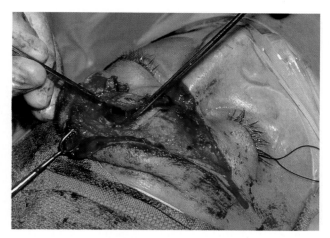

FIG. 37. Broad osteotome used to greenstick fracture the flap at the orbital roofs.

polypoid degeneration of the mucosa, and often considerable pus (Fig. 39). A sample is taken for aerobic and anaerobic infection evaluation.

All mucosa or mucocele lining is removed with a sharp elevator (Fig. 40). The drill is used to remove all vestiges of mucosa by drilling away the inner cortical layer of bone (Fig. 41). Research has shown that this step is essential to remove all mucosa. Anything less than a thorough cutting away of bone by the bur may result in recurrent disease. Our experiments in cats have shown that this bone removal is essential to ensure mucosal eradication (44). The extremities of the sinus narrow down to mere cracks in many cases.

Since the posterior wall and orbital roof are thin, drilling must be done to widen these areas in the expense of the thickness of the anterior wall. Often small diamond burs and magnification with loupes or the operating microscope are needed. Exposure of periorbita and even orbital fat may occur. This is no problem in terms of subsequent fat graft survival. Even exposure of the orbital ethmoid sinuses does not pose a threat to fat graft survival provided the sinus mucosa is eliminated. The mucosa of the frontonasal duct is inverted on itself into the nose. Continuous irrigation with saline is done during the bone removal with the bur in order to prevent excessive heating of the bone and to encourage the bleeding that is essential for nourishment of the fat graft.

The fat graft is procured from the left side of the abdomen in order not to confuse the situation in the future event of a possible appendicitis. The graft is taken as close to the time of implantation as possible. Meticulous care is devoted to the atraumatic dissection of the fat. No cautery is employed and hemostasis is obtained with fine absorbable ligatures. A fat graft whose size is as close to the sinus volume as possible is placed in the sinus (Fig. 42). Small recesses are packed with smaller pieces as thoroughly as possible. The fat remains as such from 50% to 100% with the absorbed portion being replaced with fibrous tissue. The fat is resistant to infection, impedes osteoneogenesis, and resists the intrusion of mucosa. It rapidly acquires a blood supply by direct inosculation of its amputated blood vessels to cut vessels in the bone. Rapid

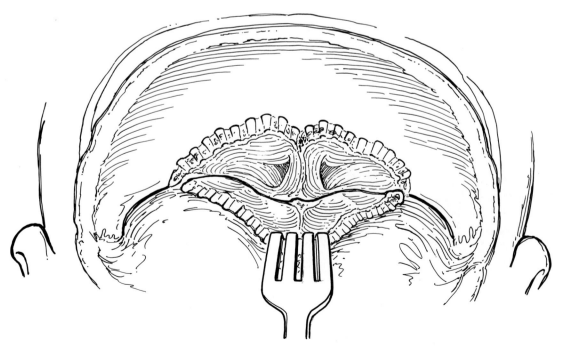

FIG. 38. Osteoplastic flap opened up and tipped forward.

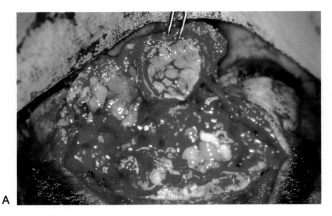

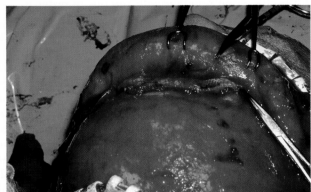

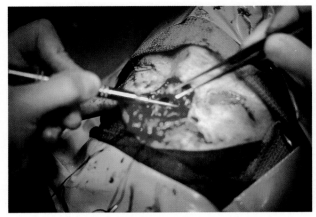

FIG. 41. Burring away inner cortical layer of bone.

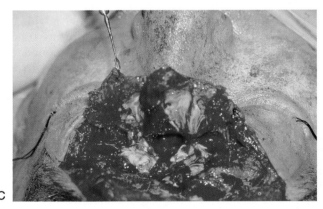

FIG. 39. Pathologic findings in frontal sinus at operation. **A:** Polypoid degeneration. **B:** Thick chocolate brown material exuding from mucocele. **C:** Copious pus in a muco-pyocele.

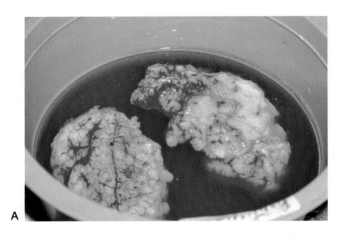

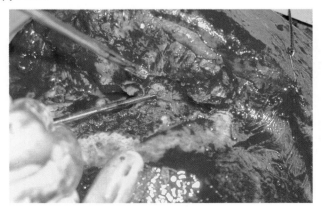

FIG. 40. Dissecting out diseased mucosa.

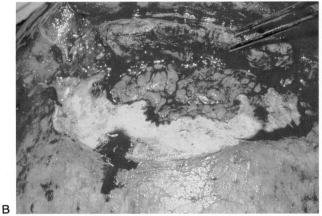

FIG. 42. A: Fat graft. **B:** Fat graft in sinus.

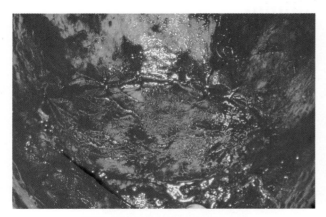

FIG. 43. Closed periosteum.

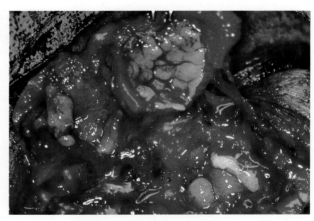

FIG. 45. Polypoid mucosa.

ingrowth of capillaries quickly revascularizes the graft. The frontonasal duct epithelium overgrows it in a short time.

The graft should just conform to the volume of the exenterated sinus. Overfilling should be avoided as should large void spaces. The periosteum is closed over the flap although this is sometimes difficult (Fig. 43). No interosseous wires or plates are required.

The skin incision is closed and a light pressure dressing is applied. The dressing is removed on the third or fourth postoperative day. Hematoma is avoided usually by the dressing. Drains are not used unless excessive oozing was present at the end of the operation.

Case 3

Patient AG is a 46-year-old man who had a lifelong history of allergic rhinosinusitis and bronchial asthma.

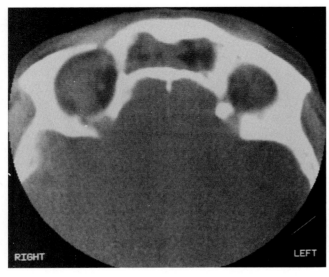

FIG. 44. Opacification of frontal sinus with polypoid mucosa and pus in chronic frontal sinusitis.

His asthma was aggravated by the purulent drainage resulting from his sinusitis. Little control was achieved by attempts at allergic desensitization. He was on continuous bronchodilators and intermittent steroids and antibiotics. One of his principal complaints was unremitting frontal headache. Radiographs showed pansinusitis with total opacification of all sinuses (Fig. 44). Bilateral Caldwell–Luc procedures were done on the maxillary sinuses with improvement of maxillary pain. External ethmoidectomies reduced the purulent nasal drainage and improved the periorbital pain.

Because of continuous frontal pain and persisting frontal sinus opacification, an osteoplastic flap and fat obliteration operation was done. At surgery, the sinus was seen to be full of purulent material and extensive polypoid degeneration of the sinus mucosa was evident (Fig. 45).

At 10 years postoperatively, he is free of frontal pain.

Case 4

Patient BC is a 33-year-old office worker who had a long history of seasonal allergic rhinitis. She presented to an ophthalmologist with displacement of her left eye in a downward and outward direction. She had complete nasal obstruction for many years. She had never had testing for inhalant allergy.

Physical examination revealed polyps in both nasal cavities and scant purulence. The left eye was slightly proptotic and deviated in an inferior and lateral direction (Fig. 46A). There was no diplopia.

Radiographs revealed thickened mucosa in the maxillary antra and opacification of the ethmoid and frontal sinuses. There was bone erosion in the left orbital roof and a soft tissue mass displacing the globe (Fig. 46B).

An osteoplastic flap was done and, at surgery, the frontal sinus mucosa was found to be thickened and a mucocele was obvious. The sinus was full of a brown-

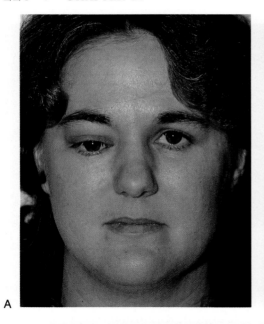

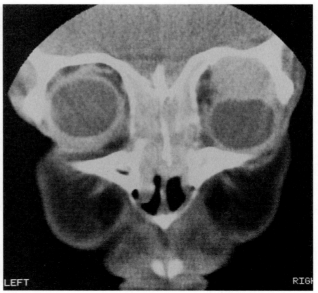

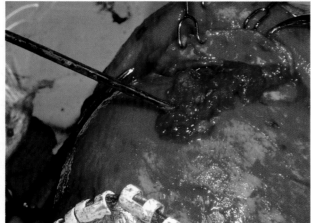

FIG. 46. A: Frontal sinus depressing left eye down and out. **B:** Coronal CAT scan showing frontal sinus mucocele displacing eye inferiorly. **C:** Intraoperative view of patient BC, illustrating frontal sinus with mucocele and glue-like purulent material.

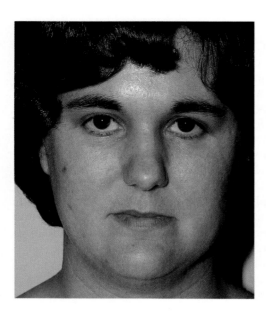

FIG. 47. Postoperative appearance after osteoplastic flap and fat obliteration.

ish semisolid material resembling silicone glue (Fig. 46C). There was a dehiscence in the frontal sinus floor. Following removal of the mucocele and drilling down the inner cortex of the sinus, the cavity was obliterated with fat.

At 8 years postoperatively, she has had an intranasal ethmoidectomy for her ethmoidal disease and has her allergic diathesis controlled with desensitization (Fig. 47). The only complication she has is slight absorption of bone at the site of her osteoplastic flap.

Case 5

Patient J is a 51-year-old teacher who had a lifelong history of rhinosinusitis. At presentation, she had a history of about 15 operations on her maxillary and ethmoid sinuses. She complained of purulent nasal drainage and headache. Examination revealed scant polypoid disease in both ethmoidectomy cavities with some purulence. Radiographs revealed thickened mucosa in the ethmoids and opacification of the frontal sinuses (Fig. 48).

Endoscopic ethmoidectomy and sphenoidotomy and opening of the maxillary ostia were done, which provided salutary relief. The frontal headache persisted, along with symptoms of maxillary sinusitis. Repeat radiographs revealed only frontal sinus opacification. An osteoplastic flap and fat obliteration operation was done through a coronal incision. The sinus mucosa was

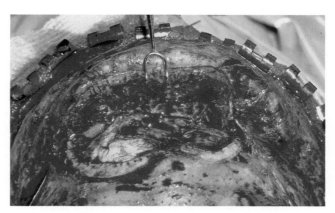

FIG. 49. Patient JM's intraopertive appearance.

grossly thickened and the sinus full of pus despite her recent prolonged course of antibiotics (Fig. 49).

She is free of disease 3 years since her frontal sinus procedure.

COMMENT

These patients are examples of severe chronic frontal sinusitis, one with a mucocele and two without. The two patients who had frontal sinusitis and had their ethmoid and maxillary disease treated first did so based on the following traditional teaching. It has long been thought that chronic and acute frontal sinusitis will clear if ethmoid and maxillary disease resolves with appropriate therapy. This dictum was obviously not true in these cases; and despite eradication of osteomeatal complex disease and active ethmoid and maxillary infection the frontal sinus disease persisted.

ACRYLIC FRONTAL OSTEOPLASTY

In cases of severe infection in which osteomyelitis of the frontal bone exists, the Riedel ablation has been done. The disease is almost always eradicated, but the residual deformity is substantial. The patient recovers for 12 to 18 months and, when stable, is then aesthetically restored with acrylic frontal osteoplasty.

The most commonly used material is a polymerized ester of methylacrylic acid: $CH_2 = C(CH_3)COOH$. A liquid monomer with an accelerator is mixed with a powder of small granules of polymerized methylacrylate that contains a catalyst. This results in a thick pourable slurry that becomes transformed into a dough-like consistency as polymerization progresses. As the dough hardens the exothermic reaction of further polymerization can produce heat of up to 100°C in vitro. However, in vivo tests in fresh femur warmed to body temperature heated to only 68°C when the polymerizing acrylic was applied (10). Although the tem-

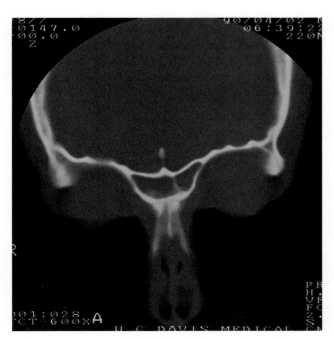

FIG. 48. Radiograph showing complete opacification of frontal sinus due to chronic sinusitis.

peratures at which body proteins denature are those in excess of 56°C, the surrounding tissues in which the acrylic is polymerized are usually cooled. The usual local reaction to methylmethacrylate is minimal (100–103), comprised of a few foreign body giant cells initially; once stabilized, a thin layer of fibrous tissue covers the implant.

The first reported use of methylmethacrylate in humans was by a German general surgeon, Zander (104), who in 1940 used it to reconstruct a cranial defect. During World War II, there was a great need for cranioplasty following surgery for the multitude of head injuries commonplace then. The early acrylics used were preformed and cured under heat and pressure. Some had the same requirement for impressions and molds needed for the metal plates in common use at the time. The use of a single-stage methacrylate cranioplasty first appeared in the literature in the 1950s (105,106).

The great advantage of this technique over the laborious two-stage process gained rapid acceptance and is still the state of the art today. The procedure is straightforward and simple, the implant can be molded in situ, and complications are few.

One of the overriding concerns is the fate of the monomer. The monomer polymer is mixed at a ratio of 1:2. Following polymerization, approximately 4% of the monomer remains. The serious hazards related to the implantation of this material have never been associated with its use in the craniofacial area. However, in orthopedics, severe hypotension, hyperpyrexia, and cardiac arrest have been reported (102,107–109). These appear to be related to the exposure of the polymerizing implant to the large raw surface areas of bare bone seen in hip surgery. Hypotension appears in part to be related to the synergism between the large blood losses and the effects of the

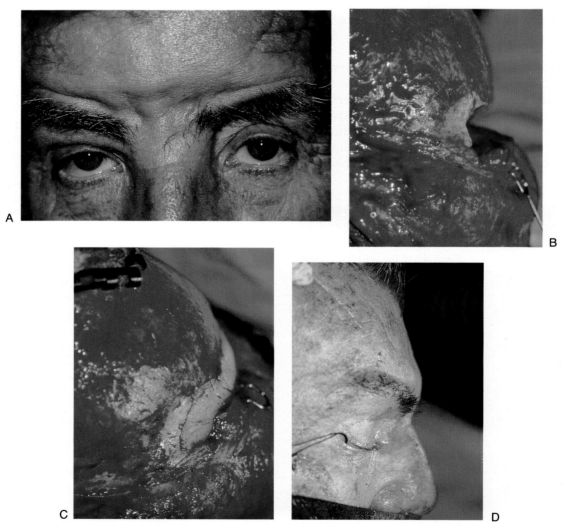

FIG. 50. Acrylic frontoplasty. A: Preoperative photograph. Patient is 1 year post-Riedel ablation. B: Frontal defect. C: Cranioplasty done. D: Postoperative profile.

monomer. Systemic reactions are thought to be due to an allergic reaction to the monomer.

The performance of acrylic frontal cranioplasty is best done 1 year after the frontal sinus infection has subsided and the skin over the frontal defect is soft and pliable. A coronal incision is the best choice in that it places the subsequent suture line at a distance from the implant. If a subperiosteal placement can be done, then a periosteal incision is made approximately 1 to 2 cm from the edge of the defect. The periosteum is elevated down to the orbits. If there was any dural exposure at the time of the initial surgery for infection, then an extraperiosteal dissection is advisable. The edges of the defect are defined. Any gross irregularities or areas of bony overgrowth are trimmed with a cutting bur. Hemostasis is essential as layers of blood tend to weaken the strength of the implant. There must be no residua of infection, granulation tissue, or mucosa at the implantation site. Additionally, there should be no connection to the nose or the other sinuses.

The monomer is added to the polymer in a metal mixing bowl. The monomer is not only sterile, but it is also bacteriostatic so it sterilizes the polymer as it is added to it. Mixing should be done with a rapid beating motion to ensure maximum wetting of the polymer. This phase should be done with the aid of a fume extractor as part of the reaction involves vaporization of the monomer, which has a noxious, objectionable odor. As mixing takes place, the consistency changes from a slurry to a tacky substance to a malleable dough. This takes about 7 minutes.

The doughy material is placed in the center of the defect and worked from the center of the defect to the periphery. Lamination and folding should be prevented, and the trapping of blood should be avoided as much as possible. The plastic is feathered over the edges of the cranium. It is better to overfill than underfill the defect. As the material hardens, which takes about the same amount of time that the mixing takes, it is molded with the fingers. Care is taken to recon-

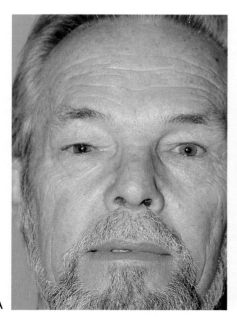
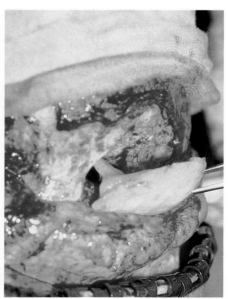

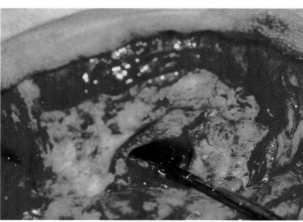

FIG. 51. Frontoethmoidal mucocele as a complication of frontocranioplasty when acrylic is exposed to ethmoid mucosa. **A:** Mucocele pushing right eye down and out. **B:** Mucopyocele surrounding acrylic plate. **C:** Hole through which acrylic extended into ethmoid block.

struct the brows and the normal bony contour to the forehead. When the doughy stage passes to the firm stage, the exothermic reaction begins to accelerate. It becomes maximum as the implant attains final hardness. Continuous irrigation of the tissues at this stage with ice cold saline will reduce tissue damage at the implant site. Some surgeons remove the implants at this point until final hardening has taken place. The problem is that the implant will often fix in situ, sticking to bone and fibrous tissue in the bed and becoming lodged within the bony undercuts at the margins. Hardening the implant without removal often precludes the necessity of wiring it into the surrounding bone.

Once in place, the edges are feathered with a cutting bur to produce a smooth transition from implant to bone (Fig. 50). Frequent checks are made with the flap turned back to ensure a normal forehead contour. If the implant is unstable, then penetrating drill holes are made in it and the adjacent bone so that the implant can be wired in place. This is infrequently necessary. If there needs to be some addition to the implant, the surface is painted with monomer and newly mixed polymer added to it.

Care must be taken that all vestiges of infection have been eliminated and that no contact with residual sinus mucosa occurs. In such instances, the complication of mucocele is uncommon (Fig. 51).

REFERENCES

1. Van Alyea OE. *Nasal sinuses: an anatomic and clinical consideration,* 2nd ed. Baltimore: Williams & Wilkins, 1951;97.
2. Ogston A. Trephining the frontal sinuses for catarrhal diseases. *Men Chron Manchester* 1884–1885;1:235.
3. Jurasz A. Ueber die Sandirung der stirnbienhohale. *Bern Klin Wochnschr* 1887;23:34.
4. Runge. As cited by Stevensen RS, Guhrie D. *A history of otolaryngology.* Baltimore: Williams & Wilkins, 1949.
5. Schaeffer JP. As cited by Sieur, Rouvillous. *Arch Int Laryngol* 1911;31:709; 32:42, 388.
6. Mermod. *Ann Mal Orville Larynx* 1986;22:337.
7. Luc H. Empyeme latent du sinus frontal duct sans cause apparante: triatemente par l'ouverture de los frontal et la currettage du foyer guerism incomplete. *Arch Int Laryngol* 1893;6:216.
8. Kuhnt H. *Uber die entzundiliche Erkrankungen der Stirnhohlen und ihre Folgezstande.* Eine Klinische Studie Wiesbaden, JF Bergman, 1895.
9. Jansen A. Neue Erfahrungen uber chronische Nebenhohlenersterungen der Nase. *Arch Ohren Nasen Kehlkopfheilk* 1902; 56:110.
10. Riedel BM. In Schenke: Inaugural Dissertation, *JENA* 1898.
11. Riedel BM. Totale resection der facialen und orbitalen sternhohlenwand. In: Denker A, Kahler O, eds. *Handbuch der Hals-Nasen-Ohren Heilkunde, vol 2.* Berlin: Springer-Verlag, 1926; 806–808.
12. Killian G. Die Killian sche radicaloperation chronischer stirnhohleneuterungen. II. Weiteres Kasuistisches Material and zusammenfassung. *Arch Laryngol Rhinol* 1903;13:59–88.
13. Ritter FN. *The Paranasal Sinuses—Anatomy & Surgical Technique,* 2nd ed. St. Louis: CV Mosby, 1978;136.
14. Knapp A. The surgical treatment of orbital complications in disease of the nasal accessory sinuses. *JAMA* 1908;51:299.
15. Lothrop HA. Frontal sinus suppuration. *Ann Surg* 1912;59: 937–957.
16. Lynch RC. The technique of a radical frontal sinus operation which has given me the best results. *Laryngoscope* 1921;31: 1–5.
17. Howarth WG. Operations of the frontal sinus. *J Laryngol* 1921; 36:417.
18. Donald PJ. Frontal sinus and nasofrontoethmoidal complex fractures. *A Self-Instructional Package #80400.* Washington, DC: American Academy of Otolaryngology–Head and Neck Surgery Foundation, 1980.
19. Boyden GL. Surgical treatment of chronic frontal sinusitis. *Ann Otol Rhinol Laryngol* 1952;61:558–566.
20. Baron SH, Dedo HH, Henry CR. The mucoperiosteal flap and frontal sinus surgery. *Laryngoscope* 1973;80:1266–1280.
21. Schonborn. Cited by Wilkop A. *Ein Beitrag zur Cauistik der Erkrankungen des sinus frontalis.* Wurzburg: F Frome, 1894.
22. Brieger. Uber chronische eiterungen des nebenhoholen der Nase. *Arch Ohren Nasen Kelkopfheilk* 1895;39:213.
23. Winkler. Beitrag zur osteoplastischen freilegung des sinus frontalis. *Verhandl Dtsch Otol Gossellsch* 1904.
24. Gussengauer. Cited by Beck JC. A new method of external frontal sinus operation without deformity. *JAMA* 1908;51:451.
25. Czerny. Cited by Beck JC. A new method of external frontal sinus operation without deformity. *JAMA* 1908;51:451.
26. Hoffman. Osteoplastic operation on the frontal sinus for chronic suppuration. *Ann Otol* 1904;13:598.
27. Beugara AR. Osteoplastic operation on the large frontal sinus in chronic suppurative sinusitis: end results. *Trans Am Acad Ophthalmol Otolaryngol* 1947;51:643.
28. Beugara AR, Itoiz AO. Present state of the surgical treatment of chronic frontal sinusitis. *AMA Arch Otolaryngol* 1955;61: 616.
29. Tato JM, Sibbald DW, Bargaglio OE. Surgical treatment of the frontal sinus by the external route. *Laryngoscope* 1954;64:504.
30. Goodale RL, Montgomery WW: Experience with the osteoplastic anterior wall approach to the frontal sinus. *Arch Otolaryngol* 1958;68:271.
31. Goodale RL, Montgomery WW. Anterior osteoplastic frontal sinus operation: five year's experience. *Ann Otol* 1961;70:860.
32. Goodale RL, Montgomery WW. Technical advances in osteoplastic frontal sinusectomy. *Arch Otolaryngol* 1964;79:522.
33. McBeth RG. The osteoplastic operation for chronic infection of the frontal sinus. *J Laryngol* 1954;68:465.
34. Bosely WR. Osteoplastic obliteration of the frontal sinuses: a review of 100 patients. *Laryngoscope* 1972;82:1463–1476.
35. Lawson W. Frontal sinus. In: Blitzer A, Lawson W, Friedman WH, eds. *Surgery of the Paranasal Sinuses.* Philadelphia: Saunders, 1985;120–148.
36. Ritter G. Enhaetung der vorderen Stirnholenwand bei der Radikaloperation. *Verh Ver Dtsch Laryngol* 1911;628.
37. Briant T. Intranasal hypophysectomy In: Paparella MM, Shumrick DA, eds. *Otolaryngology,* vol III, 2nd ed. Philadelphia: Saunders, 1980;2913.
38. Sewall EC. External operation of the ethmosphenoidal group of sinuses under local anesthesia. *Arch Otolaryngol* 1926;4(5): 377.
39. Lang J. *Clinical anatomy of the nose, nasal cavity and paranasal sinuses.* New York: Thieme Medical Publishers, 1989; 82–83.
40. Kirchner JA, Yanagiswa E, Crelin ES. Surgical anatomy of the ethmoid arteries. *Arch Otolaryngol* 1961;74:382.
41. Lotta JS, Schell RF. The histology of the epithelium of the paranasal sinuses under various conditions. *Ann Otol Rhinol Laryngol* 1934;43:945.
42. Schenk NL. Frontal sinus disease III. Experimental and clinical factors in failure of the osteoplastic flap operation. *Laryngoscope* 1975;85:76.
43. Ettin M, Donald PJ. The safety of frontal sinus fat obliteration when sinus walls are missing. *Laryngoscope* 1986;96:190.
44. Donald PJ. Tenacity of frontal sinus mucosa. *Otolaryngol Head Neck Surg* 1979;87:557–566.
45. Williams HL, Holman CB. The causes and avoidance of failure in surgery for chronic suppuration of the frontoethmoid-sphenoid complex of sinuses: with a previously unreported anomaly which produces chronicity and recurrence and the description

of a surgical technique usually producing a cure of the disease. *Laryngoscope* 1962;72:1179.

46. Scharfe EE. The use of tantalum. *Otolaryngology* 1953;58:133.
47. McNally WJ, Stuart EA. A 30-year review of frontal sinusitis treated by external operation. *Ann Otol* 1954;63:651.
48. Goodale RL. The use of tantalum in radical frontal sinus surgery. *Ann Otol* 1945;54:757.
49. Harris HE. The use of tantalum tubes in frontal sinus surgery. *Cleve Clin Q* 1948;15:129.
50. Erich JB, New GB. An acrylic obturator employed in the repair of an obstructed frontonasal duct. *Trans Am Acad Ophthalmol Otolaryngol* 1947;51:628.
51. Wolfowitz BL, Solomon A. Mucoceles of the frontal and ethmoid sinuses. *J Laryngol Otol* 1972;86:79–82.
52. Ingals EF. New operation and instruments for draining the frontal sinus. *Trans Am Laryngol Rhinol Otol Soc* 1905;2:183.
53. Anthony DH. Use of Ingal's gold tube in frontal sinus operations. *South Med J* 1940;33:949.
54. Lyman EH. The place of the obliterative operation in frontal sinus surgery. *Laryngoscope* 1950;60:407.
55. Barton RT. Dacron prosthesis in frontal sinus surgery. *Laryngoscope* 1972;82:1799–1805.
56. Neel HB, Whicker JH, Lake CF. Thin rubber sheeting in frontal sinus surgery: animal and clinical studies. *Laryngoscope* 1976;86:524–536.
57. Barton RT. The use of synthetic implant materials in osteoplastic frontal sinusotomy. *Laryngoscope* 1980;90:47–52.
58. Mihoefer W. External operation on the frontal sinus: critical review. *Arch Otolaryngol* 1928;7:133.
59. Negus VE. The surgical treatment of chronic frontal sinusitis. *Br Med J* 1947;1:135.
60. Smith F. Chronic sinus disease—its present status. *JAMA* 1933;100:402.
61. Smith F. Management of chronic sinus disease. *Arch Otolaryngol* 1934;19:157.
62. Simpson WH. The ethmosphenofrontal operation. *Arch Otolaryngol* 1937;26:270.
63. McNaught RC. A refinement of the external frontoethmosphenoid operation. A new nasofrontal pedicle flap. *Arch Otolaryngol* 1936;23:544–549.
64. Boyden GL. Surgical treatment of chronic frontal sinusitis. *Ann Otol Rhinol Laryngol* 1952;61:558–566.
65. Boyden GL. Chronic frontal sinusitis. *Trans Am Acad Ophthalmol Otolaryngol* 1957;558–591.
66. McNally WJ, Stuart EA. A 30-year review of frontal sinusitis treated by external operation. *Ann Otol Rhinol Laryngol* 1954;63:651–686.
67. Ogura JH, Watson RK, Jurema AA. Frontal sinus surgery. The use of a mucoperiosteal flap for reconstruction of a nasofrontal duct. *Laryngoscope* 1960;70:1229–1243.
68. Dokianakis GS, Helidonis E, Karamitos D, Papazoglou G: Use of a new mucoperiosteal flap from the lateral nasal wall in frontal sinus surgery. *Otolaryngol Head Neck Surg* 1981;89:912–916.
69. Goodale RL. Some causes for failure in frontal sinus surgery. *Ann Otol* 1912;51:648.
70. Beck JC. A new method of external frontal sinus operation without deformity. *JAMA* 1908;51:451.
71. Beugara AR, Itoiz OA. Estudia experimental de sobre las evoluciones del autoinjerto de grasa en el seno frontal del perro. *Rev Argent ORL* 1951;3:184–192.
72. Tato JM. Neumocranio extradural postraumantico mediatio origivado en el seno frontal y coincidiendo con un osteoma del mismo seno. *Rev Otolaringol* 1950;2.
73. Tato JM. Adipose tissue graft in otorhinolaryngology. *Arch Otolaryngol* 1974;100:467–469.
74. Marx G. Cited by Williams HL, Holman CB. The causes and avoidance of failure in surgery for chronic suppuration of the frontoethmoid-sphenoid complex of sinuses: with a previously unreported anomaly which produces chronicity and recurrence and the description of a surgical technique usually producing a cure of the disease. *Laryngoscope* 1962;72:1179.
75. Montgomery WW, Pierce DL. Anterior osteoplastic fat obliteration for frontal sinus: clinical experience and animal studies. *Trans Am Acad Ophthalmol Otolaryngol* 1963;67:46.
76. Montgomery WW, van Orman P. Inhibitory effect of adipose tissue on osteoneogenesis. *Ann Otol* 1967;76:988–997.
77. Montgomery WW. *Surgery of the Upper Respiratory System*, vol 2, 2nd ed. Philadelphia: Lea & Febiger, 1979;129–133.
78. McNeil RA. Surgical obliteration of the maxillary sinus. *Laryngoscope* 1967;77:202–217.
79. McBeth RG. The osteoplastic operation for chronic infection of the frontal sinus. *J Laryngol* 1954;68:465.
80. Samolineko A. Obliteration post-operatoire des sinus frontaux. *Arch Int Laryngol* 1913;35:336–358.
81. Hilding A. Experimental surgery of the nose and sinuses. III. Results following partial and complete removal of the mucous membrane lining from the frontal sinus of the dog. *Arch Otolaryngol* 1933;17:760–768.
82. Walsh TE. Experimental surgery of the frontal sinus: the role of the ostium and nasofrontal duct in postoperative healing. *Laryngoscope* 1943;53:75–92.
83. Abramson AL, Eason RL. Experimental frontal sinus obliteration: long term results following removal of the mucous membrane lining. *Laryngoscope* 1977;87:1066–1073.
84. Woodham JD. Safe endoscopic approaches and resections for chronic sinusitis. Presented at 44th annual meeting of the Canadian Society of Otolaryngology–Head & Neck Surgery, Montreal, June 26, 1990.
85. Sessions RB, Alford BR, Stratton C, et al: Current concepts of frontal sinus surgery. An appraisal of the osteoplastic flap–fat obliteration operation. *Laryngoscope* 1972;82:918–930.
86. Abramson AL, Eason RL, Pryor WH. Experimental results of autogenous cancellous bone chips transplanted into the infected canine frontal sinus cavity. *Trans Am Acad Ophthalmol Otolaryngol* 1976;82:148–158.
87. Lierle DM, Huffman WC. A simplified method of obliterating frontal bone defects. *Laryngoscope* 1949;59:61.
88. Knouff HA. Single stage frontal sinus obliteration. *Arch Otolaryngol* 1963;78:707.
89. Wolfe AS, Johnson P. Frontal sinus injuries: primary care and management of late complications. *Plast Reconstr Surg* 1988;82:781–789.
90. Luce AE. Discussion of Wolfe AS, Johnson P. Frontal sinus injuries: primary care and management of late complications. *Plast Reconstr Surg* 1988;82:790–791.
91. Naumann HH. Gedunken zun gegenartingen Stund der Stirnhohlen–Chirurgie. *Z Laryngol* 1961;40:733.
92. Siirala U. Obliteration of the frontal sinus with ossar. *Int Surg* 1967;47:425–427.
93. Beeson WH. Plaster of Paris as an alloplastic implant in the frontal sinus. *Arch Otolaryngol* 1981;107:664–669.
94. Coetzee AS. Regeneration of bone in the presence of calcium sulphate. *Arch Otolaryngol* 1980;106:405–409.
95. Dickson R, Hohmann A. The fate of exogenous materials placed in the middle ear and frontal sinus of cats. *Laryngoscope* 1971;81:216–231.
96. Janeke JB, Komora RM, Cohn AM. Proplast in cavity obliteration and soft tissue augmentation. *Arch Otolaryngol* 1974;100:24..
97. Schenk NL, Tomlinson JM, Ridgley CD. Experimental evaluation of a new implant material in frontal sinus obliteration. *Arch Otolaryngol* 1976;102:321.
98. Failla A. Operative management of injuries involving the frontal sinus: a study of 18 operated cases. *Laryngoscope* 1968;78:1833.
99. Montgomery WW. Frontal sinus and anterior cranial fossa. Presented at Symposium on Skull Base Surgery, June 2, 1980.
100. Hardy JM, Montgomery WW. Osteoplastic frontal sinusotomy: an analysis of 250 operations. *Ann Otol Rhinol Laryngol* 1976;85:523–532.
101. Iida M, Furuya K, Kawachis, et al: New improved bone cement (MMA-TTB). *Clin Orthop* 1974;100:279–286.
102. Charnley L. *Acrylic Cement in Orthopedic Surgery*. Baltimore: Williams & Wilkins, 1970.

103. Shultz RC. Reconstruction of facial deformities using silicones and acrylics. In: Rubin LR, ed. *Biomaterials in Reconstructive Surgery*. St Louis: CV Mosby, 1963;439.

104. Zander. Cited by Cabanela ME, Coventry MB, MacCarty CS, et al. The fate of patients with methyl methacrylate cranioplasty. *J Bone Joint Surg [Am]* 1972;54A(2):278–281.

105. Rietz K. The one stage method of cranioplasty with acrylic plastic. *J Neurosurg* 1958;15:176–182.

106. Spence WT. Form fitting cranioplasty. *J Neurosurg* 1954;11:219–225.

107. Kirwah WO. Systemic phenomena and bone cement. *Irish J Med Sci* 1973;142:342.

108. Milne IS. Hazards of acrylic bone cement. *Anesthesia* 1973;28:538–543.

109. Peebles DJ, Ellis RN, Stride SD, et al. Cardiovascular effects of methylmethacrylate cement. *Br Med J* 1972;1:349–351.

CHAPTER 18

Conventional Surgery for Ethmoid and Sphenoid Sinusitis

Paul J. Donald

The recent flurry of enthusiasm over endoscopic sinus surgery has produced not only a deemphasis on conventional surgery for ethmoid and sphenoid sinusitis but the potential for the premature obsolescence of these important procedures. Frontoethmoidectomy and ethmosphenoidectomy have been developed over a century and have evolved into an effective means of dealing with chronic sinus disease. Although some may argue to the contrary, these techniques will generally provide a more complete excision of the ethmoid block than endoscopic surgery. The supraorbital cells are especially difficult to completely marsupialize and exenterate endoscopically. The agger nasi presents a difficult angle for excision with the endoscope and in the sphenoid the most lateral recesses, although visible with an angled telescope, are difficult to resect safely.

The intranasal ethmoidectomy, a procedure taught at only a few training programs in the past, is quickly going out of fashion but was the forerunner of endoscopic sinus surgery. The other procedures to be described are now more often used in tumor surgery or for approaches to the orbit, but they are also used for cases of ethmoiditis and sphenoiditis that are refractory to endoscopic surgery and commonly when there is sinusitis with a complication. In my opinion, endoscopic surgery is infrequently suited to the management of most complications of chronic ethmoid and sphenoid sinusitis. At times, however, both endoscopic and classical procedures may be complementary.

Although the intranasal ethmoidectomy is traditionally done under local anesthesia, currently most external conventional procedures are performed using general anesthesia. It is important to augment the general anesthetic with the application of intranasal cocaine and the injection of subepithelial xylocaine with epinephrine for hemostasis.

During the draping of the patient, it is important to keep the eyes exposed in the field. Even in purely intranasal procedures, it is important because the mid-pupillary line marks the approximate location of the level of the cribriform plate. The eyes are protected either with a corneal shield or by the placement of temporary tarsorrhaphy sutures (Fig. 1).

A pack of 0.5-inch ribbon gauze soaked in a solution of 1% xylocaine with 1/180,000 epinephrine (a so-called Hibb's pack) is kept handy to be used in the exenterated cavity for hemostasis. The bipolar cautery is also helpful in this regard.

INDICATIONS

The indications for surgery of the ethmoid and sphenoid sinuses in inflammatory disease are principally resistance to medical therapy or the presence of a complication. The judgment concerning when to operate on a patient with refractory chronic ethmoid or sphenoid sinusitis involves the presumption that appropriate therapy has been instituted. This implies that suitable antibiotics have been administered to which the offending bacteria are sensitive in adequate dosages for a sufficient period of time. Possibly, the greatest oversight in the medical management of chronic sinusitis is the administration of antibiotics for too short a duration. Recalcitrant cases caused by a tenacious organism may require 6 weeks or more of continuous antibiotics to produce resolution. Great care is taken to ensure that antibiotic resistance has not occurred. Adjunctive medical measures involving mucosal shrinkage with local astringents and antihistamine–decongestant medication must be employed with the usual restrictive caveat regarding prolonged use of mucosal astringents. Allergic management should be paid close attention

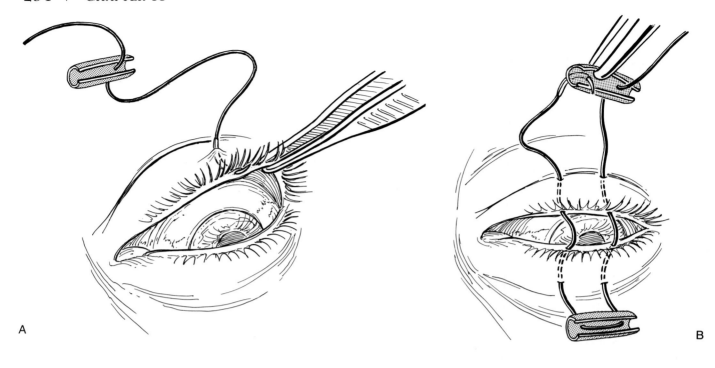

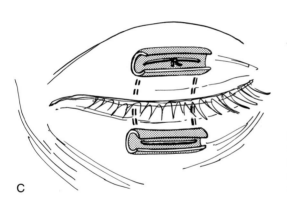

FIG. 1. Temporary tarsorrhaphy suture (Frost sutures). **A:** 5-0 Silk suture placed through approximately 1 cm of skin and pretarsal orbicularis muscle exiting at grayline of upper eyelid. **B:** The suture placed through grayline of lower lid and sutures passed through a catheter cut in half as a bolster. **C:** Sutures in place.

and even the occasional use of steroids may be indicated in the most resistant cases. The frequently neglected technique of repeated antral irrigation for a maxillary sinus fluid level should be considered. The release of pus from the antra often goes a long way to resolve persistent ethmoid sinusitis.

Although surgery is not based exclusively on radiographic findings, the persistence of opacification of the ethmoid and sphenoid sinuses coupled with the grumbling on of symptoms of sinusitis is a strong indicator of the need for surgery. How long a time period a patient should be encouraged to endure the nagging pain, fatigue, and malaise of recalcitrant sinusitis is not an easy question to answer. Symptoms and radiographic signs

that do not resolve following 6 to 8 weeks of vigorous therapy usually require surgical intervention for amelioration of symptoms.

The presence of a complication should be treated acutely by hospitalization and the immediate institution of intravenous antibiotics. Worsening or only minor improvement of symptoms once a loading dose has been achieved usually mandates surgery. Vigorous attention to symptoms of possible meningitis or ocular dysfunction must be monitored carefully and emergency intervention initiated prior to irrevocable change. Frequent observation of consciousness levels, neurological signs, and visual acuity are imperative. Specifics regarding the management of central compli-

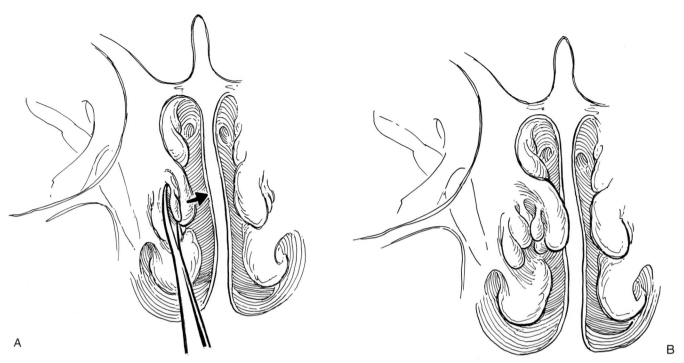

FIG. 2. A: Infracturing of middle turbinate to improve visualization of ethmoid block. **B:** Improved view of middle meatus and ethmoidal polyps.

cations are found in the chapter by Gluckman and Freije, entitled Intracranial Complications of Sinusitis, and orbital complications are found in the chapter by Donald, entitled Orbital Complications of Sinusitis.

INTRANASAL ETHMOIDECTOMY

Of all the traditional surgical procedures done for chronic inflammatory disease, this runs the greatest chance of being eliminated from the armamentarium of the sinus surgeon and likely justifiably so. As previously mentioned, endoscopic sinus surgery evolved from this operation and transformed it from a difficult and hazardous undertaking done with poor visualization to a safe procedure with excellent, albeit narrow field, exposure. However, endoscopic instruments are expensive and their use requires practice usually begun at an endoscopic sinus surgery course.

Both procedures require the operator to have a precise understanding of the highly variable anatomy of the ethmoid complex. A three-dimensional mental construct of this complex labyrinth cannot be achieved without extensive study, dissection, then practice in the anatomy lab or autopsy suite.

The procedure is best done in the semi-sitting position, mainly to create a situation where the cribriform plate is more difficult to injure. With the patient lying flat, an inadvertent breach through the cribriform area is much easier. The head-up position also diminishes blood loss by virtue of decreased venous pressure. Preoperatively, the vibrissae are trimmed to improve visualization.

Most patients who require intranasal ethmoidectomy have extensive polypoid disease. Polypectomy, often done as an office procedure, had accompanying it, either by design or accident, a limited ethmoidectomy. Since anterior ethmoid polyps are commonest and certainly most accessible transnasally, a small amount of the anterior ethmoid complex was removed with the polyps. The success of the anterior ethmoidectomy in eliminating disease in the osteomeatal complex speaks to the efficacy, albeit often temporary, of polypectomy. The often transient amelioration of disease is more of a reflection of the recalcitrance of the polypoid disease, usually of allergic origin, than the worthiness of the procedure.

Intranasal ethmoidectomy then begins with the removal of polyps that not only obstruct the airway but preclude a view of the operative field. Often an infracturing of the turbinate widens the visualization (Fig. 2). Biting forceps such as the Blaskesley and Takahashi, Wildes, and Luc forceps are used to remove both polypoid disease and involved ethmoid cells. At the beginning of the operation, all attempts possible are made to preserve the middle turbinate. By staying lateral to it, the operator is prevented from going through the cribriform plate. Since polyps commonly emanate from the lateral side of the turbinate, it is "hollowed out," removing the lateral wall and all the cells contained therein, but taking great care to leave an all-important residual medial lamina.

The ethmoid bulla and polyps are now removed (Fig. 3). Resection anterior to the uncinate process exposes the agger nasi. Gradually, tissue removal proceeds in a posterior direction under cover of the middle turbinate lamina. Visualization now often becomes progressively more difficult. If the view is obscured by bleeding, the Hibb's pack is placed for approximately 5 min until hemostasis is secured. As resection advances posteriorly, the sides rather than the point of the forceps are used. It is important to develop "the feel" of the various bony "plates" that comprise the limits of the ethmoid block. This is especially important concerning the lamina papyracea and the floor of the anterior cranial fossa. A margin of safety is added by using the Coakly curet to remove remaining remnants of cells and diseased mucosa (Fig. 4). By using a gentle sweeping motion, this residual tissue is excised and the plates are exposed. Although the cribriform is usually at the level of the interpupillary line, the orbital and supraorbital ethmoids can extend considerably higher (Fig. 5). This can be appreciated as the operator proceeds with the dissection lateral to the middle turbinate and the small superior turbinate. The width of the ethmoid block and the relative relationships of the level of the cribriform to that of the anterior fossa floor on the coronal cut computer-assisted tomography (CAT) scan or Caldwell view radiograph are frequently checked by the operator to help maintain this orientation.

As the dissection proceeds posteriorly, the grand lamina of the middle turbinate is encountered. This separation of the anterior from the posterior ethmoids brings the operator into larger cells and a wider part of the ethmoid block. The lamina papyracea now begins to curve more laterally as the equator of the globe is passed and the posterior limits of the ethmoid block are being reached. A limited resection of the posterior cells laterally is encouraged because of the proximity of the optic nerve at the back end of the ethmoid. Indeed, an Onodi cell when present commonly encompasses the nerve and its canal is frequently dehiscent (see chapter by Donald, Anatomy and Histology).

Once the posterior cells have been exenterated, the sphenoid rostrum comes into view. The position of the sphenoid sinus ostium in the face of this bone is identified (Fig. 6). It is vital at this juncture to recall that the planum sphenoidale above has the optic chiasm resting on it. Gentle palpation along the sphenoid rostrum superiorly will identify this important landmark. The utmost care is taken to avoid injury to the bone at this

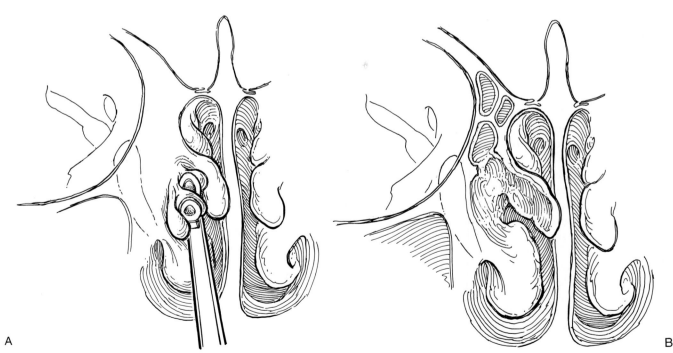

A   B

FIG. 3. A: Blaskesley forceps are used to remove polyps in middle meatus and from ethmoid bulla. **B:** Ethmoid bulla and cells of middle concha removed.

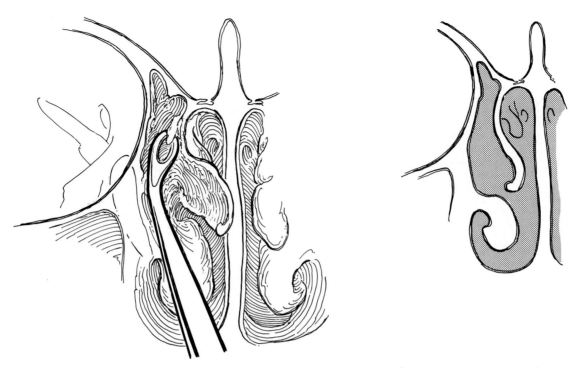

FIG. 4. Coakly curet used to gently remove cell remnants and diseased mucosa from ethmoid plates.

site. With one blade of the Blaskesley forceps in a sphenoid ostium and the other without, a sphenoidotomy is done. The sphenoid sinus is opened with the understanding that the nasopalatine artery runs a variable distance below the ostium (Fig. 7).

If the artery is cut, bleeding can be arrested with bipolar cautery or packing. A generous opening into the sphenoid sinus is recommended. Patients suffering from chronic sinus disease have a marked tendency to stenose the opening and develop recurrent infection.

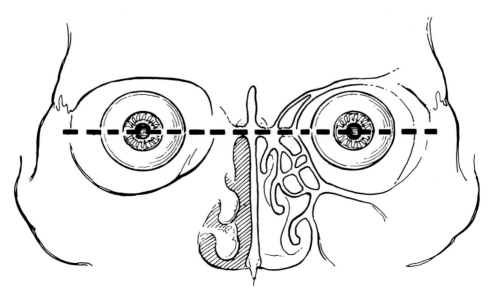

FIG. 5. Cribriform plate at the level of the interpupillary line. Supraorbital cells extend above the roof of the orbit.

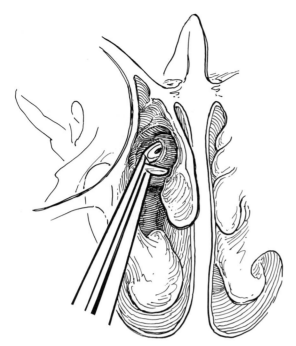

FIG. 6. Posterior cells have been exenterated and sphenoid rostrum is now in view. Anterior face of sphenoid opened with one blade of Blaskesley forceps in sphenoid ostium and the other without.

At the completion of the procedure, the side that has been operated on is packed with a Hibb's pack and attention is diverted to the opposite side. Once that side has been divested of disease, it is packed and attention is redirected to the first. The pack is removed on the initial side and the initial resection checked. This is a vitally important step as the view of the cavity now greatly enhanced by hemostasis will reveal any evidence of diseased tissues still remaining. This cavity is then repacked and the same routine conducted on the opposing side.

Unfortunately, most ethmoidectomy cavities done this way require packing, another disadvantage compared to endoscopic sinus surgery. The packing should be removed at about 48 hr to prevent bleeding.

The nose is suctioned every 48 to 72 hr for the next 10 to 12 days to remove excess mucus, crusting, coagulated blood, and, most especially, fibrin clots. These have a tendency to develop bridges between the septum and the lateral nasal wall that are the forerunners of synechiae.

It should be noted that no mention has been made concerning the management of a deviated septum that may be obstructing the intranasal view. Despite the popularity of performing septoplasty concurrently with ethmoidectomy, I believe that septoplasty in the face of active suppuration puts the patient at significant risk for postoperative septal infection. Septal abscess commonly causes quadrilateral cartilage necrosis with its aesthetically devastating consequence of saddle nose deformity. With polypoid disease and no evidence of pus, septoplasty can be done with relative safety.

A way of enhancing exposure in the patient with septal deformity and active suppuration is by the method euphemistically referred to by Lierle *(personal communication)* as the "Bulgarian maneuver." This is simply done by placing a stout elevator such as the Ballen-

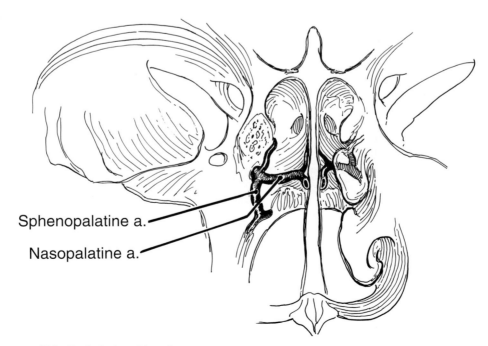

FIG. 7. Relationship of nasopalatine artery to ostium of sphenoid sinus.

Sphenopalatine a.

Nasopalatine a.

ger or the Gillies against the deflected septum and exerting sufficient pressure to bring it more toward the midline. This is often successful and avoids the portals of entry of infection facilitated by an open septal operation.

EXTERNAL ETHMOIDECTOMY

The external ethmoidectomy has been the workhorse operation of paranasal sinus disease for over 100 years. It continues to remain the most efficacious method to provide maximal exenteration of the ethmoid cells. It is a direct approach to the ethmoid block and can be complemented by either intranasal or endo-

scopic assistance. In my opinion, it provides the opportunity to perform the most thorough and complete ethmoidectomy.

A Lynch or modified Chiari incision is made with a #15 scalpel blade. The beginning of the incision is in the inferior hairs of the medial aspect of the brow. The blade is angled obliquely in the direction of the hair follicles and sweeps through an arc in the nasal ocular fold that passes through a point midway between the midline of the nose and the inner canthus of the eye. The incision is continued in this curve about 1 cm below this point (Fig. 8A). The modified Chiari incision introduces a horizontal component in the form of a step at this midpoint in order to avoid the potential for scar

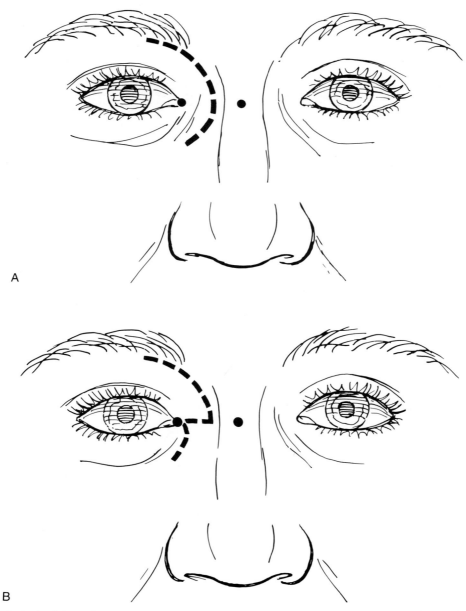

FIG. 8. Incisions for external ethmoidectomy. **A:** Lynch incision. **B:** Chiari incision.

contracture at this site (Fig. 8B). Skin and subcutaneous tissue are incised down to periosteum. Care is taken during the upper half of the incision to identify the angular artery and vein. They are incised and ligated and a subperiosteal dissection is carried toward the inner surface of the orbit. The superiormost attachment of the medial canthal tendon is elevated from its insertion on the frontal process of the maxilla and the anterior lacrimal crest. The lacrimal sac is elevated from its place in the lacrimal fossa, retracted, and the remaining medial canthal tendon elevated from the posterior lacrimal crest (Fig. 9). Superior dissection often requires the prizing off of the trochlea from its

fossa on the supermedial aspect of the orbit. This often leads to transient diplopia postoperatively that almost always corrects itself within a few weeks.

The periorbita is now relatively freely dissectable from the medial and superior orbital walls. Retraction is done with a Sewell retractor placed medially and laterally by a subcutaneously placed silk suture weighted by a hemostat. About 14 to 18 mm posterior to the lacrimal crest (1), usually along the suture line between the orbital process of the frontal bone and the lamina papyracea, the anterior ethmoidal artery is found. Hemostasis is secured by the use of two small vascular clips or the bipolar cautery (Fig. 10). Dissec-

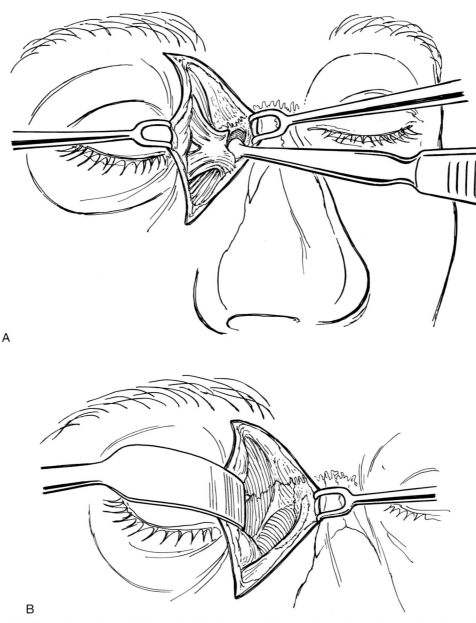

A

B

FIG. 9. A: Dissection of medial canthal tendon and lacrimal sac from the lacrimal crests and lacrimal fossa, respectively. **B:** Lacrimal fossa and anterior portion of lamina papyracea excised.

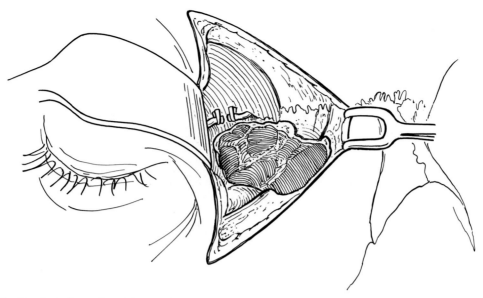

FIG. 10. Anterior ethmoid artery controlled by the placement of two small vascular clips.

tion proceeds posteriorly for a further 10 to 11 mm, where the posterior ethmoidal artery is usually encountered. During the posterior periorbital elevation, the middle or tertiary ethmoidal artery may be encountered. It is located usually about 7 mm from the anterior artery and is present in about 30% of cases.

Dissection usually ends at the level of the posterior artery. It is about 4 to 7 mm from the optic foramen, but never less than 2 mm from this structure (2). At the level of the posterior ethmoidal artery, the equator of the globe is usually passed and the medial orbital plate curves laterally.

The actual resection of the ethmoid now begins anteriorly with excision of the lacrimal fossa and lacrimal bone. This provides entry into the more anteriorly located ethmoid cells (Fig. 11). Further anterior resec-

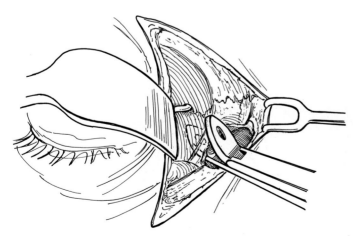

FIG. 11. Entrance into the anterior ethmoid block is done by excision of the lacrimal fossa.

tion now proceeds by biting away the bone of the frontal process of the maxilla and even occasionally some nasal bone with the Kerrison bone biting forceps (Fig. 12). The latter maneuver opens the agger nasi cells and thus complete exenteration can be accomplished. Now the removal of the ethmoid cells can be done safely with excellent visualization afforded by lateral retraction of the eye and the use of a headlight. Retraction of the orbital contents must be relaxed about every 45 to 90 sec to avoid the possible compromise of retinal circulation. This responsibility is placed on the surgical assistant, whose duty it is to remind the surgeon when this relaxation time is required.

Cells are removed with the Blaskesley forceps, proceeding in like manner to the intranasal ethmoidectomy. Visualization is far superior to the latter operation so progress is quicker and more precise. The medial lamina of the middle turbinate is preserved as an added precaution to prevent injury to the cribriform plate superiorly.

If there are no supraorbital cells present, resection has its superior limit at the frontoethmoidal suture. When these cells are encountered, the inferior aspect of the frontal bones' contribution to the medial wall of the orbit is removed. The supraorbital ethmoid cells are first identified on the radiographs then confirmed in the patient by gentle superior palpation with the up-biting Wildes forceps. Blind excision superiorly is inadvisable and progressive removal of the medial wall of the orbit is carried posteriorly until the posterior ethmoid artery is identified (Fig. 13). Removal of the posterior ethmoid cells beyond this level is carried out gingerly. The close proximity of the optic nerve requires the utmost caution. Posterior ethmoid cell re-

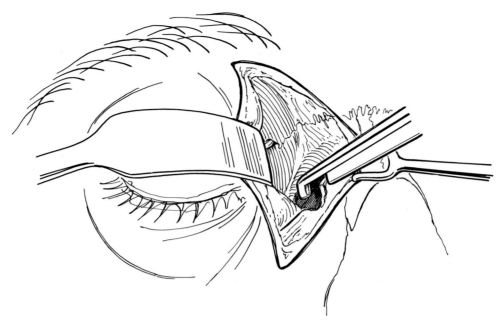

FIG. 12. Kerrison bone biting forceps used to expand exposure into agger nasi.

moval continues, but the remainder of the medial orbital wall is left intact and resection is done medial to it. The equator of the globe is now passed and diseased tissue is removed as the medial orbital wall curves laterally toward the orbital apex. Awareness of the possible presence of a dehiscent optic canal must be kept continuously in mind.

Soon dissection brings the operator to the anterior wall of the sphenoid sinus.

SPHENOIDECTOMY

Sphenoidectomy is usually included as a terminal part of each different method or approach to ethmoidectomy. I have opted to place it in a separate category, recognizing that a variety of approaches have been designed to tackle this geographically difficult sinus. The transseptal, intranasal, and external ethmoidectomy approaches as well as the endoscopic approach are

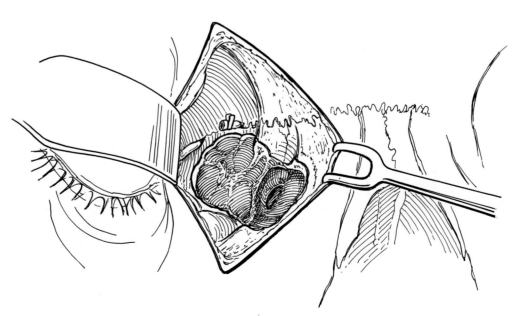

FIG. 13. Complete removal of anterior ethmoid cells and a good portion of posterior ethmoid cells is done. Note posterior ethmoidal artery at the end of excision.

commonest. In selected cases, a transoral–transpalatal and even infratemporal fossa approach may be used, but usually only in the case of neoplasm.

The transseptal route will not be discussed because it is detailed in the chapter by Pearson, entitled Transseptal–Sphenoidal Hypophysectomy. It should be added that not only does the sublabial approach provide excellent access to both sides of the sinus simultaneously, but it enables a much more efficacious means to utilize the sinus endoscope. The elimination of the impediment of the nasal septum allows much more freedom with the operating telescope. The lateral recesses of the sinus can be seen more clearly and the 30° telescope, which can be used for surgery after some practice, can be employed. This is especially important for the clearing of loculated infection that may be confined by an incomplete lateral septation. It is also especially useful in the management of laterally located cerebrospinal fluid leaks.

Using the traditional intranasal ethmoidectomy–sphenoidectomy is sometimes quite hazardous. A deviated nasal septum, a small nasal cavity, or persistent oozing all lead to an obtundation of vision, which prohibits adequate visualization. In many of these procedures, a small sphenoidotomy is all that is safe. Unfortunately, in the patient with chronic sinusitis, there is a marked tendency for cicatrization that closes this drainage hole. External ethmoidectomy and usually endoscopic surgery provide far superior visualization of the sphenoid.

All six walls of the sinus may be removed if required, but this is seldom if ever necessary. The structures most vulnerable to injury are in the sphenoid roof (see the chapter by Rice, entitled Embryology). The anterior fossa dura of the planum sphenoidale, the optic chiasm, and posteriorly the pituitary gland are separated from the cavity by a thin plate of bone. Seldom is bone at this site diseased enough to require excision. Even malignancies rarely transgress this area. The next most vulnerable region is the lateral wall. The cranial side is lined by the thickened dura of the cavernous sinus. However, directly adjacent to this dura and even invaginating the sphenoid sinus wall are (in a superior to inferior direction) the optic nerve, the abducens nerve, and the internal carotid artery. Thickened, infected mucus in the lateral recesses may be troublesome to remove and obscure areas of dehiscent bone.

The posterior wall can be removed with impunity in most instances because the thick marrow bone of the clivus is usually present in profusion. However, in cases of marked postsellar pneumatization, the cortical surface of the posterior sphenoid sinus wall may approximate the adjacent cortex of the intracranial side. In cases of invasive neoplasm or mucocele, it may be eroded down to pontine dura (Fig. 14). In a case in my experience, removal of the posterior wall of a sphenoid sinus mucocele resulted in a cerebrospinal fluid leak from a small rent in the pontine dura.

The anterior wall and floor of the sinus are the most amenable to excision. The caveats attendant to re-

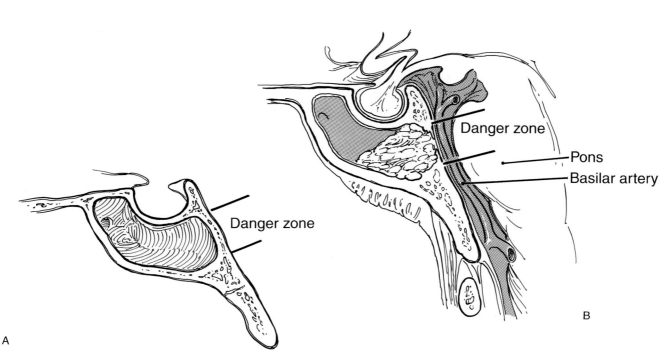

FIG. 14. A: Region of the posterior wall of the sphenoid sinus, the potential danger zone. **B:** Mucocele eroding posterior wall of sphenoid sinus exposing pontine dura.

moval of the anterior wall address the possible presence of a dehiscent optic nerve canal at the superolateral extremity of the anterior sinus wall and the nasopalatine artery traversing the face of the sphenoid rostrum. The artery can be cauterized or clipped and is usually no great problem. The optic nerve is obviously assiduously avoided. The anterior wall should be removed as completely as possible. This is extremely difficult to do with the conventional intranasal ethmoidectomy but can be done with the external ethmoidectomy sublabial or endoscopic approach. A wide removal is advised because of the frequency of scarring and closure of more conservative excisions. A small ostium will provide scant aeration or drainage in a chronically infected sphenoid sinus. Finally, the management of the sphenoid sinus floor is addressed. For some curious reason, the sphenoid floor is rarely removed by most surgeons, yet its complete excision offers the best opportunity to marsupialize the sinus. The floor is composed of a portion of the basisphenoid contribution to the clivus. It is also the anterior roof of the nasopharynx. In extensively pneumatized sphenoid sinuses, the position of the internal carotid arteries posterolaterally to the medial pterygoid plate in the foramen lacerum needs to be kept in mind. The artery is rarely a problem in that the foramen exists in the suture line between the petrous apex and the lateral body of the sphenoid. Moreover, the most inferior extent of it is obturated by a cartilage plug. Only the most vigorous drilling and dissection from this approach will produce injury to the internal carotid unless under the most unusual of circumstances. In removing the sphenoid floor, which I now do in recalcitrant recurrent chronic sphenoiditis, the pituitary drill can be employed. This can be done endoscopically through a sublabial approach, which is the easiest, or through an external ethmoidectomy. It can also be done transnasally but is much more difficult because of the restricted space. The bone of the floor is simply burred away until flush with the posterior wall (Fig. 15). The soft tissue of the anterior nasopharyngeal roof remaining following bone removal is removed by sharp dissection. This helps to eliminate the possibility of prolapse of this tissue into the sphenoid cavity and later possibly loculating infection. Diseased mucosa and infected bone are removed from the sinus and the area is packed, usually with a combination of anterior and posterior packs. The packs are removed 5 to 7 days later and the nose is periodically suctioned until healing has taken place. The endoscopic approach usually does not require packing in most instances but, with excision of the floor, it is not uncommonly needed.

COMPLICATIONS

The commonest complication of surgery for ethmoid and sphenoid inflammatory disease is recurrence of the disease. Severe chronic sinusitis is one of the most refractory to treatment of any of the diseases of the head and neck. The successful management of allergic diatheses when present by avoidance, immune ther-

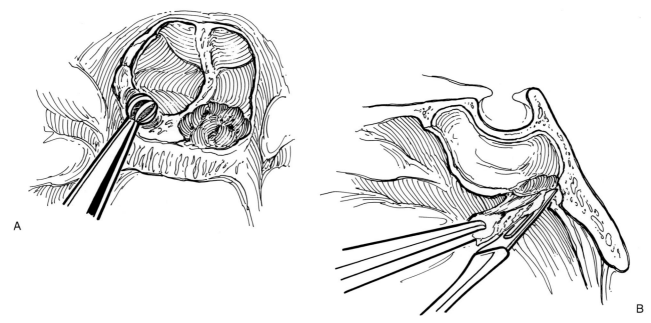

FIG. 15. A: Bone of the floor of the sphenoid sinus removed with cutting bur. **B:** Underlying nasopharyngeal mucosa and basipharyngeal fascia excised in order to adequately marsupialize sinus.

apy, antihistamines, decongestants, and steroids coupled with the appropriate administration of microorganism-specific antibiotics for a sufficient length of time is essential for adequate control. Cognizance of the aspirin-sensitive asthma (ASA), asthma, polyposis triad and the role of cystic fibrosis and ciliary dysfunction syndromes is necessary for appropriate treatment. Patients should be warned that surgery may only provide temporary relief that may last 6 months or 6 years.

Since the advent of endoscopic sinus surgery, there have been a plethora of complications—most likely reflective of the inexperience of the operator. In Stankiewicz's original report (3) on this procedure, he quoted a 29% incidence of complications in his first group of 90, including one case of cerebrospinal fluid leak, one case of blindness (fortunately temporary), and five cases of hemorrhage, two of which lost 1200 cc of blood. In the second half of patients in this series, the complication rate dropped to 2% (3).

Table 1 is a compilation of complications from various sources (3,4).

One of the commonest is cerebrospinal fluid rhinorrhea. This complication is dealt with in the chapter by Pearson, entitled Cerebrospinal Fluid Rhinorrhea. It is important to understand that about 20% of cerebrospinal fluid fistulas develop meningitis. The controversy over the use of prophylactic antibiotics continues. It is my choice not to place such patients on antibiotic therapy. The dripping of crystal clear watery fluid from the nose especially on bending over is classic. The sensation of a salty or salty–sweet postnasal discharge is also a common symptom. Headache may be a prominent feature but is often absent. A collection of the fluid that is positive for glucose and especially β-transferrin clinches the diagnosis. Identification by metrizamide contrast computed tomography (CT) and fluorescein staining of intranasal pledgets or radioimmunosorbent assay (RISA) scanning is too often unrewarding.

TABLE 1. *Complications of endoscopic sinus surgery*

Complication	Wigand (4) (M = 220) (%)	Stankiewicz (3) (M = 90) (%)
Neuralgia, face and head	1.8	1.0
Postoperative anosmia	0.9	0
CSF leak	0.9	1
Orbital hematoma	0.5	7
Ethmoid mucocele	0.5	0
Death	0	0
Blindness	0	1 (temporary)
Diplopia	0	0
Meningitis	0	0
Ozena	0	0
Synechiae	0	8
Hemorrhage	0	7

Orbital symptoms vary from a periorbital hematoma to blindness. When the periorbita is violated during endoscopic surgery or intranasal ethmoidectomy, it is not uncommon for the patient to suffer a periorbital hematoma. It is usually not severe, with the only symptom being a scant amount of ecchymosis in the eyelid or periorbital skin. They resolve without sequellae. Massive hematoma is decidedly rare and is a threat to vision on the basis of increased intraorbital pressure. Treatment is lateral canthotomy and drainage of the hematoma.

Injury to the optic nerve is probably the most dire of all complications of ethmoid or sphenoid surgery. This can occur with any ethmoid or sphenoid operation. Even a too vigorous opening of the Cushing–Landau retractor in the sublabial transseptal operation can cause a fracture across the optic canal, injuring the nerve. The frequent occurrence of a dehiscent canal in an Onodi cell has been referred to before. The presence of this cell places the nerve at great danger during posterior ethmoidectomy and sphenoidectomy. Review of the CT scans prior to surgery is essential in anticipation of this potential complication. Amaurosis on awakening from surgery should be followed by immediate optic nerve decompression (see the chapter by Rice, entitled Fractures of the Orbital Apex). An argument for initial treatment with high-dose steroids could be made, but in my opinion emergency release of any possible constricting hematoma should be done. Nerve severance or vascular shearing (see the chapter by Rice, entitled Fractures of the Orbital Apex) sounds the death knell for that nerve.

Lateral rectus palsy may follow surgery on the sphenoid sinus. Even though the abducent nerve is located in the lateral adventitia of the internal carotid artery, it still may be damaged. For a mysterious reason, the sixth cranial nerve is the most susceptible to injury of all the cranial nerves. Treatment is expectant using a short course of high-dose steroids. Most spontaneously resolve.

Transient diplopia may occur after external ethmoidectomy because of trochlear dislodgement. This is almost always transient as the trochlea reattaches and the normal action of the superior oblique muscle resumes. Very rarely a Brown's syndrome (see the chapter by Trevino, Food Allergies and Hypersensitivities) may occur secondary to inflammatory changes and scarring in this delicate apparatus. Diplopia in upward and inward gaze is the classic symptom.

Hypertrophic scar formation may occur in either the Lynch or modified Chiari incision. The Chiari incision is less susceptible to this by virtue of the horizontal component opposite the medial canthus. Such scars often resolve with intralesional steroid injection with a compound such as triamcinolone 40. Persistent scars will often form a web and these can be managed easily with one or two Z-plasties. One of the great concerns of ethmoidectomy, especially if accompanied by middle turbinectomy, is atrophic rhinitis. This is an uncommon complication in my experience because of the patient's continued hypersecretion brought about by an underlying allergy or vasomotor rhinitis. In the initial phases of healing, some dryness and crusting are common and should be treated with saline irrigations, often as frequently as four times per day. Hourly nasal spray with a saline solution or a combination of 10% propylene glycol in saline creates a suitably moist intranasal environment. With the passage of time, the nose appears to regain its innate ability to moisten its mucosa and no moisturization is required. Although complica-

tions following ethmoid and sphenoid surgery may and will occur, in the best and most experienced hands their frequency appears to be somewhat less among those individuals that have a thorough understanding of the anatomy of this complex area.

REFERENCES

1. Kirchner JA, Yanagisamwa E, Crelin ES. Surgical anatomy of the ethmoid arteries. *Arch Otolaryngol* 1961;74:382.
2. Lang J. *Clinical anatomy of the nose, nasal cavity and paranasal sinuses.* New York: G Thieme, 1989;82.
3. Stankiewicz JA. Complications of endoscopic intranasal ethmoidectomy. *Laryngoscope* 1987;97:1270.
4. Wigand EM. *Endoscopic surgery of the paranasal sinuses and anterior skull base.* New York: G Thieme, 1990;139.

CHAPTER 19

Conventional Surgery for Infection of the Maxillary Sinus

Jack L. Gluckman

Recently, the surgical approaches for sinus infecitions have shifted from conventional to endoscopic techniques. There is little doubt, however, that as the love affair with the technology and technique of functional endoscopic sinus surgery runs its course, there will be a resurgence of interest in the more conventional techniques. Certainly an expertise in both approaches is needed for the practice of contemporary rhinology.

The conventional techniques that will be discussed are simple, safe, tried and trusted, and remarkably effective in the vast majority of cases. They are here to stay and the practicing otolaryngologist and trainee are well advised to remain familiar with these procedures.

ANTRAL LAVAGE

General Considerations

While this relatively simple technique can hardly be regarded as a true surgical procedure, it does have an important role in the management of maxillary sinusitis and therefore warrants discussion in some detail.

Indications

Diagnostic

1. Evaluation of radiographic evidence of an opaque maxillary antrum.
2. To obtain material for culture and sensitivity in acute, relapsing, and chronic maxillary sinusitis.
3. To obtain material for cytology in suspected malignancy of the maxillary sinus.

Therapeutic

1. Drainage of an empyema of the maxillary sinus, which has failed conservative therapy.

Technique

There are three approaches for antral lavage of the maxillary sinus: via the natural ostium, via the inferior meatus, and sublabially through the canine fossa (Fig. 1).

Via the Natural Ostium

This approach is not commonly utilized because of the concern that it may induce fibrosis of the natural

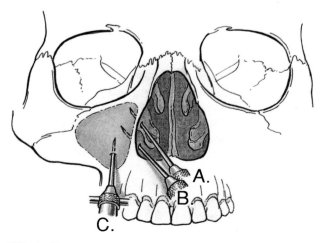

FIG. 1. Techniques for antral lavage. A: Via the natural ostium. B: Via the inferior meatus. C: Via the canine fossa.

247

ostium with subsequent stenosis. There is also an increased likelihood of inadvertently damaging the orbital floor.

Via the Inferior Meatus

This is the most common technique. The key to success of this procedure is to prepare the patient adequately as to what to expect and to allay the natural fear of a large needle being stuck through the nose into the sinus! This fear is usually fueled by horror stories dredged up from a distant past or from some acquaintance who barely survived this procedure and lived to tell the tale! The time spent explaining the procedure in intricate detail is well spent and reassurance should continue throughout the procedure.

In children this procedure should be performed under a general anesthetic but in adults, local anesthesia will usually suffice. Four percent cocaine, liquid or paste, or any other combination of a vasoconstrictor and local anesthetic can be used. The best technique is to first paint the anterior aspect of the inferior turbinate and inferior meatus as well as the anterior aspect of the nasal septum with the cotton carrier in order to facilitate the subsequent insertion of the carrier along the length of the inferior meatus. The anterior aspect of the nasal septum should be anesthetized as pressure will be exerted on this area when inserting the trocar and cannula into the sinus. At least 10 min should be allowed for the local anesthetic to achieve the desired effect.

Once suitable anesthesia has been achieved, the patient should be placed in a sitting position and a waterproof protector placed over the shoulders and upper chest. A Lichtwitz trocar and cannula is then used to puncture the maxillary sinus. This is placed in the inferior meatus and the optimal site of puncture determined by running the instrument along the inferior aspect of the attachment of the inferior turbinate until the genu is palpated. This is the point at which the bone is thinnest. The trocar is then angled toward the lateral canthus of the eye; the patient's head is steadied with the other hand while the instrument is advanced through the medial wall of the maxillary antrum. The patient is advised that a crack will be felt prior to performing the procedure. Once in the sinus, the trocar is withdrawn and the cannula further advanced.

The patient is now asked to sit forward with the mouth open and the head held over a basin in order to collect the irrigated material. A 30 cc syringe filled with normal saline is connected to the cannula by intravenous tubing. The sinus should first be aspirated to ensure that the cannula is in the sinus cavity. Either air or secretion should be aspirated with ease. If aspiration is not possible, the cannula may be misplaced or the

sinus filled with a solid mass. Once the correct position has been established, the sinus is gently irrigated forcing the saline into the sinus. The patient will experience an initial sense of pressure, which is relieved as the material is extruded through the natural ostium. The irrigation is continued until the return from the sinus is clear. The cannula is then withdrawn and the specimen is sent for culture and sensitivity or cytology depending on the indication.

Complications

1. Pain and discomfort while performing the puncture. This is usually because of inadequate anesthesia but may be due to excessive thickness of the antral wall. If a puncture cannot be performed, this approach should be aborted and the sublabial approach attempted.
2. Malposition of the cannula. Occasionally, insertion through the posterior wall into the pterygomaxillary fissure may occur as a result of performing the puncture too posteriorly or at the wrong angle. Likewise, the trocar may be inserted through the roof of the antrum into the orbit and irrigation will result in immediate periorbital swelling. This unfortunate event may occur even if the cannula is correctly placed within the sinus, if a congenital or post-traumatic dehiscence of the floor of the orbit exists. The anterior wall of the maxillary sinus may be perforated, resulting in subcutaneous swelling.
3. Pain on antral lavage. This occurs when the natural ostium is occluded by polypoid material or stenosis. The patient will experience intense pressure and even pain on irrigation. In this situation, the saline should be aspirated or a second cannula inserted to facilitate adequate irrigation.

Via Sublabial Approach

This technique is preferred by many otolaryngologists because it is simple to perform and the bone over the canine fossa is extremely thin.

Anesthesia is achieved by injecting local anesthetic in the gingivobuccal sulcus over the canine fossa. Once a suitable level of anesthesia has been obtained, the trocar and cannula is inserted through the canine fossa, being careful to avoid the apices of the teeth. Irrigation is performed in the usual manner and the saline collected through the nose as it is expelled through the natural ostium.

Complications

1. Cellulitis of the cheek secondary to contamination by the infected contents of the maxillary sinus.
2. Subcutaneous emphysema particularly if the pa-

tient sneezes or blows the nose in the immediate postoperative period. This usually spontaneously resolves over a few hours to days.

In conclusion, maxillary sinus lavage is an excellent technique especially for draining an acute empyema, which has failed to respond to conservative therapy. If repeated punctures are envisaged, it is preferable to insert an indwelling catheter through the cannula, enabling the antrum to be irrigated repeatedly over the course of the day. This is particularly useful in a child.

NASOANTRAL WINDOW (INTRANASAL ANTROSTOMY)

General Considerations

Drainage procedures for the maxillary sinus were first described in the latter half of the 19th century with the dominant controversy even then being whether the antrostomy should be created in the inferior meatus, to enable the sinus to drain by gravity, or in the middle meatus, which even then was regarded as the more physiologic approach. This debate continues to this day with proponents and detractors of both approaches: the functional endoscopists having universally adopted the middle meatal approach while the conventional sinus surgeons, the inferior approach.

For the purposes of this chapter, however, only the inferior meatal approach will be discussed as the role of the middle meatomy will be covered in the chapter, "Endoscopic Sinus Surgery," by Rice.

The inferior meatus antrostomy, which permits ventilation and drainage of the maxillary sinus, is a tried and trusted technique for maxillary sinusitis. Its role, however, is somewhat controversial, being regarded as valueless by some authors (1) and extremely effective by others (2). It fulfills many of the criteria of an ideal operation: that is, it is quick and simple and easily taught and learned and is remarkably effective in the vast majority of cases.

The bone of the inferior meatus is thinnest at its central superior area, where the bone is predominantly lamellar bone. This represents the optimal site for creating the antrostomy, that is, appropriately 2 cm from the pyriform aperture (Fig. 2). This corresponds to the genu of the attachment of the inferior turbinate and is the site of the maximal height of the inferior meatus. It should be remembered that the floor of the maxillary sinus is always lower than the floor of the nose, with this difference ranging from 5 to 16 mm, and therefore no matter how low the antrostomy, it will always be higher than the floor of the maxillary sinus.

A further limiting factor to the creation of a wide antrostomy is a constant branch of the lateral sphenopalatine artery, which enters the inferior meatus 4 to

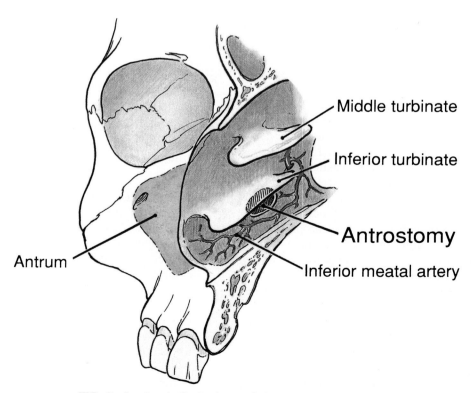

FIG. 2. Anatomic limitations of the nasoantral window.

5 cm from the pyriform aperture, descends below the level of the palate, and then ascends anteriorly in the meatus (3). The site and size of the antrostomy are therefore limited by the attachment to the inferior turbinate superiorly, the floor of the nose inferiorly, and the inferior meatal artery together with the sloping inferior turbinate attachment anteriorly and posteriorly.

Indications

Therapeutic

1. Chronic or relapsing maxillary sinusitis, which has proved refractory to conservative therapy, particularly if the mucosa has not undergone irreversible hyperplastic change.
2. Vacuum headache due to impaired aeration of the maxillary sinus.
3. Removal of a foreign body.
4. Drainage of a mucocele.

Diagnostic

1. Biopsy of lesions of the maxillary sinus.

Preoperative Evaluation

A decision needs to be made to determine whether to perform this procedure under local or general anesthesia. In addition, an x-ray of the sinus or better still a computed tomography (CT) scan should be obtained to evaluate the extent of the disease process and to determine the pneumatization of the sinuses.

Technique

While this procedure can certainly quite easily be performed under local anesthesia, it is infinitely more comfortable for the patient to have the procedure performed under a short general anesthetic. Even if general anesthesia is used, a suitable vasoconstricting agent should be placed in the inferior meatus to aid in hemostasis. If local anesthesia is to be used, cocaine pledgets augmented with the injection of local anesthesia, with or without epinephrine, should be placed in the inferior meatus and along the under surface of the inferior turbinate. After waiting the obligatory 10 min, during which the patient is draped in the routine manner, the nose is carefully inspected, particularly the middle meatus, in an attempt to identify any obvious treatable pathology that may be occluding the natural ostium of the maxillary sinus. This should be removed if feasible.

The inferior meatus is exposed by in-fracturing the inferior turbinate using either a periosteal elevator or knife handle and the turbinate held in its new position with a medium sized nasal speculum positioned in the inferior meatus (Fig. 3).

The optimal site to perform the antrostomy is at the genu of the attachment of the inferior turbinate, which is approximately 2 cm posterior to the anterior aspect of its attachment to the wall of the nose. The bone is thinnest at this point. The antrostomy is then created under direct visualization using any one of a wide variety of instruments varying from a curved clamp to a specifically designed harpoon or a back-biting forceps. The instrument is directed to the lateral canthus of the eye. Once the initial opening has been created, it should be enlarged to a dimension of approximately 2.0 cm in length and 1 cm in height by any combination of forward and back-biting bone forceps given the anatomic limitations already discussed. The turbinate should then be gently relocated to its original position and packing placed in the inferior meatus only if needed for hemostasis. This can usually be removed within the hour.

Postoperative Care

The patient should be advised that there may be some bleeding and therefore he/she should refrain from blowing the nose vigorously for 48 hr. The patient may also be informed that clots of blood may be expected on blowing the nose over the next week or two. Analgesics are rarely necessary. Topical decongestant and saline solution for irrigation are helpful in decreasing postoperative nasal congestion and should be administered for 5 days.

Results

If performed for the appropriate indications, this is an extremely effective procedure, particularly for chronic and relapsing maxillary sinusitis. Occasionally, however, it is ineffectual for the following reasons:

1. The infected mucosa of the maxillary sinus has undergone chronic hyperplastic change and fails to resolve after drainage and aeration of the sinus. This mucosa needs to be removed and this is performed more effectively via a Caldwell–Luc procedure.
2. The mucociliary flow continues to direct the sinus secretions to the natural ostium, rendering the inferior meatal antrostomy ineffective. While experimentally this may occur (4,5), this does not appear to be a problem in the majority of cases.
3. Premature closure of the nasoantral window. This is particularly a problem in younger adults and children (3). The reasons for premature closure in-

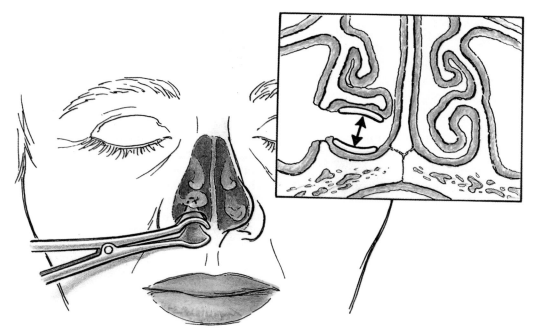

FIG. 3. Nasoantral window. The turbinate is in-fractured and the inferior meatus exposed using a nasal speculum.

clude inadequate initial size and the formation of adhesions, usually because fragments of bone have been left in the meatus with secondary osteomyelitis, which encourages scarring (2). If the antrostomy remains open at one year, it is liable to remain open long term (3). The antrostomy should therefore be created as widely and cleanly as possible.

Complications

1. Hemorrhage. Usually minimal hemorrhage is encountered. If, however, the antrostomy is created too far posteriorly, the inferior meatal artery can be traumatized and this may lead to significant hemorrhage, necessitating cauterization and/or packing.
2. Orbital damage secondary to perforating the thin orbital floor. Performing the antrostomy under direct visualization will prevent this.
3. Osteomyelitis. In the older literature it is stated that the nasoantral window should not be performed in the presence of acute infection because of the danger of developing osteomyelitis. In this day and age of adequate antibiotic coverage this does not appear to be a valid concern.
4. Dental injury, particularly in the pediatric patients.
5. It has been suggested that the creation of the antrostomy may actually predispose the sinus mucosa to an increased incidence of infection (6). There is no clinical evidence that this is a valid concept (2).

6. Damage to the superior alveolar nerves if the antrostomy is created too far anteriorly (4), with resultant impaired sensation of the teeth (2).
7. Scarring between the inferior turbinate and meatomy (7).

CALDWELL–LUC PROCEDURE

General Considerations

Although a number of surgeons were performing similar operations at that time, it was George Caldwell of New York who, in 1893, first described the procedure as we know it. Four years later Henri Luc, in Paris, described an identical operation. Today in the English literature, the procedure is called the Caldwell–Luc operation, while in the French literature the term is Luc–Caldwell! By definition this procedure consists of an exploration of the maxillary antrum by an anterior antrostomy together with the creation of a nasoantral window.

Indications

Diagnostic

1. Evaluation of intrasinus pathology particularly if a neoplasm is suspected.

Therapeutic

1. Treatment of chronic hyperplastic sinusitis that has proved refractory to more conservative measures.

2. Removal of a foreign body.
3. Removal of cysts, benign tumors, and antrocho-anal polyps.
4. Closure of large oroantral fistula.
5. Reduction and fixation of maxillary fractures. This approach is rarely used today.

An Approach To:

1. Ethmoid sinuses (i.e., transantral ethmoide-ctomy).
2. Orbit (transantral orbital decompression).
3. Pterygomaxillary fossa (transantral ligation of the internal maxillary artery and vidian neurectomy).

Technique

Anesthesia

While this procedure can be performed under local anesthesia, it is certainly easier to perform under general anesthesia. If local anesthesia is to be used, the patient should be sedated adequately prior to commencing the procedure. The gingivobuccal sulcus should be infiltrated with local anesthesia and topical anesthesia placed in the inferior meatus. The infraorbital nerve should also be blocked with local anesthesia.

Even if performed under general anesthesia, the sulcus should be infiltrated with local anesthesia combined with a vasoconstrictor to improve hemostasis and, in addition, a vasoconstrictor placed intranasally above and below the inferior turbinate. The pharynx should be packed to prevent any aspiration of blood. The ipsilateral eye should not be taped or sutured, permitting the surgeon to observe the eye, particularly while working on the roof of the antrum, thereby avoiding any inadvertent damage to the orbital contents.

An incision is made just inferior to the gingivobuccal sulcus extending from the lateral incisor to the second molar. The initial cut should be made just through the mucosa, ensuring that the curvature of the sulcus is followed and that the parotid duct is not traumatized

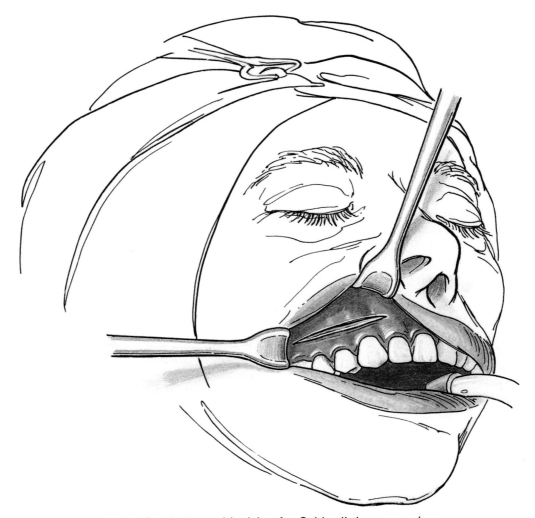

FIG. 4. Gingivobuccal incision for Caldwell–Luc procedure.

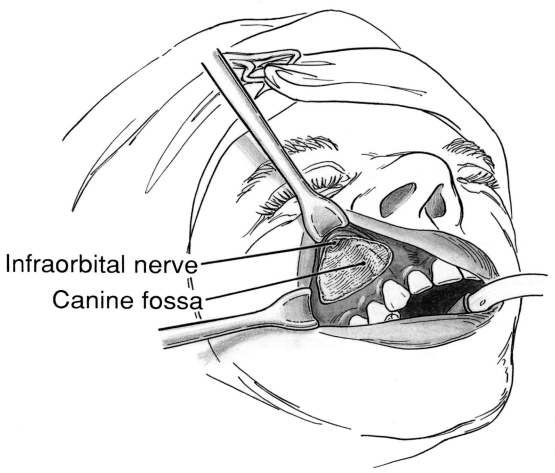

FIG. 5. Exposure of the anterior face of the maxillary antrum.

in any way (Fig. 4). The incision is then deepened through the periosteum down to bone. A limited inferior flap is developed to facilitate adequate closure at the termination of the procedure. The dissection is then performed by elevating subperiosteally and exposing the anterior face of the maxillary antrum (Fig. 5). This should be continued to the infraorbital foramen, ensuring that the nerve is not unduly stretched by retraction or directly damaged.

The anterior face of the antrum is then fenestrated in the canine fossa using either a hammer and gouge, chisel, or drill. When using a gouge or chisel, care should be taken to remove a square-shaped segment of bone in a controlled manner and not to inadvertently fracture into the infraorbital canal or dental apices (Fig. 6A). The antrostomy is then widened using a Kerrison punch until the entire contents of the maxillary antrum can be visualized adequately (Fig. 6B). The pathology encountered is then managed in the appropriate manner. If there is evidence of chronic hyperplastic sinus mucosa, this should be stripped using an elevator or curette and removed using a cup forceps. When removing the mucosa on the roof of the antrum, the assistant

should expose the eye to prevent any inadvertent injury to the orbital contents.

Finally, the nasoantral window is created into the inferior meatus. This is technically easier when performing a Caldwell–Luc as the edges of the antrostomy can be debrided of redundant mucosa or fragments of bone.

The incision is then closed using interrupted absorbable suture, ensuring that the knots are buried. The nose is usually packed loosely, but if there is any significant oozing the sinus can be packed through the nose. This is rarely necessary.

Postoperatively, the patient should use a cold compress over the cheek to minimize the swelling and have a soft diet for a few days. Some degree of anesthesia over the cheek and of the teeth is a normal sequela and gradually recovers. The patient should be warned to expect this.

Results

This procedure is extremely useful diagnostically, therapeutically, and as an approach to regional areas.

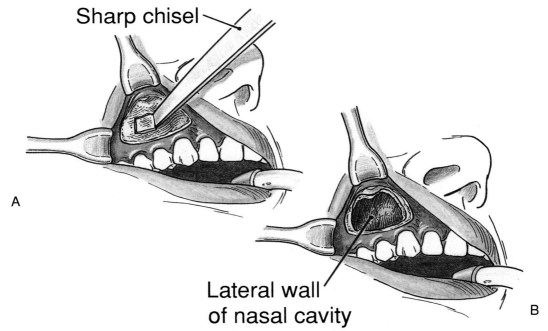

Sharp chisel

A

Lateral wall
of nasal cavity

B

FIG. 6. A: Removal of the anterior face of the maxillary sinus using a hammer and chisel. **B:** Exposure obtained of the maxillary sinus via the Caldwell–Luc approach.

Its role in managing chronic maxillary sinusitis is somewhat controversial especially in this age of more conservative sinus surgery. It does, however, in my mind, remain the mainstay for the treatment of chronic refractory sinusitis with hyperplastic mucosa.

Complications

1. Persistent oroantral fistula. This is a rare occurrence, particularly if the mucosal incision is not sutured or if chronic infection of the sinus persists.
2. Persistent anesthesia in the distribution of the infraorbital nerve. This invariably results from extending the dissection too high and directly injuring the nerve or due to excessive traction being placed on the nerve. Great care should be taken to avoid this complication.
3. Injury to the orbit due to inadvertent perforation of the roof of the antrum, particularly if there is a congenital or post-traumatic dehiscence. For this reason the surgeon should always directly visualize the eye when the roof of the antrum is being dissected.

4. Damage to tooth roots if the anterior antrostomy is extended too inferiorly.
5. Hemorrhage. If significant, it can be controlled by packing.

In conclusion, knowledge of these simple surgical procedures remains important to the management of chronic maxillary sinus infections, and if properly performed they remain exceedingly useful.

REFERENCES

1. Macbeth R. Caldwell–Luc operation 1952–1966. *Arch Otolaryngol* 1968;87:630–635.
2. Mann W, Beck C. Inferior meatal antrostomy in chronic maxillary sinusitis. *Arch Otorhinolaryngol* 1978;221:289–295.
3. Lund VJ. Fundamental considerations of the design and function of intranasal antrostomies. *J R Soc Med* 1986;79:646–649.
4. Hilding AC. Experimental surgery of the nose and sinuses. Changes in the morphology of the epithelium following variations in ventilation. *Arch Otolaryngol* 1932;16:9–17.
5. Proetz AW. *Essays on the applied physiology of the nose*. St Louis: Annals Publishing, 1941.
6. Capps FCW. Observations on the treatment of infections of the maxillary antrum. *J Laryngol Otol* 1952;66:199–210.
7. Lavelle RJ, Harrison MS. Infection of the maxillary sinus: the case for the middle meatal antrostomy. *Laryngoscope* 1971;81: 90–106.

CHAPTER 20

Endoscopic Sinus Surgery

Dale H. Rice

Over the past two decades there has developed a considerable interest in endoscopic surgery of the paranasal sinuses. This began as an outgrowth of the work of Messerklinger and Wigand. While both were interested in the rehabilitation of the sinus mucosa, they approached the problem quite differently. Messerklinger studied intently the mucociliary flow patterns in the nose and sinuses under normal and pathologic conditions and demonstrated that in the majority of cases chronic sinusitis was a result of obstruction in the anterior ethmoid sinuses (1). Wigand, on the other hand, dealt clinically with patients with pansinusitis and found that the quickest and safest way to eliminate the disease process and reaerate the sinuses was to widely open all the sinuses in conjunction with a complete ethmoidectomy (2,3). Both stressed that clearing the obstruction would allow the mucosa to return to normal. Another concurrent development was that of the endonasal endoscopes using Hopkins optics. These instruments allowed excellent visualization within the nose and sinuses with their straight and angled lenses. In conjunction with this, the instrument companies developed small, long-handled instruments appropriate for work in the nasal cavity and sinuses under direct visual control (Figs. 1 and 2).

Another development that aided in the popularization of this technique was computed tomography (CT). Coronal CT is particularly good at showing the fine bony architecture of the paranasal sinuses as well as areas of mucosal obstruction. Thus one can examine the nasal cavity more precisely than ever before using the endoscopes in the office and then see within the sinuses in a much more detailed fashion with CT scans (Fig. 3).

Early in the development, Messerklinger stressed a limited anterior ethmoidectomy and middle meatal antrostomy as the procedure of choice, while Wigand stressed the total frontosphenoethmoidectomy and middle meatal antrostomy. Experience has taught that neither operation works every time and that the extent of surgery must match the severity of the patient's disease. From a practical standpoint, the Messerklinger technique is the more commonly used and works well in most patients. It is an anterior-to-posterior approach and allows one to stop when normal mucosa is reached. For the patient with severe pansinusitis, however, or the patient who has been operated on before, particularly with absent landmarks, the posterior-to-anterior approach may be somewhat safer. This latter technique begins with identification of the sphenoid sinus and skull base as the initial step.

PATIENT SELECTION

The ideal patient for endoscopic sinus surgery is one with a clear history of chronic or recurrent bacterial sinusitis. Patients who respond briefly to antibiotics or who fail to respond may be expected to do well with this surgery. Patients with allergies as a complicating factor will do less well. The infections may be markedly improved or even controlled, but the allergies will continue. Smokers or those who are exposed to other nasal irritants will also continue to have nasal symptoms, although infections may not be prominent after successful surgery.

The place of endoscopic sinus surgery in other sinus disorders is uncertain at present. Patients with bilateral nasal polyps will continue to get recurrent polyps regardless of the technique, although the rate of recurrence is of course unpredictable. Endoscopic sinus surgery is a useful adjunct in children with immunologic abnormalities or immotile cilia syndromes but the surgery is not curative for the *primary* disorder.

Patients having the proper history should be examined thoroughly. For many, the nasal exam need not be more complicated than routine anterior rhinoscopy.

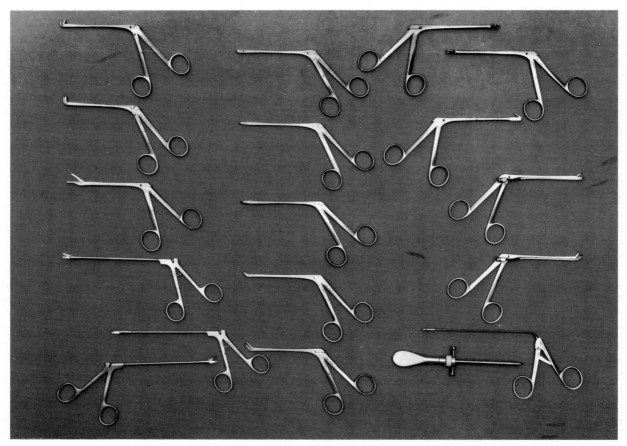

FIG. 1. Instruments available for endoscopic sinus surgery.

If the abnormalities are obvious, no further nasal examination is necessary at that time. If the examination is grossly normal, or otherwise inadequate, office nasal endoscopy should be performed. This use of the nasal endoscopes may be the single biggest practical advance in endoscopic sinus surgery. Nasal endoscopy is best performed by first using a topical vasoconstrictor and anesthetic agent and allowing it ample time to work. Following this, it is generally an easy matter to systematically examine the nasal cavity using a 2.7 mm endoscope with either a 25° or 30° wide angle lens. The entire nasal cavity should be examined, including the nasopharynx, with particular attention paid to the middle meatus, where it is likely the main abnormality will be found (Figs. 4 and 5).

Even if the office nasal endoscopy is normal, in a patient with the appropriate history, a coronal CT scan without contrast media should be obtained. This should generally be obtained when the patient is in the best possible medical condition so as to highlight the basic underlying abnormality. In the majority of cases, the CT scan will show abnormalities in the anterior ethmoids and maxillary sinuses (Figs. 6 and 7). The other sinuses should also be evaluated carefully and the appropriate operative approach planned.

OPERATIVE TECHNIQUE

For the typical patient with chronic or recurrent sinusitis, the operation may be performed under either local or general anesthesia. The operation is performed on an outpatient basis. It is wise to have the patient spray his or her nose with a vasoconstrictive agent on call to the operating room. Many drugs used in general anesthesia today are vasodilators and getting the vasoconstriction started early is worthwhile. Once the patient is in the operating room, and after successful induction, the nasal cavity should be packed with cottonoids soaked in either 4% cocaine, 1% xylocaine with 1/100,000 epinephrine, or some other vasoconstrictor. These should be allowed to remain in the nasal cavity for approximately 5 to 10 min. The onset of action for cocaine is 4 min. Upon removal, it is wise to systematically reexamine the nasal cavity with the endoscope to be certain that the original plan of surgery is still appropriate (Fig. 8). Following this, the middle turbinate and the lateral nasal wall adjacent to the middle turbinate should be injected judiciously with small amounts of 1% xylocaine with 1/100,000 epinephrine including the uncinate and bulla, if they can be visualized. Following this, an additional cottonoid soaked

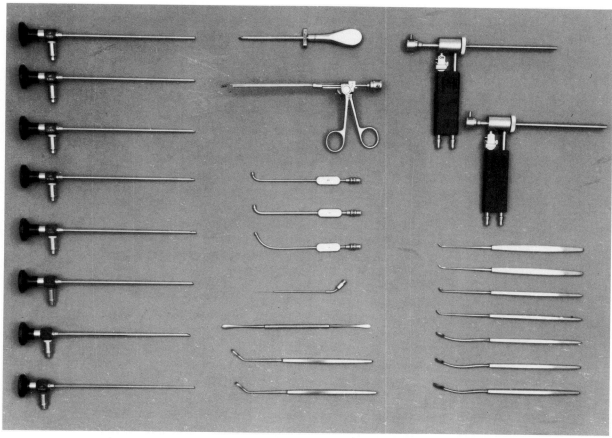

FIG. 2. Additional instruments and the endoscopes available for endoscopic sinus surgery.

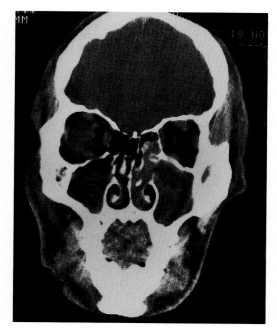

FIG. 3. Coronal CT scan showing ethmoid and maxillary sinusitis on the right and a mucus retention cyst of the maxillary sinus on the left.

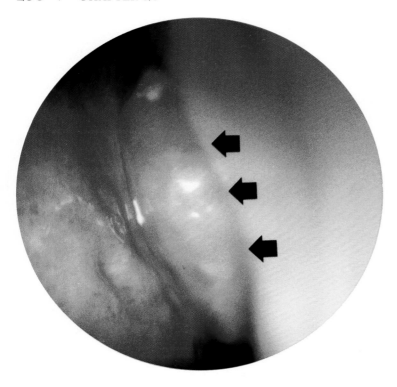

FIG. 4. Endoscopic view of ethmoid polyp *(arrows)* within middle meatus.

in 1% xylocaine with 1/100,000 epinephrine should be inserted directly into the middle meatus. This is best done with bayonet forceps without teeth to make it easy to release the cottonoid upon placement. An additional 5 min should be allowed to pass. If the patient has significant polyps, they may be removed at this

time either with the headlight in the traditional manner or with the endoscopes. Furthermore, if a septoplasty is needed to gain access to the middle meatus, it should be performed at this time.

Again, the nasal cavity should be inspected and the procedure initiated. In the usual patient, an incision is

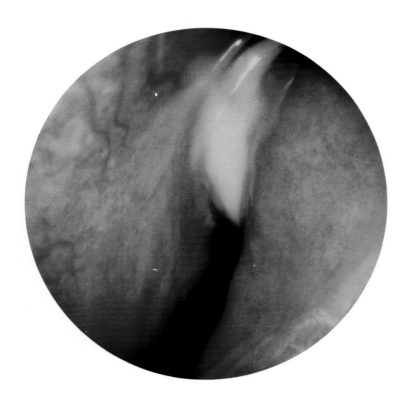

FIG. 5. Endoscopic view of mucopurulent drainage in the middle meatus.

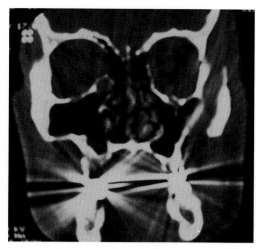

FIG. 6. Coronal CT scan showing opacified bulla ethmoidalis on left. Patient had recurrent left facial pain at the medial canthus that responded to antibiotics, only to recur afterward. Endoscopic drainage of the bulla resulted in a permanent cure.

made in the base of the uncinate from superior to inferior with a sickle knife and it is pushed medially. It is then grasped with the Blakesley forceps and removed (Fig. 9). This will establish the initial lateral plane of dissection, which is the lamina papyracea. Bear in mind that the anterior ethmoids are approximately 0.5 cm wide. Next, the forceps should be used to remove the remainder of the uncinate if any remains from the frontal recess area superiorly to the insertion of the inferior turbinate inferiorly. This maneuver will decompress the hiatus similunaris and infundibulum anteriorly. To decompress it posteriorly, the bulla ethmoid-

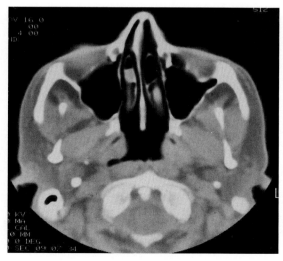

FIG. 7. Axial CT scan showing air–fluid level in right concha bullosa. Patient had history similar to the patient in Fig. 6.

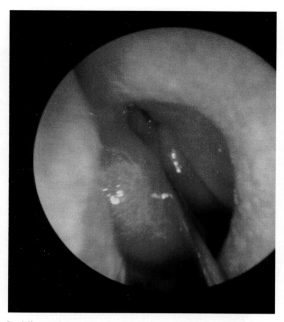

FIG. 8. View through endoscope of normal middle meatus. Middle turbinate is being pushed medially with a Freer elevator. The uncinate process and bulla ethmoidalis can be seen clearly to the right of the turbinate.

alis is next removed (Fig. 10). During this maneuver, the forceps blades should be opened and closed vertically. Thus the blades will be parallel to the lamina papyracea rather than pointing toward it. This likewise is removed from the fovea to the top of the inferior turbinate (Fig. 11). This may expose the natural ostium of the maxillary sinus. Often it will not, however, because the amount of mucosal disease may be such that the opening is visually obscured.

In the rare case where the ostium seems open and adequate in size, it need not be manipulated. In the more typical case, however, it can be identified by palpation with either the angled Blakesley forceps or the curved olive-tipped antrum suction cannula. Once it is identified, using the angled forceps the mucosa in the vicinity of the ostium can gently be removed until it is readily visualized. At this point the ostium can be enlarged in one of two ways. Using the reverse cutting forceps, the anterior margin may be enlarged anteriorly (Fig. 12). Occasionally, it is just as easy to enlarge it posteriorly with the angled forceps. In this situation, direct visualization will allow placement of one jaw of the forceps into the maxillary sinus while one remains in the middle meatus and the posterior margin of the ostium is enlarged. It is as yet unclear as to the optimum size of the natural ostium once the ethmoids have been removed. Some evidence would suggest that it needs be approximately 0.5 to 1.5 cm in diameter. If there is an accessory ostium, it should be connected to the natural ostium to prevent mucus from draining

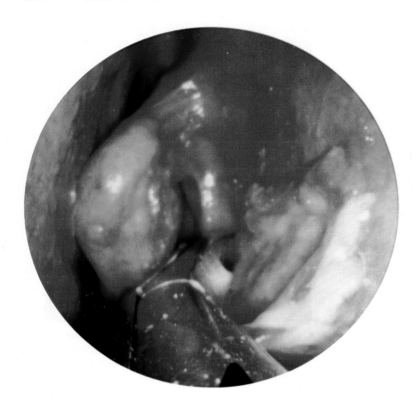

FIG. 9. Endoscopic view of uncinate process being removed by 45° Weil–Blakesley forceps.

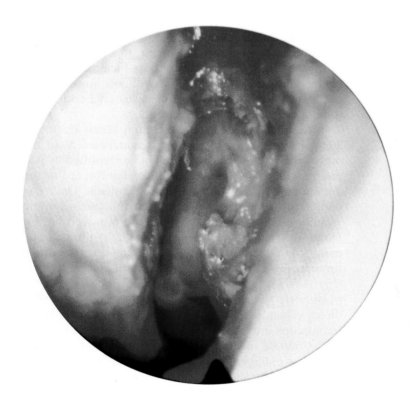

FIG. 10. Endoscopic view of bulla ethmoidalis following removal of uncinate process.

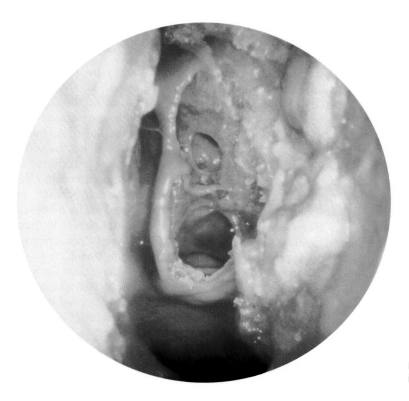

FIG. 11. Endoscopic view of basal lamella following removal of bulla ethmoidalis.

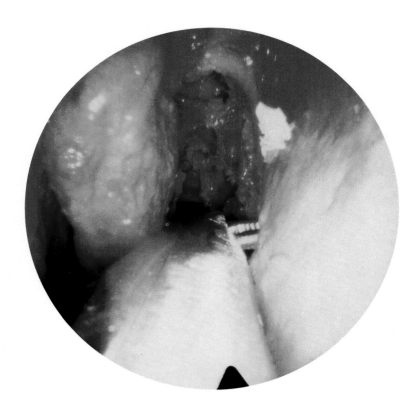

FIG. 12. Endoscopic view of reverse cutting forceps within natural ostium of maxillary sinus.

out the natural ostium and back through the accessory ostium into the sinus forming a circular, never-ending draining pattern.

If one is completely unable to identify the natural ostium even by palpation, the safest maneuver is to make one in the fontanelle. This should be done just above the insertion of the inferior turbinate approximately halfway between the anterior and posterior ends of the inferior turbinate. When in doubt, it is safest to go more posterior as the floor of the orbit is further from the medial antral wall posteriorly than it is anteriorly. Once the sinus has been entered, it can then be enlarged safely while visualizing the orbital floor.

At this point one should have a clear view of the maxillary sinus (Fig. 13) and should have removed the anterior ethmoid cells such that the posterior boundary of this space is now the basal lamella. In the patient with the usual anterior ethmoid–maxillary sinus disease, the operation is complete at this time. If the patient has more extensive disease, further dissection should be performed. If the patient has posterior ethmoid and sphenoid disease, the dissection can proceed through the basal lamella. This is done most safely by staying close to the lateral edge of the middle turbinate until the sphenoid is reached (Fig. 14). The sphenoid can be entered and its ostium enlarged. It is generally wise to do little or no dissection within the sphenoid unless it is absolutely necessary. This is particularly true in superior and lateral directions where one might encounter the optic nerve or the carotid artery. Fur-

thermore, enlarging the ostium too far inferiorly may transect a branch of the sphenoethmoid artery and lead to annoying pulsatile bleeding.

A complete ethmoidectomy should be performed using preestablished landmarks as a guide. One is the fovea ethmoidalis, the superior aspect of the dissection. The lamina papyracea is on the same parasagittal plane as the natural ostium of the maxillary sinus and dissection lateral to this should not be done. In addition, the sphenoid ostium establishes the posteriormost aspect of the dissection. Again, once a complete ethmoidectomy has been performed, the procedure is complete unless the patient has frontal sinus disease.

For frontal sinus disease, the frontal recess is then inspected. Dissection here is immediately posterior to the superior attachment of the middle turbinate (Fig. 15). One needs to use the angled Blakesley forceps and often will need an angled telescope. The dissection should be directly vertical, immediately behind the anterior attachment of the middle turbinate. If one proceeds gently in this direction, removing only mucosa and eggshell bone, one will encounter the floor of the frontal sinus (which will have a definite hard feeling) and its natural ostium. At this point, the natural ostium of the frontal sinus should be visualized readily and any obstructing mucosa should be removed gently (Fig. 16). If need be, the ostium to the frontal sinus may be enlarged but this is rarely necessary (Fig. 17).

Some patients have a concha bullosa in the middle turbinate, which should be opened in either of two circumstances—if it is part of the disease process or if it

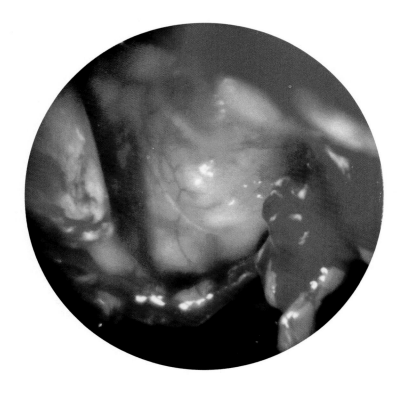

FIG. 13. Endoscopic view of maxillary sinus through enlarged natural ostium.

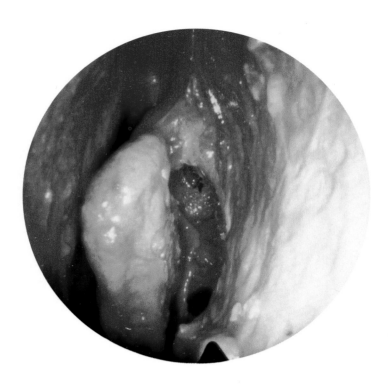

FIG. 14. Endoscopic view of anterior face of the sphenoid sinus.

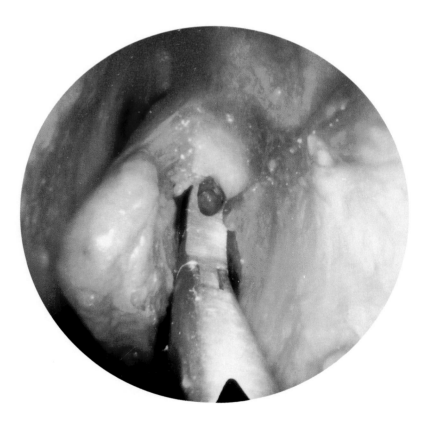

FIG. 15. Endoscopic view of the 45° Weil–Blakesley forceps entering the frontal recess area.

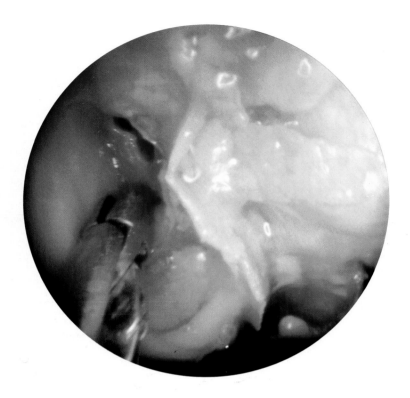

FIG. 16. Endoscopic view of the frontal sinus ostium.

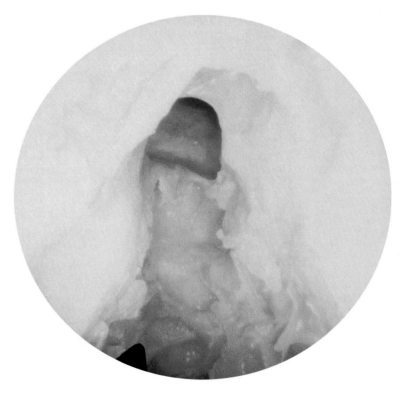

FIG. 17. Endoscopic view of the frontal sinus following removal of obstructing frontal recess mucosa.

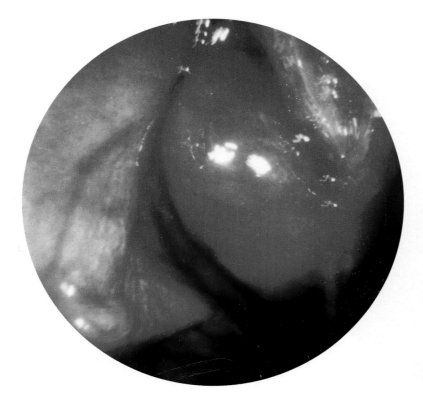

FIG. 18. Endoscopic view of expanded middle turbinate because of concha bullosa.

has expanded into the middle turbinate such that the turbinate itself encroaches on the middle meatus (Fig. 18). Using the sickle knife, an incision is made in the anterior end of the middle turbinate to expose the air cell. Using the straight biting forceps, the lateral lamella of the middle turbinate is then removed sufficiently to provide adequate drainage and to enlarge the middle meatus (Fig. 19).

In general, chronically infected mucosa of the sinuses will return to normal once satisfactory drainage has been established. This may take some time, however, and thick drainage is generally the last symptom to disappear, long after symptoms of pain and pressure have abated. Occasionally, work will need to be done within the maxillary sinus itself. If so, it can often be done through a very large middle meatal antrostomy. If this is inadequate, an inferior nasoantral window can be made. One can then view the sinus through one ostium and insert the instrument through the other.

If the patient has only a maxillary sinus problem that needs to be biopsied or drained, a canine fossa puncture can be performed with the antral trocar. The lesion can then be identified by inserting the telescope through the trocar sheath. The sheath is then pointed directly at the lesion, the telescope is removed, and the forceps is inserted for tissue removal. If necessary, the optical forceps can be used through the sheath, but this can be quite tedious.

Occasionally, one is faced with a patient who has had multiple previous operations, often a Caldwell–Luc with transantral and transnasal ethmoidectomy, which has failed. Frequently, these patients can also be managed by endoscopic sinus surgery, but occasionally it is prudent to do this with a different technique. This is particularly true if the middle turbinate has been resected and therefore is lost as a valuable landmark. These patients generally need a total sphenoethmoidectomy. Patients with massive polyposis, recurrent pansinusitis, cystic fibrosis, and those being considered for lung transplant also fall into this group.

The initial steps of this procedure are similar to the one discussed already in terms of obtaining optimum vasoconstriction. However, since the middle turbinate is often missing and that important landmark is absent, one needs to proceed more cautiously. It is best to establish the remaining important landmarks early in the dissection. The two safest to establish are the natural ostium of the maxillary sinus, which can be done low and posterior along the superior part of the inferior turbinate and the lamina papyracea, which is on the same parasagittal plane and the sphenoid ostium. One should be particularly careful when dissecting in this parasagittal plane. One can then identify directly the natural ostium of the sphenoid sinus posteriorly approximately 1 cm from the nasal septum. This will establish the posterior boundary of the dissection. Once these two landmarks are established, one can carefully work superiorly to identify the fovea ethmoidalis and

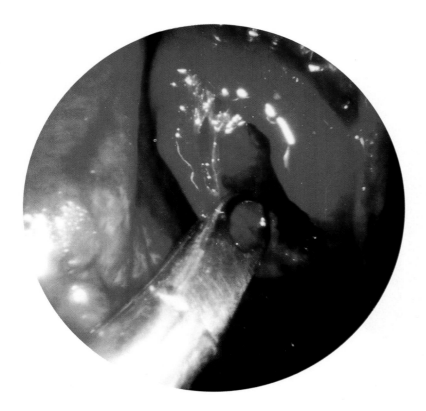

FIG. 19. Endoscopic view of lateral lamella of middle turbinate (concha bullosa) being removed.

then do a complete ethmoidectomy under direct visualization.

Upon completion of the ethmoidectomy, the maxillary sinus ostium is enlarged as before. If the sphenoid ostium has not already been enlarged, it should be done at this time. Finally, the frontal recess and frontal sinus can be addressed.

POSTOPERATIVE CARE

The postoperative care is quite important in these patients and can be done in one of several ways. One technique is to see the patient on a daily or near daily basis to manually clean the middle meatus of crusts, scabs, and inspissated mucus. Others prefer to see the patients less frequently, once or twice a week, while having the patient perform nasal irrigations with normal saline multiple times, usually three, per day. Still others prefer to pack the middle meatus and remove the packing anywhere from 1 to 7 days postoperatively and begin cleaning at that time. All these techniques work quite well if carefully adhered to. The basic key is to keep the operative site as clean as possible to allow healing to progress as rapidly as possible. This degree of postoperative cleaning should continue until the operative site is mucosally covered. In addition, the patient should be on perioperative antibiotics and should be started on steroid nasal sprays in the early postoperative period. It is probably wise in those patients who have perennial allergies to continue lifelong irrigations and nasal sprays. Those patients who have no secondary problems, other than chronic infection, can stop these once healing has occurred.

In general, symptoms of pain and pressure will be relieved in the very early postoperative period while thick postnasal drainage will continue until the mucosa within the sinuses has returned to normal. This may take weeks to months depending on the severity of the disease and the rapidity of healing. The patient should be warned of this preoperatively. The irrigation should be done as often as necessary to keep the site free of clots and crusts and may be done effectively with a nasal irrigator attached to a dental irrigator or with a rubber bulb ear syringe.

Despite all this postoperative care, failure, when it does occur, usually occurs early. In general, if the patient is symptom-free for several weeks to a month or two and then begins to have recurrent symptoms, failure is imminent and in general even intensive office care fails to prevent this. It is generally better to admit failure and plan revision surgery early. Late failure is uncommon, excluding those patients who have allergies, recurrent polyps, or other underlying uncorrectable problems.

COMPLICATIONS

Complications with endoscopic sinus surgery should be few and are usually minor. This technique takes careful study in learning and increasing experience increases confidence. Throughout the dissection, every maneuver should be done under direct visualization and one should constantly be aware of the depth and angle of penetration. The potential complications of an operation performed with endoscopes are no different than the complications performed without them. The eye and the brain have the same unchanging relationships to the sinuses. Dissection too superiorly may lead to a cerebrospinal fluid leak. If this is recognized intraoperatively, it should be repaired endoscopically with fascia and a mucosal flap with tissue glue and packing. If it is recognized postoperatively, conservative treatment should be instituted unless it is clearly too large to seal spontaneously. If it fails to close spontaneously, reoperation either endoscopically or externally should be performed.

Dissection too laterally may lead to a breach of the lamina papyracea. One should be constantly aware of material in the middle meatus and should cease dissecting immediately if fat is encountered. In general, if this is done there will be no adverse affects on the eye. The fat should be neither removed nor pushed back into the orbit but merely left in place and the dissection continued around it. The eye should be observed throughout the procedure and the eyelids should in fact not be taped shut. An ophthalmologic consultation should be obtained in the recovery room. In general, there will be no adverse effect other than some ecchymosis in the area of the medial canthus and the medial lower eyelid. More posterior entry into the orbit may result in damage to the medial rectus muscle or to the optic nerve and again if this possibility occurs immediate ophthalmologic consultation should be obtained. One should always be prepared to do an orbital decompression should sudden bleeding occur within the orbit. This is most quickly obtained by doing a lateral canthotomy. If one is still in the operating room, complete medial decompression can easily be done endoscopically by removing the entire lamina papyracea and even the medial floor of the orbit.

Dissection too anteriorly can lead to damage to the nasolacrimal apparatus. Damage to the nasolacrimal apparatus probably occurs more frequently than realized (4). It is probable that many times when the duct is transected it will fistulize spontaneously into the nasal cavity without obstruction. Should obstruction occur, however, it can generally be repaired through endoscopic intranasal dacryocystorhinostomy as first described by Rice (5).

The most devasting complication of endoscopic sinus surgery is penetration of the dura through the fovea ethmoidalis or cribriform plate. This complication frequently leads to a rapidly fatal outcome secondary to hemorrhage from the anterior communicating artery or one of its branches. Should this complication occur and be recognized, an immediate neurosurgical consultation should be obtained.

ANCILLARY PROCEDURES

Several ancillary procedures have been described using these instruments. One just mentioned is the intranasal dacryocystorhinostomy. The basic technique involves removing the mucosa over the lacrimal bone 1 to 1.5 cm anterior to the base of the uncinate process. The underlying bone can then be removed with a variety of instruments such as the back-biting forceps from the base of the uncinate or perhaps with a curet or a drill. This removed mucous membrane and bone should be directly lateral to the anterior aspect of the middle turbinate just inferior to its superior attachment (Fig. 20). Once the bone is removed, the lacrimal sac will be exposed. To confirm this, a lacrimal probe should be inserted through the inferior punctum and canaliculus into the sac. Intranasally, the sac will be seen to be tented by the probe, confirming its location. The medial wall of the sac should then be incised with a sickle knife, exposing the lacrimal probe, and most of the medial wall of the sac should then be removed with the Weil–Blakesley forceps.

It is also possible to endoscopically repair some cerebrospinal fluid fistulas. In general, the fistula should be no larger than 1 cm in greatest diameter. If the fistula is difficult to identify, 0.2 ml of 5% fluorescein mixed in 5 to 10 ml of cerebrospinal fluid should be injected slowly into the lumbar subarachnoid space (6). Once the site of the fistula is identified, the mucous membrane around it should be removed backward for several millimeters. Next, a fascia graft should be obtained from any convenient site. Ideally, the graft should then be placed over the dura and bone and tucked under the surrounding mucosa if possible. At this point, tissue adhesives can be used to hold the mucosal graft in place. The graft is then held in place with Gelfoam, coated with an antibiotic ointment.

Subperiosteal orbital abscesses can also be managed endoscopically in experienced hands. Hypotensive anesthesia is advisable. The initial step is to perform a complete ethmoidectomy as described previously. Complete hemostasis must be obtained at the end of this procedure. Next, the lamina papyracea should be breached anteriorly and dissection continued until there is free drainage of the abscess. Only the minimal amount of bone should be removed to satisfactorily

Periorbita   Orbital fat   Medial rectus muscle   Frontal sinus

Posterior
ethmoid
cell

Nasolacrimal
duct

Inferior
oblique
muscle

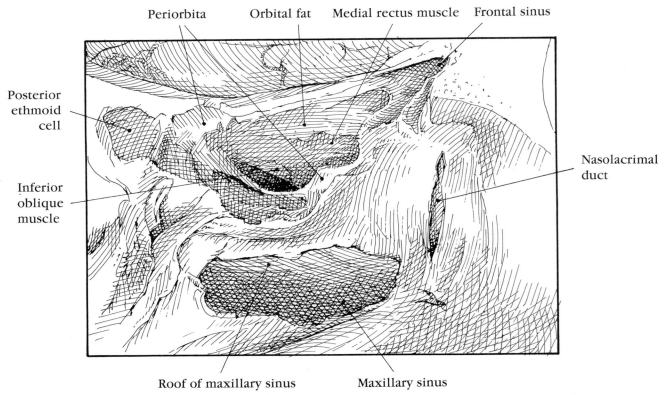

Roof of maxillary sinus   Maxillary sinus

FIG. 20. Drawing of relevant anatomy.

drain the abscess. Great care should be taken to avoid penetration of the periorbita. The patient should be observed carefully in the postoperative period to be certain that the abscess has been drained in its entirety. Should there be any doubt, a CT scan should be obtained immediately.

Orbital decompression can also be performed endoscopically. This technique has much in common with that described above for drainage of a subperiorbital abscess but calls for complete removal of the lamina papyracea as well as the medial orbital floor. An early step should involve making a very large maxillary antrostomy in the middle meatus to allow excellent visualization of the orbital floor and its juncture with the lamina papyracea. Care must be taken to preserve the bone in the area of the frontal recess to avoid obstructing the frontal sinus and to preserve the bone in the region of the optic canal to provide protection of the optic nerve. It is also critical not to open the periorbita until all bone has been removed (7). The periorbital incisions are performed radially in a posterior-to-anterior direction with the orbital floor incisions beginning in the most lateral aspect and proceeding medially. Likewise, the incisions of the periorbita underlying the lamina papyracea proceed from superior to inferior. The degree of decompression is assessed by gentle manual pressure on the globe.

The final ancillary procedure is optic nerve de-

compression. The utility of optic nerve decompression for fractures involving the optic canal are greatly debated, but should the procedure be indicated, it can be performed endoscopically. The first step is a total sphenoethmoidectomy as described above. Again, meticulous hemostasis is necessary before beginning with the actual decompression. In this case, the posterior half of the lamina papyracea is removed in an anterior-to-posterior direction with care being taken to avoid injury to or penetration of the periorbita. Penetration of the periorbita may lead to herniation of fat into the operative field, which may seriously compromise exposure. Dissection proceeds posteriorly along the medial wall of the orbit toward the orbital apex. The posterior ethmoid artery may be recognized as it penetrates the medial orbital wall at the level of the cribriform plate and as is well known is approximately 5 mm anterior to the optic nerve. The contribution of the sphenoid bone to the optic canal must be removed using J-curets, sinus forceps, and occasionally Kerrison rongeurs while entering the superior–lateral aspect of the sphenoid sinus. The fracture line may be visible at this point. The periosteum surrounding the optic nerve is incised radially along the medial aspect of the nerve using a Beaver sickle knife. Cerebrospinal fluid usually is seen at this point as the sheath of the optic nerve is contiguous with the dura. This completes the decompression. The patient should receive perioperative antibiotics and systemic steroids, if both have not already been started.

RESULTS OF ENDOSCOPIC SINUS SURGERY

In carefully selected patients with no complicating factors, results of endoscopic sinus surgery are usually gratifying. Figure 21 shows the preoperative and postoperative results in a patient with recurrent right maxillary sinusitis, which would respond only briefly to antibiotics.

The same is true in children who have no underlying incurable medical problem. Figure 22 shows the preoperative and postoperative scans of an 8-year-old girl with a 3 year history of nearly constant bilateral purulent rhinorrhea. She had missed a great deal of school in the preceding 2 years and had been on nearly constant antibiotics. Complete immunologic and allergic workups were normal. She underwent a simple bilateral anterior ethmoidectomy and middle meatal antrostomy.

Even more complicated patients can be managed successfully with good technique and compulsive postoperative care. Figure 23 shows the axial CT scans of a patient with classic allergic fungal sinusitis. This

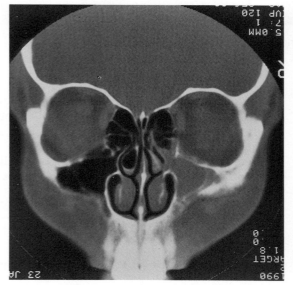
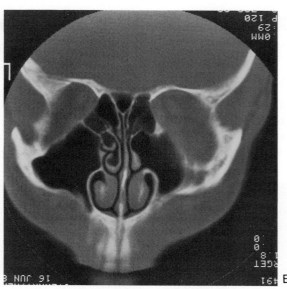

FIG. 21. A: Preoperative coronal CT scan showing ostiomeatal obstruction on the right. **B:** Postoperative CT scan of same patient.

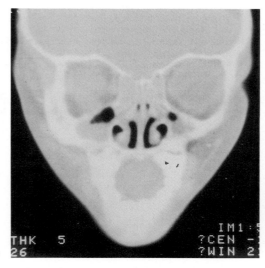
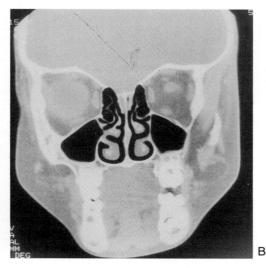

FIG. 22. A: Preoperative CT scan of 8-year-old girl with 3 year history of constant bilateral purulent rhinorrhea. **B:** Postoperative view of the same patient.

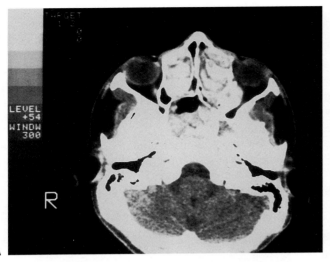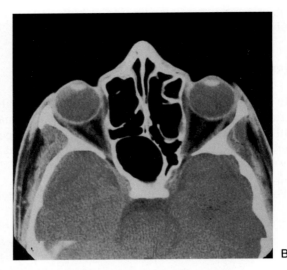

FIG. 23. A: Preoperative axial CT scan showing the classic appearance of allergic fungal sinusitis. **B:** Postoperative scan of the same patient.

patient required a complete frontosphenoethmoidectomy to achieve this result.

Clearly, not all patients will get a perfect result. Patients with allergies (recognized or unrecognized), pa-

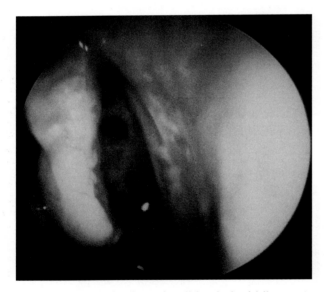

FIG. 24. Endoscopic view of well-healed middle meatus.

tients who smoke, patients who form polyps, and patients with severely scarred mucosa will do much less well. Revision surgery is common over time and can be quite challenging.

Figure 24 shows an endoscopic view of a well-healed postoperative result—the result one strives for in every patient.

REFERENCES

1. Messerklinger W. Endoskopische diagnose und chirurgie des residivierdes sinusitis. In: Krajna Z, ed. *Advances in nose and sinus surgery*. Zagrab: Zagreb University, 1985.
2. Wigand ME, Steiner W, Jaumann MP. Endonasal sinus surgery with endoscopical control: from radical operation to rehabilitation of the mucosa. *Endoscopy* 1978;10:255–260.
3. Lusk RP, Muntz HR. Endoscopic sinus surgery in children with chronic sinusitis: a pilot study. *Laryngoscope* 1990;100:654–658.
4. Wigand ME. Transnasal ethmoidectomy under endoscopic control. *Rhinology* 1981;19:7–15.
5. Rice DH. Endoscopic intranasal dacryocystorhinostomy. *Am J Rhinol* 1988;2:127–128.
6. Mattox DE, Kennedy DW. Endoscopic management of cerebrospinal fluid leaks and encephaloceles. *Laryngoscope* 1990;100:857–862.
7. Kennedy DW, Goodstein ML, Miller NR, Zinreich SJ. Endoscopic transnasal orbital decompression. *Arch Otolaryngol Head Neck Surg* 1990;116:275–282.

CHAPTER 21

Fungal Infections of the Sinuses

Paul J. Donald

Fungal infections of the paranasal sinuses are relatively uncommon. Although sinusitis afflicts up to 20% of individuals during the course of their lives, very few contract fungal sinusitis. The first reported case of fungal sinusitis was by Plaignaud (1) in 1791. An actual detailed clinical description of *Aspergillus fumigatus* of the nasal cavity was first described in 1885 by Schubert (2). Maxillary sinusitis specifically identified as *A. fumigatus* was initially delineated by Zarniko (3) in 1891. The first case described in the United States was by MacKenzie (4) but it wasn't until 1961 that the first actual series of cases were described in a literature review by Sevetsky and Waltner (5). In 1978, Titche (6) presented a literature search of 110 cases that included 25 cases from the Sudan, where a particularly aggressive form of the disease is seen with *Aspergillus flavus* being the commonest cause. Depending on the virulence of the organism and the susceptibility of the host, the resultant disease process can vary from an indolent almost asymptomatic nuisance to a devastating, rapidly progressive, fatal disease.

Fungal sinusitis has emerged as a more vital health problem in modern times because of the rising incidence of immune deficient states such as acquired immunodeficiency syndrome (AIDS), immunosuppression secondary to the treatment of leukemia, and that induced in transplant patients, uncontrolled diabetics, and patients who are undergoing broad spectrum antibiotic therapy. In addition, the frequency of travel into endemic areas and the increased mobility of foreigners who emigrate from these countries are ever increasing relevant factors. Improved means of clinical detection and laboratory diagnosis have more clearly identified affected individuals.

MYCOLOGY

Fungi are found mainly in air, dust, soil, plants, and decaying organic matter. They adhere to dust particles and are thus inhaled in inspired air and deposited on the nasal and paranasal sinus mucosa. They are ubiquitously found in the environment but rarely ever become pathogenic. The warm moist environment of the upper respiratory tract is an ideal environment for the proliferation of fungi, but host resistance is high, except under favorable growth conditions in highly susceptible individuals.

Fungi are closely related to bacteria; some such as the Actinomycetales and *Nocardia asteroides* are transitional types possessing characteristics of both types of organism (7). The Actinomycetales branch like fungi but also assume bacillary and coccoid forms. *Nocardia* stains acid-fast like the tubercle bacillus.

Fungi possess a unique property among microorganisms called dimorphism, meaning that they may exist both as a spore form and as a branching, mycelial form. The form the organism takes is usually influenced by varying environmental conditions. Unlike bacteria, their cell walls are composed of chitin, mannans, and occasionally cellulose. Although some fungi exist purely as spores or hyphae, most of the human pathogens are dimorphic. There is a wide range of morphologic types of both spores and branching patterns. In particular, the presence or absence of segmentations or septa of the hyphae will often distinguish one species from another (Fig. 1). The fungi are thus broadly categorized as septated or nonseptated types. The pathogenic variety tend to be dimorphic and of the septate variety (8); they also principally reproduce by asexual reproduction. The hyphae branch like a tree from a central stem or from a common node such as *Rhizopus*. The terminal buds have a varying morphology such as spherical sporangia or are arrayed in clusters like the conidiophores of *Aspergillus*. These fungi appear to grow best on Sabouraud's dextrose agar at 20 to 37 °C. They are, however, difficult to grow and it may take weeks to produce identifiable colonies.

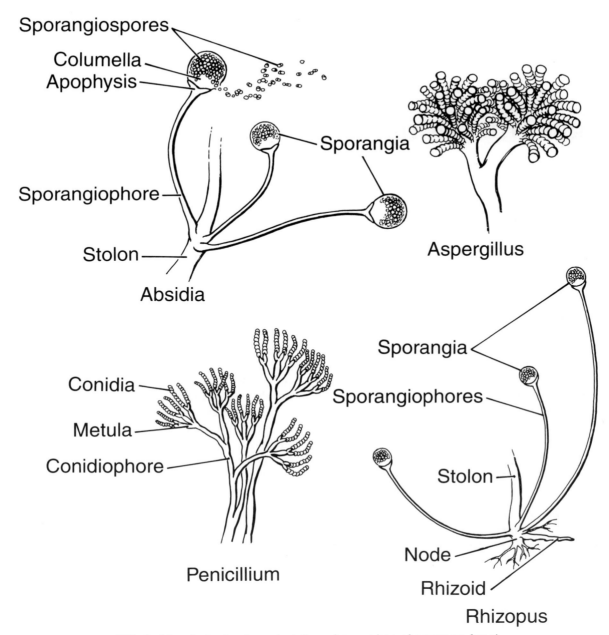

FIG. 1. Morphologic characteristics of a number of common fungi.

The taxonomy of fungi is very confusing mainly because of recent problems of precise identification of specific organisms. The suggestion of Manning et al. (9) to divide the fungi into those that are pathogenic to humans, such as *Aspergillus* and *Mucor*, and those that are common saprophytes and usual laboratory contaminants that only very rarely infect humans appears quite reasonable and convenient.

Table 1 lists the most important genera of pathogenic mycotic organisms that afflict the nose and paranasal sinuses (8,10). The list is rather staggering but the most commonly seen in clinical practice in the Western

TABLE 1. *Genera of mycotic organisms*

Aspergillus	*Cladosporium*	*Mucor*
Entomophthora	*Candida*	*Histoplasma*
Drechslera	*Sporothrix*	*Blastomyces*
Alternaria	*Rhinosporidium*	*Paracoccidioides*
Pseudoallescharia	*Rhizopus*	*Coccidioides*
Schizophyllum	*Cunninghamella*	*Cryptococcus*
Bipolaris	*Conidiobolus*	*Paecilomyces*
Exerohilum	*Basidiobolus*	
Curvularia	*Absidia*	

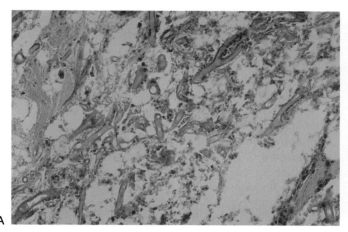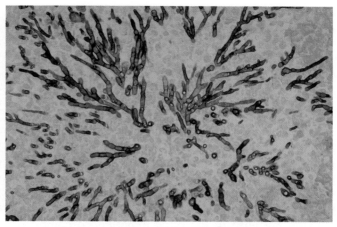

A   B

FIG. 2. A: Photomicrograph of hyphae from mucormycosis (H&E, × 200). **B:** Photomicrograph of hypha from *Aspergillus* (methenamine silver, × 100).

world are *Aspergillus, Mucor, Rhizopus,* and *Alternaria.*

Diagnosis is best made by tissue biopsy, staining of the specimen followed by microscopic examination and culture in Sabouraud's agar. Sometimes a smear may be stained and examined, thereby precluding the need for biopsy. Even potassium hydroxide preparations can sometimes produce identification of the organism. Fungal specific stains such as Grocot's methenamine silver (GMS), Gridley, or periodic acid–Schiff (PAS) are most often necessary for definitive diagnosis of the organisms (Fig. 2).

PATHOPHYSIOLOGY

As previously mentioned, the ubiquitous distribution of fungi and the rarity of disease speak to the low virulence of these organisms. With the exception of aflatoxin, produced by *Aspergillus flavus,* the fungi do not produce toxins but induce a hypersensitivity to the chemical constituents in their cell walls. This is especially exemplified in allergic *Aspergillus* sinusitis, wherein an actual immunoglobulin E (IgE) mediated type of hypersensitivity is induced. The activity of this organism is also enhanced by a hypoxic environment. Other than direct invasiveness, the mechanism of tissue destruction is unknown.

The nonspecific defense against fungi is provided by leukocytes, which phagocytose the organisms and kill them via various intracellular mechanisms. The specific immune response to mycotic organisms can be either humoral or cell fixed in type. The humoral response activates lymphocytes and macrophages through lymphokines and other mediators, stimulating increasing phagocytosis and fungal death. The subsequent formation of a granuloma of the noncaseating

type is the typical reaction of the cellular defense. The antigens released by the fungi can also result in a brisk inflammatory response (8).

Although the most usual means of acquisition of the fungus is by the nasal route via dust-bound spores, another putative cause is from dental fillings. *Aspergillus* grows easily in the zinc oxide and paraformaldehyde used in endodontic treatment (11,12). Even if the affected tooth is eventually removed, the organisms tend to remain.

Aspergillus can also be acquired by smoking marijuana (13). In a study by Kagan (13), 11 of 12 marijuana cigarettes tested cultured positive for *Aspergillus.* In addition, a test for precipitins to *Aspergillus* was done in blood samples of 21 marijuana smokers. Eleven of 21 showed a positive reaction compared to only one of ten nonsmoking controls.

CLINICAL MANIFESTATION

Aspergillosis

The most common fungal infection encountered in the nose and paranasal sinuses is that caused by the fungus of the genus *Aspergillus.* The most prevalent species are *A. fumigatus, A. flavus,* and *A. niger.* The country that reports sinus aspergillosis most frequently is the Sudan. The passage of the spores of the organism is facilitated by its hot, dusty climate. Particularly characteristic here is the fulminant invasive form of the disease commonly caused there by *A. fumigatus* and *A. niger.*

Aspergillosis can take on three forms of pathophysiological activity, resulting in three rather different disease states. These are (a) the mycetoma form, (b) the invasive fulminant form, and (c) the allergic form.

Mycetoma

The mycetoma form is the least troublesome and simplest to handle. The patient is often a victim of chronic sinusitis and not infrequently has had prior surgery. The onset of the infectious process by this saprophytic organism is often facilitated by the patient's placement on long-term antibiotic therapy. The fungal spores floating on dust particles are inhaled through the nose and adhere to the nasal and paranasal sinus mucosa. Because of the often experienced combination of obstruction to the sinus ostia, poor ciliary clearance, and lack of competition from the usual resident organisms due to chronic antibiotic therapy, the fungi proliferate. *Aspergillus fumigatus* is the most common organism involved because it lacks the ability to actually invade the sinus mucosa. It tends to sit on the mucosal surface and create problems by its local effects. The hyphae stimulate a primary inflammatory reaction by the host as a first nonspecific immune defense. A purulent exudate forms, but the literally unopposed fungi continue to proliferate, producing a tangle of mycelia with entrapped mucus and exudate. This produces the so-called mycetoma pathognomonic of this form of the disease. The fungus ball sits in the sinus, slowly enlarging, and over time can result in expansion and then erosion of the bone of the sinus walls. Obstruction of sinus egress will produce secondary bacterial infection of the isolated sinus.

Radiographs may reveal the signs of underlying predisposing sinus disease such as mucosal thickening or polyp formation. The mycetoma appears on computed tomography (CT) scanning as an opacification of the sinus that is isodense with the surrounding soft tissue. It lacks homogeneity and may appear to have an "onion skin" type of conformation interspersed with areas of radiopacity that have a similar density to bone (Fig. 3). Stammberger (14) and Klopp et al. (15) attributed the density of these bodies to deposits of calcium phosphate and calcium sulfate in necrotic areas of the mycetoma. Zinnreich et al. (16) showed that these concretions not only contained calcium but also significant quantities of iron, magnesium, and manganese.

Treatment consists of total excision of the fungus ball, removal of diseased mucosa, and the assurance of adequate sinus drainage. During the procedure, copious irrigation of the sinus cavity is recommended. A solution of an antifungal agent such as ketoconazole may be instilled within the sinus as added protection against recurrence.

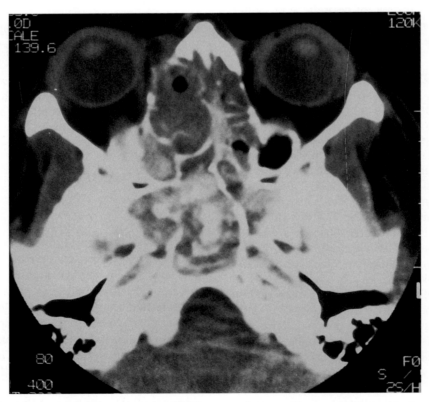

FIG. 3. Computer-assisted tomography (CAT) scan of aspergilloma of sphenoid sinus showing onion skin appearance and numerous hyperdense concretions.

Invasive Aspergillosis

Invasive aspergillosis is a usually rapidly spreading, virulent form of the disease that invades sinus mucosa and adjacent bone and may spread to the soft tissue in the adjacent area. This disease usually attacks the immunologically compromised host such as patients with AIDS or those who are on immunosuppressive therapy after transplantation. Hematologic malignancies and their treatment that impair immunocompetence may also predispose patients to this invasive variety of the disease. This latter scenario is the most common in my experience. A neutropenia and depressed T-cell function are common predisposing factors creating this vulnerability. Invasive aspergillosis of the sinuses is a fulminant and sometimes rapidly fatal disease causing widespread necrosis and marked systemic symptoms (Fig. 4). The invasion of local tissue often mimics malignancy. A necrotizing mucoperiostitis with rapid penetration of the sinus walls occurs. Facial swelling and erythema follow. Proptosis is seen in approximately 60% of cases (Fig. 5). Rapid intracranial invasion may occur along veins and arteries, with the formation of a mycotic aneurysm. Death may follow in a few hours to a few days. Intracranial invasion is a very poor prognostic sign. However, occasionally some patients may undergo a slower more protracted course.

Treatment involves radical surgical debridement of all necrotic tissue. In some instances, the eye may infarct or be irreversibly invaded and require full exenteration (Fig. 6). All involved sinuses require extensive

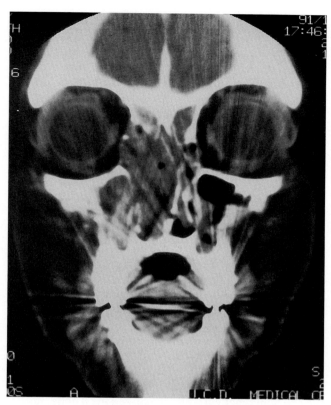

FIG. 5. Coronal CAT scan showing orbital invasion of invasive aspergillosis. Patient presented with proptosis.

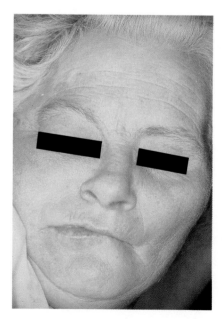

FIG. 4. Elderly, debilitated woman with invasive aspergillosis of the maxillary sinus masking as a sinus malignancy.

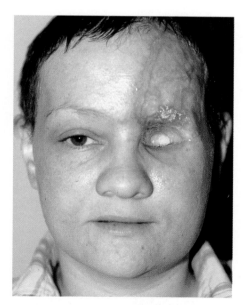

FIG. 6. Young woman with ketoacidosis secondary to diabetes mellitus who required orbital exenteration. Riedel frontal sinus ablation and frontal craniectomy for invasive aspergillosis of the frontal sinus.

resection and wide drainage. There is no place for conservative endoscopic surgery. Wide exposure and complete sinus removal are the rules. Systemic antifungal agents, specifically, appropriate doses of amphotericin B in amounts of up to 2 g total in divided doses, are administered intravenously.

Repeated debridement may be necessary for continuing necrosis. Lavage of the surgical cavities with solutions of amphotericin B may be helpful.

Allergic Aspergillus Sinusitis

Allergic *Aspergillus* sinusitis was first described in 1983 by Katzenstein (17) as a new disease entity in seven patients. Allergic *Aspergillus* bronchopulmonary disease had been characterized earlier and the reaction of the sinus mucosa was discovered to be identical to that in the bronchi. Although the pathophysiology is speculative, it appears likely to be analogous to the bronchopulmonary variety of the disease. It is thought the reaction is a combination of a type I Gell and Coombs (IgE mediated) and type III (immune complex type) reaction (18). Following the adherence of dust-borne spores to nasal mucus, fungal antigens on the cell wall react with IgE sensitized mast cells, initiating the immunologic cascade. This produces a copious outpouring of characteristic allergic mucin, often with eosinophils. The mucus is thick, is filled with hyphae (Fig. 7), and often displays Charcot–Leyden crystals (Fig. 8), which are thought to be the product of eosinophil granule degradation (10). The resultant contents of the affected sinuses are a characteristic thick, tenacious, gelatinous, greasy green material often with brownish-green concretions. The underlying mucosa is thick and often polypoid. Multiple sinuses may be involved.

Patients present with nasal obstruction and anterior green rhinorrhea often with brownish-green concretions. There is often thickened mucosa and not uncommonly nasal polyps. There may be a past history or family history of allergy. A search must be made for the possibility of the concomitant presence of the allergic bronchopulmonary form of the disease. The duration of the disease has been quoted to be from 3 months to 21 years (19).

The radiographs show sinus opacification with occasionally erosion or in some cases bowing of the sinus walls (Fig. 9). The concretions of calcium, manganese, and magnesium salts show up as irregular radiodense bodies (Fig. 10). A layered appearance to the opacification of the sinus may be seen. The intraorbital and in-

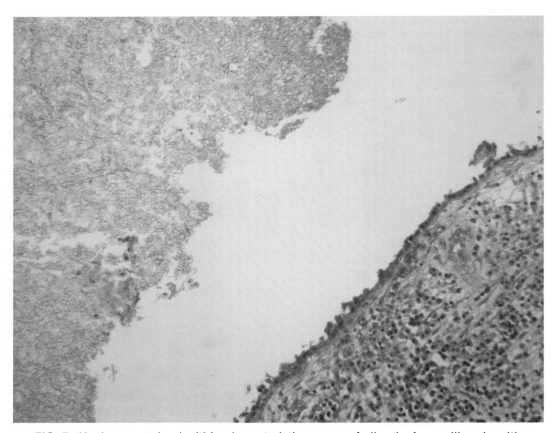

FIG. 7. Hyphae contained within characteristic mucus of allergic *Aspergillus* sinusitis.

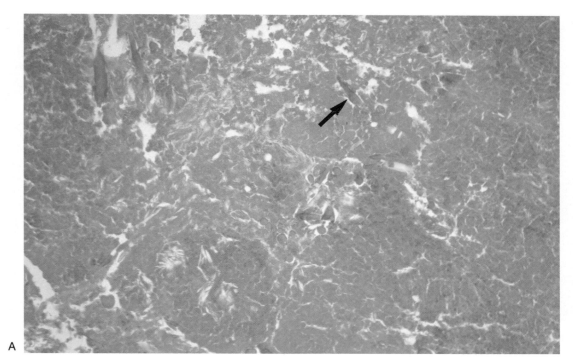

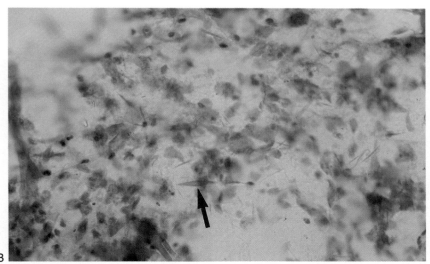

FIG. 8. A: Charcot–Leyden crystals in allergic fungal sinusitis (H&E, ×100) (see *arrows*). **B:** Charcot–Leyden crystals in mucus smear (Papanicolaou, ×100).

tracranial invasion not too uncommonly seen suggests malignancy (20) (Fig. 11).

Diagnosis is usually made on staining the mucosa to look for the characteristic organism and the possible appearance of Charcot–Leyden crystals. Since the fungi do not invade the mucosa in allergic fungal sinusitis, biopsies of the sinus lining do not demonstrate the organism within the tissues. The most effective stains are the Gemori and Grocott's methenamine silver (GMS) stain, PAS, and Gridley. The GMS is most commonly used. They demonstrate the septated hyphae of *Aspergillus* with 45 degree angled branching. Occasionally, the conidiophores are identified (Fig. 12). Eosinophils are commonly seen within nasal secretions and a mild eosinophilia is manifest in the peripheral blood. Patients are usually skin test positive to *Aspergillus*.

Manning et al. (9) have shown in a series of 22 cases of allergic fungal sinusitis that a number of other fungi are also involved in the pathogenesis of this form of the disease (Fig. 13). Indeed, only one patient cultured out *Aspergillus* and the commonest organism was *Bi-*

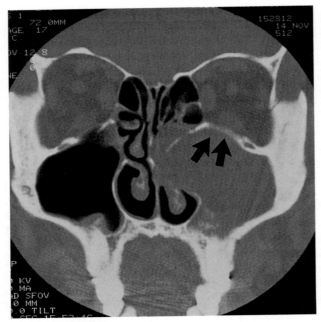

FIG. 9. Axial CAT scan of sinuses showing bowing of the maxillary sinus wall by allergic aspergillosis.

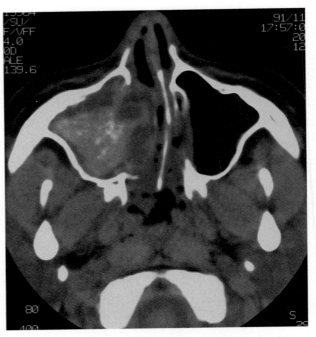

FIG. 10. CAT scan of sinuses in the axial plane demonstrating irregular radiodense bodies characteristic of the concretions of allergic *Aspergillus* sinusitis.

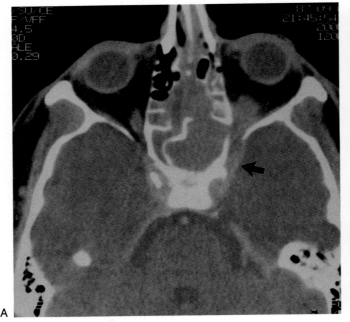

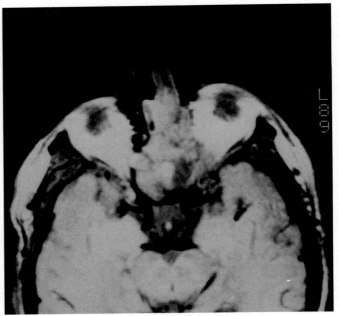

FIG. 11. Intraorbital and intracranial opacification emanating from the maxillary and ethmoid sinuses suggesting malignancy, but actually representing *Aspergillus* sinusitis. **A:** CAT scan (*arrow* points to middle fossa extension). **B:** MRI.

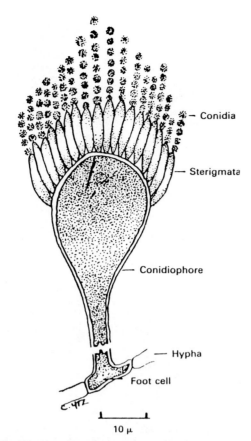

FIG. 12. Diagram of vegetative form of *A. fumigatus* illustrating conidiophore and conidia. (From ref. 21, with permission.)

Labels on figure: Conidia, Sterigmata, Conidiophore, Hypha, Foot cell, 10 μ

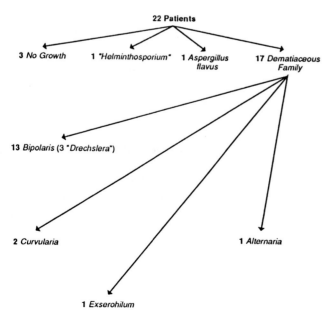

FIG. 13. Culture results of 22 patients with allergic fungal sinusitis illustrating the variety of etiological agents. (From ref. 9, with permission.)

Labels on figure: 22 Patients; 3 *No Growth*; 1 *"Helminthosporium"*; 1 *Aspergillus flavus*; 17 *Dematiaceous Family*; 13 *Bipolaris* (3 *"Drechslera"*); 2 *Curvularia*; 1 *Alternaria*; 1 *Exserohilum*

polaris (13/22). On staining *Biopolaris*, *Curvularia* sp. and *Drechslera* sp. have the same septate hyphae with the same angled branching pattern.

Treatment consists of surgical debridement of the affected sinuses, removal of all polypoid mucosa, and relief of septal obstruction and other impediments to sinus drainage. Corticosteroids are somewhat controversial but many authorities believe that effective control of the disease cannot be adequately achieved without them. Although topical steroids in the form of nasal inhalations have been attempted, they are generally ineffective (22). Safirstein et al. (22) demonstrated an 80% incidence of clinical improvement on prednisone. This reduces the inflammatory response and slows the outpouring of mucus. The recommended regimen is an initial 2-week dose of prednisone 0.5 mg/kg/day followed by alternate day therapy for 3 to 6 months, then a slow tapering dose. If a recrudescence of symptoms appears, then the steroids are reintroduced. In Waxman's series (18), the outcome of the patients fell into three distinct groups: (a) a group that responded immediately to one single surgical treatment; (b) another that was resistant to treatment and required repeated procedures; and (c) a final group who had delayed recurrence of disease often years after initial treatment. Long-term antifungal medication in this disorder has been found to be of no benefit.

It is important to reemphasize that other fungal agents such as *Curvularia, Alternaria,* and *Drechslera* can also cause allergic fungal sinusitis not too dissimilar to that caused by *Aspergillus.*

Mucormycosis

Probably the most devastating of the mycological diseases of the head and neck is rhinocerebral mucormycosis. The disease was first described in diabetic patients in ketoacidosis. The etiological organisms belong to the class Phycomycetes (also called Zygomycetes, hence the more correct term for the disease is zygomycosis) and the order Mucorales. The family Mucoraceae includes the most commonly found genera in mucormycosis, including mainly *Mucor, Rhizopus,* and *Absidia.* The other family Entomophthoraceae that also occupies this order is pathogenic to humans and found in tropical climates. It produces chronic, indolent subcutaneous masses and in contrast to mucormycosis usually attacks healthy hosts. It has not been implicated in rhinocerebral disease. Although the genera *Rhizopus* is most commonly the etiological agent, the genera *Cunninghamella* in the family Cunninghamellaceae have also been reported (21).

Mucormycosis can cause disease processes in many other body systems. Pulmonary and disseminated forms are seen in patients with diabetes and hematological malignancies. Immunocompromised patients are commonly victims of the disseminated form of the disease. Burn patients may also fall victim to this type. Pulmonary lesions often occur as a consequence of superinfection in an area of preexisting bacterial pulmonary infection. This results in areas of infarction, lung abscess, cavitation, and pleural effusion. Virtually any organ system can be involved. The fungus can even affect needle tracks and has been reported along the path of polyethylene implants injected for breast enlargement (21).

The pathophysiology of the disease is brought about by the invasion of blood vessel walls, the plugging of small vessels by fungal mycelia, and the manifestations of the infarction that subsequently ensue. This invasive character is enhanced by ketoacidosis in diabetics. In an experiment in rabbits, the animals were found to be far more susceptible in the ketoacidotic state than when in hyperglycemia with acidosis (23). However, *Rhizopus*, which has an active ketone reductase system, thrives in an environment that is both acidic and hyperglycemic (23). The effects of diabetic ketoacidosis in diminishing the chemotactic response of leukocytes in the human ketoacidotic patient may in part explain this phenomenon (21). In addition, the hyphae are too large for engulfment by host phagocytes, which tend to align along these processes, killing the organism through humoral mechanisms principally via the myeloperoxidase pathway. *Rhizopus* tends to thrive in a hypoxic environment promoted by the poor perfusion secondary to the small vessel disease in the diabetic patient.

The fulminant form of the disease with a frequently fatal outcome is the variety familiar to most practitioners. A mild, more indolent form is now becoming more apparent that does not have the devastating course of the commonest type.

Mucormycosis patients are mostly diabetic and in a state of ketoacidosis, but they may be immunocompromised by the aforementioned disease processes. The clinical picture usually begins with headache, low-grade fever, lethargy and malaise, nasal obstruction, and nasal drainage that is often bloody. In the rapidly progressive variety, the course quickly progresses in a downhill fashion. Diplopia, visual loss, and palatal, nasal, and facial necrosis rapidly ensue. Initial presentation of the patient in the comatose state is a common manner in which the patient is first seen. The rapid progression of the disease is exemplified by the patient in Fig. 14. His facial necrosis progressed quickly from some discoloration of his palate on his arrival in the emergency suite to total palatal infarction, bilateral blindness, and necrosis of the nose and adjacent facial skin by the time his surgery began.

The classical finding on physical examination is the black necrosis of septum or turbinates seen on intra-

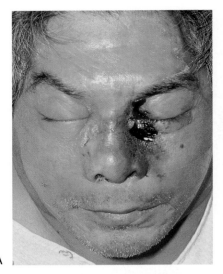

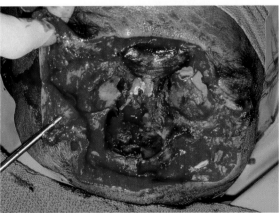

FIG. 14. Patient with rapidly advancing mucormycosis. **A:** Within 2 hr, he infarcted his facial skin, eyes, palate, and nose. **B:** Extensive facial resection including bilateral orbital exenteration was done as a life-saving procedure.

nasal examination. Mycelial thrombi and the vasculitis induced by the fungus results in the infarction characteristic of zygomycosis. Purulence and bleeding may also be seen.

Ocular findings run the gamut from eye pain and ophthalmoplegia to blindness and ocular infarction. A relatively early sign is external and internal ophthalmoplegia brought about by inflammatory change and invasion of the contents of the superior orbital fissure. In addition to diplopia, blurred vision ensues because of retinal edema. When the ophthalmic vein is affected, increased venous pressure produces chemosis and proptosis. As the disease process progresses, the oculomotor function is ablated and a fixed frozen eye results. The retina becomes devascularized from either venous or arterial thrombosis or both and retinoscopy reveals a grey, infarcted retina, absence of venous pulsations and layering of blood in the arterioles with resultant complete blindness.

Infarction of both eyes may eventuate either from progression of disease from the opposing ethmoid sinuses or via cavernous sinus thrombosis. Since the ophthalmic veins of each side drain into their respective cavernous sinus and the sinuses are connected across the midline via the circular sinus around the pituitary stalk and the basilar plexus overlying the intracranial aspect of the clivus, the organisms can affect both sinuses and thereby infarct both eyes. Once one cavernous sinus is infected, the disease process spreads rapidly to the opposite side. When both eyes are affected, cavernous sinus thrombosis is highly suspect.

Although unilateral involvement can occur and remain as such, it is distinctly uncommon. Despite the fact that mucormycosis always begins in the sinuses, the disease spreads intracranially very quickly, hence the common assignation rhinocerebral mucormycosis. Unfortunately, once the disease extends intracranially the prognosis drops considerably. In a literature review by Anand et al. (24) of 230 cases of mucormycosis, 55% were found to have intracranial extension of disease. The mortality rate at this stage, once 100%, has recently improved to 67%.

A variation to the usual fulminant, prostrating form of the disease that is becoming more apparent recently is a more benign indolent variety (Figs. 15 and 16). These patients are not in coma although they may be hyperglycemic and in poor diabetic control. This less aggressive type is more commonly seen in patients with AIDS or leukemia, and those who are otherwise immu-nocompromised. They are usually afebrile or present with a low-grade temperature and the mucosa is variably very pale or initially erythematous. Purplish or black turbinates or septum may also be seen, but much less commonly so. The disease is more slowly aggressive. Purulence and bleeding are usual and a high index of suspicion is essential in susceptible individuals in order to make the diagnosis. Biopsy proven nonseptate hyphae with vascular invasion leaves little doubt as to the etiology (Fig. 17). The patient in Fig. 15 presented as a diabetic with low-grade fever, proptosis, and mild facial pain. Examination revealed pale nasal mucosa with swelling, but no infarction. Despite vigorous therapy, he infarcted both eyes, requiring bilateral exenteration. He responded to amphoteracin B and hyperbaric oxygen and made a full recovery. Although he presented in a subacute fashion, the disease proved to be quite aggressive, requiring extensive surgical and intensive medical therapy to effect a cure.

The main elements of treatment for mucormycosis are control of the diabetes and coma, surgical debridement, general physiological support, amphotericin B, and, in some cases, hyperbaric oxygen.

The often florid hyperglycemia is treated with insulin. Management of dehydration, metabolic acidosis, and electrolyte imbalance is critical. The patient is best managed in an intensive care unit with a medical intensivist closely monitoring these parameters. Since many of these patients have other organ failures secondary to their primary disease process, these must be thoroughly treated as well.

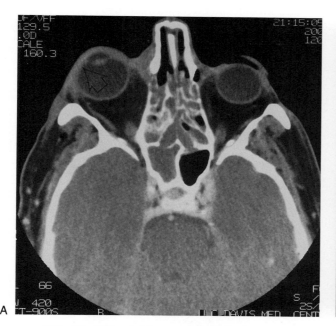

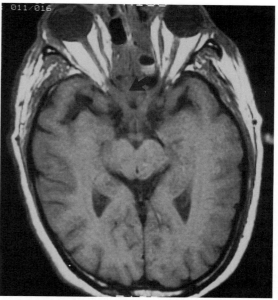

FIG. 15. Fifty-eight-year-old diabetic man with indolent form of mucormycosis. **A:** CAT scan shows diffuse patchy ethmoidal opacification bilaterally, proptosis of right eye, and preseptal cellulitis *(arrow)*. **B:** MRI shows opacification of ethmoids and soft tissue swelling around optic nerve of right eye (see *black arrow*).

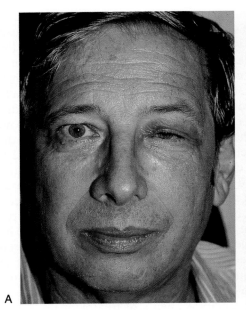
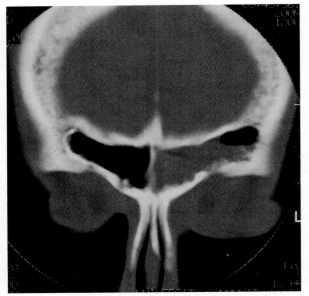

A

B

FIG. 16. Indolent form of mucormycosis. **A:** Ambulatory patient with a swollen red eye and ophthalmoplegia. **B:** Frontal sinus opacification that turned out to be mucormycosis.

The essential surgical element in treating these patients is adequate debridement of all infarcted, necrotic tissue. This often requires a very aggressive approach, otherwise the patient will surely die of the disease. All nonviable tissue is excised because the lack of blood supply to these tissues has eliminated the ability of antifungal chemotherapy to reach the disease process. All dead material must be removed back to healthy surrounding bone and soft tissue. This often entails orbital exenteration, sinus excision, and even partial rhinectomy and facial skin excision (Fig. 14B). The criterion of adequate excision is to resect until bleeding bone and soft tissue are achieved. Anything less will leave viable fungi within the nonliving tissues of the host that will thus render the patient refractory to further medical therapy. Complete external ethmoidectomy with sphenoidotomy, wide frontal sinusotomy, and medial maxillectomy are usually the rules. If the

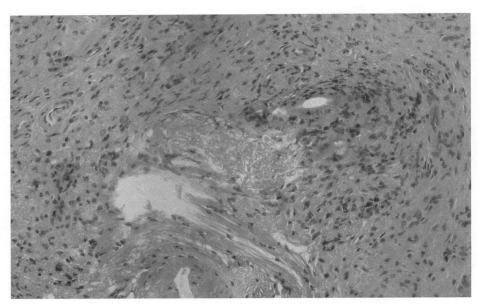

FIG. 17. Tissue samples from patient with mucormycosis demonstrating invasion of maxillary sinus by organisms with nonseptated hyphae pathognomonic of the disease (H&E, ×100).

palate is involved, it is removed. The nasal septum is commonly involved, and it is completely excised unless a dorsal and caudal strut of uninvolved cartilage for structural support can safely be preserved. Wide opening of the sinuses permits easy drainage and facilitates irrigation of the cavities to keep them free of debris. Packing of the sinus cavity is avoided if possible. Packing is employed when necessary to control bleeding, but it is removed as soon postoperatively as possible, usually in about 48 hr.

In the past, craniotomy for cerebral extension has been controversial. Since 1980 (24) craniotomy for this advanced form of the disease has changed the mortality rate from 20% to 75%. Cranial bone, dural, and direct cerebral invasions require resection. Frontal abscesses require drainage. Reconstruction of dura and calvarium should employ vascularized flaps as much as possible. Free grafts, especially alloplastic materials and cadaveric material such as lyodura, must be avoided. The use of newly developed skull base resection techniques (see the chapter, Skull Base Surgery for Sinus Neoplasms, by Donald) should be used in those patients with cavernous sinus and internal carotid artery involvement.

Since 1955, when it first became available (25), the mainstay of medical therapy has been the administration of the antifungal agent amphotericin B. The total dosage is somewhat variable depending to a large degree on the response of the patient. The total dose on average is usually around 2 g. A considerable amount of mystique and myth has evolved concerning dosing of this toxic antimicrobial. Since it has a half-life of 24 hr, once the desired blood level of 2.0 to 2.5 μg/ml has been reached by administering daily doses, the dosing schedule can be done on alternate days. An initial single dose of 0.25 mg/kg body weight is given intravenously over a 45- to 60-min period on the first day of treatment. On the second day, the dose is increased to 0.5 mg/kg and the third day 0.75 mg/kg. Alternate day dosing at 0.75 mg/kg is done from then on and the dosage is adjusted by periodic blood level checks 2 hr posttreatment. For a detailed protocol of amphotericin B administration, see Table 2.

The drug should be given intravenously via catheter because of its highly irritating character to vessel walls and thrombophlebitic potential. Certain precautions are advisable. Using a large vein and an indwelling catheter will help to prevent this complication. A central venous line is best because of the rapid dilution consequent to the high blood flow at this site. Damage to the peripheral vessels can be diminished by diluting the drug to less than 10 mg/cc and adjusting the pH to 6.0 to 6.5. The addition of heparin 50 μ/ml will also help to obviate the problem. Steroids should not be used as glucocorticoids alter the structure of amphotericin B, thus eliminating its effectiveness.

Unfortunately, this drug has a number of side effects, most temporary, but some permanent. Almost all patients develop nausea and vomiting after administration but some tolerance does occur. Pretreatment with an antiemetic is helpful, as is slow administration over an hour, adequate dilution, and instillation in a large vessel. Such prophylaxis can also diminish the other usual temporary side effects of headache, fever, and chills. Prolonged administration over many hours does little to diminish these distressful symptoms.

Anemia develops in 75% of patients occasionally with a thrombocytopenia. Direct suppression of erythropoiesis and, in some, attendant renal failure are responsible for this. Once the therapy has stopped, the anemia usually self-corrects. The two other organ systems adversely affected by amphotericin B are the renal and neurological systems. Renal toxicity is usually proportional to duration of treatment. If the total dose does not exceed 2 g, approximately 30 mg/kg body weight, then less than 15% of patients will have renal damage. This, although not debilitating, is permanent. However, when total doses exceed 5 g or about 75 mg/kg body weight, 80% of patients will have permanent, severe renal impairment. There is serious injury to both the glomerulus as well as the tubules. Some protection can be afforded by ensuring that the patient has a normal serum sodium from the outset of treatment and to alkalinize the urine. Osmotic diuretics like mannitol give no protection.

A manifold constellation of neuropathic conditions may occur that include hyperthermia, hypotension, confusion, delirium, incoherence, depression, psychotic behavior, tremors or convulsions, blurred vision, hearing loss, quadraparesis, and brachial plexus dysfunction. Intrathecal injections may lead to radiculitis and arachnoiditis as well as central effects.

The medication is highly toxic but very effective and is the only entirely reliable drug available at the present time. Its use at a lower, less toxic level combined with rifampin or 5-fluorocytosine as yet needs to be tested. The favorable reports of these latter two agents in managing *Aspergillus* sp. and *Rhizopus* sp. lend some optimism (26–28).

Because the fungi of the Zygomycetes thrive in an oxygen-poor environment, the addition of hyperbaric oxygen to the regimen has a theoretical advantage. Hyperbaric oxygen is emerging as an increasingly more important arm of the therapy. Proponents of this modality enthusiastically support its use based on limited, but highly favorable, experimental work and clinical experience (29–32). As reported by Anand et al. (24) of the 13 patients thus far treated with adjunctive hyperbaric oxygen, 8 of whom had intracranial disease, 70% survived. Our own favorable but limited experience lends further support to the efficacy of this modality.

TABLE 2. *A protocol for the intravenous administration of amphotericin B*

Pharmacy preparation
1. The desired dose is added to sufficient 5% glucose solution for iv injection to provide a final concentration of ≤10 mg/dl (peripheral vein, may be 15 to 20 mg/dl for infusion in a central vein).
2. Sufficient heparin solution is added to yield a final concentration of 50 U/dl.

Premedication—given 30 min before giving amphotericin B
1. Aspirin (or acetaminophen), 15 to 20 mg/kg body wt, po (repeat dose every 3 hr for two additional doses).
2. One of the following (repeat dose once, 4 hr after initial dose):
   a. Prochlorpromazine, 0.2 to 0.3 mg/kg body wt, po or iv.
   b. Metaclopramide, 2.0 mg/kg body wt, po or iv.
   c. Meperidine, 0.5 to 1.0 mg/kg body wt, po or im.

Injection
1. The patient should be supine in bed.
2. The temperature, pulse, and blood pressure must be recorded before starting treatment.
3. The infusion assembly should incude a Y tube or similar arrangement (to provide access to both 5% glucose solution without additives and the dose of amphotericin B) and an infusion pump.
4. First day—0.25 mg/kg body wt:
   a. Inject 5 to 10 mg over a period of 5 min, then switch to the 5% glucose solution without additives.
   b. Measure blood pressure at 5 min, 15 min, and 30 min.
      (1) If there has been no fall in blood pressure, give the remainder of the dose of amphotericin B within 20 min.
      (2) If there has been a fall in blood pressure
         (a) Without symptoms:
             Elevate the foot of the bed, inject 0.9% NaCl solution (10 ml/kg body wt) over 30 min, and give the remainder of the dose of amphotericin B within 45 min.
         (b) With symptoms:
             Elevate the foot of the bed, inject 0.9% NaCl solution (10 ml/kg body wt) over 30 min, and give ephedrine, 0.3 to 0.6 mg/kg by im injection.
             If there is prompt restoration of the bood pressure and subsidence of symptoms, repeat the 5 to 10 mg dose.
             i. If hypotension does not recur, give the remainder of the dose over 45 min.
             ii. If hypotension recurs, put off therapy for 2 to 3 days before trying again.
5. Second day—0.50 mg/kg body wt:
   a. If there was no hypotension with the first dose, inject the second dose over a period of 30 to 45 min (measure the blood pressure at 5 min, 15 min, 45 min).
   b. If there was transient hypotension with the first dose, again assess the effect of injection of 5 to 10 mg, as with the first dose, before giving all of the second dose.
6. Third day—0.75 mg/kg body wt:
   If there was no hypotension with the second dose, inject the third dose over a period of 45 to 60 min (measure the blood pressure at 5 min, 15 min, 45 min).
7. Fourth day—no amphotericin B.
8. Fifth day—0.75 mg/kg body wt.
9. Sixth day—no amphotericin B.
10. Seventh day—0.75 mg/kg body wt
   a. Pretherapy, obtain blood (low or trough specimen) for assay of the concentration of amphotericin B.
   b. Inject dose, noting exact duration of administration.
   c. Two hours after therapy obtain blood (high or peak specimen) for assay of the concentration of amphotericin B.
11. Continue alternate-day of regimen treatment, adjusting the dose to yield a 2 hr postdose concentration of 2.0 to 3.0 μg/ml serum (trough of 0.5 to 1.0 μg/ml).
12. When the appropriate dose is determined, continue therapy on alternate days for inpatients and thrice weekly (Monday, Wednesday, Friday) for outpatients.

Surveillance (in addition to clinical evaluations)
1. Before therapy:
   a. Obtain pictures of lesions; radiographic, radionuclide, and ultrasound examinations; cultures; and serologic studies within 1 week before treatment.
   b. Determine creatinine clearance, urea nitrogen, creatinine, K^+, and Mg^{2+} within 48 hr before treatment.
   c. Carry out urinalysis and complete blood count on the day treatment is started.
2. During therapy:
   a. Weekly—perform studies of 1-b and 1-c above. If treatment goes smoothly, shift to biweekly to monthly observations after 4 weeks of therapy.
   b. Monthly—perform studies of 1-a above, plus assays of peak/trough concentrations of amphotericin B in blood.
3. After therapy:
   The studies of 1-a, 1-b, and 1-c above should be repeated monthly for 3 months, then quarterly for 6 months, and finally semiannually for a period of years appropriate for the mycosis.

REFERENCES

1. Plaignaud M. Observation sur un fongus du sinus maxillaire. *J Chir* 1791;1:111–116.
2. Schubert J. Zum Kasiustick des Aspergillus-mykosen. *Deutsch Arch Klin Med* 1885;36:162.
3. Zarniko C. Aspergilusmykose der Kieferhole. *Deutsch Med Wochenschr* 1891;17:1222.
4. MacKenzie JJ. Preliminary report on *Aspergillus* mycosis of the antrum maxillare. *Johns Hopkins Med J* 1893;4:9.
5. Sevetsky L, Waltner J. Aspergillosis of the maxillary antrum. *Arch Otolaryngol* 1961;74:695.
6. Titche LL. Aspergillosis of the maxillary sinus. *Ear, Nose Throat J* 1978;57:398.
7. Baude AI. Diseases caused by fungi. In: Thorn GW, Adams RW, Braunwold E, Isselbacher KJ, Petersdorf RG, ed. *Harrison's principles of internal medicine,* 8th ed. New York: McGraw-Hill 1977;937–953.
8. Shugar MA. Mycotic infections of the nose and paranasal sinuses. In: Goldman JL, ed. *The principles and practice of rhinology.* New York: Wiley, 1987;717–734.
9. Manning SC, Schaefer SD, Close LG, Viutch F. Culture positive allergic fungal sinusitis. *Arch Otolaryngol* 1991;117:174–178.
10. Corey JP, Romberger CF, Shaw GY. Fungal diseases of the sinuses. *Otolaryngol Head Neck Surg* 1990;103:1012–1015.
11. Beck-Mannageta J, Necek D, Grazzerbauer M. Zahn argliche Aspekte der solitaren Kieferholen—Aspergillose. *Z Stomatol* 1986;83:283–315.
12. Beck-Mannageta J, Necek D. Radiological findings in aspergillosis of the maxillary sinus. *Oral Surg Oral Med Oral Pathol* 1986; 62:345–349.
13. Kagan S. *Aspergillus:* an inhalable contaminant of marijuana. *N Engl J Med* 1981;304:483–484.
14. Stammberger H. Endoscopic surgery for mycotic and chronic recurring sinusitis II. *Ann Otorhinolaryngol* (Suppl 119) 1985; 94:3–10.
15. Klopp W, Fotter R, Steiner H, Beaufort I, Stammberger H. Aspergillosis of the paranasal sinuses. *Radiology* 1985;156: 715–716.
16. Zinnrich JS, Kennedy DW, Malat J, et al. Fungal sinusitis: diagnosis with CT and MR imaging. *Radiology* 1988;169:439–444.
17. Katzenstein AA, Sale SR, Greenberger PA. Pathologic findings in allergic *Aspergillus* sinusitis. *Am J Surg Pathol* 1983;7: 439–443.
18. Waxman JE, Sale SR, Spector JG, Katzenstein ALA. Allergic *Aspergillus* sinusitis: concepts in diagnosis and treatment of a new clinical entity. *Laryngoscope* 1987;97:261–266.
19. Allphin AL. Allergic fungal sinusitis: problems in diagnosis and treatment. *Laryngoscope* 1991;101:815–820.
20. Sarti EJ, Blaugrund SM, Camins MB, Lin PT. Paranasal sinus disease with intracranial extension: aspergillosis versus malignancy. *Laryngoscope* 1988;98:632–635.
21. Edwards JE. Lyomycosis. In: Hoeprich PD, Jordan MC, eds. *Infectious diseases,* 5th ed. Philadelphia: Lippincott 1989; 1192–1199.
22. Safirstein B, D'Souza M, Simon G, et al. Five year follow-up of allergic bronchopulmonary aspergillosis. *Am Rev Respir Dis* 1973;108:450–459.
23. Blitzer A, Lawson W. Mycotic infections of the nose and paranasal sinuses. In: English GM, ed. *Otolaryngology.* Philadelphia: Lippincott, 1991;1–18.
24. Anand VK, Gilbert A, Alemar G, Griswold JA. Intracranial mucormycosis: an experimental model and clinical review. *Laryngoscope* 1992;102:656–662.
25. Hoeprich PD, Rinaldi MG. Candidosis. In: Hoeprich PD, Jordan MC, eds. 5th ed. *Infections Diseases,* Philadelphia: Lippincott, 1989;474–478.
26. Arroyo J, Medoff G, Kobayashi GS. Therapy of murine aspergillosis with amphotericin B in combination with Rifampin or 5-fluorocystosine. *Antimicrob Agents Chemo* 1977;11:21–25.
27. Christenson JC, Shalit I, Welch DF, et al. Synergistic action of amphotericin B and Rifampin against rhizopus specius. *Antimicrob Agents Chemo* 1987;31:1775–1778.
28. Hughes CE, Harris C, Moody JA, et al. In vitro activities of amphotericin B in combination with four antifungal agents and Rifampin against aspergillus sp. *Antimicrob Agents Chemo* 1984; 25:560–562.
29. Couch L, Theilen F, Mader JT. Rhinocerebral mucormycosis with cerebral extension successfully treated with adjunctive hyperbaric oxygen therapy. *Arch Otol Head Neck Surg* 1988;114: 791–794.
30. Ferguson BJ, Mitchell TG, Moon R, et al. Adjunctive hyperbaric oxygen for the treatment of rhinocerebral mucormycosis. *Rev Infect Dis* 1988;10:551–559.
31. Price JC, Stevens DL. Hyperbaric oxygen in the treatment of rhinocerebral mucormycosis. *Laryngoscope* 1980;90:737–747.
32. Cairney WJ. The effect of hyperbaric oxygen on certain growth features of four dermatophytes. *Frank J Seiby Res Lab Tech Rep* 1980;80–88.

PART III

Trauma

CHAPTER 22

Maxillary Fractures

Paul J. Donald

Fractures of the midfacial area commonly transgress both the maxillary and ethmoid sinuses. As elucidated by Le Fort (1,2), these injuries are commonly bilateral. In 1901, French physician Rene Le Fort did about 40 experiments in which he struck the faces of human cadavers with a wooden club or threw the face against the edge of an autopsy table. He applied the blows from different directions, supported the head with a resisting board, or struck the head unsupported. He found that the fractures generally aligned themselves in a somewhat predictable pattern. However, he did state that often variations occurred that were dependent on the direction of the blow and the method of its delivery.

The three basic patterns of fracture he described have continued to carry his name to the present time. The Le Fort I fracture (Fig. 1) is a low fracture traversing the maxilla and nasal septum just above the alveolar ridge and usually missing the pterygoid plates. This was first described by Guerin in 1866 (3). The Le Fort II or pyramidal fracture (Fig. 2) goes across the nose and descends steeply across the maxillae, crosses the lower maxillary walls, and goes through the pterygoid plates. The most severe maxillary fracture, the Le Fort III, separates the maxillae and nose from the cranial base, the so-called craniofacial dysfunction (Fig. 3). This fracture goes through the nasal bones and septum through the medial and lateral walls and floors of both orbits, then through the arches of the zygomata. The fracture goes through the infratemporal fossae and the pterygoid plates. Associated injuries to the eyes, lacrimal apparatus, and medial canthal tendons are not uncommon. Fractures that separate one or both zygomata from the facial skeleton are also often seen.

Although these fractures are most often bilateral, they are uncommonly symmetrical. It is then not uncommon to have a Le Fort I on one side and a Le Fort III on the other. Furthermore, in an asymmetric fracture, the zygoma may be fractured away from the maxillary skeleton. Finally, on rare occasions, a hemimaxillary fracture may occur (Fig. 4). In this instance, the maxilla, usually complete with the zygoma, is fractured away from the rest of the face.

PATHOPHYSIOLOGY

To understand the pathophysiology of the signs and symptoms of maxillary fractures, it is necessary to appreciate some of the biophysical characteristics of the midfacial skeleton. The maxilla is interposed between two strong craniofacial bony structures—the cranial base and the mandible. Although the maxilla is comprised of relatively thin bone, with the notable exception of the alveolar ridge, the arch configuration and its series of interlocking trusses provide strength.

The midfacial skeleton has evolved into a magnificently architecturally designed stress-resisting structure by virtue of a series of trusses and braces (4). In engineering terms, a truss is a structure comprised of beams, rods, or stress bearers arranged in a triangle, or combination of triangles, to form a rigid framework that will support a load over a wide area on any of its sides or points. The inherent structure of a truss renders it highly resistant to forces brought to bear upon it at any angle to its sides or corners. If additional members are added to this basic structure and the geometric configuration is lost with transformation into a square or other figure, then strength is lost and the structure will collapse under similar circumstances of stress. The addition of additional struts to the basic truss to transform the triangular configuration to a pyramid creates a series of three interlocking triangles. The flat triangular configuration of a truss is then transmuted into the three planes of space.

The middle third of the face is comprised of a series of trusses arranged in all three planes. The trusses are

289

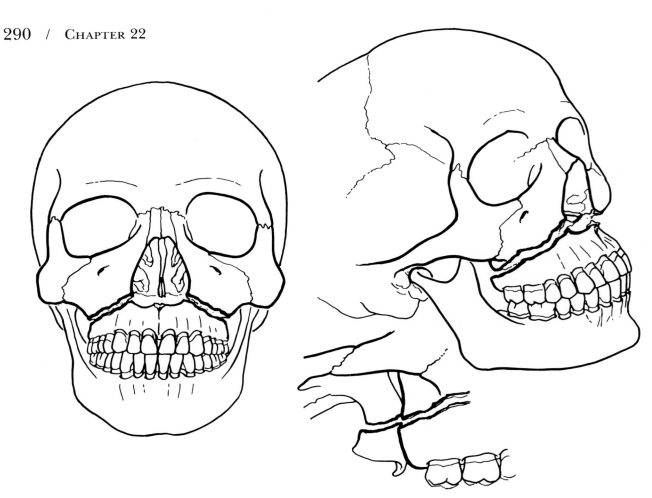

FIG. 1. Le Fort I fracture.

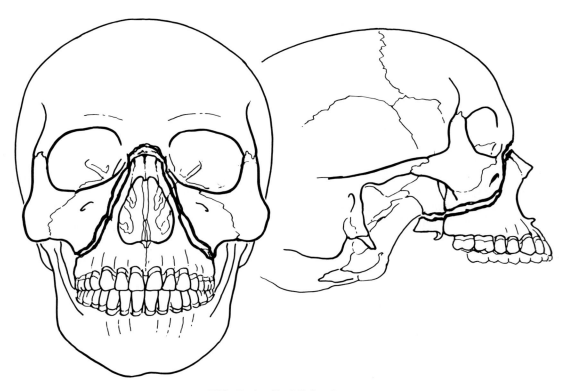

FIG. 2. Le Fort II fracture.

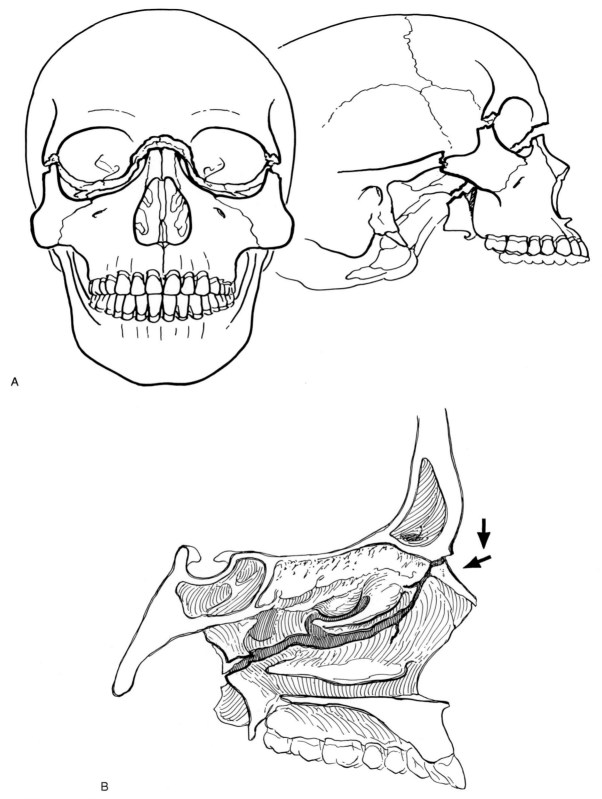

A

B

FIG. 3. Le Fort III fracture. **A:** Posterior–anterior and lateral views. **B:** Sagittal section through lateral nasal wall.

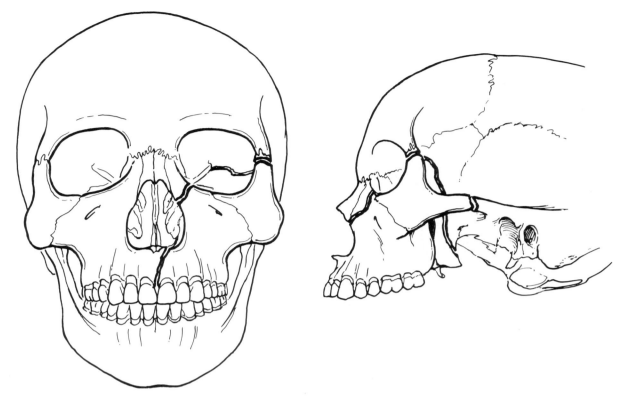

FIG. 4. Hemimaxillary fracture.

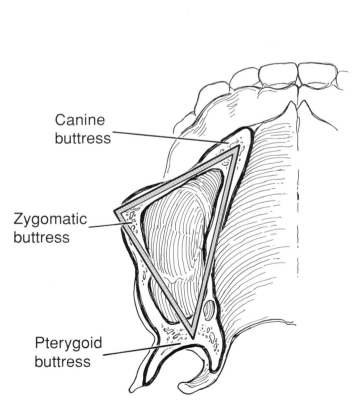

Canine buttress

Zygomatic buttress

Pterygoid buttress

FIG. 5. Series of interlocking trusses comprising the supports of the central face.

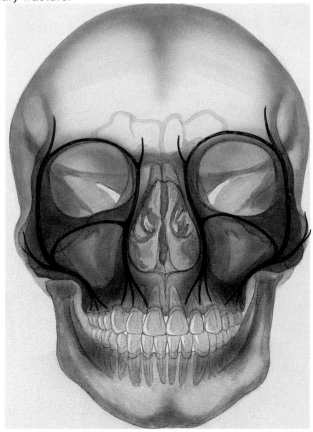

FIG. 6. Biomechanical stress curves of the middle one-third of the face.

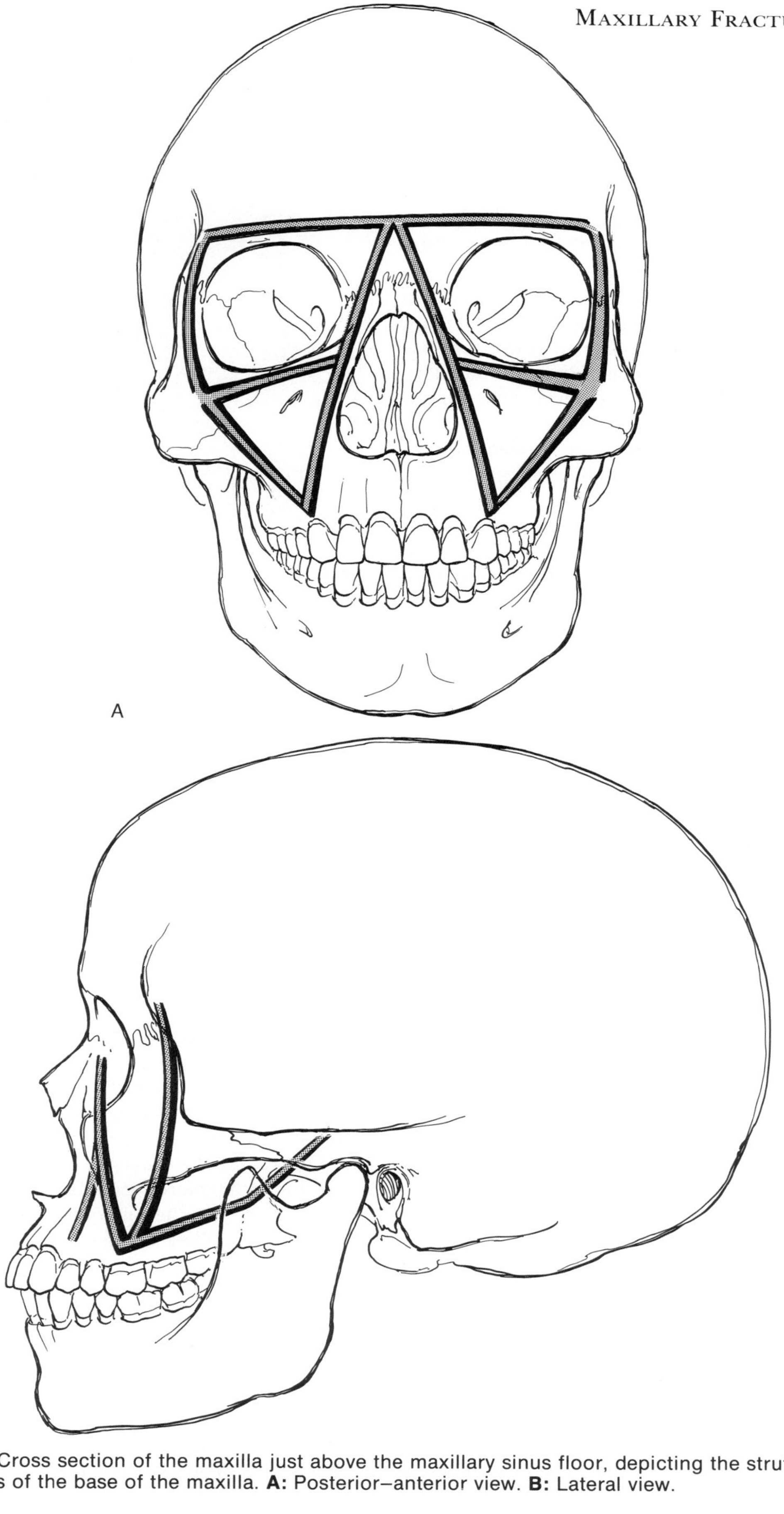

FIG. 7. Cross section of the maxilla just above the maxillary sinus floor, depicting the struts of the truss of the base of the maxilla. **A:** Posterior–anterior view. **B:** Lateral view.

made up of braces of thickened bone that are arranged around thin areas of bone as seen in Fig. 5.

These trusses are responsible for the form of the bio-mechanical stress curves of the central facial skeleton (Fig. 6). These buttresses ascend first from the alveolar ridge anteriorly over the stout bone of the pyriform ridge and then split to extend superiorly along the medial orbital rim and laterally along the inferior orbital rim. The second buttress extends from the lateral alveolar ridge curving under the malar eminence with a smaller component extending along the more lateral aspect of the infraorbital rim. The final buttress extends from the posterior alveolar ridge and maxillary tuberosity area up through the posterior wall superiorly. The pterygoid plates act as a form of flying buttress, attaching posteriorly at the stout maxillary tuberosity and the lateral aspect of the basisphenoid at the base of the skull.

A typical example of the triangular configuration of stress-bearing components of the midface is shown in Fig. 7. The thickened bone seen as the component bars of the truss configuration are the canine buttress, zygomatic buttress, and the maxillary tuberosity–pterygoid buttress.

Two of the principal muscles of mastication attach to the pterygoid plates. These plates are not part of the maxilla per se but, because of their intimate contact with the posterior maxillary wall and their property of

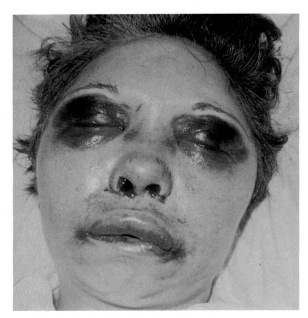

FIG. 9. Patient blind in both eyes after a Le Fort III fracture passing through orbital apices.

being one of the major stress points of the midface skeleton, are commonly disrupted in maxillary fractures. Whereas the medial pterygoid muscle is the major distracting force in vertically unfavorable fractures of the mandible, this muscle serves equally as a major distracting force in midfacial fractures. There is a tendency then for this muscle to rotate the maxillary fragment in an inferoposterior direction (Fig. 8) as it displaces the maxilla toward its insertion on the mandible.

Because the maxilla comprises the major portion of the orbital floor, high fractures often produce severe comminution of the floor. The intraocular and orbital signs produced are similar to those of the fractured zygoma as described by Donald in Fractures of the Zygoma. In addition, because of the severity of the injury, fracture lines extending into the orbital apex and the optic canal may occur, producing diminished vision or blindness (Figs. 9 and 10).

Due to the bilaterality of Le Fort fractures, the connection of the paired maxillae by the intervening nasal bones mandates their involvement in all Le Fort II and III fractures. They may be compound and comminuted (Fig. 11) and the nasal dorsum is often displaced. Dorsal flattening is not uncommon due to the frontal direction of the injuring force (Fig. 11). The septum is always fractured and deviation is not uncommon.

Occasionally, the palate will be split, creating two disconnected floating facial fragments (Fig. 12). This is much more uncommon in Le Fort I than the other fractures. In the hemimaxillary fracture, in which only the maxilla of one side is broken, a hemipalatal fracture

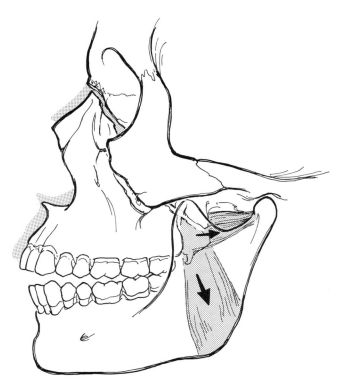

FIG. 8. The vertical pull of the medial pterygoid muscle forces the fractured maxilla toward the mandible, producing premature contact between the distal molar teeth.

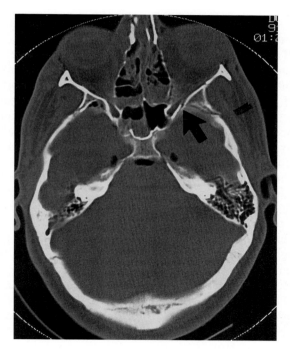

FIG. 10. Computed axial tomography (CAT) scan of patient, demonstrating orbital apex fracture producing blindness.

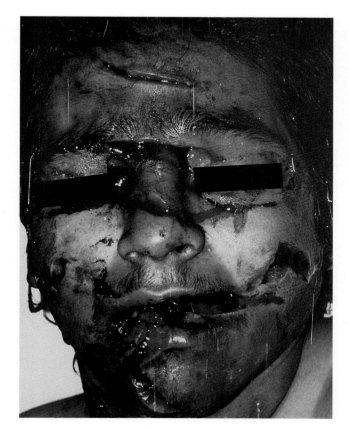

FIG. 11. Compound nasal fracture involved in Le Fort III fracture.

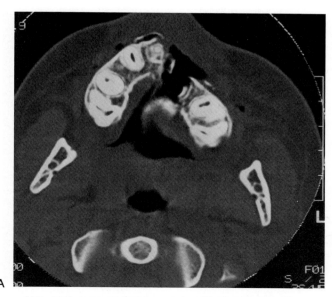

A

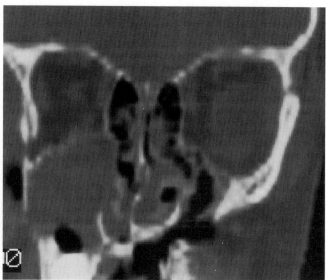

B

FIG. 12. Site of palatal fracture usually seen in an asymmetric fashion through the nasal floor. A: Axial CAT scan showing massive midpalatal fracture angling through the left hemipalate. B: Coronal reconstruction.

occurs. The fracture almost never goes through the midline suture and usually goes through one nasal floor or the other. This was well established by Le Fort's studies (1,2). The vertically fractured palate presents particular problems in maintaining stability.

The fracture lines in the Le Fort II and especially Le Fort III fractures pass through the ethmoid bloc. In doing so, it is not uncommon for the fractures to pass high, fracturing the fovea ethmoidalis and cribriform plate and producing a cerebrospinal fluid (CSF) leak. These leaks occur in at least 25% of all Le Fort II and III fractures (5).

In Le Fort III fractures, the zygomata are a part

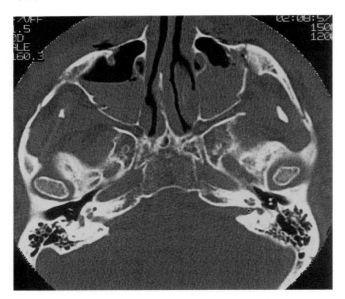

FIG. 13. CAT scan of unusual fracture of both zygomata but not connected across midline. This is therefore not a Le Fort fracture.

of the fracture fragment. The injury will occasionally result in a fracturing of the zygoma separately from the attached maxilla. This may produce all the symptoms associated with a tripod fracture of the zygoma (Fig. 13).

CLINICAL PRESENTATION

These patients are always the victims of major trauma. A force of significant magnitude is required to fracture the midface from the rest of the cranial skeleton. Motor vehicle accidents, gunshot wounds, and industrial mishaps comprise most of the etiological scenarios. They are often patients who have suffered injuries to a number of systems. Concomitant head injury is very common, but abdominal and thoracic trauma and extremity fractures may be present alone or in combination.

Airway distress may be the presenting problem because of the downward and backward displacement of the maxilla due to the pull of the pterygoid muscles. This may be compounded by hematoma, edema, and contusion in the palatal and pharyngeal area as well as the possible problems of broken dentures or teeth in the airway. This is especially true in gunshot wounds to the face, especially those from a shotgun (Fig. 14). The oral cavity must be carefully suctioned and cleared of debris immediately on entering the emergency treatment area. If a fractured mandible has also been sustained by the patient, the prolapse of a comminuted body fracture will further obstruct the airway. Pulling the tongue forward with an oral airway may remedy

the situation especially if the patient is in coma, a not uncommon problem in this group of patients.

If alert, the patient will obviously complain of generalized pain over the midface. Numbness over the infraorbital nerve distribution is often seen in Le Fort II and III patients and those with concomitant zygoma fractures. Severe trismus and pain on approximating the teeth are usual. The patient may feel the palate move on biting down. The patient will complain of malocclusion, which often takes the form of an anterior open bite brought about by the distraction force of the medial pterygoid muscles (Fig. 8). As the posterior inferior rotation is brought about by the pull of this muscle toward the mandibular angle, the molar teeth will be brought into premature contact. This so-called gagging of the distal dentition will result in the open bite seen anteriorly (Figs. 15 and 16). In addition to the effects on dentition, the distracting force of the muscle will cause an elongation of the face. This is often not appreciated early after the accident because of the severe facial swelling that is the usual accompaniment of this injury. However, once this swelling subsides, not only is the facial elongation apparent (Fig. 17) (the "horse-face" appearance), but a flattened or "dish-face" appearance may be obvious as well. This retrusive effect of the medial and lateral pterygoids produces the characteristic visage exemplified in Fig. 18. In the early stages of the injury the "purple pumpkin" appearance of the face so characteristic of the Le Fort fractures obscures the discrepancies in bony configuration rendered by the various fractures (Fig. 9). This distortion obscures visualization of fracture step-offs, which are often difficult to palpate.

The unique and ubiquitously pathognomonic sign of

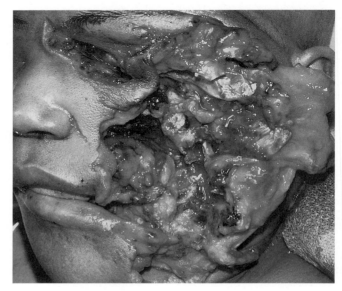

FIG. 14. Massive injury to face caused by self-inflicted gunshot wound resulting in Le Fort fracture of maxilla.

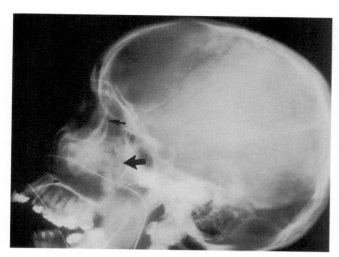

FIG. 15. Lateral radiograph of patient with a Le Fort III fracture of maxilla, demonstrating an open bite produced by gagging of the molar teeth resulting from the downward and backward rotation of the maxilla.

Le Fort fractures is the "floating palate." With the thumb over the anterior alveolar ridge and anterior nasal spine and fingers against the palate, a rocking of the palate can be appreciated (Fig. 19). With the fingers of the opposite hand, palpation along the low maxillary face will detect the characteristic motion of the Le Fort I fracture. Palpation over the nasal dorsum and perhaps the medial orbital rims will reveal the motion indicating a Le Fort II fracture. A Le Fort III fracture will demonstrate motion at the lateral orbital rims or at the inferior

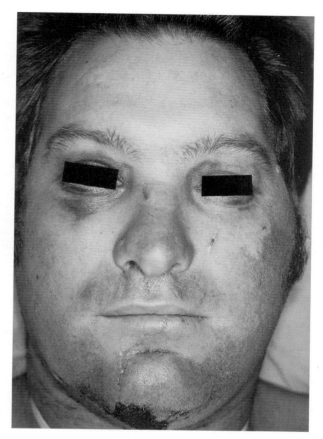

FIG. 17. Facial elongation produced secondary to a Le Fort fracture.

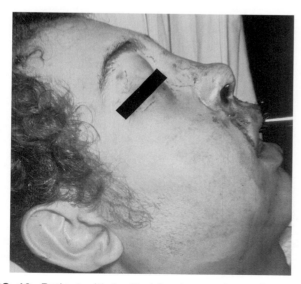

FIG. 16. Patient with Le Fort fracture and anterior open bite.

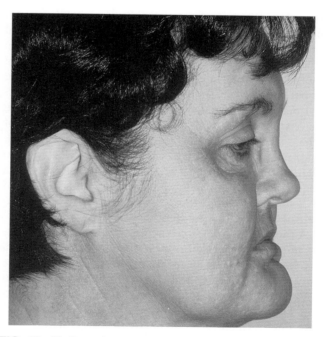

FIG. 18. Flattened or "dish-face" deformity brought on by a Le Fort II fracture with inadequate fixation.

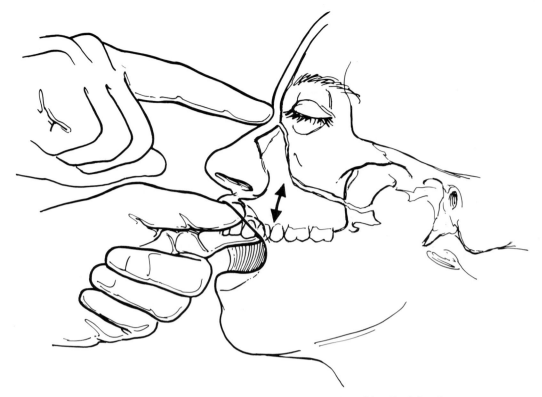

FIG. 19. Rocking of the palate, pathognomonic of Le Fort fractures.

orbital rim if there is an associated isolated zygoma fracture. The latter injury will demonstrate the usual zygomaticofrontal suture step-off and zygomatic arch defect.

Many Le Fort fractures have other associated injuries. Alveolar ridge fractures containing teeth are not uncommon. Moreover, large anterior alveolar–dental segmental fractures are occasionally confused with Le Fort I fractures. It is important when testing for palatal mobility that the anterior nasal spine is included in the grasp and the fingers are placed well in the palate.

Epistaxis is usually seen because of the fracture across the nasal dorsum and septum. The presence of a halo sign if the nose is bleeding or of a pure CSF leak once it has stopped must be sought (Fig. 20). The halo sign, brought about by a mixture of CSF and blood, is seen when a drop of blood is gathered on a towel and a clear halo double the width of the clot is seen to spread at the clot's periphery.

Although some minor bleeding from the nose or associated facial lacerations or breaks in the oral mucosa are frequently seen, occasionally massive hemorrhage may occur. This usually arises from one of two sources: the internal maxillary or internal carotid arteries. The internal carotid artery may be torn by a fracture line through the basisphenoid or lateral sphenoid sinus wall. This is a devastating injury with a high mortality rate. The diagnosis is not always easy to make

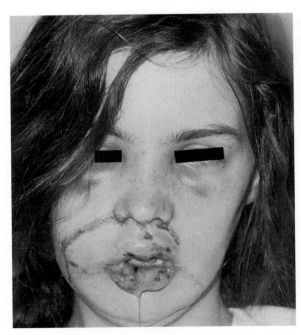

FIG. 20. Patient with bilateral CSF rhinorrhea following Le Fort III fracture. Note streaks on face from a mixture of blood and CSF.

and treatment is difficult. Vigorous nasal packing is about the only treatment that can be invoked in the early emergency situation. If early control is successful, permanent control can be achieved by the use of detachable balloons placed using invasive angiographic techniques. Operative intervention is achieved via the transeptal route or a lateral infratemporal fossa–middle fossa approach. The second and more common site of bleeding is from one or both descending palatine or internal maxillary arteries. Once identified, these vessels can be ligated with nonabsorbable suture or clipped with locking hemeclips. A patient in my experience lost 20 units of blood before bleeding sites were identified from the internal maxillary arteries and hemostasis secured with clips.

Intraoral palpation will reveal bony disruption along the lateral face of the maxilla in Le Fort I fractures and a rising defect from the posterior maxillary face ascending superiorly in Le Fort II and III fractures.

RADIOGRAPHIC EVALUATION

For many years, the x-ray diagnosis of midfacial fractures was dependent on an analysis of standard sinus films. For many such fractures, these plane films will often suffice. The Caldwell, Waters, lateral, and submentovertex views comprise the standard series. Unfortunately, manipulation of the head to produce these views often has to await neurosurgical clearance, ensuring the absence of injury to the cervical spine. A solution to this dilemma has been the development of an excellent screening technique called panoramic zonography (6,7). This technique employs technology

similar to panoramic radiographs of the mandible. It produces an image of uniform clarity throughout the midface including the pterygoid plates (Fig. 21). This can be done without changes in the patient's head position.

A series of radiographic signs can be identified when reviewing these films that will indicate a fracture. Delbalso et al. (7) outline the four "S's" of facial fractures: sinus, soft tissue, symmetry, and sharpness. Alterations in the configuration of the sinus walls, sinus opacification, or abnormal linear densities within the sinus cavities denote fracture. The "S" for soft tissue may be represented by swelling of the facial skin and subcutaneous tissue overlying the facial bones or a swelling under the mucosa of the sinus lining represented by a hematoma. The third "S" stands for symmetry. A check is made on each side of the face of bony prominences and significant skeletal landmarks to ensure that they are the same configuration on both sides. Step-offs along otherwise normal bony ridges then become more obvious. The final "S" is for sharpness. This describes an abnormal sharpness of image created by a fractured bone edge. This phenomenon brings about a number of characteristic radiographic signs such as the "railway track sign." This sign is caused by a bony fragment that is turned and produces an abnormal linear density paralleling a known skeletal landmark such as the lateral orbital rim (Fig. 22). At this site, the sign is produced by rotation of the zygoma. The "trap-door sign" is characteristic of orbital floor fractures when the floor hangs down into the maxillary sinus. There may be one or two trap doors, depending on the configuration of the fracture. The "bright light"

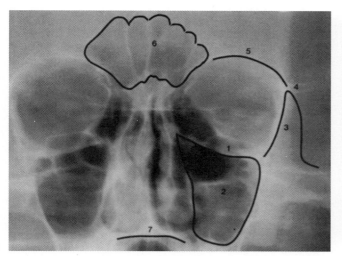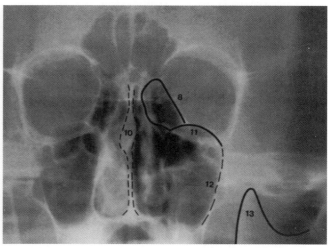

A   B

FIG. 21. Panoramic zonography of the midface, illustrating the clarity of detail of the maxillary skeleton obtained without changing the patient's head position. **A:** 1, orbital floor; 2, maxillary sinus; 3, lateral orbital rim; 4, lesser wing of sphenoid; 5, superior orbital rim; 6, frontal sinus; 7, palate/nasal floor. **B:** 8, lesser wing sphenoid; 9, ethmoid sinus; 10, septum; 11, orbital floor; 12, lateral wall of maxillary sinus; 13, coronoid process of mandible. (From ref. 7, with permission.)

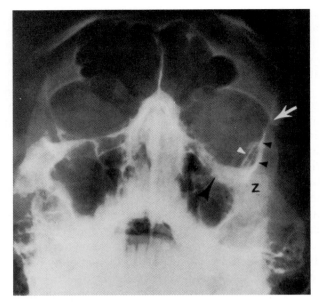

FIG. 22. "Railway track" sign in lateral orbital wall. The *arrows* point to fracture lines.

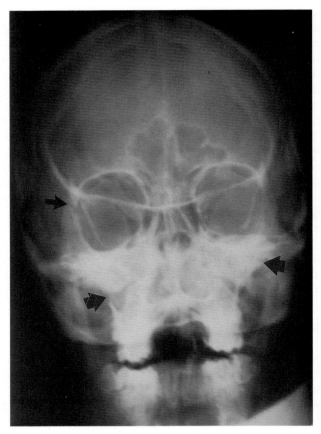

FIG. 23. Caldwell view showing fractures in the lateral maxillary walls (*large arrows*) and at the right zygomatico-frontal suture (*small arrows*) in a Le Fort I and right Le Fort III fracture combination.

sign indicates the presence of a fracture fragment in the sinus cavity. An important landmark to visualize is an alteration in the smooth lateral wall of the maxillary sinus as it blends into the undersurface of the zygoma as seen in the Caldwell view (Fig. 23). Alterations in symmetry clearly indicate a fracture into the maxillary sinus or a fracture of the zygoma. Disruptions through the pterygoid plates and lateral walls of the maxillary sinus are seen on the lateral view (Fig. 15). Fracture lines through lateral sinus walls, the nasal dorsum, and septum, coupled with disruption of normal linear densities seen through the maxillary sinuses on the poster-oanterior, Towne (Fig. 25), Waters (Fig. 22), and Caldwell (Fig. 23) views, are highly suggestive of the diagnosis. Craniofacial separation is also usually obvious on these latter views. Skull fractures and cerebral contusion are much more common than the cervical spine fractures for which we usually assiduously search.

In recent years, the computed axial tomography (CAT) scan has largely supplanted plane films in the diagnosis of midface fractures. The detail and accuracy are far superior to plane film radiography. The axial views are most revealing although valuable additional information can sometimes be obtained with coronal cuts. Coronal cuts, however, are difficult to obtain because of the positioning required by the fracture patient. The degree of disruption in the pterygoid region, the maxillary walls, the zygomata, ethmoids, and nasal skeleton are exquisitely portrayed by the axial CT scan (Figs. 24, 26, and 27). Additionally, both axial and coronal cuts will demonstrate the presence of any associated optic canal fracture (Fig. 13). Sites of fracture,

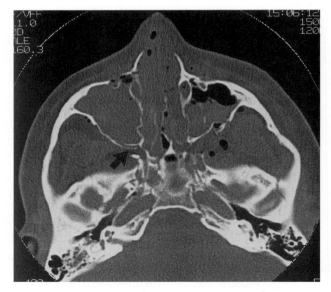

FIG. 24. Fracture of the right pterygoid plate (*arrow*) in a right Le Fort III and II fracture combination.

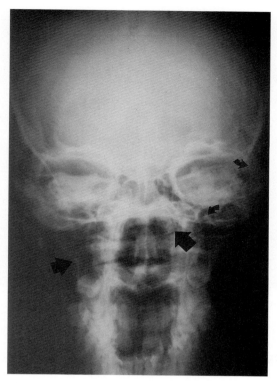

FIG. 25. Towne view shows fracture through pyriform rims of nose and maxilla (*arrow*). Also visible are fracture lines through the left orbital floor and left zygomatico-frontal suture line.

degrees of displacement, extent of comminution, and adjacent skull base and mandibular fractures are well demonstrated. The addition of three-dimensional rendering of the images further enhances the display of the lines of fracture, displacement, and degree of comminution (Fig. 28).

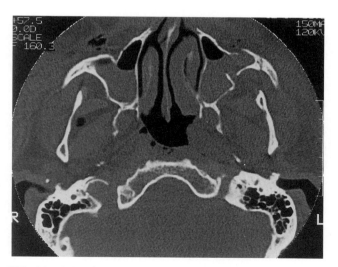

FIG. 26. Axial CT scan of Le Fort III fracture on the *left* and a Le Fort II on the *right*.

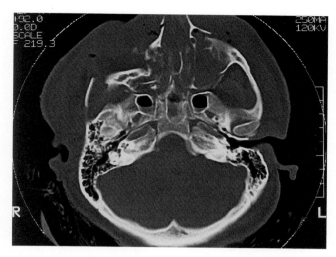

FIG. 27. Axial CAT scan showing Le Fort III fracture on *right* and Le Fort II on *left*.

Careful inspection for cranial floor fractures should be done as these are potential sites for CSF leakage.

TREATMENT

Early treatment initially requires securing the airway and controlling nasal and oral bleeding. As previously mentioned, the patient may present in the emergency room in airway distress and require immediate intubation or urgent cricothyroidotomy. Oral intubation is preferred over nasotracheal intubation because of the danger of accidental passage of the tube into the intracranial cavity if a comminuted skull base fracture exists when the nasal route is employed. If such fractures are present, even if the tube is not passed intracranially, there can be aggravation of existing fractures and dural tears. Moreover, the continued presence of this foreign body may set the stage for meningitis.

Oral intubation should not be attempted if a high index of suspicion exists regarding either a cervical spine fracture or a fractured larynx. In these cases, a cricothyroidotomy should be performed to secure a safe airway. In most instances of Le Fort fracture, a tracheostomy will be required on a temporary basis. Some Le Fort I fractures may not need this procedure especially when rigid fixation is used, but most patients with these fractures are not safe without it.

Intracranial injuries or trauma to the chest or abdomen may preclude immediate definitive repair of midface fractures. Treatment is often limited to tracheostomy, closure of facial lacerations and the placement of arch bars with intermaxillary fixation and elastic traction, procedures that can be done simultaneously while surgical control of other injuries can be performed. Restoration of premorbid dental occlusion can

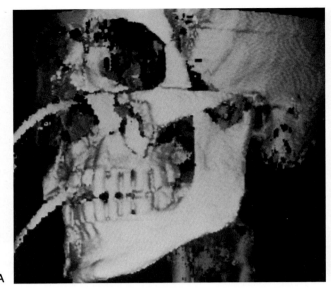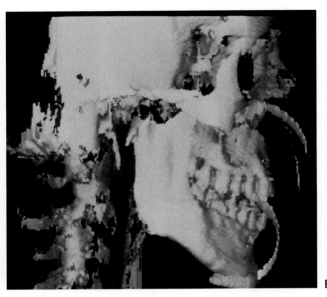

A

B

FIG. 28. Three-dimensional imaging showing a combination Le Fort II and III fracture. **A:** Three-quarter view on *left*. **B:** Lateral view on *right*.

be accomplished with strategically placed elastic traction during the subsequent period while surgical clearance is awaited. Cerebral injury, adult respiratory distress syndrome (ARDS) and other complications of surgical shock, and stabilization of chest and abdominal injuries may delay definitive surgical intervention for as long as 2 weeks. During this time, resolution of facial swelling aids somewhat in the eventual correction of the deformity. It is good practice during this waiting period to obtain dental records and preinjury photos of the patient to guide the restoration of preinjury dental occlusion and the normal facial configuration of that individual. For instance, if the patient has a premorbid cross-bite, this should be reestablished at the time of definitive repair. As another example, it is important to know that a patient with a Le Fort III fracture and nasoethmoidal complex fracture prior to the fracture had a flattened nasal dorsum. Fracture repair is no time to attempt orthognathic correction or cosmetic rhinoplasty.

Since the introduction of intraosseous wiring of facial fractures by Milton Adams in 1942 (8), reestablishment of midfacial continuity has traditionally been done by the ligation of key bony fragments with stainless steel wire, placing the patient in intermaxillary fixation, and suspending the facial skeleton from the cranium. This is a tried and true method that gives reproducible good results when correctly utilized. About 20 years ago, European maxillofacial surgeons began to utilize systems of plates and screws for the rigid fixation of these fractures. Fixation with plates in the first decades of use were accompanied by a high incidence of infection. In 1949, a Belgian surgeon named Danis (9) introduced the principle of axial bone

compression to enhance healing of fractures. The Swiss Association for the Study of Internal Fixation (ASIF) developed this system for the treatment of extremity fractures, but it was Luhr (10) who in 1968 first reported successfully using a compression system for facial fractures. Within a year, Allgower et al. (11) and Spiessl (12) reported on compression plating using the ASIF system.

Independent of the method of fixation, certain key principles must be adhered to in order to produce an acceptable functional and aesthetic result. The critical functional component of the maxilla that requires precise restoration is the dental arch. In the dentulous patient, the aim is the reestablishment of the premorbid occlusion. Even minor deviations from this are noticeable by the patient and can be a great source of annoyance and discomfort. Orbital floors must carefully be reconstituted and an attempt must be made to achieve the premorbid orbital volume to prevent enophthalmos and ocular muscle dysfunction. The reconstitution of the orbital rims to their normal symmetry and configuration is a vital aesthetic consideration.

The nose should be reduced to its normal projection when possible and straightened. The septum should be placed in the midline. Often lead plates will be required for the severely shattered nose to maintain projection. This fracture is often accompanied by tears to one or both medial canthal tendons. For repairs of these structures, see the chapter by Donald entitled Frontal and Ethmoid Complex Fractures.

The critical aesthetic feature to reestablish in these patients is vertical height; prevention of retrusion of the maxilla is also important. This can be achieved by plating, interosseous wires, or a combination of both.

WIRING

Interosseous wires or plates can be placed by elevating a bicoronal scalp flap or a combination of well placed small facial incisions. Selected intraoral incisions may be needed as well. The bicoronal incision begins about 1 to 2 cm behind the hairline and extends down to a point about the level of the root of the auricular helix (see the chapter, Frontal Sinus Fractures, by Donald, Fig. 19B). The flap is elevated in the subgaleal but extraperiosteal plane. Periosteum is elevated over the lateral orbital rims at the fracture sites and carried for a short distance into the infratemporal fossa by a narrow dissection of the temporalis muscle, enough to accommodate a malleable retractor. This latter maneuver is not necessary if plates are to be used. The zygomaticofrontal area, the usual site of lateral orbital rim fractures, is identified and holes are drilled

for wires or plates. One hole on either side of the fracture line is sufficient to pass an intraosseous wire, but a minimum of two holes per side are required if a straight miniplate is to be affixed. For plating, the holes should be drilled slowly with a 1.5-mm penetrating bur. A malleable retractor is inserted between the temporalis muscle and the rim to prevent catching any soft tissue in the drill. Copious irrigation is used during the drilling process with frequent clearing of the drill from the hole to prevent bone dust from building up within it. If wiring is used, a 26-gauge wire is passed through the drill holes and secured loosely. If a Le Fort III fracture is present, then a second larger hole that will accommodate a 24-gauge suspension wire is drilled above the fixation wire hole. If there is a lateral skull fracture or the lateral and superior orbital rim are also fractured, the suspension wire may need to be placed through an outer calvarial drill hole (Fig. 29) or anchored around

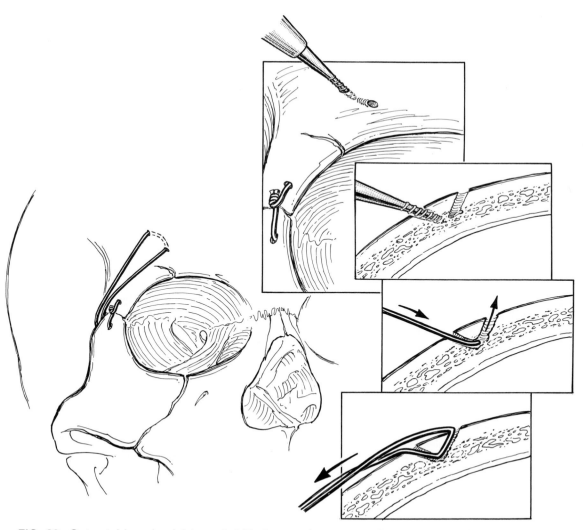

FIG. 29. Outer table calvarial tunnel drilled to anchor suspension wire in cases in which a Le Fort III and calvarial fracture coexist.

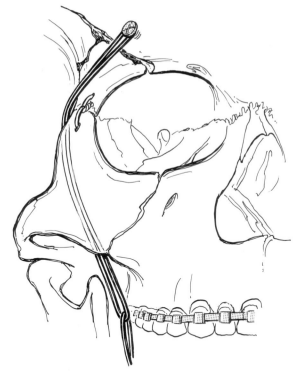

FIG. 30. As an alternative to problem outlined in Fig. 28, a calvarial screw may be used as an anchor for the suspension wire.

a screw placed in the calvarium (Fig. 30). A pullout wire is placed around the calvarial tunnel wire. However, if a screw anchor is used, it should be removed at the same time that the suspension wire is pulled.

The bony work in the region of the lateral orbital rim can also be done through a lateral brow incision (Fig. 31). This incision is much easier and faster to do and leaves a barely perceptible scar in most patients.

In almost all Le Fort III fractures and all Le Fort II fractures with attendant zygoma fractures, the floor of the orbit should be explored. The fractures of the infraorbital rim are best managed with either a subciliary or infraorbital crease incision (Fig. 32). Any facial lacerations that will provide adequate access are obviously utilized instead of the aforementioned incisions. The incisions usually are centered over the palpable fracture. An infraorbital crease incision should not extend the width of the eye for fear of producing lid edema from scar contracture. Subciliary incisions must be stair-stepped to avoid ectropion. Great care is taken not to violate the septum orbitale. A linear incision is made in the infraorbital rim periosteum. This layer is elevated and dissected along the floor of the orbit, avoiding penetration of the periorbita. All prolapsed orbital soft tissue is gently elevated out of the maxillary sinus. Dissection beyond the equator of the globe is only done exercising the greatest of caution.

Fortunately, little prolapse of tissue is usually encountered beyond this point. Orbital dissection, indeed any manipulation of the maxilla, is highly questionable if the patient has only monocular vision. A detailed review of the radiographs is essential to rule out the presence of an orbital apex fracture. Despite this, occult intraocular injuries may go undetected and may become manifest only after aggravation by orbital dissection produces postoperative blindness. Preoperative consultation by an ophthalmologist is mandated in all Le Fort II and III fractures.

The orbital floor is restored by a packing of medicated gauze through the antrum if the fragments are large and not too badly displaced. When extensive comminution exists, the implantation of a floor graft of anterior maxillary wall, nasal septum, split calvarium, or carved irradiated cartilage can be done. Alloplasts should be avoided. A three-point support is necessary to maintain the graft in position. The graft should not be placed much beyond the equator of the globe because of danger to the optic apex. Additional support may be provided by antral packing.

The infraorbital rim can be restored by placing obliquely angled drill holes on either side of each fragment and wiring in place with either 26- or 28-gauge wires. A tight anatomical reduction is not essential, but an apposition of fragments that aesthetically restores the continuity of the infraorbital rim is required. The skin of the lid requires protection from the drill shaft during hole placement. The Shirley retractor provides an excellent shield during this maneuver. The wire is threaded through the hole in the smallest fragment. A folded-over 28- or 30-gauge wire may need to be passed through the largest fragment in order to capture the osteosynthesis wire and pull it through. The wire is loosely secured (Fig. 32B,C).

Once the lateral orbital and infraorbital rims are loosely connected with interosseous wires and the nose has been reduced, suspension wires are now passed. The wires are passed either over the zygomatic arches in Le Fort I and II fractures, or through a high lateral orbital rim drill hole or calvarial drill or screw hole in the case of Le Fort III fractures. The wires are passed with an awl (Fig. 33) deep to the zygomatic arch and close to the maxillary bone to exit opposite the first maxillary molar tooth. These 24- to 22-gauge wires are twisted upon themselves and formed into a button so that a second wire passed through the loop thus made can be anchored to the lower arch bar (Fig. 34). All irregular wire surfaces are covered with dental wax.

The Rowe–Killey maxillary disimpaction forceps are now placed to reduce the fracture, with the straight blade of each forcep placed through the nose and the curved blade directed around the alveolar ridge (Fig. 35). A forward distracting force is applied to disimpact the maxillary fragment. A force of slowly increasing,

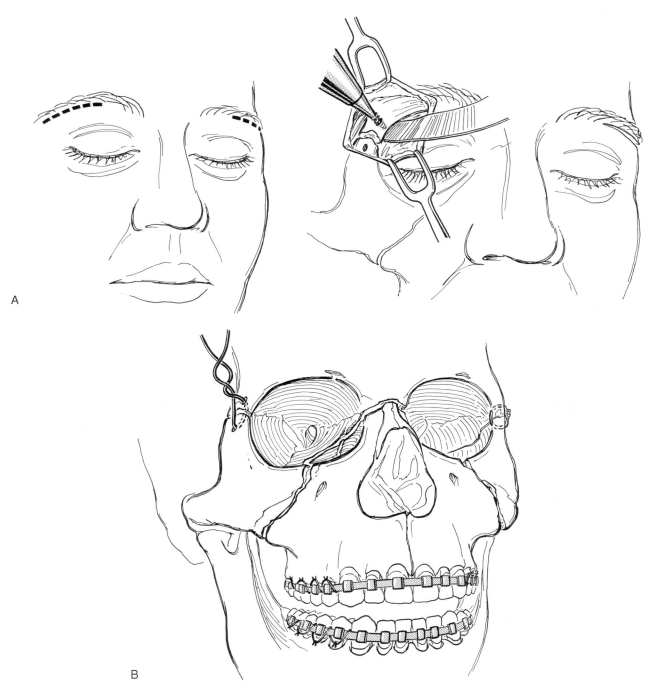

FIG. 31. Lateral orbital wall approach. **A:** Incision line and holes drilled. **B:** Fixation wire loosely placed.

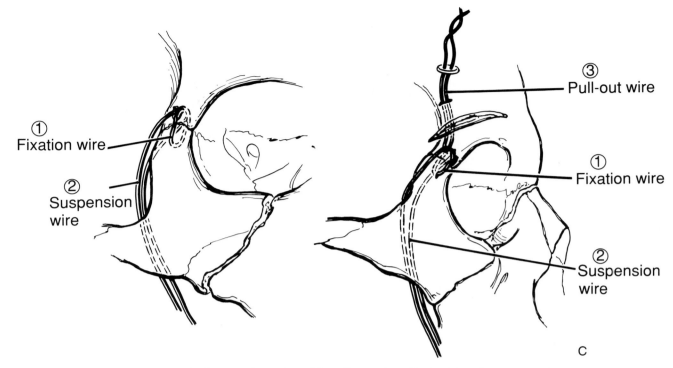

FIG. 31. *Continued.* **C:** Suspension wire with pullout wire attached has been passed.

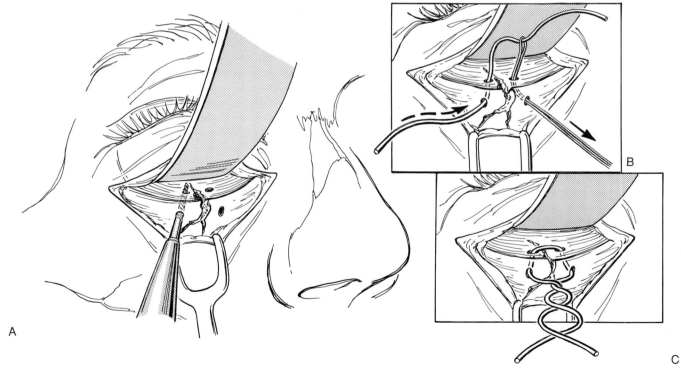

FIG. 32. Infraorbital approach. **A:** Incision line. **B:** Holes drilled and wire passed through one fragment. Capture wire shown through second drill hole. **C:** Wire lightly secured.

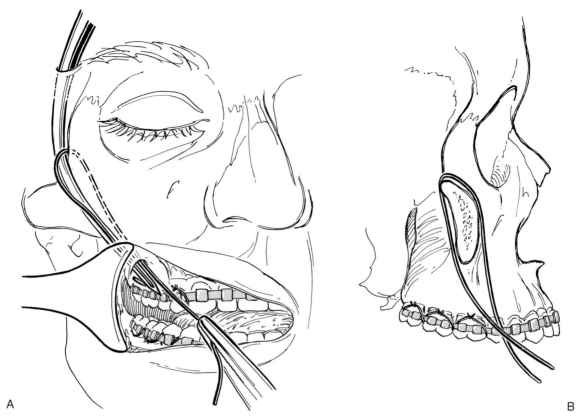

FIG. 33. Use of suspension wire. **A:** Suspension wire passed deep to zygoma. One end is secured while the other end is passed over the arch. **B:** Lateral view showing circumzygomatic wire ready for suspension.

firm, steady pressure is required. A slight downward and upward motion is occasionally needed to loosen the fragment. Little to none of this disimpaction may be necessary if the patient has been pulled into occlusion by elastic traction. Occlusion and facial proportions are frequently checked until enough distraction has been done to achieve satisfactory reduction. All interosseous wires are then tightened, the suspension wires are fixed to the lower arch bar opposite the first molar or second premolar tooth, the nose is packed, and the wounds are closed. Great care is exercised not to "overreduce" the middle one-third of the face. If excessive upward force is applied during reduction or too much traction is exerted by the suspension wires, a considerable risk of shortening the middle one-third of the face exists (13). When careful attention to reduction and fixation is exercised, midface shortening rarely, if ever, occurs.

In Le Fort II fractures, if the infraorbital rims are fractured, then interosseous wires are used. Otherwise, reestablishment of pretrauma occlusion and reduction of nasal position coupled with suspension wire immobilization will reduce and fix the fracture.

In Le Fort I fractures, occlusal restoration with arch bars and maxillary suspension can be combined with intraosseous wiring to produce a stable reduction. Through a gingival buccal sulcus incision, the pyriform rim and lateral maxillary sinus wall can be exposed. Drill holes in the maxillary bone attached to the alveolar process and the adjacent pyriform rim will anchor the fragment in place (Fig. 36). Additional stability can be provided with circumzygomatic suspension wires.

PLATING

Plate fixation has revolutionized the management of midfacial fractures. Plating systems offer some distinct advantages over interosseous wires. If sufficient bone exists, some degree of compression can be induced at the fracture site. If so, then an opportunity for primary bone healing by the ingrowth of osteons across the fracture site can be achieved. This is a more rapid and stable form of healing in contrast to the indirect healing by callus formation, which usually occurs at the sites of wire fixation. Wire exerts its force against bone over a narrow area, compared to the five times greater surface area of exposure resulting from a 2-mm screw. Bone adjacent to the wire often undergoes a minor degree of absorption sufficient to loosen the approxima-

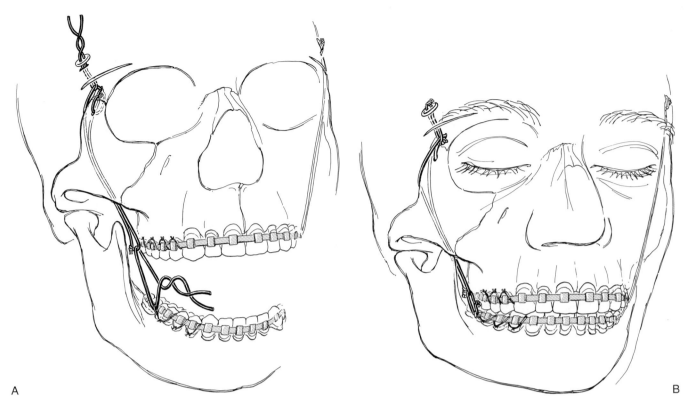

A   B

FIG. 34. A: When zygoma is not intact, both wires are passed deep to the arch after anchoring to lateral orbital rim. **B:** Wire button is formed so that second wire is secured to lower arch bar. Fixation is tightened and patient occlusion is reestablished.

tion between fragment, thus markedly reducing rigidity of fixation (13). The miniplates of such systems as Luhr and AO type can be bent to conform to the normal anatomical curves of the maxilla and zygoma. They are fixed in place with self-tapping screws. The screws are 2 mm in diameter and only require 2 mm of bony thickness to gain a firm hold. Screws are available that are as small as 1.5 mm in length. At least two screws must be placed in each fragment to provide enough stability to avoid intermaxillary fixation. If cross or square plates are used only one hole is required.

In areas where sufficient bony thickness permits, dynamic compression can be done by virtue of eccentrically drilled holes in the plates. The screw holes are drilled at the furthest distance from fracture in the eccentric plate holes. If the AO system is used, a 1.5-mm drill is used for a 2-mm screw and a 1.1-mm drill for a 1.5-mm screw diameter. A tap inserted through the tap guide is used to cut the threads for the AO screws and the screws are inserted. If the Luhr system is used, the screws are self-tapping and a 1.5-mm twist drill is used to create the bone holes to accommodate a 2-mm diameter screw. Each screw is inserted until the screw shoulder begins to engage the plate. The screws with a 30 degree angled shoulder will then slide

down the inclined plane of the plate as they are gradually alternately tightened (Fig. 37), compressing the bone fragments together. Once the compression screws are tightened in place, then the fixation screws are placed on either side. Although an excellent principle thinness of the maxilla precludes adequate compression at most sites.

Plates are placed to support the stress buttresses. The biomechanical appropriateness of the plating systems is the strongest argument in their support. The zygomaticofrontal buttress at the lateral orbital rims provides the strongest fixation point in the reconstruction because it possesses the thickest bone (varying from 3.9 to 6.5 mm) (Fig. 38) (14). Plate osteosynthesis at this point provides a stable point of fixation between the midface and the cranium. Disruptions of the Le Fort II type require alveolar ridge to pyriform crest plating as well as fixation between the frontal bone and the nose. Posterolateral fixation of the maxillozygomatic buttress is one of the most difficult to achieve (Fig. 41). Once reduction has been obtained, the continuity of the orbital rims is supported by curved miniplates of sufficient length to bridge all fractures (Fig. 39). Careful bending of the plate is essential so that the plate molds to the bone rather than the bone accommo-

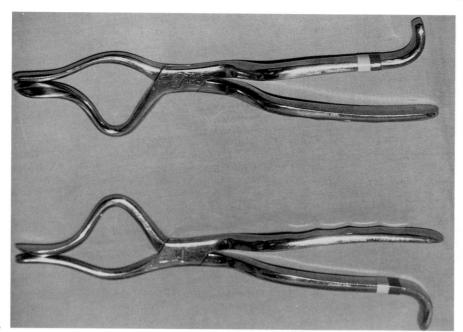

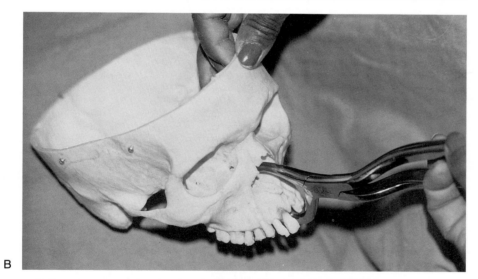

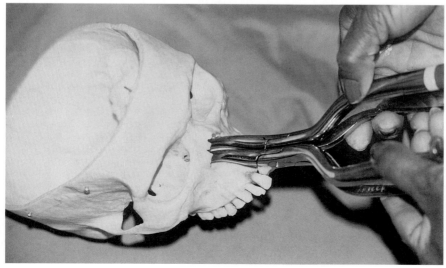

FIG. 35. Maxillary disimpaction using Rowe–Killey forceps. **A:** Pair forceps. **B:** Forceps applied on one side. **C:** Forceps applied on both sides.

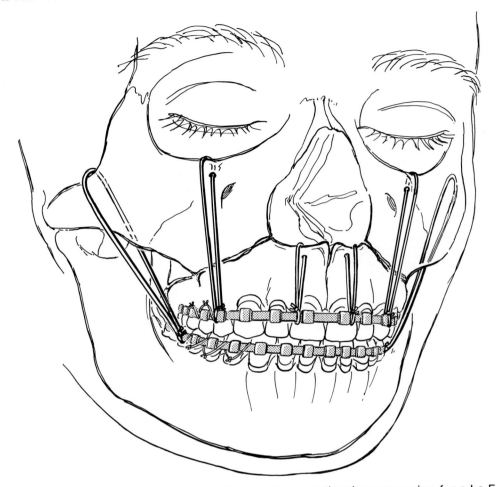

FIG. 36. Wire fixation between alveolar ridge and zygomatic wire suspension for a Le Fort I.

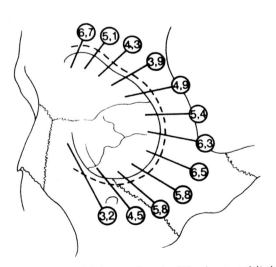

FIG. 37. Average thickness (mm) of the bony orbital rim. (From ref. 14, with permission.)

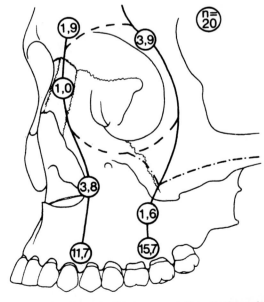

FIG. 38. Average bony thickness at the plating sites for reestablishing the stress buttresses of the midface. (From ref. 14, with permission.)

cured airway should be maintained in the early days postreduction.

Complex Le Fort fractures may require both wire and plate fixation. Suspension wires can almost always be avoided but some fragments are too small and unstable to even accommodate a microplate. Long

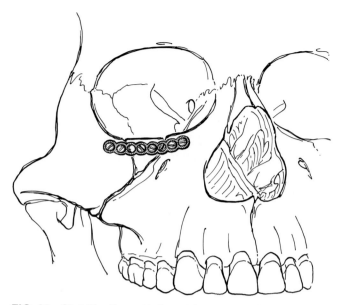

FIG. 39. Stabilization of infraorbital rims with miniplates.

dating the plate. To restore the posterior stress buttresses, plates are placed between the alveolar ridge and the pyriform rim in Le Fort I fractures (Fig. 40), between the alveolar process and the undersurface of the zygoma in Le Fort II fractures (Fig. 41A) and between the ridge and the posterior maxilla near the pterygoid plates in Le Fort III fractures (Fig. 41B). No suspension wires are necessary. The vertical height of the face is rigidly fixed and patients often come out of intermaxillary fixation in the first postoperative week. Some authorities even claim that tracheostomy is unnecessary. Although plating usually permits the early discontinuance of tracheostomy, I believe that this se-

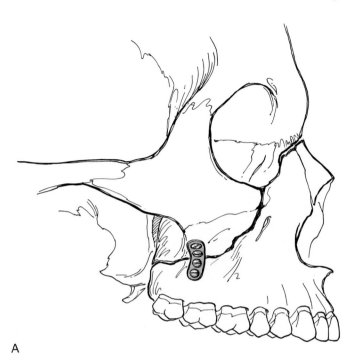

A

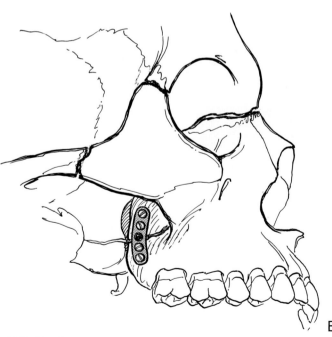

B

FIG. 41. Stress buttress plates between alveolar process and maxilla. A: Le Fort II fractures between alveolar ridge and zygomatic buttress. B: Le Fort III fractures between alveolar ridge and maxilla adjacent to pterygoid plates.

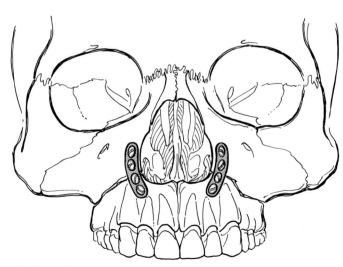

FIG. 40. Plates placed in Le Fort I fracture from pyriform rims to alveolar ridges.

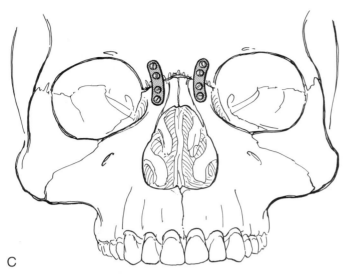

C

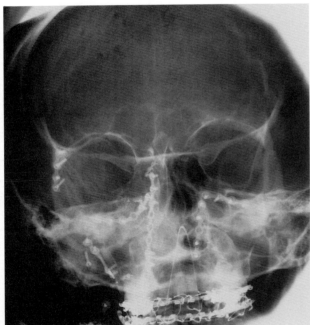

D

FIG. 41. *Continued.* **C:** Plate between frontal process maxilla and frontal bone. **D:** Caldwell radiographic view showing multiple plates and lag screw to repair a right Le Fort III and Le Fort II fracture.

bridging plates can be used with two-hole fixation at the two extremes of the plate and one hole in each intervening fragment to restore continuity.

Finally, in defense of the interosseous wiring system, it must be said that, in contrast to the reports of some authors who present cases with midfacial shortening after the use of suspension wires, I have never had this happen in a 20-year experience of at least 500 maxillary fractures treated in this fashion. Wiring is reliable and effective but plating is more biophysically sound and allows the patient to go without intermaxillary fixation.

REFERENCES

1. Le Fort R. Experimental study of fractures of the upper jaw: I, II. *Rev Chir Paris* 1901;23:208–360.
2. Le Fort R. Experimental study of fractures of the upper jaw: III. *Rev Chir Paris* 1901;23:479.
3. Sullivan WG. Maxillary fractures. In: Foster CA, Sherman JE, eds. *Surgery of facial bone fractures.* New York: Churchill Livingstone, 1987;151.
4. DuBrul EL, ed. *Sicher's oral anatomy,* 8th ed. St Louis: CV Mosby, 1988;54–60.
5. Morgan GDG, Madan OK, Bergerat JPC. Fractures of the middle third of the face: a review of 300 cases. *Br J Plast Surg* 1972; 25:147.
6. Hallikainen D, Paukker P. Panoramic zonography. In: Delbalso AM, ed. *Maxillofacial imaging.* Philadelphia: Saunders, 1990; 1–33.
7. Delbalso AM, Hall RE, Margarone JE. Radiographic evaluation of maxillofacial trauma. In: Delbalso AM, ed. *Maxillofacial imaging.* Philadelphia: Saunders, 1990;37.
8. Adams WM. Internal wire fixation of facial fractures. *Am J Surg* 1956;92:12.
9. Danis R. *Theorie et practique de l'osteosynthese.* Paris: Masson, 1949.
10. Luhr HG. Zur stabilen osteosynthese bei unterkiefer fracturne. *Deutsch Zahnartztl Z* 1968;23:754.
11. Allgower M, Ehrsam R, Ganz R, et al. Clinical experience with a new compression plate "DCP." *Acta Orthop Scand Suppl* 1969;125:45–61.
12. Spiessl B. Experience with the ASIF instrument set in treatment of mandibular fractures. *Schweiz Monatsschr Zahnartztl* 1969; 79:112m.
13. Kellman RM, Schilli W. Plate fixation of fractures of the mid and upper face. *Otolaryngol Clin North Am* 1987;20:559–571.
14. Schilli W, Niederdellmann H. Internal fixation of zygomatic and midface fractures by means of miniplates and lag screws. In: Kruger E, Schilli W, eds. *Oral & maxillofacial traumatology,* vol 2. Chicago: Quintessence Publishing, 1986;177–196.

CHAPTER 23

Fractures of the Zygoma

Paul J. Donald

There are certain prominences or protuberant features in the face that present almost as target areas for trauma. These are the nose, the mentum of the mandible, and the malar eminence of the zygoma. It is not surprising then that they are the commonest areas in the face that become fractured.

The zygoma is the second most commonly fractured facial bone; only the nose is broken more frequently. In a series of 1900 facial fractures seen at Los Angeles County Hospital (1), 1200 involved the zygoma. Schuchardt and co-workers (2), from Dusseldorf, found that 22% of all midface fractures were of the zygoma. About 85% of all fractures of this type occur in males and 80% occur between the ages of 18 and 45 (3). In my own experience of approximately 4500 facial fractures, the mandible is the most commonly fractured bone, followed by the zygoma, and then the nose. This may simply reflect our referral pattern.

Reduction and often fixation are required because of disturbance of both function and aesthetic balance to the face. The prominence of the malar eminence is an extremely important aesthetic landmark. Because high cheekbones are considered a mark of beauty, any dissymmetry of this important facial feature is extremely noticeable and will mar an otherwise beautiful countenance.

In urban America, motor vehicle accidents are the commonest cause of these fractures. However, in Europe and Great Britain, altercations, falls, industrial accents, or sporting events are most commonly the cause (4,5). Cranial injuries and fractures of the cervical spine must be ruled out in all cases, but they are not as commonly found with malar fractures as with maxillary fractures.

ANATOMY

The zygoma, or malar bone, comprises the lateral buttress of the middle one-third of the face. It makes a significant contribution to the orbital and maxillary sinus walls and forms the superior part of the medial wall of the infratemporal fossa.

The bone is comprised of a central body with three processes: orbital, maxillary, and temporal (Fig. 1). The orbital process extends superiorly to articulate with the orbital process of the frontal bone. Its thickened anterior aspect contributes the inferior two-thirds of the lateral orbital rim. Posteriorly, it thins out to a vertical platelike structure making up much of the lateral orbital wall, which articulates posteriorly with the sphenoid bone near the orbital apex. A small but important bony outcropping on the medial surface of the lateral orbital rim of the zygoma is Whitnall's tubercle (Fig. 2). It is located 10 mm below the frontozygomatic suture and 2 mm inside the rim (7). This forms the attachment of Lockwood's suspensory ligament of the eye. With inferior displacement of the zygoma during fracture, the lateral aspect of the globe is carried downward because of this attachment, producing diplopia and, in some, an anti-mongoloid slant.

The orbital plate extends horizontally for a short distance medially, where it articulates in the orbital floor with the orbital process of the maxilla. The orbital floor contribution of the zygoma thickens anteriorly to form part of the infraorbital rim. The infraorbital rim is situated at a higher level than the orbital floor. The floor tends to slope inferiorly in a gentle concavity as it extends posteriorly. In addition, the floor slopes somewhat inferiorly in the medial to lateral direction. From the orbital apex anteriorly, the infraorbital fissure insinuates itself between the zygomatic and maxillary contributions to the orbital floor. The fissure ends approximately 15 mm from the infraorbital rim; but about 5 mm behind this point, the infraorbital nerve, which has been traveling in the fissure, makes a right-angled bend medially and assumes a more inferior declination as it enters the infraorbital canal. It exits the bone at the

313

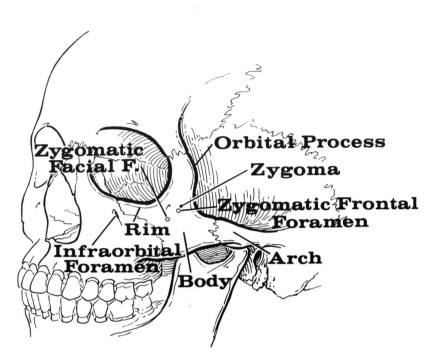

FIG. 1. Illustration showing processes of zygoma.

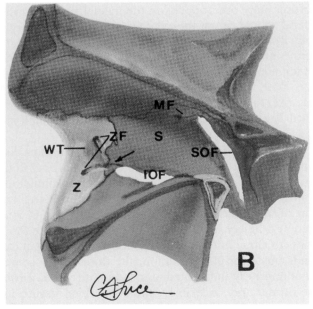

FIG. 2. Lateral wall of orbit demonstrating Whitnall's tubercle (WT) that forms the attachment of Lockwood's suspensory ligament of the eye. Z, zygoma; IOF, inferior orbital fissure; SOF, superior orbital fissure; ZF, zygomaticofacial and zygomaticotemporal canals; S, sphenoid; MF, middle meningeal foramen. (From ref. 6, with permission.)

infraorbital foramen and ramifies, supplying the skin of the anterior aspect of the middle third of the face (Figs. 2 and 3). Although all the orbital walls are thin, the floor is the thinnest and by far the most vulnerable to fracture.

The maxillary process extends inferiorly from the infraorbital rim and inferolaterally to articulate with the maxilla and make up a small part of the anterior and lateral walls of the maxillary sinus (Fig. 1). It is in the proximity of the suture line that many of the zygoma fractures occur. On its lateral face and as it becomes the orbital process, the maxillary process forms for a short distance the deep surface of the anteriormost aspect of the infratemporal fossa.

The temporal process of the zygoma extends from the lateral–posterior aspect of the zygomatic body, curving outward to articulate in a synostosis with the zygomatic process of the temporal bone. These two processes make up the zygomatic arch, a notable landmark of the upper lateral skull projecting like a handle from each side. Although the contribution of the zygoma to this arch is rather small, it forms the thickest part.

The body of the zygoma is a thick bone whose convex configuration produces the characteristic malar eminence of the cheek. The medial surface of this portion of the bone is excavated to a varying degree by the maxillary sinus. Two foramina penetrate this region to provide exit for the zygomaticofrontal and zygomaticofacial nerves, which supply sensation to the skin overlying the malar eminence.

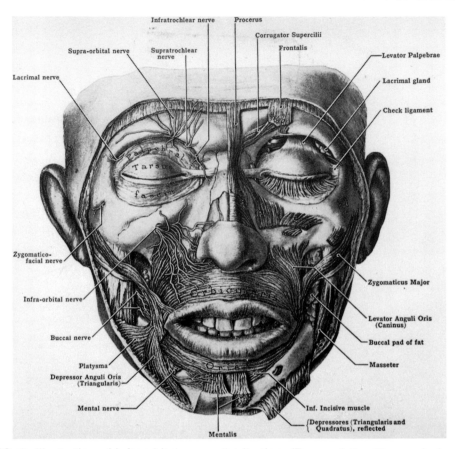

FIG. 3. Illustration of infraorbital nerve distribution. (From ref. 8, with permission.)

The most important structure related to the zygoma is the eye. The malar bone makes up most of the lateral orbital wall and about one-fifth of the floor. Signs and symptoms related to eye function are the most significant clinical features of zygoma fractures. In a review of 720 patients by Jelks and La Trenta (7), intraocular injury was present in 14% to 40% of zygomatic fractures that involved the orbital floor.

The muscles related to the zygoma are many and varied (Fig. 4). The orbicularis oculi is attached in its orbital part over the orbital rims. Its significance lies in its provision of route of access to the repair of zygoma fractures. The temporalis muscle takes origin in the temporal fossa of the lateral skull and then traverses inferiorly under the zygomatic arch to insert on the coronoid process of the mandible. The masseter muscle takes origin on the lateral surface of the mandibular body and ramus near the angle. The zygomaticus major and minor take origin on the zygomatic body but are of little clinical significance in zygoma fractures.

The infraorbital nerve exits the infraorbital foramen and supplies sensation to the cheek, lower eyelid, lateral nose, and upper lip (Fig. 3). Numbness in this distribution following zygoma fracture is one of the commonest symptoms.

PATHOPHYSIOLOGY

The body of the zygoma is the thickest and strongest part of the bone; the orbital plates are the thinnest and most vulnerable. The zygoma contributes along the adjacent maxillary wall an integrated series of buttresses, which are in part responsible for the structural integrity and strength of the facial skeleton (Fig. 5). These lines of strength offer resistance to fracture when force is imposed thereon. Figure 6 illustrates the thinnest and most fragile regions of the zygoma in the transilluminated skull. The zygomatic arch is cushioned between muscle layers with the masseter muscle emerging from its inferior and inferomedial surface and the temporalis muscle coursing deep to it through the infratemporal fossa to insert on the coronoid process. Despite this, scant soft tissue separates the arch from the overlying skin.

The amount of force required to fracture the different components of the zygoma obviously varies somewhat with the thickness of the bone. It is apparent that far less force is required to fracture the arch than the body. Body fractures require about 930 to 3470 newtons whereas the arch requires 911 to 2120 newtons (9).

Facial trauma is obviously the etiologic factor re-

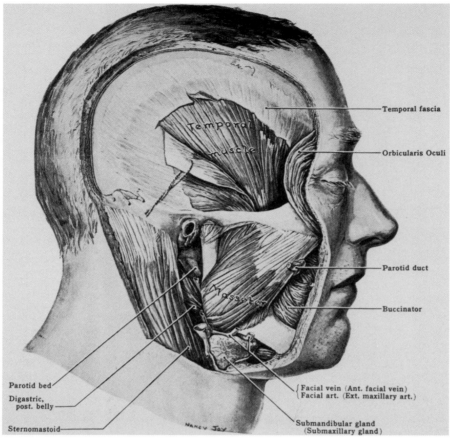

FIG. 4. Muscles related to the zygoma. (From ref. 8, with permission.)

sponsible for zygoma fractures. The blow may arise from motor vehicle accident, industrial accident, altercation, bullet, or fall.

In the literature, the most prevalent cause appears to be more dependent on the setting of the hospital doing the reporting than anything else. For example, Matsunaga and Simpson (1) from L. A. County/USC Medical Center reported a high percentage of zygoma fractures resulting from auto accidents, which is consistent with their proximity to local freeways. On the other hand, Winstanley (10) from England found only 8% of the fractures he saw were caused by auto accidents, with the majority of the remainder from assaults and sporting events. Our own experience is about equal between motor vehicle trauma and personal assault, the hospital being a major trauma center, close to a number of major highways and in an area with a high rate of violent crime.

CLINICAL PRESENTATION

The zygoma fracture may be merely one of a constellation of facial fractures. Fractures of the maxilla are the commonest to accompany a zygoma fracture. The classical pattern of the Le Fort fracture is not always followed by the fracture line, and the zygoma is commonly fractured independently. For example, the zygoma may be part of a Le Fort I fracture or in continuity with a Le Fort II or hemimaxillary fracture.

The fractures may be undisplaced with minimal symptoms or badly displaced and comminuted, presenting with symptoms arising as a result of the compromise of function of adjacent anatomical structures.

A classification of zygoma fractures helps in both anticipation of clinical signs and symptoms and also assists in the planning of the appropriate surgical procedure for correction. Simply classified, fractures of the zygoma are:

1. Arch
2. Rim
3. Tripod
4. Body

Figure 7 illustrates each type of fracture. They may be displaced or nondisplaced, simple or compound, simple or comminuted.

Although classification systems are designed to improve the understanding of clinical entities, the evolu-

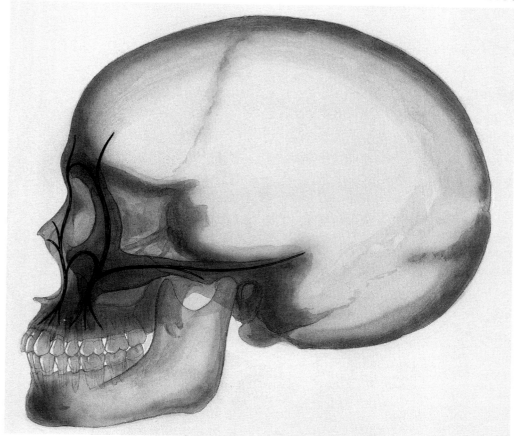

FIG. 5. The zygomatic buttress contributions to the structural integrity of the facial skeleton.

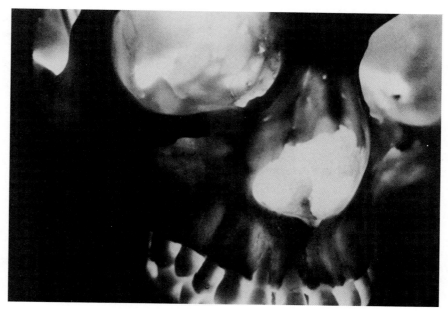

FIG. 6. Transilluminated view of skull.

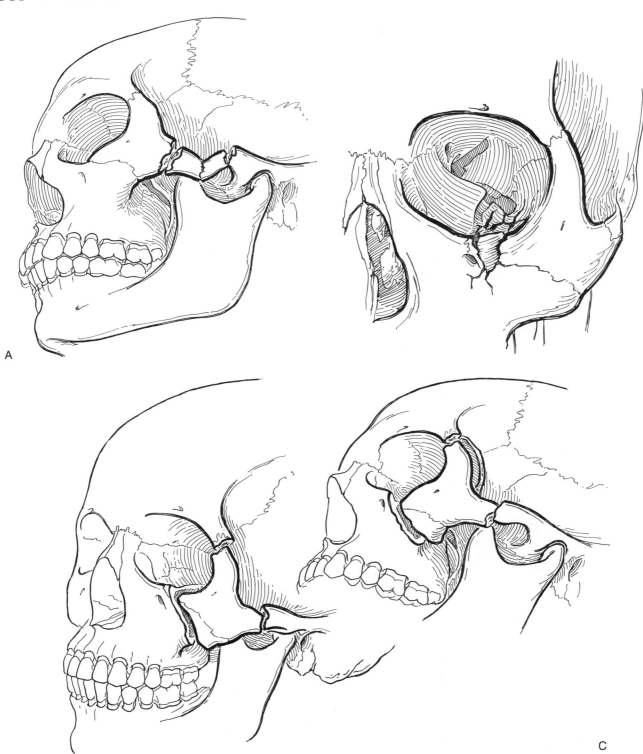

FIG. 7. Various types of zygoma fracture. **A:** Arch. **B:** Rim. **C:** Tripod. **D:** Body. (From ref. 11, with permission.)

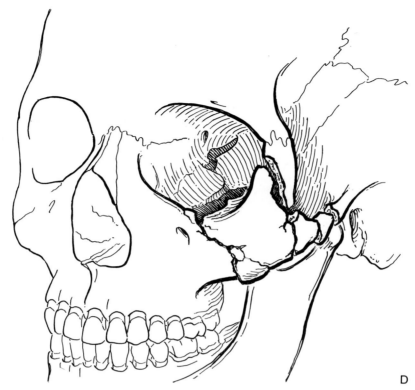

D

FIG. 7. *Continued.*

tion of the organization of zygoma fractures into distinct groups has increased in complexity to the point where it confounds rather than clarifies. The original classification by Knight and North (12) succinctly described by Dingman and Natvig (13), is further modified by Rowe and Killey (14). Yanigasawa (15) added another dimension when he pointed out that the fractures may not only rotate on a vertical axis but on a longitudinal one as well. Feinstein and Krizek (4) do an admirable job of amalgamating these systems in an attempt to bring order out of chaos, as seen in Fig. 8.

ZYGOMATIC ARCH

The arch generally fractures in two places and the fractured segment is displaced medially. The pain of the injury that results from the disruption of the bone is compounded by trismus. This in turn arises from two factors. First, the impingement on the coronoid process of the mandible on the depressed zygomatic arch fragment causes both pain and obstruction of jaw opening. Second, because of the origin of the masseter muscle on the arch, any opening of the mandible will cause pain by pulling on the broken bone. A notable depression can be seen and felt over the arch area. Although the defect often fills in with hematoma in the early post-traumatic period, the defect is usually quite

apparent to palpation and is eventually clearly visible once the hematoma has resolved (Fig. 9).

A base view is the best radiograph to manifest this fracture, and a special cone-down view on the arch will clearly delineate it (Fig. 10). Its relationship to the coronoid process will easily be appreciated, as will any impingement of this process onto the fractured arch.

TRIPOD FRACTURE

The tripod fracture is the commonest fracture of the malar bone. The zygoma is completely fractured away from the facial skeleton. The tripod fractures are so named because of their characteristic three major radiographic findings. Fractures of the lateral orbital rim, arch, and infraorbital rim are pathognomonic, but indeed the fracture extends from the infraorbital rim through the anterior and lateral walls of the maxillary sinus, into the infratemporal fossa and through both lateral and inferior orbital walls. Finally, the arch is fractured in one or more places (Fig. 7C). The usual displacement of the fragment is inferiorly, medially, and posteriorly. There is often a medial rotatory component as well.

In tripod fractures, the orbital floor is always fractured. The fracture may vary from a simple crack to a comminuted fracture that is displaced into the antrum

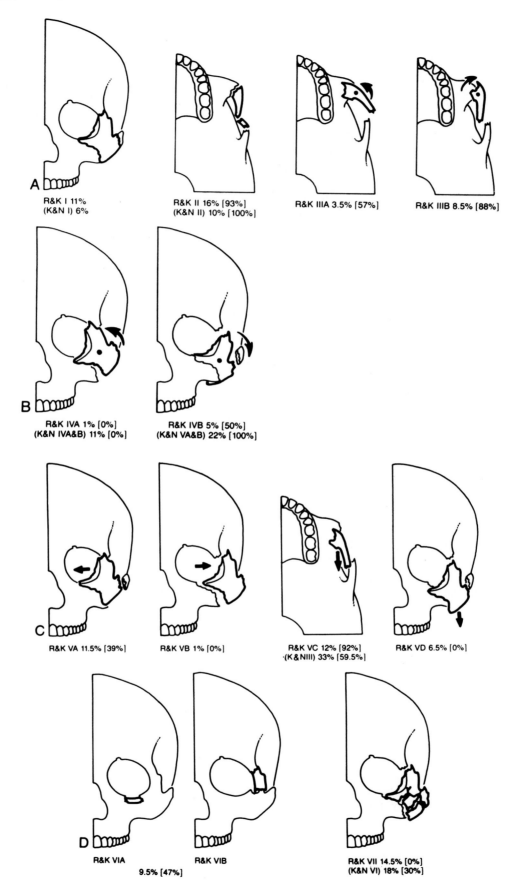

R&K I 11%
(K&N I) 6%

R&K II 16% [93%]
(K&N II) 10% [100%]

R&K IIIA 3.5% [57%]

R&K IIIB 8.5% [88%]

R&K IVA 1% [0%]
(K&N IVA&B) 11% [0%]

R&K IVB 5% [50%]
(K&N VA&B) 22% [100%]

R&K VA 11.5% [39%]

R&K VB 1% [0%]

R&K VC 12% [92%]
·(K&NIII) 33% [59.5%]

R&K VD 6.5% [0%]

R&K VIA

R&K VIB

9.5% [47%]

R&K VII 14.5% [0%]
(K&N VI) 18% [30%]

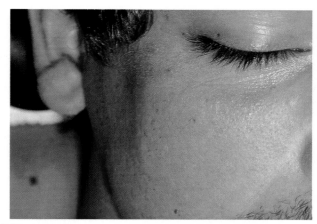

FIG. 9. Defect on side of face resulting from depressed zygomatic arch fracture. (From ref. 11, with permission.)

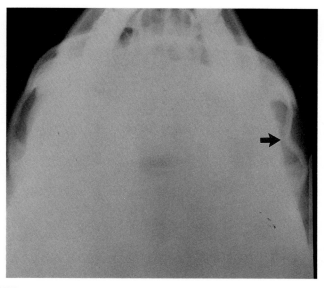

FIG. 10. Base view of zygomatic arch showing fracture on right side (see *arrow*).

in a fashion similar to an orbital blow-out fracture. The degree of comminution and displacement will determine whether orbital prolapse, with possible resultant periorbital soft tissue entrapment, occurs. The fracture passes through the infraorbital foramen, producing dysfunction of that nerve with symptoms of numbness over the cheek, upper lip, and lateral nose.

Ophthalmic symptoms are often prominent in tripod fractures. Not only are intraocular injuries common, but disturbances of the walls as they relate to the globe can produce disturbances in vision. In a review of 1524 midfacial fractures from a number of series, Feinstein and Krisek (4) found a 28% incidence of severe orbital floor injuries in 720 cases of intraocular injuries. These injuries included in the anterior chamber: corneal abrasion and laceration, hyphema, and anterior chamber recession or disruption; in the posterior chamber: iridodialysis, iris sphincter rupture, ciliary body rupture, lens subluxation or dislocation; and finally, in the back of the globe: vitreous hemorrhage, choroidal rupture, retinal detachment, commotio retinae, retrobulbar hemorrhage, scleral laceration, and optic nerve contusion, hematoma, and laceration.

The lateral attachment of the suspensory ligament of the eye, Lockwood's ligament, is through the lateral canthal tendon to Whitnall's tubercle on the orbital

process of the zygoma. With inferior displacement of the zygoma, the eye is carried downward, producing diplopia on straight ahead gaze. This change in visual axis is often compensated for by a tilting of the head to regain fusion of visual images (Fig. 11). Immediately following the injury, diplopia can also be produced by orbital hematoma and edema. This is transitory and will usually resolve within 24 hr. Another cause of diplopia is inferior displacement of the globe into the maxillary sinus through a traumatically induced dehiscence of the orbital floor (Fig. 12). Initially, no diplopia on straight ahead gaze may occur with the orbital floor fracture because of intraocular swelling or edema. As the swelling abates, enophthalmos occurs, sometimes with diplopia on straight ahead gaze. Usually, both signs will be present, but they are dependent on the amount of orbital content prolapse.

One of the major signs of orbital floor fracture is entrapment on upward gaze. Either periorbital fat and connective tissue or the inferior rectus muscle becomes impaled on fracture fragments as the eye begins to roll upward (Fig. 13). Sometimes the inferior rectus

---

FIG. 8. Comparison of modified Rowe and Killey (R&K) classification of zygoma fractures with that proposed by Knight and North (K&N) (%, incidence of fracture type; %, postreduction stability). **A:** R&K I and K&N I, nondisplaced fractures; R&K II and K&N II, zygomatic arch fractures; R&K III A, medial rotation around vertical axis; R&K III B, lateral rotation around vertical axis. **B:** R&K IV A, medial rotation around longitudinal axis; K&N IV A, medial rotation upward at the infraorbital margin; K&N IV B, medial rotation inward at the frontal malar suture; R&K IV B, lateral rotation upward at the infraorbital margin, K&N V A,B, lateral rotation outward at the frontal malar suture. **C:** R&K V A, medial displacement without rotation; R&K V B, lateral displacement without rotation; R&K V C, posterior displacement without rotation; K&N III, unrotated fractured bodies; R&K V D, inferior displacement without rotation. **D:** R&K VI A, B, rim fracture; R&K VII, complex fractures; K&N VI, complex fractures. (From ref. 16, with permission.)

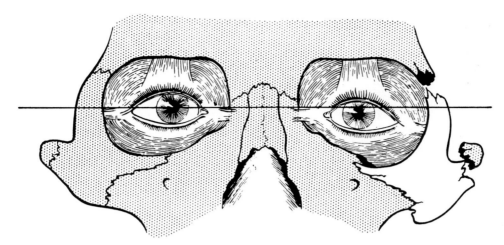

FIG. 11. Inferior displacement of eye on fractured side by virtue of attachment of Lockwood's suspensory ligament to zygoma. Visual axis is disordered and patient develops diplopia. (From ref. 13, with permission.)

muscle becomes irritated by the fracture fragments and instead of being actually physically entrapped is put into spasm, preventing the muscle forces of the superior rectus and inferior oblique from rotating the eye skyward. The best method of testing entrapment is the so-called forced duction test. A drop of topical anesthetic is placed in the inferior conjunctival fornix of the eye. The eye is grasped with a fine-toothed forceps, either directly by the inferior rectus muscle via the conjunctiva or by the sclera at the corneal limbus, and an attempt to roll the eye upward is made. The affected side is compared to the normal side. Failure to roll the eye superiorly, or marked resistance to this maneuver, constitutes a positive test indicating significant entrapment.

Subscleral hemorrhage is common, but it is indicative only of intraocular trauma. Enophthalmos, although effaced early in the post-trauma period by periorbital swelling, becomes more apparent as edema recedes. This produces a deepened supratarsal fold and the appearance of recession of the globe into the socket (Fig. 14). Inferior displacement of the eye may give an anti-mongoloid slant to the palpebral fissure. With the

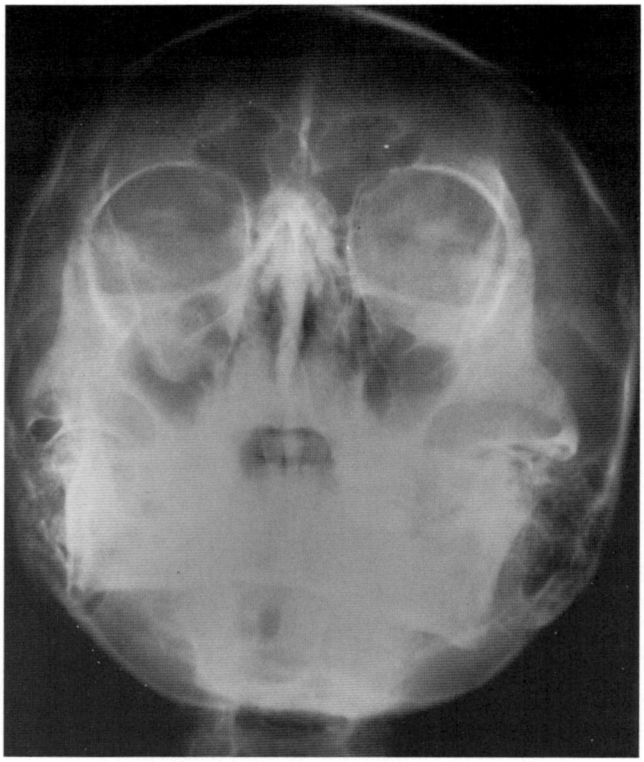

FIG. 12. Posterior–anterior view radiograph illustrating prolapse of orbital contents into maxillary antrum. (From ref. 11, with permission.)

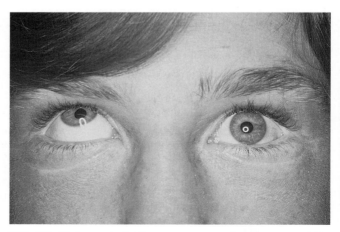

FIG. 13. Entrapment of eye on upward gaze caused by fracture of the orbital floor. (From ref. 11, with permission.)

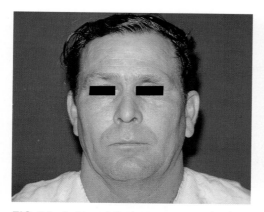 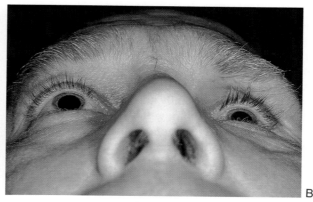

FIG. 14. A: Enophthalmos as a result of zygoma fracture with periorbital fat absorption. Illustrates a deepened supratarsal fold and orbital recession. **B:** In addition to orbital recession, there is lateral depression of malar eminence. (From ref. 11, with permission.)

distraction of the septum orbitale accompanying this inferior fragment, there may be an ectropion because the tarsal plate is pulled away from the sclera.

In displaced tripod fractures, the malar eminence is usually flattened (Fig. 14). But in some instances, the zygomatic body is rotated medially in the vertical axis and the malar eminence becomes more prominent (Fig. 15). In these cases, the zygomatic arch portion attached to the body is usually rotated laterally, that is, a clockwise rotation if the left zygoma is involved, producing an unnatural prominence in the upper lateral face. Malar flattening, however, is by far the commonest finding and frequently is the only reason for fracture reduction. The best way to assess this is to stand behind the patient who is seated in the examination chair. The head is tilted backward and the relative prominence of the malar eminences visualized. A finger is pushed over each eminence so that the effect of overlying soft tissue swelling can be eliminated. The

examiner's line of sight is dropped until the finger tip to malar eminence interface is at the horizon of view over the brow of the patient's extended head. The interfaces normally should be at the same level, but if not, zygomatic depression can be appreciated and even quantitated. Swelling of the brow or bony asymmetry of the supraorbital ridges will interfere with interpretation of this test.

Palpable step-offs and tenderness at the zygomaticofrontal and zygomaticomaxillary suture lines are pathognomonic of a tripod fracture of the zygoma. The infraorbital rim defect is usually located in its medial half. The arch fracture is often difficult to palpate because of overlying swelling as well as the relative thickness of the skin and subcutis of this area. It is not uncommon to have comminution at this site so that there is a wide gap palpable. The arch fracture, if not palpable, can be determined by placing the palms of the hands over the posterior portion of the arch near the temporal bone and applying a compressing force. Pain will be elicited at the fracture site.

Epistaxis will occur if the maxillary sinus mucosa is torn; however, the bleeding is often scant. Subcutaneous emphysema occasionally may occur as well, and crepitus can sometimes be palpated as far down as the clavicles. Trismus is often present, but the limitation of mandibular opening is transient. Trismus will be more persistent if there is much displacement of the zygomatic arch. Pain is elicited by the action of the masseter at its origin on the arch, and problems of mandibular dysfunction may result from the impingement of the coronoid process on the depressed arch as previously described in arch fractures. Crepitation, displacement, and ecchymosis along the gingival buccal sulcus line is palpated and visualized on intraoral examination. Placing the intraoral finger more superiorly and laterally along the gingival buccal sulcus will permit pal-

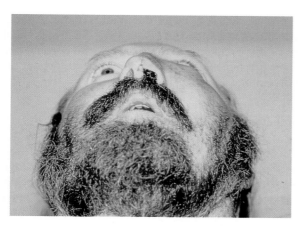

FIG. 15. Badly displaced tripod fracture of zygoma. Rotation of fragment produces a prominence rather than a depression over the malar eminence. (From ref. 11, with permission.)

pation of the undersurface of the arch and tenderness as well as displacement will readily be appreciated.

Testing with alternating pinprick and soft touch over the distribution of the infraorbital nerve will verify its involvement in the injury. The patient may also experience numbness in the teeth of the upper quadrant on the affected side. This is usually transient. Epistaxis is confirmed on intranasal exam with blood emanating from the middle meatus. Subcutaneous emphysema will be detected by palpation of crepitations in the skin over the maxillary sinus.

Body Fracture

A variant of the tripod fracture is the "body" fracture. This injury, instead of having its most lateral component on the arch, is fractured through the zygomatic body. These fractures usually are the result of trauma of considerable force (Fig. 7D).

The signs and symptoms differ little from those of the tripod fracture. There is no trismus unless the arch is fractured, and both the arch and the body may be involved. Malar depression usually is very severe because the fracture is through the eminence.

Careful review of the radiographs is necessary to establish the presence of the body fracture. The CAT scan gives a more accurate depiction of this injury.

Radiographs

The standard sinus views—the Waters, Caldwell, lateral, and submentovertex—are usually sufficient to make the diagnosis of tripod fracture. A cone-down view of the arches helps to make the diagnosis of the arch component (Fig. 10). Although computer-assisted tomography (CAT) scanning (Figs. 16 and 17A) and three-dimensional reconstruction (Fig. 17B) of zygoma fractures are more definitive than plane views, they are much more expensive and, in most cases, are unnecessary either to make the diagnosis or to plan the therapy. Three-dimensional reconstruction from CAT scan images, despite the obvious appeal, has limited value.

On plane radiographs, the Waters view is probably the most informative. Zygomaticofrontal separations and separations of the rim are usually clearly seen. Segmental fractures of the rim are best seen with this view. Opacification of the maxillary sinus indicates bleeding into the sinus, usually from rupture of the sinus roof mucosa, but can result from tears in the anterior or lateral wall lining. Prolapse of the globe into the sinus can be seen on the Waters projection but is best delineated by polytomography or coronal CAT scan. Fractures in the orbital floor are most clearly seen with this latter technique (Fig. 18). The presence of an ab-

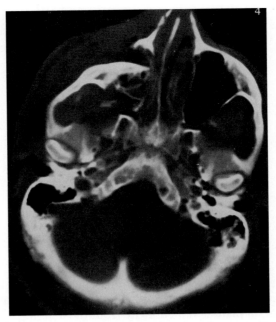

FIG. 16. CAT scan of markedly depressed zygomatic fracture. (From ref. 11, with permission.)

normal linear density in the sinus indicates either the orbital floor or lateral sinus wall is fractured.

Displacement of the fracture can be appreciated radiographically, although it does not always correlate well with the degree of displacement seen at surgery. This is probably due to the difficulty of displaying a three-dimensional event on a two-dimensional radiograph. The degree of fragment rotation often is the principal cause of this distortion. Comminution is displayed on the plane films but is clearly best illustrated on the CAT scan. This is also true for displacement. The Caldwell view best depicts the zygomaticofrontal suture separations, and the submentovertex view most clearly illustrates the arch fractures. These two sites are not as clearly seen in the Waters view. Although the axial view on the CAT scan best illustrates the degree of displacement of the zygoma, the coronal plane images are necessary to best demonstrate orbital floor involvement.

Ophthalmological Assessment

It is essential in most cases of zygomatic fracture to have a preoperative assessment by an ophthalmologist. This is especially mandated in those patients with eye signs or symptoms. Even without these, occult injuries may be detected only by a meticulous eye exam. A preoperative vision check may reveal a previously undetected amblyopia in the unaffected eye. This may produce some hesitation in reducing the fracture on the side of the best eye. A careful screening of the

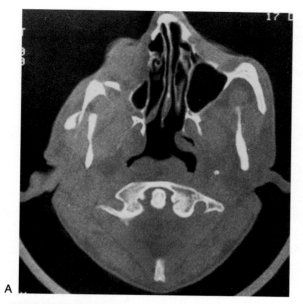

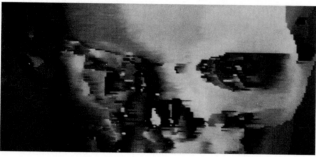

FIG. 17. Severely fractured zygoma. **A:** CAT scan. **B:** Three-dimensional reconstruction of CAT scan showing degree of displacement of fracture fragments. (From ref. 11, with permission.)

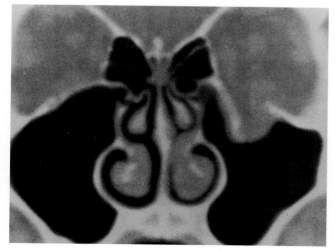

FIG. 18. Coronal CAT scan showing clearly the fracture of the orbital floor and prolapsed contents. (From ref. 17, with permission.)

radiographs may reveal additional fractures in the orbital apex that may endanger the optic nerve during reduction. Any sign of intraocular injury should delay repair until a time when the ophthalmologist gives clearance.

SURGICAL REPAIR

Arch Fractures

Fractures to the zygomatic arch can be managed surgically under either general or local anesthesia. After premedication with an analgesic such as morphine and a sedative such as Nembutal or diazepam, local infiltration at the site of incision and at the fracture site(s) is all that is required.

The Gillies technique is the one most commonly employed. A 1.5 to 2 cm incision is made in the temporal scalp approximately 2 to 3 cm above the hairline (Fig. 19). Incision, then dissection, is carried through the superficial layer of temporalis fascia. A tunnel is created with a periosteal elevator under the depressed arch fragment. A Boies elevator or Cottle skin elevator is placed under the fracture fragment and the arch is elevated into position. Care is taken not to lever the bone into position as the pressure of the elevator against the fulcrum point on the underlying calvarium may cause a skull fracture. A strong lifting force is usually required to reposition the fractured arch segment. Once it slides into place, no further splinting or fracture fixation is needed because of the splinting action of the underlying temporalis muscle.

In some resistant fractures, either those with impaction of fragments or those whose operative treatment has been delayed longer than 7 to 10 days, reduction may be quite difficult. The Rowe–Killey elevator (Fig. 20) will allow the application of substantial force through its design as a third-class lever. The blade is under the arch, the fulcrum against the operator's hip, and the handle positioned above the blade (Fig. 20). Any fracture, except one that has become ossified, can be reduced with this instrument. Firm countertraction is exerted by the surgeon's assistant holding the patient's head in order for reduction to occur.

Postoperatively, once the wound is sutured, a protective splint is constructed from a bent finger splint taped to the head and positioned over the reduced arch (Fig. 21). This will prevent redislocation of the fragment if the patient should inadvertently strike it or roll over on it in bed.

In rare instances, reduction of the arch will not be maintained favorably by the splinting action of the temporalis muscle. In these instances, packing with a Penrose drain covered in antibiotic ointment will maintain reduction. The pack is removed in 10 to 14 days.

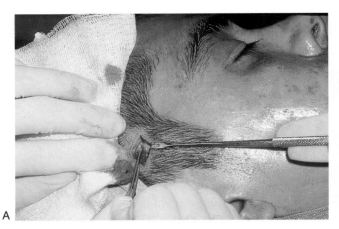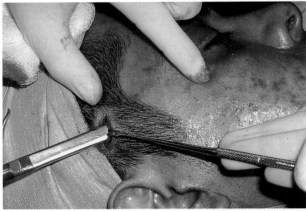

FIG. 19. A: Incision is made in hairline for reduction of zygomatic arch fracture using the Gillies technique. **B:** Boies elevator is placed under the fractured arch to lift fractured segments into position. (From ref. 11, with permission.)

Tripod Fracture

A host of methods have been described to reduce and fix tripod fractures. Interosseous wiring, introduced by Adams (18) in 1942, is still used successfully. This is my preferred method, and it has been effective in the management of over 400 zygoma fractures. In most cases, a two-point fixation is all that is required, and although the advocates of the Steinman pin fixation technique are enthusiastic about their results (1), the problem of possible rotation around a single point of fixation jeopardizes the maintenance of correct fragment alignment.

Incisions of approximately 1.5 cm in length are made in the brow and the infraorbital regions. The brow incision begins in the lateral aspect of the brow with the blade angled obliquely to carry the cut in the direction

of the follicles of the eyebrow hairs (Fig. 22). Periosteum is incised and, with retraction superiorly and then inferiorly, the length of the lateral orbital rim can be explored. The commonest site of fracture is the zygomaticofrontal suture area. Occasionally, there may be two fractures with an intervening floating segment. Once the fracture sites have been identified, the perios-

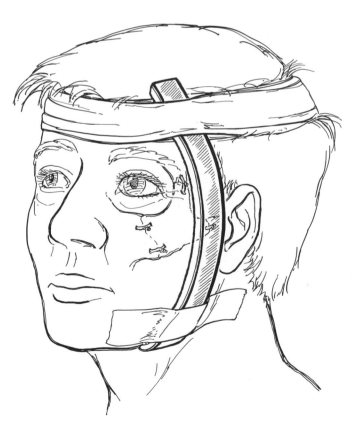

FIG. 20. Reduction of zygomatic arch fracture using the Rowe–Killey elevator. Elevator is inserted under arch and the arch is levered into position with the fulcrum at the operator's hip; upward pressure is exerted with the handle. (From ref. 11, with permission.)

FIG. 21. A protective finger splint is taped over the fracture site. (From ref. 11, with permission.)

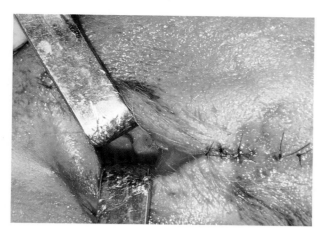

FIG. 22. Lateral brow incision 1.5 cm in length is used for lateral orbital rim exposure. Fracture is visualized in wound. (From ref. 11, with permission.)

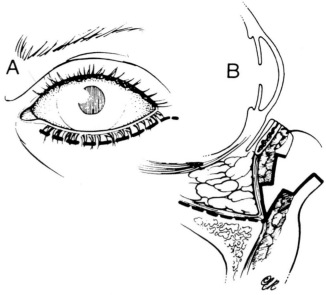

FIG. 24. **A:** Subciliary incision. **B:** Infraorbital incision is stair-stepped through the skin and orbicularis oculi muscle to prevent scar contracture to septum orbitale. (From ref. 16, with permission.)

teum is cleared with just enough room to drill the holes for wire fixation. Dissection is carried into the infratemporal fossa posteriorly to the rim. Penetrating bur holes are placed on either side of the fracture into the fossa, and a 26-gauge wire is passed through both holes and loosely secured (Fig. 23). Attention is then directed to the infraorbital rim.

Selection of incisions include a choice between a subciliary or blepharoplasty incision, an incision in a natural crease in the "eye bag" area, or one through the transconjunctival route. In my own hands, the blepharoplasty incision is too often accompanied by ectropion, which, although temporary, is disturbing to the patient. The transconjunctival route, although a very direct approach to the infraorbital rim, gives a limited exposure to the orbital floor. One great advantage of this incision is the avoidance of incision through

the septum orbitale, thus avoiding one of the major causes of postoperative ectropion.

In making the infraorbital incision, it is important to remember to stair-step the incision (Fig. 24). This is absolutely essential to prevent the direct adherence of the skin incision to the septum orbitale or the maxillary periosteum, which causes the phenomenon of ectropion in these cases. Care is taken to make the incision over the fracture site and not to encompass the entire length of the lower lid as a long incision often results in a trapdoor deformity creating an edematous lid (Fig. 25). Once the skin incision is made in the crease, the

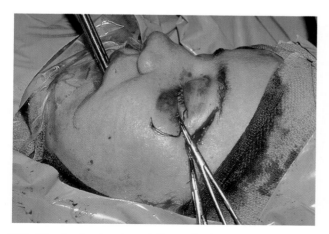

FIG. 23. A wire is placed through the lateral orbital rim fractures and kept loose until the fracture is reduced. (From ref. 11, with permission.)

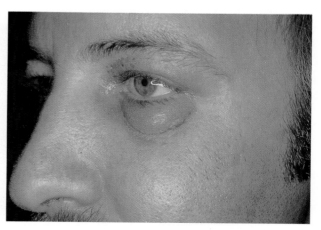

FIG. 25. Edematous lower lid produced as a consequence of making an infraorbital crease incision the length of the eye. (From ref. 11, with permission.)

skin is elevated inferiorly for approximately 3 mm. This flap is retracted and the iris scissors are used to penetrate the orbicularis oculi muscle through to the underlying maxillary and zygomatic periosteum. Before splitting the muscle in the plane of the fibers, blunt palpation through the muscle is done to ensure the ensuing incision will be over bone and not over septum orbitale. Retraction of the muscle is done with the Shirley retractors and the fracture line is exposed. The periosteum over the fracture area is cut and the dissection is carried onto the orbital floor. As the inferior orbital rim is reached, it must be noted that the floor slopes rather abruptly inferiorly away from the rim as one proceeds in a posterior direction into the orbit. If a straight back approach is taken, the periorbita will be ruptured and orbital fat will prolapse into the wound.

The amount of orbital floor comminution is assessed. Simple crack fractures with minimal displacement need no attention. Comminuted fractures and those with displacement require accurate reconstitution of the floor. A number of techniques have been described to accomplish this goal. A popular method of floor reconstruction is the use of an alloplastic material such as supramid mesh, Silastic sheeting, acrylic, titanium mesh, or proplast. Although this is successful in the majority of cases, there is a significant incidence of graft extrusion (Fig. 26). As a rule, I avoid alloplasts. If the floor fragments are large enough, they can be pulled back into position by the use of small hooks (while the eye is protected with an orbital retractor). Alternatively, the fragments can be replaced by packing placed into the maxillary antrum via an antral–meatal window or a Caldwell–Luc antrostomy. This is done while the floor is viewed by direct visualization through the infraorbital rim incision. With the packing in place for 2 weeks, the floor becomes solid enough to support itself when the packing is withdrawn. Approximately 50% of depressed orbital floor fractures

can be managed in this latter fashion without the use of a graft.

If extensive comminution exists or missing bone results during debridement and cleansing of the wound, then the gap in the floor is bridged with a graft. Suitable materials are nasal septum, rib, hip, split calvarium, or irradiated cartilage. The most exquisite graft is a carefully procured graft of the maxillary face. It has the thinness required and has a concavity that closely resembles the orbital floor. If an autograft is not possible, my next graft of preference is thinly carved irradiated costal cartilage. The graft must be well supported on three sides. It is not necessary to cover any floor dehiscences much behind the equator of the globe. In fact, placing a graft in the posterior part of the orbit jeopardizes the optic nerve.

The fracture of the rim is now attended to. Drill holes are made through the rim on either side of the fracture going from the face of the maxilla and zygoma into the orbital floor. These holes are by nature obliquely angled and the infraorbital skin requires protection by a metal retractor while they are being placed. A 26-gauge wire is placed through both holes and loosely secured (Fig. 27).

A Boies elevator or, in the case of a badly impacted fracture, the Rowe–Killey elevator is placed through the brow incision under the body of the zygoma and the fracture is reduced into the correct alignment. With the fracture in position, the brown and rim wires are tightened into place. If the orbital floor has been fractured and is prolapsed, it can be repositioned and kept in place with an antral pack placed either through an antral–meatal window or a limited maxillary antrostomy. However, if an orbital floor graft has been placed, packing is usually unnecessary and is used only if there is any question as to its stability

The wounds are all closed in meticulous fashion with a 4-0 or 5-0 absorbable suture in the deep layers and

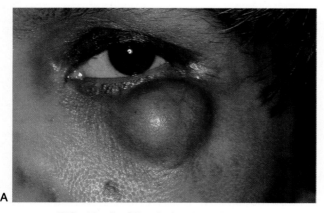
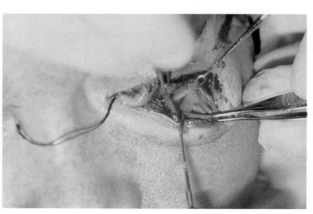

A

B

FIG. 26. A: Silastic implant in orbital floor with overlying cyst. Graft is becoming extruded. **B:** Silastic fragment extruding. Note fibrous capsule surrounding implant. (From ref. 11, with permission.)

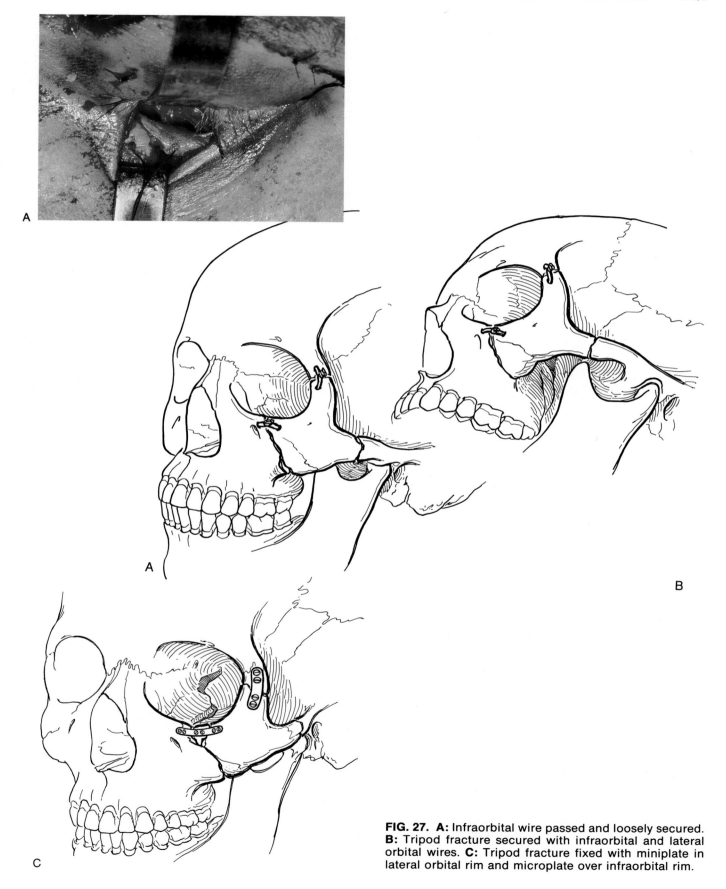

FIG. 27. A: Infraorbital wire passed and loosely secured. **B:** Tripod fracture secured with infraorbital and lateral orbital wires. **C:** Tripod fracture fixed with miniplate in lateral orbital rim and microplate over infraorbital rim.

5-0 or 6-0 monofilament suture in the skin. In repairing the infraorbital incision, closure of the skin is all that is necessary. The perosteum and orbicularis muscles do not require suturing. A finger splint is then placed over the area of repaired bone.

Body Fracture

A fracture through the zygomatic body is very similar to a tripod fracture and is often considered the same, despite the fact that the most posterior fracture, in these cases, is usually through the malar body, rather than the zygomatic arch. Body fractures deserve special attention because of their common tendency to relapse. Although they may be accompanied by a fracture of the arch, a separate fracture line traverses the zygomatic body from the lateral extent of the orbital floor down through the lateral maxillary sinus wall. Commonly the result of considerable force, they usually present with marked malar flattening.

Reduction is difficult because of the loss of purchase by the elevator with the fracture being anterior to the zygomatic arch. The elevator in the infratemporal fossa just cannot reach the displaced fragment. A large urethral sound placed through an antral–meatal window provides the force and leverage against the inner surface of the zygomatic recess necessary for adequate reduction (Fig. 28).

Once reduction has been achieved, fixation presents another problem. The usual two-point wire fixation employed in the tripod fracture will not be effective in body fractures. The support of the anterior aspect of the reduced arch given by the temporalis muscle in the tripod fracture is lost in those of the malar body. Consequently, a three-point fixation is required. In addition, the only fracture through the lateral orbital rim may be where it gains the orbital floor, making the

placement of the drill holes and insertion of fixation wire difficult. Additional exposure may be obtained by extending the brow incision into a crow's foot laterally, creating a triangular skin flap through which to work (Fig. 29A). The third point of fixation is at the lateral maxillary wall inferiorly, done via a Caldwell–Luc incision. Drill holes through the lateral maxillary wall attached to the fragment and through that portion connected to the alveolar ridge are done and a fixation wire is placed through both (Fig. 29B). This is difficult to do but forms a firm anchor point inferiorly. If much comminution exists at this site, a bone graft may have to be interposed in order to maintain adequate fragment position. The best solution to fractures of the zygomatic body is the use of plating. The miniplates designed for the maxilla are best. A Y-plate is utilized in the orbital fracture and an X-plate for the body fracture (Fig. 29C).

Finally, a firm antral pack is placed to shore up the repair. The pack is left in for 2 to 3 weeks; however, if it becomes infected it is withdrawn sooner. In some instances, the pack can substitute for the antral wire; however, the wire forms the best support. Without these precautions, relapse is very common in this group of fractures.

PLATING PROCEDURE

An increasingly popular alternative to the wiring of facial fractures is the use of metal plates. Various alloys have been used, but currently the most popular appears to be those containing titanium. The plates come in multiple sizes and shapes; and one system has mandibular, mini, and micro sets. The screws are of variable length and many are self-tapping. The mini set is most adaptable to the zygoma (Fig. 30). Accurate bending of the plate is essential so that it will conform

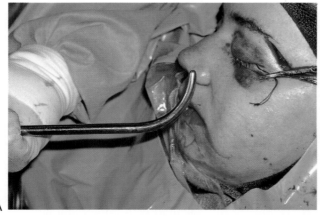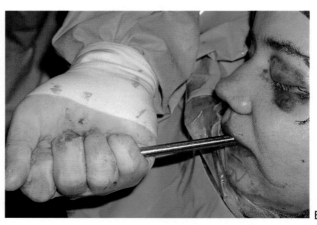

FIG. 28. A: A urethral sound introduced through a Caldwell–Luc incision. **B:** Upward and lateral pressure is used to reduce zygomatic body fracture. (From ref. 11, with permission.)

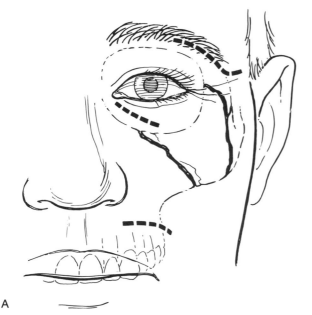

A

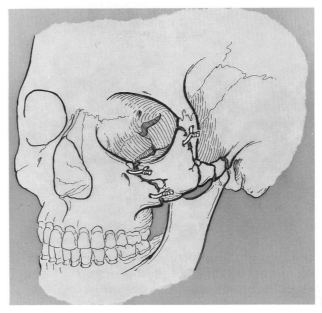

B

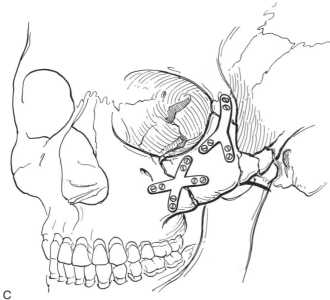

C

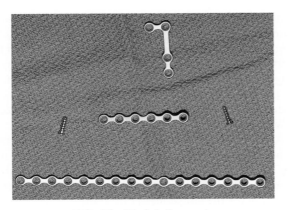

FIG. 30. Miniplating set.

FIG. 29. **A:** Incisions for approach to zygomatic body. Note extension of brow incision into "crow's foot" crease laterally. **B:** Fixation wires placed to maintain fracture reduction. **C:** Miniplates used for fixation. Y-plate is used at orbitozygomatic suture and X-plate stabilizes body. (From ref. 11, with permission.)

to the curve of the bony surface. Errors in conformation of the plate to the bone will be translated into a permanent malposition of the fracture fragment. At least two screws are placed in each fragment. Only one plate is usually necessary. It is placed over the lateral orbital rim and onto the zygomatic body. Drilling the holes slowly, using an in-and-out motion, at a low speed with constant irrigation will prevent burning of the bone with later osteonecrosis and loosening of the screws. A depth gauge is provided to measure screw length. A wide selection of screws in even numbered lengths is provided.

In comminuted fractures of the infraorbital rim, bony continuity can be provided with wiring or the use of microplates (Fig. 31). The microplates have short self-

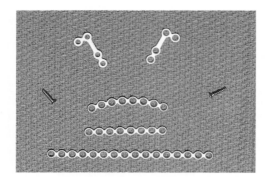

FIG. 31. Microplating set.

tapping screws, are lightweight, and are barely palpable under the skin.

In fractures of the zygomatic body, a plate may be required to connect the lateral orbital rim to the malar eminence, but an additional curved plate between the alveolar ridge and the body may be required as well. This will reinforce the posterior buttress of the midface (Fig. 29C).

The main advantage of plating is the rigid stability provided with fixation at a single site. The disadvantages are the precision required to accurately bend the plate to the appropriate shape and the complaints of pain or being able to feel the plate postoperatively.

OLD FRACTURES

The management of old unrepaired fractures is much more difficult than handling them when fresh. Once 10 to 14 days have passed, the fracture begins to heal. At this stage, it is difficult or impossible to reduce the fracture even with the sturdy Rowe–Killey elevator and maximum force. An osteotome placed in the fracture sites with refracturing throughout the circumference of the fracture is often necessary to loosen the fragment.

Fractures that are 6 to 12 months old, or older, present quite a different problem (Fig. 14). The small fragments impacted at the fracture edges that resulted from the medial displacement of the zygoma during the initial traumatic episode absorb during the healing period. On the other hand, the usual downward displacement of the fragment produces a gap at the zygomaticofrontal suture area. This gap subsequently fills in with fibrous tissue that slowly ossifies. The overlying skin and soft tissue contract in against the displaced bone, producing, in many instances, a hideous deformity (Fig. 32).

The assessment of these fractures in anticipation of repair must involve a consideration of the soft tissue as well as skeletal elements. Many of these patients have enophthalmos as a result of trauma to the perior-

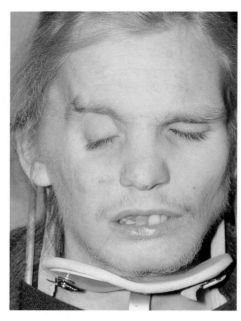

FIG. 32. Hideous deformity resulting from 12-month-old unrepaired zygomatic fracture with marked displacement. (From ref. 11, with permission.)

bital fat with absorption and/or prolapse of orbital tissues into the maxillary antrum. Depressed, widened, or hypertrophic scars may overlie the site of injury. The management of these will be discussed in the section on complications.

Radiographic assessment of the deformity can be done by plane films, CAT scanning, and three-dimensional reconstruction of the CAT scan. The Waters view will depict the amount of lengthening of the lateral orbital wall on the fracture side. A line drawn obliquely through the normal orbit will be considerably shorter than this line drawn through that of the fractured side. Calculations can be made to help predict how much lateral wall bone removal will be necessary to restore the normal orbit size (Fig. 33). The CAT scan will portray accurately the degree of displacement of the fragment in the posterior–anterior and medial–lateral planes (Fig. 16). Three-dimensional reconstruction is an exciting innovation, presently in its infancy, that reproduces from the data stored on the CAT scan tape a three-dimensional image in any projection desired (Fig. 17B). Also, using this technology, an implant can be produced that will fill the defect or that can act as a template to produce a graft of alloplastic or homograft material for this purpose.

A facial moulage may be done by taking a facial impression with an algenate compound and then making a cast in stone (Fig. 34). An acrylic implant can then be made by waxing in the defect to produce the template for the subsequent fabrication of the alloplast. The facial moulage is a simple technique that produces

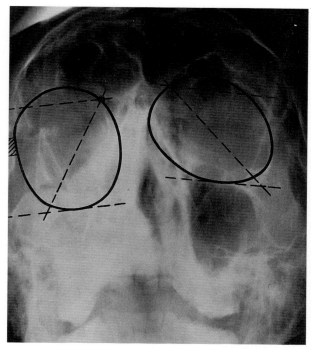

FIG. 33. Waters view showing, on the fracture side, the increased length of an oblique line drawn from the superior–medial to the lateral–inferior border of the orbit. Triangulation reveals the elongation on the fracture side. (From ref. 11, with permission.)

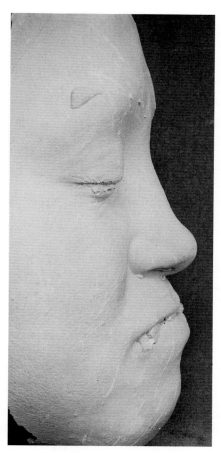

FIG. 34. Facial moulage of patient with facial fracture. (From ref. 11, with permission.)

an accurate three-dimensional, visible, and palpable reproduction of the defect. It is extremely valuable in any proposed facial skeletal reconstructive effort. Facial moiré photography (19) is another method of depicting the deformity and an excellent way of producing a photographic comparison of pre- and post-operative results.

The reconstruction of a malunion of a displaced zygoma fracture can be done by bony repositioning or onlay grafting. The method I prefer is zygomatic osteotomy and iliac crest bone grafting. At times, the nature of the fracture is so severe that the osteotomy and repositioning technique will need augmentation with onlay grafts.

Bernstein (20) has best described the technique of the osteotomy treatment of delayed fractures. This technique involves osseous incision of the entire zygomatic fracture with an osteotome, excision of a portion of the lateral orbital rim, and the interpositional bone grafting in the maxillary osteotomy site.

The approach is through three incisions: the brow, the infraorbital region, and the gingival–buccal sulcus (Fig. 29). An alternative incision is through a coronal scalp flap. The fracture site in the lateral orbital rim is exposed. The previously calculated height of bone is removed in a rectangular piece with a power saw, cutting bur, or osteotome. Once the periorbita is elevated

and the eye is protected by a retractor, the saw cut is carried down to the infraorbital fissure through the same incision. Using the infraorbital incision, the fracture site in the inferior orbital rim is identified and the osteotome is driven through the rim at this site and carried back to the anterior aspect of the infraorbital groove. Subperiosteal dissection along the fracture line inferiorly proceeds along the face of the maxilla and around its side laterally. The osteotomy proceeds on the face of the maxilla from the infraorbital rim along the fracture site to as far as possible into the infratemporal fossa. A gingival–buccal sulcus incision completes the exposure and the osteotomy cut in the anterolateral maxillary wall is connected to that in the lateral orbital wall in the infratemporal fossa. The arch is cut across from above, and care is taken to see if one or two fractures exist at this latter site.

The fracture is mobilized with the Rowe–Killey forceps and lifted into position. Drill holes are placed in the lateral orbital and infraorbital rims, and wires are passed through them or a miniplate is used. As the fracture is reduced, a gap opens in the inferior aspect of the fracture. This gap in the anterior and lateral walls

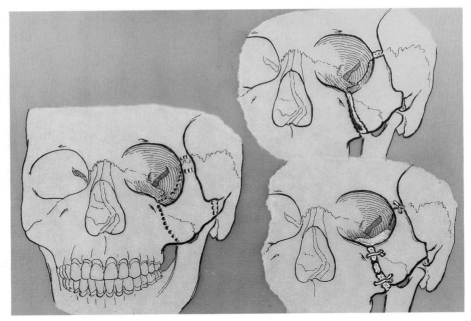

FIG. 35. Osteotomy and repositioning of old zygoma fracture. **Left:** Lines of osteotomy and area of osteotomy from lateral orbital rim. **Right:** Reduction of fracture with interposition of bone grafts. (From ref. 11, with permission.)

of the maxillary sinus needs to be filled with a bone graft either from the iliac crest or split calvarium (Fig. 35). Fixation can also be done using plates and screws.

If the zygoma has been crushed during the prior traumatic event, the reduced zygoma may yet still be inadequate to provide the correct projection at the malar eminence. Some form of onlay grafting will be required. A host of alloplasts and tissues are available for implantation. My preference is irradiated cartilage, because it suffers relatively little absorption where overlying muscle exerts pressure on it and it is easy to carve. Split calvarium works well also.

A simpler method of remediation of these deformities is with the use of an onlay graft. Either homologous grafts or alloplastic materials can be used. Materials such as acrylic, Silastic rubber, proplasts, and supramid mesh are among a few of the implants commonly used. I avoid the use of alloplastic materials because of their general lack of biointegration, a tendency to slip, and a propensity for extrusion. Although many biological implants tend to absorb to a greater or lesser degree, they tend to conform to the requirements of the local tissues, become fixed in situ by fibrous tissue, are easy to carve, and have a low incidence of infection or extrusion. Iliac crest, rib, and split calvarium are the most commonly used bone grafts. Autologous or preserved costal cartilage grafts are easiest to carve, but the fresh material tends to warp after carving. Irradiated cartilage has a long history of successful usage (21), although a recent report

indicates a high incidence of absorption over the long term (22).

A pocket is created over the defect through a brow incision extended into a crow's foot. The pocket should only be deep enough and wide enough to accommodate the implant and is made subperiosteally. The graft is carved to accommodate the defect being sure to allow for extension from the zygomatic body onto the lateral orbital rim and the infraorbital rim if deficiencies exist there. The graft should be made too large to start with and then is trimmed and sculpted until the desired shape is attained. For both the lateral and infraorbital rim extension, care is taken to feather the edges to avoid an obvious step-off at the recipient bone–graft interface. A well contoured onlay graft will restore excellent facial symmetry and balance.

COMPLICATIONS

Ophthalmologic

The most serious complications of zygomatic fractures are those associated with ocular dysfunction. Earlier in this chapter, the types of ocular injury are described. If not treated, any of them could cause permanent damage. The gravest problem, of course, is permanent blindness. This can arise as the result of injury to the optic nerve, retrobulbar hemorrhage, rupture of the globe, serious injury to the vitreous body, retinal tears, or massive injury to the anterior chamber.

Although the blindness may occur at the time of injury, it may also occur during the reduction. In Karlan's (22) review of the literature, he found fewer than 20 cases of blindness reported following reduction of zygomatic fractures. The first case was reported by Gordon and McCrae (23) in 1950. Dingman *(personal communication)* described three cases in which blindness occurred following transantral reduction through a Caldwell–Luc approach. However, Crumley et al. (24), in a series of 160 patients with orbital floor fractures, reported no instance of blindness following reduction. In my own experience, there have been no instances of postoperative blindness. During my training, however, a colleague repaired a zygoma fracture that had been sustained some 15 years prior and then had the patient awaken with blindness in the ipsilateral eye.

Blindness occurring during the repair of a zygoma fracture can result either from the aggravation of a previously undiagnosed intraocular problem or from the impaction of bony fracture fragments into the optic nerve. A thorough preoperative ophthalmologic exam is essential. Additionally, a careful inspection of the radiographs is done to rule out a fracture near the orbital apex. Fractures in this vital region definitely rule out malar fracture reduction unless the eye is already blinded. Even onlay grafting is dangerous. If, on the CAT scan, a bony fragment is seen impinging on the optic nerve and there is evidence of failing vision, operative decompression of the optic canal is indicated. Although some controversy exists concerning the use of steroids and observation versus operative intervention, I feel that the presence of a spicule within the optic canal mitigates decompression, especially in the case of progressively failing vision.

In the early postoperative period vigilance for postreduction hematoma is essential as retro-orbital hematoma is another important cause of blindness. Proptosis, pain, ptosis, increasing intraocular tension, and especially diminished visual acuity are important warning signs. Bleeding from the anterior and posterior ethmoid vessels, as well as intraorbital vessels, results in a hematoma causing optic nerve compression. Restriction of fluid administration and immediate decompression of the orbit into the maxillary antrum, ethmoid bloc, or both, will often alleviate the problem.

Diminished visual acuity was seen postoperatively in 30% of patients in the Crumley et al. (24) series. However, 28% of the patients improved and only 2% became worse.

Persistent diplopia is probably the commonest ophthalmologic complication following zygomatic repair. In Karlan's (22) review, approximately 7% of patients had this complication. Diplopia in primary gaze is exceedingly rare after fracture reduction, but in extremes of gaze, especially in the superior fields, it is not uncommon. Because these fields of gaze are infrequently

used, this complication is not debilitating and usually goes unnoticed by the patient. Harley (25) states that if the inferior rectus and inferior oblique muscles are entrapped for longer than 2 months, the chances of persistent diplopia in these patients is high. Because neuropraxia and direct muscle trauma can result in muscle impairment for up to 6 months (6), such a delay is necessary prior to the consideration of any muscle balance surgery.

Enophthalmos may result from either fat absorption or persistent prolapse of orbital contents either into the antrum or, to a much lesser extent, into the ethmoid or frontal sinuses. The so-called blow-in fracture of the ethmoid sinuses is very uncommon and rarely results in prolapse of fat and permanent enophthalmos. If the actual orbital size is increased by an unrepaired or poorly reduced zygoma fracture, then enophthalmos will result. Harley (25) reported an 11% incidence of persistent marked enophthalmos and a 12% incidence of a minor degree of the deformity for a total of 23% after zygoma fracture reduction. Atonen et al. (26) reported a total incidence of 41% with 15% marked and 26% minor enophthalmos. If the fracture had lost its reduction and the orbital volume is excessive, a refracture as previously described will reduce orbital size and help in correction. A prolapsed floor, even if markedly displaced when reduced, will produce significant improvement (Fig. 36).

Lost volume from fat absorption is a particularly vexing problem. Although surgical correction by the implantation of glass beads (27) or other materials has been recommended, the real danger of inducing blindness in an otherwise healthy eye renders these procedures extremely hazardous. This technique is usually limited to an orbit with a nonseeing eye. Orbitotomies and insertions of bone grafts through the lateral, inferior, or superior walls have been described (6). The most popular is the insertion of a split calvarial graft next to the lateral orbital wall. Finally, the use of the craniofacial techniques developed by Tessier have been modified to do circumferential orbitotomies, strip resection, and orbital volume reduction—a prodigous surgical undertaking to solve a comparatively minor aesthetic problem.

Infraorbital Nerve Symptoms

The fracture line frequently passes through the infraorbital canal and foramen. One of the annoying complications is persistent anesthesia or hypoesthesia over the distribution of the infraorbital nerve, or persistent neuralgia following fracture repair. It may result from the blow responsible for the injury or the impingement of fracture fragments. Table 1 describes the incidence in three large series of persistent neurosensory disturb-

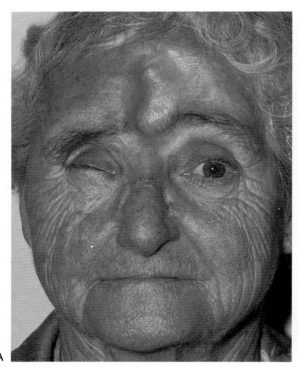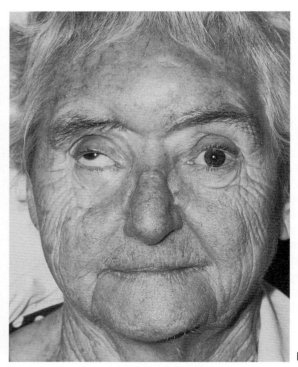

A   B

FIG. 36. A: Elderly woman with old zygoma fracture and marked disruption of orbital floor with prolapse of globe into the maxillary sinus. **B:** Postoperative appearance after placement of large irradiated cartilage graft in orbital floor. This patient also had cranioplasty to repair a forehead defect. (From ref. 11, with permission.)

ance following open and closed reduction. This high incidence is rather alarming, but most of the symptoms are of reduced sensibility. Neuralgia, which is fortunately uncommon, is exceedingly difficult to manage. Although surgical decompression has been recommended by some, the results are highly unpredictable. Prior to any surgical attempt, an exhaustive discussion with the patient concerning the variability of success in these cases is mandatory. Various forms of nerve ablation also have limited success.

Ectropion

Ectropion can result from an unrepaired fracture when the prolapsed globe pulls away from the lower

eyelid. In repaired fractures, ectropion most commonly results from fibrous adhesion of the cutaneous scar from the infraorbital incision to the bony infraorbital rim (Fig. 37). This is most often the result of neglecting to "stair-step" the incision from the skin through the orbicularis oculi and onto the upper maxilla. When the incision goes straight through to the rim, the cutaneous incision often adheres to the septum orbitale, which in turn cicatrizes down to the underlying bone. This is more commonly experienced when the incision is made in an infraciliary crease than when made lower down on the lid (31).

Unless the orbital floor is poorly repaired or marked fat absorption has resulted in severe enophthalmos, the ectropion secondary to globe retraction will be reversed by repair of the fracture. Most ectropion resulting from the infraorbital incision will disappear with time as the process of healing progresses with absorption of edema fluid and maturation of the scar. Massaging of the scar daily will greatly enhance this process.

In those cases in which ectropion secondary to scar formation does not remit, the scar will require revision. The binding of the soft tissues to the septum orbitale and to the rim is incised and released, then each layer is closed individually. The incision of course must be "stair-stepped" in order to avoid relapse of the defor-

TABLE 1. *Neurosensory disturbances persisting after surgery*

Series	Incidence of open reduction	Incidence of closed reduction
Lund (29)	65%	40%
Altonen et al. (26)	57%	27%
Hardt and Steinhauser (30)	22%	20%

From ref. 28, with permission.

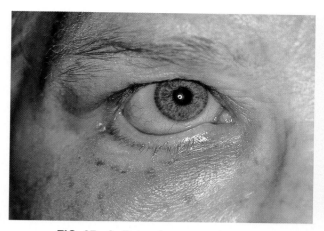
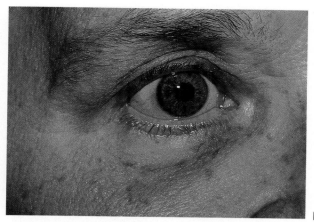

FIG. 37. A: Ectropion secondary to scarring of subciliary incision to septum orbitale. **B:** This was corrected over time by vigorous massage. (From ref. 11, with permission.)

mity. On rare occasions, a full thickness skin graft from the upper lid may be needed to correct the deformity.

Lid Edema

Lower lid edema most commonly results from an incision in the inferior infraorbital crease that has extended the entire width of the eye (Fig. 25). The important pathophysiological factors appear to be the obstruction to lymphatic drainage from the eyelid and scar contracture of the slightly trapdoor-shaped scar. Much of the edema spontaneously resolves as exemplified in the modified Khunt–Szymanowski flap seen in Fig. 38, which was used for reconstructing a midfacial defect.

Lack of spontaneous correction may then be remedied by the use of a couple of Z-plasties to break up the line and reduce the cicatricial element of the deformity.

Coronoid Process Ankylosis

The problems related to unreduced or improperly reduced zygomatic fractures are not only reflected in the malar bone per se but also to its effect on the mandible. Specifically, the lack of adequate reduction of the zygomatic arch can lead not only to impingement of the coronoid process on the arch but to actual fibrous or fibro-osseous ankylosis of these two osseous structures (Fig. 39). This obviously causes marked restriction of jaw opening, with pain and difficulty in eating. Attempts to correct this by actively manipulating the mandible to forcibly open it are generally ineffective. However, if there is merely early fibrosis and edema, manipulation may be successful.

If only impingement exists, correction is effected by osteotomy of the zygomatic arch. This can be done through an extension of the so-called Gillies incision in the scalp. The osteotome is slid in the subtemporalis plane onto the arch. Osteotomies are created at the three points of fracture and a stout elevator is used to lift the arch out laterally. If there is much in the way of fibrosis to adjacent soft tissues, considerable sharp dissection may be necessary before mobilization of the fragments can be achieved. Once the arch is in position, packing is needed to keep the arch out. A rolled up Penrose drain covered in antibiotic ointment or a pack of iodoform ribbon gauze is placed in the infratemporal fossa and under the arch, giving it support. The packing is removed 10 to 14 days later.

Ankylosis of the coronoid process of the mandible to the arch presents a difficult problem. This ankylosis may be fibrous or bony and prohibits any significant motion of the jaw. Diagnosis is made on the clinical presentation and confirmed radiographically. An axial CAT scan and polytomography in the coronal plane will usually delineate the problem. The approach to the amelioration of this problem is done by a more direct route than the Gillies approach for the uncomplicated arch fracture. Either an intraoral or preauricular incision is used, supplemented by a lateral brow incision if necessary. The preauricular incision is carried onto the scalp and carried forward in a hockey-stick fashion (Fig. 40). A small skin flap is elevated anteriorly. A short incision (4 to 6 mm long) over the zygomatic arch periosteum allows a subperiosteal dissection over the posterior aspect of the arch and carries the elevator inferiorly to the fracture site, where its attachment to the coronoid process can be visualized. Although formerly coronoid resection was advised (15), this is no longer done. The fractured arch is freed up from the coronoid with sharp dissection or, if necessary, by osteotomy. An intraoral approach may best expose the coronoid process and provide the most advantageous

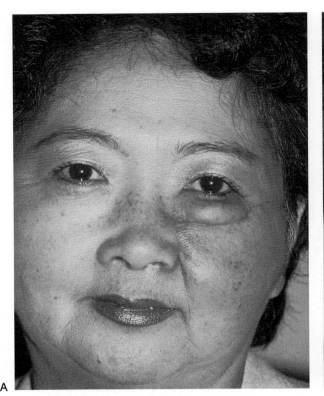
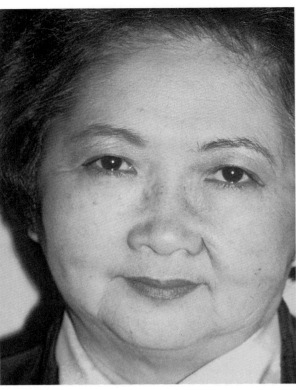

A   B

FIG. 38. A: Patient with marked lid edema 2 months following an infraorbital incision that extended the width of the palpebral fissure and beyond as part of a Khunt–Szymanowski flap reconstruction of the face. **B:** Resolution 7 months later after treatment with vigorous massage. (From ref. 11, with permission.)

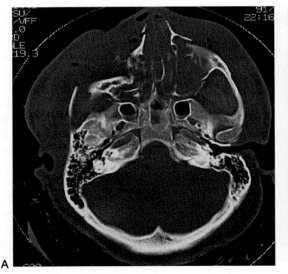
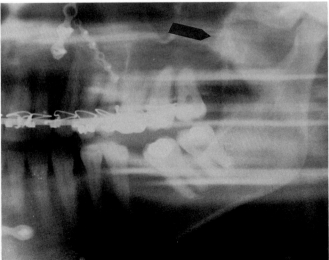

A   B

FIG. 39. A: Preoperative axial CT scan of young woman with a severely comminuted Le Fort II and III fracture and badly depressed zygomatic component. **B:** Postoperatively, she developed bony ankylosis between the coronoid process of the mandible and the zygomatic arch. (*Arrow* points to region of ankylosis.)

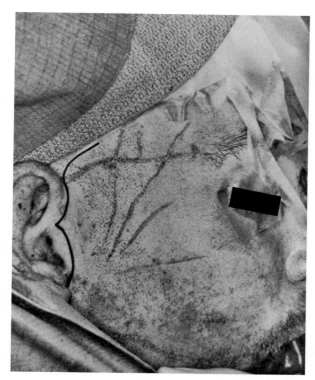

FIG. 40. Preauricular incision used as an approach to the coronoid process. The temporal branch of the facial nerve is marked out on the face. (From ref. 11, with permission.)

route for osteotomy. The coronoid and arch are separated and the arch is restored to its normal anatomical position. Once the coronoid is free, it may be advisable to place a sheet of Silastic between the process and the replaced arch that now lies lateral to it. The arch is packed into position and the packing removed in 10 to 14 days. Once the packing is removed, vigorous jaw exercises are necessary to restore effective opening.

REFERENCES

1. Matsunaga RS, Simpson W. Simplified protocol for the treatment of malar fractures. *Arch Otolaryngol* 1977;103:535.
2. Schuchardt K, Schwenzer N, Rottke B, Lentrodt J. Ursachen Haufigkeit und Lokalisation der Frakturen desGesichsschadels. *Fortschr Kiefer Gesichtschia* 1966;11:1.
3. Shumrick DA. Malar zygomatic fractures in maxillofacial trauma. In: Mathog RN, ed. *Maxillofacial trauma.* Baltimore: Williams & Wilkins, 1984;340–349.
4. Fienstein RF, Krizek TJ. Fractures of the zygoma and zygomatic arch in surgery of facial bone fractures. In: Foster CA, Sherman JE, eds. *Surgery of facial bone fractures.* New York: Churchill Livingstone, 1987.
5. Lentrodt J. Maxillofacial injuries—statistics and causes of accidents. In: Kriger E, Schilli W, eds. *Oral and maxillofacial traumatology,* vol. I. Chicago: Quintessence Publishing Company, 1982;43–47.
6. Zide BM, Jelks GW. *Surgical anatomy of the orbit.* New York: Raven Press, 1985;5.
7. Jelks GW, La Trenta G. Orbital fractures. In: Foster CA, Sherman JE, eds. *Surgery of facial bone fractures.* New York: Churchill Livingstone, 1987;67–91.
8. Grant JB. *Grant's atlas of anatomy,* 6th ed. Baltimore: Williams & Wilkins, 1972.
9. Nahum AM, Gatts JD, Gadd WE, et al. Impact tolerance of the skull and face. In: *Proceedings of the 12th Stop Car Crash Conference.* Warrendale, PA: Society of Automotive Engineers, 1988;302–316.
10. Winstanley RD. The management of fractures of zygoma. *Int J Oral Surg* 1981;10(5):235.
11. Donald PJ. Zygomatic fractures. In: English GM, ed. *Otolaryngology.* Philadelphia: Lippincott, 1990.
12. Knight JS, North JF. The classification of malar fractures: an analysis of displacement as a guide to treatment. *Br J Plast Surg* 1961;13:325–339.
13. Dingman RO, Natvig P. *Surgery of facial fractures.* Philadelphia: Saunders, 1969;212–213.
14. Rowe NL, Killey HC. *Fractures of the facial skeleton,* 2nd ed. Edinburgh: E&S Livingstone, 1970;276–344.
15. Yanigasawa E. Symposium on maxillofacial trauma. III. Pitfalls in the management of zygomatic fractures. *Laryngoscope* 1973;83:527.
16. Foster CA, Sherman JE, eds. *Surgery of facial bone fractures.* New York: Churchill Livingstone, 1987.
17. Dolan KD, Jacoby CG, Wendy RKS. *Radiology of facial injury.* Philadelphia: Field & Wood, 1988.
18. Adams WM. Internal wiring fixation of facial fractures. *Surgery* 1942;12:523–540.
19. Karlan MS. Contour analysis in plastic and reconstructive surgery. *Arch Otolaryngol* 1979;105:670–679.
20. Bernstein L. Delayed management of facial fractures. *Laryngoscope* 1970;80:1323–1341.
21. Donald PJ. Cartilage grafting in facial reconstruction with special consideration of irradiated grafts. *Laryngoscope* 1986;96:786–807.
22. Karlan MS. Complications of malar fractures. In: Mathog RN, ed. *Maxillofacial trauma.* Baltimore: Williams & Wilkins, 1984;350–359.
23. Gordon S, McCrae II. Monocular blindness as a complication of the treatment of a malar fracture. *Plast Reconstr Surg* 1981;68:94–99.
24. Crumley RL, Leibsohn J, Krause CJ, Burton TC. Fractures of the orbital floor. *Laryngoscope* 1977;87:934–947.
25. Harley RD. Surgical management of persistent diplopia in blow-out fractures of the orbit. *Ann Ophthalmol* 1975;7:1621.
26. Altonen M, Kohonen A, Dickhoff K. Treatment of zygoma fractures: internal wiring, antral packing, reposition without fixation. *J Oral Maxillofac Surg* 1976;4:107.
27. Taiara C, Smith BM. Correction of enophthalmos and deep sulcus by posterior subperiosteal glass bead implantation. *Br J Ophthalmol* 1973;75:741–746.
28. Mathog RH. *Maxillofacial trauma.* Baltimore: Williams & Wilkins. 1984;358.
29. Lund K. Fractures of zygoma: a follow-up study of 62 patients. *J Oral Surg* 1971;29:557.
30. Hardt H, Steinhauser EW. Treatment results after zygomatic orbital fractures. *Schweiz Monatsschr Fahnheilkd* 1976;86:825.
31. Shray RC, Holtmann B, Ribando JM, et al. A comparison of conjunctival and subciliary incisions for orbital fractures. *Br J Plast Surg* 1977;30:142.

CHAPTER 24

Orbital Blow-out Fractures

Dwight R. Kulwin and Robert C. Kersten

A blow-out fracture of the orbit is defined as an isolated fracture of an orbital wall not involving the orbital rim. Such fractures typically involve the orbital floor and/or medial wall.

In the vast majority of circumstances, the fracture is displaced away from the orbital cavity. Thus the orbital floor is "blown-out" into the maxillary sinus, the medial wall is "blown-out" into the ethmoid sinus, the orbital roof is "blown-out" into the frontal sinus and/or intracranial cavity, and the lateral wall is "blown-out" into the temporalis fossa.

Upon occasion, rather than being displaced away from the orbit, an orbital wall may be displaced into the orbital cavity. While such fractures are termed "blown-in" fractures, rather than "blow-out" fractures, the mechanism of injury is similar.

RELEVANT CLINICAL ANATOMY

The orbit is pyramidal in shape with its apex directed posteriorly, superiorly, and medially toward the optic foramen. The base of the pyramid (the orbital rim) is in the frontal plane of the face. The orbital rims are composed of the frontal bone superiorly, the zygoma laterally, the frontal process of the maxilla medially, and the maxilla inferiorly.

The orbit has four walls. The medial wall (from anterior to posterior) is formed by the frontal process of the maxillary bone, the lacrimal bone, the lamina papyracea of the ethmoid bone, and the lesser wing of the sphenoid. The orbital floor is composed of the maxillary bone, the zygomatic bone (laterally), and the palatine bone. The lateral wall is composed entirely of the zygomatic bone, and the roof is defined by the frontal bone.

The lateral wall of the orbit is the thickest of the four walls and rarely is involved in an orbital blow-out fracture. Similarly, the orbital roof is a rather sturdy structure and susceptible to being blown-out only in those individuals with extremely large and extensive frontal sinuses, who tend to have a thinner than average orbital roof.

While the medial wall of the orbit is actually thinner (0.5 mm in thickness) than the orbital floor (1 mm in thickness), it is functionally stronger as it is supported by the many fine bony septations of the ethmoid sinus.

The orbital floor is by far the weakest of the four orbital walls. Not only is it quite thin, but it is virtually unsupported across its entire span and is further weakened by a central dehiscence, the infraorbital groove and canal.

The four rectus (superior, inferior, medial, and lateral) and the superior oblique muscles arise in the posterior portion of the orbit from the annulus of Zinn that surrounds the optical canal. The inferior oblique muscle arises from the posterior lacrimal crest. Together, these six muscles surround the eye. Between them is a fibrous network, the intermuscular septum. This effectively separates the orbit into two compartments, an intraconal (intramuscular) space and the extraconal space.

Both the intraconal and extraconal spaces have their respective fat pads, which serve to cushion and protect the eye. These fat pads are actually collections of variously sized fat globules, which are held in place by a fine fibrous meshwork extending throughout the orbit, attaching to various bony structures, the intermuscular septum, the extraocular muscles, and the orbital septum. There is little, if any, fat between the medial rectus and the medial orbital wall, while there is a large amount of fat around the inferior rectus and between it and the orbital floor.

Coursing from posterior to anterior along the orbital floor, and arising in the inferior orbital fissure, is the infraorbital neurovascular bundle. Posteriorly, it lies in a groove in the superior portion of the orbital floor.

As the bundle gently angles inferiorly it becomes covered with bone to form a canal, finally emerging onto the anterior maxillary face 4 mm below the inferior orbital rim. In addition to supplying sensory innervation to its facial dermatome, the infraorbital nerve, through small, delicate dentate branches, provides sensation to the ipsilateral upper gum and teeth.

In completing our discussion of orbital anatomy relevant to understanding orbital wall fractures, one must mention several vessels that perforate the orbital walls. At the top of the medial orbital wall, at the ethmoidal–frontal suture line, lie the anterior and posterior ethmoidal vessels. When disrupted, these large, high-pressure vessels can be a significant source of orbital hemorrhage. Similarly, along the orbital floor, disruption of the infraorbital neurovascular bundle can be a significant source of orbital bleeding. Approximately halfway along its course from posterior to anterior, a large orbital perforating vessel arises from the infraorbital artery, passing up through the intermuscular septum. When disrupted, this can cause significant orbital, and even intramuscle, conal hemorrhage.

PATHOPHYSIOLOGY OF ORBITAL FRACTURES

There are two prevailing theories as to the physiology of isolated orbital wall fractures. The commonly discussed "hydraulic theory" suggests that when a force (fist, ball, high-pressure air or water stream, etc.) with a diameter smaller than the opening of the orbital rim hits the eye, this results in a marked increase in orbital pressure due to acute posterior movement of the eye. This force is then transmitted to the relatively thin orbital walls, causing them to give way and fracture outward, as the force required to rupture the eye itself is usually greater than that required to blow-out the orbital wall.

The alternative "buckling theory" suggests that force applied to the orbital rims may cause them to deform, without actually fracturing. This force is transmitted to the thin orbital walls, causing them to buckle and fracture. This theory is consistent with case reports of isolated orbital wall fractures in which eye protection is worn at the time of insult, or cases in which laterality of the traumatic force rules out the hydraulic theory.

It may well be a combination of both mechanisms, or additional unknown causes, that explains the universe of orbital blow-out fractures.

DIAGNOSIS OF ORBITAL WALL FRACTURES

Symptoms and Signs of Orbital Wall Fractures

The symptoms and signs caused by an orbital blow-out fracture depend on the particular anatomic structures involved.

Soft tissue injury, as manifested by edema and ecchymosis, is seen in the vast majority of such injuries. As a rule, the greater the degree of swelling and bruising, the greater the likelihood of a fracture. However, one can see a tremendous degree of soft tissue change without a fracture, especially if a superficial subcutaneous vessel is disrupted. Similarly, on occasion, we have seen total orbital floor fractures in which little, if any, soft tissue change was present.

As previously discussed, the weakest portion of the orbital floor is along the infraorbital groove and canal. Thus hypesthesia along the distribution of the infraorbital nerve is an invariable finding in fractures of the orbital floor, as virtually all such orbital floor fractures involve this location. Findings can vary from near total anesthesia of the entire dermatome to a history of transient numbness of the teeth and lip. The latter location is the single most sensitive area to check for sensory changes, as the fine dentate branches of the nerve coursing down through the maxillary sinus to the gums and teeth are the nerve structures most easily damaged.

On occasion, we have seen a patient with orbital trauma and infraorbital hypesthesia, in which the orbital computed tomography (CT) scan effectively rules out a floor fracture. In such cases we theorize that a direct blow to the infraorbital nerve at the site of its exit from the infraorbital foramen onto the anterior maxillary face has occurred.

Restricted range of motion of the eye is a frequent consequence of an orbital wall fracture. This may be manifested by an inability to fully move the eye in all directions, diplopia, and pain with eye movement. This is seen most commonly in fractures of the floor and occasionally in fractures of the medial wall. Very rarely do fractures of the other two walls cause decreased range of motion of the eye. Causes of restricted range of motion following orbital trauma may be mechanical, neurologic, myopathic, or combined.

In a patient with orbital trauma, if significant orbital edema and/or hemorrhage develops, the orbit may become rather tight. This may result in a mechanical inability of the eye muscles to fully move the eye. In addition, if significant displacement of the globe occurs secondary to edema and hemorrhage, double vision may develop due to anatomic misalignment of the eyes.

Herniation of orbital tissues through orbital fractures is a common occurrence. This is seen with either pathophysiologic mechanism of injury. Tissue entrapment tends to occur in small to medium blow-out fractures. Tissue may become adherent to the orbital fracture, or a trapdoor fracture may allow passage of tissue through the fracture, and then the bone may spontaneously pop back into position, trapping the tissue. In large, broad-based fractures, the entire wall is fractured and bent into the sinuses. In such cases, tissue entrapment is uncommon and a restriction of gaze is rare. Herniation of orbital fat through an orbital wall fracture is seen most commonly in orbital floor fractures and rarely in other wall fractures, for the reasons previously discussed.

Entrapment of the various fibrosepta that surround the orbital fat, be they trapped in the fracture line or adherent to the raw surface of the fracture, can mechanically inhibit normal movement of the eye, as the septa also attach to the extraocular muscles and the intermuscular septum. True entrapment of an extraocular muscle itself is much less commonly seen.

Entrapment of the interior rectus muscle and surrounding septa will inhibit vertical movement of the eye, causing vertical diplopia (double vision with images superimposed on top of each other). Similarly, entrapment of the medial rectus muscle and surrounding septa will inhibit horizontal movement of the eye, causing horizontal diplopia (double vision with images superimposed side-by-side). Initially, such tissue entrapment causes pain with movement of the involved tissues; however, this usually subsides within a few days.

The site of entrapment along the anterior/posterior plane of the orbit determines the type of motility disturbance present. Anterior entrapment (sometimes referred to as anterior tether) results in an inability of the patient to look up. If the entrapment is tight enough, the eye may be fixed and totally unable to move. In such cases, the eye may be fixed in straight-ahead gaze, or even in downgaze, depending on the mechanism of injury.

Posterior entrapment (posterior tether) tends to allow reasonably normal passive range of motion of the globe (forced ductions). Frequently, in such cases the contractile properties of the inferior rectus are diminished either mechanically or from a myopathy of the rectus at the site where the muscle fractured through the orbital wall. All this may result in a seemingly paradoxical ability of the eye to move upward or even to be fixed in an angled upward position, but the patient is unable to look down.

Entrapment of orbital tissues along a broad base or in the middle of the orbital floor will result in a combination of these findings.

In the hydraulic mechanism of blow-out fracture, as orbital pressure increases it is transmitted to the orbital walls through the orbital structures, fracturing them outward. The structure that actually presses against the wall causing it to fracture is frequently the rectus muscle. Such a blow to the muscle may result in a significant enough injury to result in at least a transient myopathy and resultant dysfunction of the muscle, causing a gaze abnormality and double vision. Post-

traumatic hemorrhage into the muscle or muscular edema may result in similar findings.

The innervation of the rectus muscles is from within the muscle cone, in the posterior one-third of the muscle. Thus a traumatic motor neuropathy is quite uncommon, although occasionally seen. A special case is when a fracture fragment penetrates the posterior portion of the intermuscular septum, injuring the nerve.

The findings in medial wall fracture entrapment are similar and analogous to those of fractures of the orbital floor.

Forced duction testing is of some value in determining the cause and site of a gaze restriction but is not as helpful as is commonly believed. If forced ductions are normal, a mechanical cause of a gaze abnormality is effectively ruled out. But even in the most experienced hands, positive forced ductions provide only a modest degree of help in differentiating between the various types and locations of mechanical restrictions.

Subcutaneous emphysema and pneumo-orbitum are indicative of a medial wall fracture. As previously stated, there is a great deal of fat in the inferior portion of the orbit. This tends to plug a floor fracture site, minimizing passage of air through the maxillary sinus into the orbit. As there is little fat between the medial rectus and the medial orbital wall, and as the lamina papyracea tend to prevent herniation of tissue into the ethmoid sinus, medial fractures tend to remain open. There is also a much more direct route for air passage into the orbit from the nasopharynx through the ethmoid sinus, than through the more circuitous route of the maxillary sinus.

Because of the aforementioned reasons, development of orbital air and subcutaneous emphysema is a much more common happenstance after medial wall fractures than orbital floor fractures.

The development of subcutaneous emphysema usually follows aggressive nose blowing by the patient. It is not uncommon for a patient to be unaware he/she has a fracture, until several days following trauma when he/she blows the nose with resultant passage of air into the eyelids and orbit, acute orbital swelling, and the development of subcutaneous emphysema. We also have seen similar circumstances in patients with facial trauma who are placed on respirators and then develop subcutaneous emphysema and pneumo-orbitum.

Another unusual circumstance resulting in subcutaneous emphysema and the development of pneumo-orbitum is the patient with a fracture of an unusually large and well-aerated frontal sinus.

Ipsilateral epistaxis is also a clinical sign of a medial wall fracture. Bleeding from a floor fracture tends to result in a maxillary hemosinus. However, in a medial wall fracture blood tends to pass spontaneously and directly into the nose. In addition, if the anterior ethmoid artery is involved in the fracture, brisk arterial bleeding may result.

This latter cause of epistaxis is important to remember, as one will see an occasional patient with a history of brisk epistaxis that will last for a short period of time, and then spontaneously stop, only to recur 5 to 10 days later. Such patients may have had a small subclinical tear of the anterior ethmoidal artery at the time of periorbital trauma, and the artery intermittently bleeds, then goes into spasm, only to bleed again when clot lysis occurs.

If there is significant enlargement of the bony orbit or diminution of orbital volume occurs from herniation of tissue into the sinuses, a change in the relationship between the size of the bony orbit and the volume of the orbital structures may occur. This is manifested by enophthalmos (posterior displacement of the eye), or hypo-ophthalmos (inferior displacement of the globe). While sometimes seen acutely, these changes usually are masked by compensatory post-traumatic edema and hemorrhage and only slowly become evident as these resolve.

Radiology of Orbital Wall Fractures

Radiographic studies of the traumatized orbit are necessary to confirm that an orbital fracture is present and to ascertain its size, location, degree of depression and evidence of tissue herniation and/or entrapment.

Plain radiographic studies may be of some value in screening patients in whom there is little evidence of an orbital wall fracture. However, one cannot ascertain to any reliable degree the size and/or degree of displacement of an orbital wall fracture from a plain film. We have seen many patients in whom plain films were normal, yet who proved on more sophisticated testing to have a very large orbital wall fracture that required treatment.

The standard Caldwell posterior/anterior frontal view is useful in evaluating the orbital rims and the superior orbital walls, the superior orbital fissure, the sphenoid ridges, and the superior portion of the orbit. The modified Waters view, with the film taken along a line parallel to the orbital floor, is best used to demonstrate the orbital floor and the maxillary sinus. Lateral views occasionally may be of some help, and of course all films should be taken in the upright position so as to best demonstrate air–fluid levels.

Computed tomography is the current radiologic gold standard for evaluation of the orbital walls. Cuts should be at 5 mm, or even better 3 mm, widths, and the views chosen should be those perpendicular to the wall one wishes to study. Therefore, when studying the orbital floor, the two best views are the direct coronal and direct sagittal scan, while in examining the medial or-

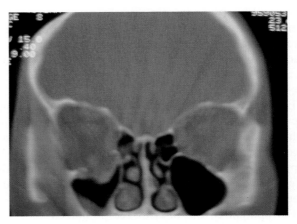

FIG. 1. Coronal orbital CT scan of large blow-out fracture.

bital wall, direct axial and direct coronal views are superior.

Both bone and soft tissue windows should be acquired, but contrast is unnecessary.

On technically good scans, one is able to accurately delineate the presence of a fracture, its size, degree of depression, and location. In addition, by using the views stated above, one can see the extraocular muscles and confirm either entrapment of the muscles or displacement of the muscles, indicative of perimuscular tissue entrapment (Figs. 1 to 4).

Technically good, clinically appropriate CT views are the *sine qua non* for thoroughly evaluating an orbital wall fracture and deciding on an appropriate treatment course.

We tend to use the following algorithm to help us decide when to order CT scans of the orbits.

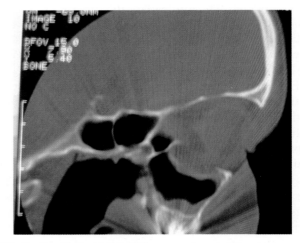

FIG. 2. Sagittal orbital CT scan of same fracture as in Fig. 1.

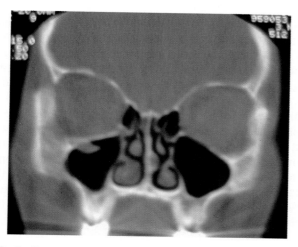

FIG. 3. Coronal orbital CT scan of same fracture as in Fig. 1 after repair with Teflon plate showing excellent reconstitution of floor.

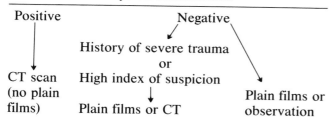

Patient with Orbital Trauma:
Physical Examination

Magnetic resonance imaging (MRI) is of little value in evaluating orbital fractures, except if one specifically wishes to look at either the optic nerve or for evidence of a significant orbital hematoma.

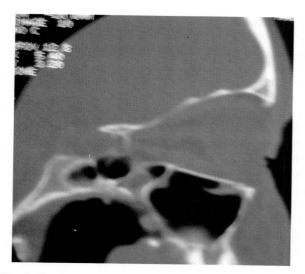

FIG. 4. Sagittal orbital CT scan of same postoperative fracture as in Fig. 1.

INITIAL MANAGEMENT

At the time of the initial evaluation, a thorough ocular examination should be performed. Significant ocular injuries have been reported to occur in 10% to 30% of patients. Corneal abrasions, anterior uveitis, lens dislocation and cataract, hyphema, glaucoma, vitreous hemorrhage, commotio retinae, retinal detachment, and traumatic neuropathy, among other pathologies, may be seen.

As the orbit is a skull base structure, a thorough neurologic evaluation is appropriate in all patients with significant orbital trauma.

Orbital evaluation is directed toward looking for the previously discussed symptoms and signs of an orbital wall fracture. In addition to the ocular evaluation, one should ascertain ocular function by measuring visual acuity, checking pupillary findings (especially looking for asymmetry or a relative afferent pupillary defect), and performing confrontational visual fields.

One must evaluate any soft tissue injury and palpate the orbital rims. Any limitation of ocular excursion should be noted and quantified, and forced ductions should be performed as appropriate. Hertel exophthalmometry measurements should be taken.

The patient is instructed to refrain from taking any aspirin-containing products or nonsteroidal anti-inflammatory drugs (because of the potential adverse effect on platelet function), in case surgery should be necessary. The patient is further advised not to blow the nose. Ice packs are employed for the first 2 to 3 days following trauma.

If there are no contraindications, oral prednisone 1 mg/kg/day may be given for 1 week. This has been shown to reduce long-term motility dysfunction as well as to more rapidly delineate those patients who will require surgery because of enophthalmos or persistent mechanical restriction of gaze. Fractures involving the medial wall have a greater incidence of orbital cellulitis. While some authors have recommended broad-spectrum antibiotic prophylaxis for 5 days' time in this subgroup, we do not routinely do so.

INDICATIONS AND TIMING FOR SURGERY

Less than 50% of patients with isolated orbital wall fractures will require surgical intervention. Indications for surgery of orbital fractures fall into two categories: (a) significant motility disturbances that are not improving and (b) a decrease in orbital volume sufficient to cause significant enophthalmos and hypo-ophthalmos.

Patients with persistent nonimproving diplopia that is clinically significant may require surgical repair. The clinical significance of a fracture can vary widely, depending on age, occupation, and the like. What is problematic for one individual may be asymptomatic for another. Surgery is indicated only for those patients in whom the restriction can be shown to be mechanical in origin (positive forced ductions) *and* can be shown radiographically to be caused by tissue entrapment in a fracture. That is, on CT scanning, one can see tissue caught in the fracture, or the rectus muscle is deviated toward the fracture side compared to the contralateral eye. Remember, there are other causes besides entrapment that can result in a mechanical restriction and positive forced ductions.

As previously stated, small to medium fractures are those most likely to result in tissue entrapment and motility disturbances. In such cases, we observe the patient every few days during the first 10 days following injury, looking for a change in extraocular motility dysfunction and forced duction testing. Surgery is best performed between 10 and 20 days following injury. Prior to this it is not possible to reliably separate out those patients requiring surgery from those who will spontaneously improve. Beyond 20 days, scar formation makes dissection more difficult. We attempt to operate on all patients with mechanical restriction of gaze within this period.

The other indication for repair of an orbital wall fracture is a fracture that has either resulted in acute enophthalmos and hypo-ophthalmos or, on CT scan, is demonstrated to be large enough to likely result in such. In these patients, CT scanning will demonstrate significant displacement (greater than 3- to 5-mm displacement of more than 50%) of an orbital wall. It has been our experience that if a patient has normal motility and a "borderline" large fracture, following the patient frequently may be reasonable; and if enophthalmos does develop, surgical intervention usually can be performed satisfactorily weeks to months later.*

SURGERY

The goals of surgery in an isolated orbital wall fracture are to elevate orbital contents out of the fracture site, to release any adhesions between orbital contents and the fracture site, to prevent any readhesion to the fracture site, and then to restore the orbital walls to a normal shape, reducing the increased orbital bony volume back to normal.

General anesthesia is used. A broad-spectrum antibiotic and dexamethasone are given intravenously at the start of the procedure. Local anesthetic with epinephrine is infiltrated across the width of the lid, prior to the surgical scrub so that 10 to 15 min will have elapsed before the incision. This allows for maximal vasoconstriction. A full face prep is performed. When draping

_____

Editor's note: This approach however, is controversial and others will opt for early intravention.

the patient, both eyes should be left exposed so that forced ductions can be performed and compared side to side. Forced ductions are performed prior to incision and additionally during the procedure, to ascertain that a complete release of any entrapment has occurred.

A number of different approaches can be used to gain access to the orbital floor. It is our preference to perform either an anterior approach through a lower lid crease incision or a posterior approach through the conjunctiva in conjunction with a lateral canthotomy and cantholysis. Either approach allows entry into the plane between orbital septum and orbicularis muscle and dissection is then carried in this plane down to the infraorbital rim (Fig. 5).

The advantage of the percutaneous approach is that it is a simpler procedure and it is not necessary to disrupt the lateral canthus. The disadvantages are that it leaves a facial scar (although this is usually almost imperceptible) and, especially in younger patients, may cause contracture of the skin muscle flap, resulting in lower lid retraction. The advantages of the conjunctival approach are the lack of visible scar and reduced risk of lid retraction. The disadvantages are that disinsertion of the lateral canthal tendon is required, and medial exposure may be more limited. More extensive canthotomy and incision of the orbicularis muscle laterally are required to fully expose medial wall fractures.

We recommend against using an infraciliary incision as there is a high incidence of postoperative eyelid retraction due to the great length of the myocutaneous flap that is elevated to reach the orbital rim.

In the lid crease approach, the lower lid crease is marked while the patient is still awake by having him look up and down. As surgery is begun, an incision is made with a scalpel and sharp dissection is carried through the orbicularis. Bipolar cautery is preferred for maintenance of hemostasis in blow-out fracture repair and other orbital surgery since unipolar cautery may be preferentially conducted along orbital nerves. Scissor dissection is then carried out inferiorly between the orbicularis muscle and the orbital septum down to the orbital rim. Every effort should be made to keep the orbital septum intact.

In the transconjunctival approach, a 3- to 5-mm lateral canthotomy is carried out with a scissor directed horizontally. The scissor is then rotated 90 degrees (inferiorly), cutting all the tissue of the lateral retinaculum (including the inferior crus of the lateral canthal tendon) between skin and conjunctiva. When this has been completed, the lateral edge of the lid can be retracted completely from the orbital rim. A scissor is used to separate the fused edge of conjunctiva, septum, and retractors, from the inferior edge of the tarsal plate, beginning at the lateral canthotomy and extending medially to the punctum. A silk suture is passed through the cut edge of conjunctiva and retractors, drawn supe-

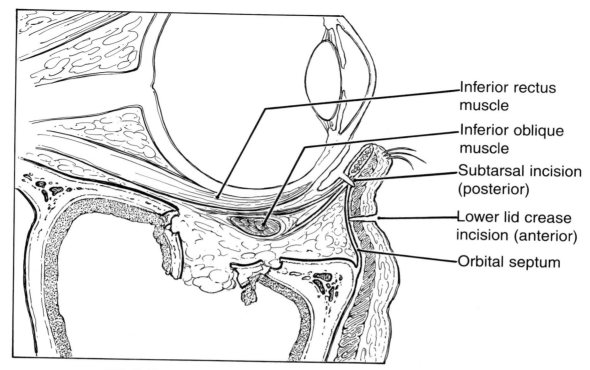

Inferior rectus muscle

Inferior oblique muscle

Subtarsal incision (posterior)

Lower lid crease incision (anterior)

Orbital septum

FIG. 5. The anterior and posterior approaches to the orbital floor.

riorly, and clamped to the drapes. This facilitates dissection between conjunctiva and retractors posteriorly and orbicularis anteriorly and also protects the cornea.

Scissor dissection is carried inferiorly between the orbicularis muscle anteriorly and the septum posteriorly down to the infraorbital rim. During dissection of the posterior approach it is important to maintain vertical traction on the lid margin to prevent folding of the skin and orbicularis, resulting in a full-thickness "button-hole" through the anterior lamella.

The plane of dissection is the same regardless of approach. The only difference is that the plane is entered posteriorly if the transconjunctival approach is used. In either approach, dissection down to the infraorbital rim is aided by frequent finger palpation to keep the position of the rim clearly in mind. Once the dissection has reached the rim, the skin muscle flap is retracted inferiorly. Soft tissue overlying the rim can be bluntly dissected until periosteum is exposed. The periosteum on the anterior edge of the rim is incised from the level of the punctum across the full width of the rim, ending just below the lateral orbital tubercle. Care must be taken to avoid straying too far inferiorly with the knife blade and so damaging the infraorbital nerve. The orbital septum can gently be held out of the way with a broad malleable retractor.

The posterior edge of the periorbita is elevated across the width of the rim with a Joseph periosteal elevator. A Freer periosteal elevator is used to elevate the periorbita posteriorly along the floor. Periorbita

overlying the floor is elevated easily except where it is entrapped by the fracture. The typical orbital fracture will be encountered 5 to 10 mm behind the rim, medially and perhaps laterally to the infraorbital neurovascular bundle. Before attempting to directly elevate the orbital contents out of the fracture, blunt dissection is carried medially and laterally around the fracture. Elevation of the uninvolved orbital contents is necessary to allow visualization and can be achieved with a malleable retractor or right angle Sewell orbital retractor. Care must be taken to relax retraction of orbital contents every few minutes to prevent ischemia of the orbital tissue or globe.

The most tedious and difficult portion of the procedure involves the elevation and disimpaction of periorbital tissues from the fracture site. The periosteal elevator is insinuated between the orbital tissue and fracture and used to pry the soft tissue from the fracture site. Two orbital retractors are helpful in lifting the prolapsed tissues in a "hand-over-hand" fashion. This is usually a frustrating and repetitive procedure as orbital contents tend to continually spill around the retractors and into the fracture. If the tissues are tightly impacted in the fracture it may be helpful to enlarge the fracture with Kerrison rongeurs in order to facilitate release of the tissues from the fracture site. With more adherent tissue or in older fractures, it may on occasion be necessary to grasp prolapsed orbital fat and fibrous tissue with a hemostat to apply traction superiorly.

There are three tissue layers that must be distin-

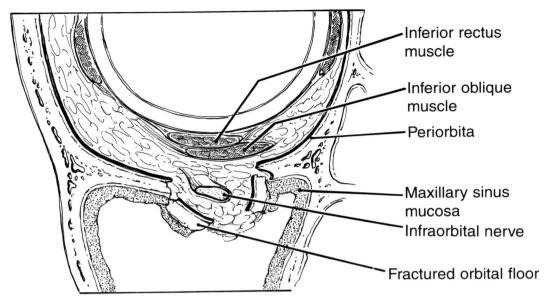

Inferior rectus
muscle

Inferior oblique
muscle

Periorbita

Maxillary sinus
mucosa

Infraorbital nerve

Fractured orbital floor

FIG. 6. There are three tissue layers that must be distinguished during the disincarceration of prolapsed orbital tissues: (a) orbital contents, superiorly; (b) maxillary sinus mucosa, inferiorly; and (c) sandwiched between these two, the infraorbital neurovascular bundle. In long-standing fractures, it can be very difficult to identify the infraorbital nerve, as the sinus mucosa and orbital contents may be adherent to it.

guished during the disincarceration of prolapsed orbital tissues: (a) orbital contents, superiorly; (b) maxillary sinus mucosa, inferiorly; and (c) sandwiched between these two, the infraorbital neurovascular bundle. In long-standing fractures it can be very difficult to identify the infraorbital nerve as the sinus mucosa and orbital contents may be adherent to it. Cautious sharp dissection may be necessary on occasion to free the nerve from adjacent scar tissue (Fig. 6).

The goal during this stage of surgery is to completely separate the orbital contents from the underlying infraorbital nerve and sinus mucosa. It is important not to incarcerate any sinus mucosa within the orbit, or an epithelial-lined cyst may develop.

The end points in this stage are the release of all adhesions between orbital tissue and the fracture and the complete elevation of the orbital contents above the plane of the fracture. This can be confirmed by direct observation of the entire floor defect and by forced ductions. Once this is achieved, attention is directed toward resurfacing the orbital floor to cover the fracture and maintain support of the orbital contents.

Orbital implants can be either alloplastic or autogenous. The vast majority of fractures can be managed nicely with alloplastic implants. We use Teflon implants, which come in three preformed sizes, for the left or right orbit. These contour nicely to the orbital floor, are stiff enough to provide adequate support, are very smooth and slippery so orbital contents will not adhere to them, and have an extremely low infection

or extrusion rate. The implants often need to be trimmed with a scissor to an appropriate contour.*

The implant is slid beneath the elevated orbital contents to cover the floor defect. The implant must be seated behind the orbital rim without impinging posteriorly on the infraorbital fissure. It needs to be sized appropriately so there is no tendency to migrate anteriorly.

Once the implant has been seated and is resting in the concavity just posterior to the infraorbital rim, forced ductions are again repeated. Occasionally, residual edema caused by the floor manipulation may cause some slight restriction compared to the contralateral side, but there should be reasonable symmetry. If there is residual restriction, the implant must be inspected closely around its entire periphery and it must be ascertained that it completely covers the fracture and that no tissue is trapped between the fracture and the implant.

For the vast majority of orbital floor fractures, no implant fixation should be necessary. The key to implant stability is to make certain the implant is large enough to completely cover the defect and yet small enough that there is no tendency to migrate anteriorly. The infraorbital rim has a natural lip, which will prevent forward migration if the implant is sized properly.

After the implant has been placed along the floor and if forced ductions are satisfactory, the periorbita is sutured to the periosteum along the infraorbital rim.

Editor's note: The senior author does not use alloplasts here because of the frequent extrusion rate in his experience.

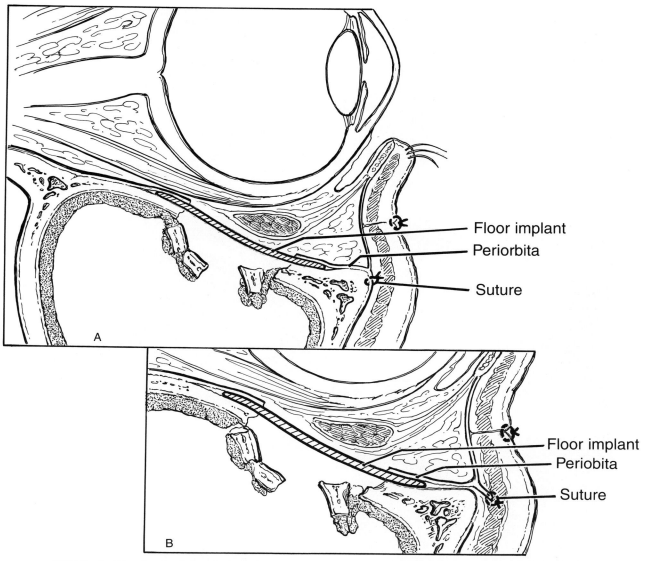

FIG. 7. A: The implant has been placed along the floor and the periorbita is sutured to the periosteum along the infraorbital rim with interrupted 5-0 Vicryl sutures. **B:** If it is impossible to suture the periorbita to the periosteum, then the suture can be passed through the orbicularis muscle overlying the periosteal edge. This will reposition the periorbita so that it will scar into satisfactory position.

Our preference is to use interrupted 5-0 Vicryl sutures. If it is not impossible to suture the periosteum over the face of the maxilla, then the suture can be passed through the orbicularis muscle directly overlying the periosteal edge (Fig. 7). This will reposition the periorbita so that it will scar into satisfactory position. After periorbital closure, forced ductions are again performed. If they show residual restriction, the periosteal suture should be released and the floor implant again inspected to ensure that it has not shifted position.

If a percutaneous approach has been used, the skin muscle flap is merely draped over the septum and the skin is closed with a 6-0 suture. A layered closure is neither necessary nor desirable, as it will tend to shorten the orbicularis layer and result in postoperative lower lid retraction.

If a transconjunctival approach is used, conjunctiva is sewn to the inferior border of the tarsus using a running 6-0 mild chromic suture.

This is begun medially. It is not necessary to bury the knot beneath the punctum as this is sufficiently medial to the cornea as to not irritate. No attempt is made to separately close the retractors as these are tightly adherent to conjunctiva and will be brought back into satisfactory position by the conjunctival closure.

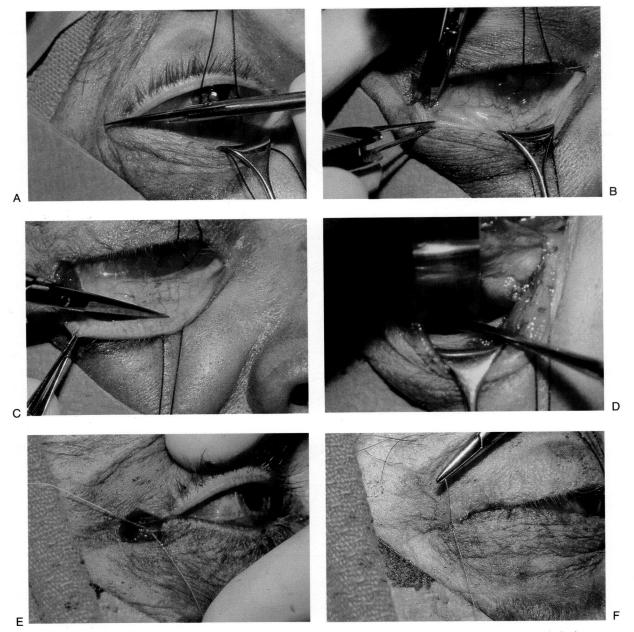

FIG. 8. Transconjunctival approach to the orbital floor. **A:** Lateral canthotomy. **B:** Lysis of inferior crus of lateral canthal tendon. **C:** Separating lower eyelid retractors from the inferior tarsal border. **D:** Elevating periorbita. **E:** Closing cantholysis. **F:** Closing canthotomy.

The inferior crus of the lateral canthal tendon at the site of the cantholysis is repaired using 5-0 Vicryl suture. The knot is buried. Next, the gray lines of the cut edge of the upper and lower lid are sutured together with a single 6-0 mild chromic suture to exactly align the canthal angle in an anterior–posterior direction (Figs. 8 and 9).

Occasionally, in the older patient, a tarsal strip procedure can be performed if significant horizontal laxity is present. The canthotomy is then closed with interrupted 6-0 mild chromic sutures.

All patients are hospitalized following surgery to allow frequent examinations in the first 24 hr after surgery. This also allows intravenous antibiotics and steroids to be continued. The patient's head is kept elevated at 45 to 60 degrees with continuous ice packs as tolerated.

In addition to looking for increasing ecchymosis or proptosis, visual acuity and pupillary checks are carried out by the nursing staff every 2 hr to allow early detection of orbital hemorrhage.

The patient is instructed to refrain from blowing the

nose for 2 weeks postoperatively. Oral antibiotics are continued for 3 to 5 days postoperatively, but not corticosteroids. Topical antibiotic ointment is applied at the end of the procedure and may be repeated postoperatively as desired by the surgeon.

One exception to our choice of Teflon as an implant material is the presence of a total floor defect in which not enough bone remains intact at the periphery to support the implant. While there are many ways to solve this problem, our choice is to use Medpore "synthetic bone" in 1.5- or 3-mm thickness. This can be heated in warm water on the surgical back table and then cut

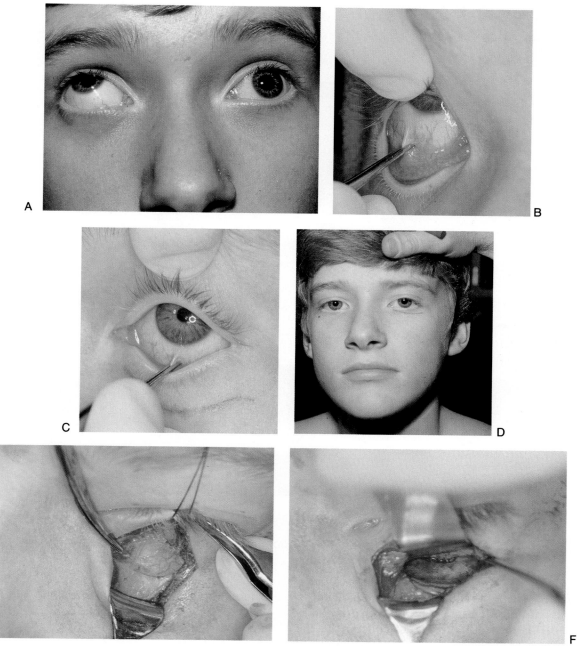

FIG. 9. Transcutaneous approach to the orbital floor. **A:** Inability to look up with left eye. **B:** Normal forced ductions of right eye. **C:** Positive forced ductions of left eye. **D:** Lower eyelid crease incision. **E:** Myocutaneous flap elevated down to the rim. **F:** Tissue incarcerated in fracture. **G:** Disimpacted fracture. **H:** Teflon plate trimmed to fit. **I:** Teflon plate in place covering floor fracture. **J:** Periorbita/periosteum closure. **K:** Skin closure. **L:** Postoperative resolution of restriction of upgaze.

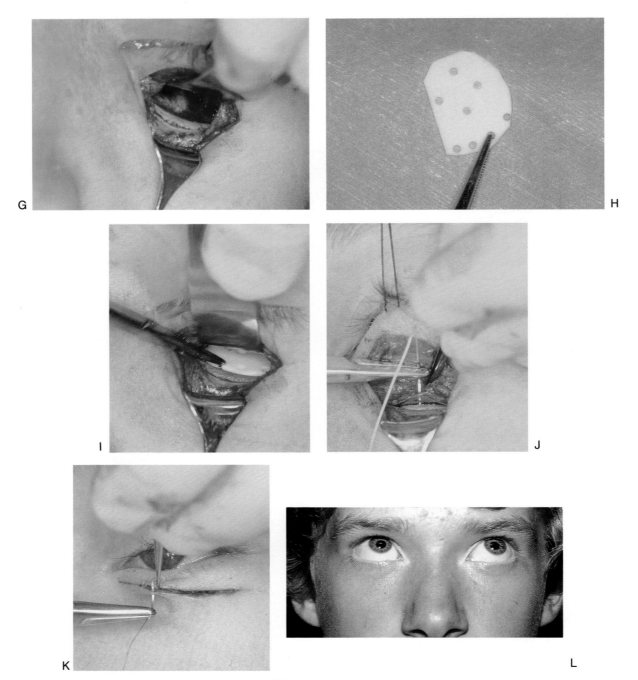

FIG. 9. *Continued.*

and molded to shape. Frequently, one can judiciously wedge this into position in the orbit so that no additional support is needed. If there is any concern that the implant will not hold, we cantilever it from the anterior orbital rim, attaching the long arm of a T-shaped microplate across the top of the implant. We then angle the plate about 70 to 80 degrees and screw the horizontal portion of the T to the orbital rim.

We prefer this technique to autogenous bone grafts, such as split calvarium, as there is no donor site and no tendency to unpredictable bony absorption with variable postoperative results.

POSTOPERATIVE COURSE AND OTHER CONSIDERATIONS

The patient is counseled preoperatively that diplopia may actually be worse in the immediate postoperative period because of swelling and manipulation of the orbital contents. Motility usually improves within the first 7 to 10 days after surgery. However, large series have shown that up to 20% of patients will have residual significant diplopia, which is probably related to fibrosis of the rectus muscle caused by damage at the time of the initial trauma. If this fails to clear, then extraocular muscle surgery may be required.

Infraorbital hypesthesia is usually better immediately postoperatively but may also be exacerbated, especially if surgery is performed on "old" fractures where significant adhesions to the infraorbital nerve exist. Sensation usually returns as long as the nerve has been left intact, but this may take several months.

Some degree of enophthalmos may persist once the postoperative swelling resolves. This may be due to fat atrophy, incomplete repositioning of herniated orbital tissues, or residual anatomic misalignment of the orbital floor with resultant residual enlargement of the bony orbital volume.

We usually do not treat a medial wall fracture, be it isolated or combined with a floor fracture, unless marked prolapse of soft tissues or entrapment is present. This is for two reasons: first, any residual globe malposition is usually clinically insignificant; second, exposure of the medial wall through a cosmetically acceptable approach is rather difficult. Additionally, implants placed along the medial orbital wall are difficult to shape and position, tend to migrate inferiorly, and may impinge on the lacrimal system and inferior oblique muscle.

If treatment of a medial wall fracture is indicated, dissection can be carried medially through the floor exposure and tissues repositioned. As previously stated, although implants can be shaped to cover both the medial wall and floor, we usually just disimpact the tissue, debride the ethmoid sinus, and leave the fracture uncovered.

In cases of severe tissue incarceration in a medial wall fracture, a direct approach to the medial wall through a "Lynch" type incision may be needed. The fracture is then treated as described for a floor fracture.

In old, large floor fractures in which treatment is indicated for enophthalmos and/or hypo-ophthalmos, the fracture should not be "repaired." Rather, our preference is to place on top of the depressed floor a Medpore implant of appropriate horizontal dimension and thickness so as to reduce the bony orbital volume to a more normal state.

BIBLIOGRAPHY

1. Aronowitz J, et al. Long term stability of Teflon orbital implants. *Plast Reconstr Surg* 1986;78:166.
2. Converse JM, Smith B. Editorial: on the treatment of blowout fractures of the orbit. *Plast Reconstr Surg* 1978;62:100.
3. Dortzbach RK, Elner VM. Which orbital floor blowout fractures need surgery? *Adv Ophthalmic Plast Reconstr Surg* 1987;6:287.
4. Fujino T. Experimental "blow-out" fracture of the orbit. *Plast Reconstr Surg* 1974;54:81.
5. Fujino T, Sato TB. Mechanism of orbital blow-out fracture: experimental study by three-dimensional eye model. *Orbit* 1987;6:237.
6. Green RP, Peters DR, et al. Force necessary to fracture the orbital floor. *Ophthal Plast Reconstr Surg* 1990;6:211.
7. Hawes MJ, Dortzbach RK. Surgery on orbital floor fractures. Influence of time of repair and fracture size. *Ophthalmology* 1983;90:1066.
8. Holtman B, Wray R. A randomized comparison of four incisions for orbital fractures. *Plast Reconstr Surg* 1981;67:731.
9. Hornblass A. Pupillary dilatation in fractures of the floor of the orbit. *Ophthal Surg* 1979;10(11):44.
10. Kersten RC. Blow-out fracture of the orbital floor with entrapment caused by isolated trauma to the orbital rim. *Am J Ophthalmol* 1987;103:215.
11. Kulwin DR, Leadbetter MG. Orbital rim trauma causing a blowout fracture. *Plast Reconstr Surg* 1984;73(6):969.
12. Kushner BJ. Paresis and restriction of the inferior rectus muscle after orbital floor fracture. *Am J Ophthalmol* 1982;94:81.
13. Leone CT, et al. Surgical repair of medial wall fracture. *Am J Ophthalmol* 1984;97:349.
14. Lyon DB, Newman SA. Evidence of direct damage to extraocular muscles as a cause of diplopia following orbital trauma. *Ophthal Plast Reconstr Surg* 1989;5:81.
15. Manson P, Clifford C, et al. Mechanisms of global support and post traumatic enophthalmos—I & II. *Plast Reconstr Surg* 1986;77:193.
16. McCord CD, Moses JL. Exposure of the inferior orbit with fornix incision and lateral canthotomy. *Ophthalmic Surg* 1979;10:53.
17. Millman AL, et al. Steroids and orbital blowout fractures—a new systematic concept in medical management and surgical decision-making. *Adv Ophthalmic Plast Reconstr Surg* 1987;6:291.
18. Norma JE, Dan NG, Rogers PA. Post-traumatic infraorbital neuropathy. *Orbit* 1982;1(4):259.
19. Nunery WR. Lateral canthal approach to repair of trimolar fractures of the zygoma. *Ophthal Plast Reconstr Surg* 1985;1:175.
20. Segrest DR, Dortzbach RK. Medial orbital wall fractures: complications and management. *Ophthal Plast Reconstr Surg* 1989;5:75.
21. Smith B, et al. Volkmann's contracture of the extraocular muscles following blowout fracture. *Plast Reconstr Surg* 1984;74(2):200.
22. Smith B, Regan WF Jr. Blow-out fracture of the orbit: mechanism and correction of internal orbital fracture. *Am J Ophthalmol* 1957;44:733.
23. Westfall CT, Shore JW. Isolated fractures of the orbital floor: risk of infection and the role of antibiotic prophylaxis. *Ophthalmic Surg* 1991;22:409.
24. Wojno TH. The incidence of extraocular muscle and cranial nerve palsy in orbital floor blow-out fractures. *Ophthalmology* 1987;94:682.

CHAPTER 25

Fractures of the Orbital Apex

Dale H. Rice

Hippocrates was the first to record the association of facial trauma with blindness (1). Twenty-three hundred years later, Berlin in 1879 performed the first scientific investigation of trauma to the optic nerve (2). He noted that facial injuries could result in a fracture of the optic canal with secondary injury to the optic nerve. Later, work by Pringle (3), Hughes (4), and Walsh (5) further elucidated the mechanisms of indirect injury to the optic nerve. In total, these authors performed over 400 postmortem examinations into the mechanism of injury to the optic nerve. They discovered that the injury was rarely directly from osseous compression, laceration of the nerve, or hemorrhage into the nerve itself. The more common mechanisms of injury were hemorrhage into the optic nerve sheath or contusion of the nerve with subsequent edema and compression. Thus the basic pathological process was an injury that led to secondary vascular compromise. These investigators also noted that, in the majority of cases, the injury was within the optic canal where the sheath is fixed to its bony surroundings.

RELEVANT ANATOMY

The keystone to the posterior bony orbit is the sphenoid bone (Fig. 1). All neurovascular structures to the orbit pass through this bone. The superior orbital fissure is a gap between the lesser and greater wings of the sphenoid. The optic canal itself is medial to the superior orbital fissure and completely within the substance of the lesser wing of the sphenoid (Fig. 2). The sphenoid bone itself is a complex bone, lying in a central position at the base of the skull. It plays a major role in connecting bones of the facial skeleton to those of the cranial base. The sphenoid contributes walls to the anterior and middle cranial fossa, to the orbit, to the nasal cavities, and to the temporal, infratemporal, and pterygoid palatine spaces (6,7). The interior articu-

lations include the cribiform plate, the perpendicular plate of the ethmoid, and the lamina papyracea (Fig. 3). It articulates posteriorly with the occiput, laterally with the temporal and parietal bones, and inferiorly with the pyramidal process and horizontal plate of the palatine bone and the vomer. The sphenoid bone does not articulate directly with the maxilla or with the mandible. However, it is separated from the maxilla by only the thin pterygoid process of the palatine bone and the portion of the ethmoid bone that forms the floor of the orbit. The bony canal is thickest as the nerve enters the canal from the orbital side, especially on the medial side adjacent to the ethmoid–sphenoid junction. This thickness has been designated the optic tubercle. The canal runs in an anterior–inferior declination to the Frankfort plane at an average angle of 15.5 degrees (Fig. 4). The canal also courses in an anterolateral angle to the midline at an average of 39.1 degrees (33 to 44.4 degrees) (8). The distance between the medial lip of the anterior extremity of the optic canal and the midsagittal plane is on average 16.1 mm on the right and 14.9 mm on the left. The intracranial distance between the medial lip of the optic canal and the midsagittal plane is 7.0 mm (Fig. 5). The shape of the canal is roughly circular at the orbital end, has a narrowing or waist at the midcanal called the isthmus, then widens at the intracranial end. It averages 4.6 mm wide and 5.1 mm high at this point (6). In contrast, the posterior limit of the canal averages 7.07 mm (5 to 9.5 mm) and the anterior opening in the orbit 4.8 mm (8). The length of the canal averages 11.67 mm in men and 10.95 mm in women on the medial side, and 11.05 mm in men and 10.38 mm in women on the lateral side. The range of canal length has been found to be 8 to 16 mm long (8) (Fig. 5). Canal wall thickness varies greatly. The most relevant dimension to decompression surgery is the medial canal wall. Much of it is in the sphenoidal sinus, producing an actual bulge in 80%

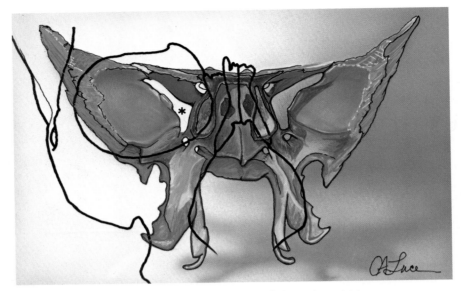

FIG. 1. Coronal representation of the sphenoid bone.

of cases. The presence of an Onodi cell also is an important determinant. According to Habal et al. (10) this occurs in 25% of individuals. In Lang's series (8), he found the same scenario in only 12%. The canal wall thickness in these individuals averages only 0.83 mm on the right and 0.95 mm on the left (Fig. 6). On the sphenoid sinus side, the wall was 0.1 mm in only 4%.

In 8% of cases, the wall was more than 8 mm in thickness and in a few cases the nerve was dehiscent into the sinus. The average length of the nerve in the sinus was 7.7 mm (Fig. 4). The location of the nerve is approximately 5 mm (1 to 11 mm) from the posterior ethmoid foramen.

The length of the optic nerve from the scleral surface

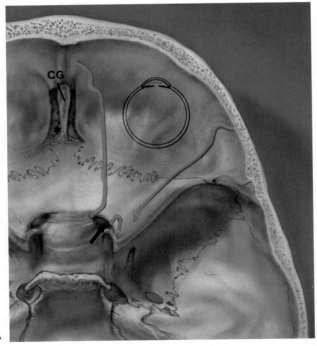

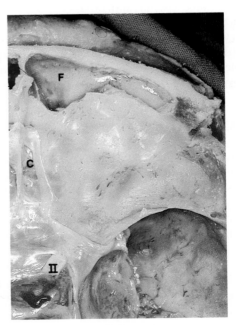

FIG. 2. A: View of floor of anterior cranial fossa. CG, crista galli; *, frontosphenoidal suture; *arrow,* optic foramen. **B:** Anatomic specimen depicting frontal sinus, cribriform plate, and floor of anterior cranial fossa. F, frontal sinus; C, crista galli; II, cranial nerve II (optic nerve).

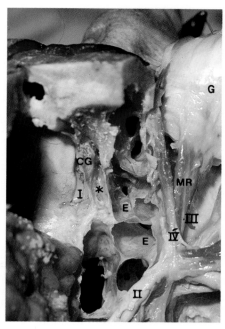

FIG. 3. Anatomic dissection showing neuromuscular structures that enter the orbit via the sphenoid bone. G, globe; CG crista galli; *, cribriform plate; I, olfactory nerve; E, ethmoid sinuses; S, sphenoidal sinuses; MR, medial rectus muscle; II, optic nerve; IV, trochlear nerve; III, oculomotor nerve.

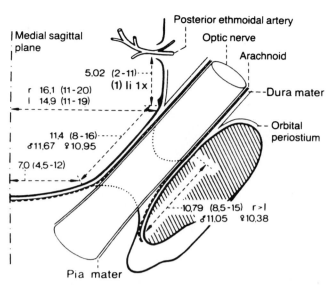

FIG. 5. Distance relationship of posterior ethmoid foramen to optic canal. Length of optic canal and distance from midline vary. (From ref. 8, with permission.)

of the globe to the chiasm is approximately 40 mm. The intracranial course is about 9 to 10 mm, the canalicular portion approximately 8 to 11 mm, and the rest in the orbit. Intracranially, the nerve is covered by pia, arachnoid, and cerebrospinal fluid (CSF). As the nerve enters the canal, the CSF is precluded to a large degree by numerous small pia and arachnoid adhesions. The

dura splits into two layers (Fig. 7) within the orbit, the outer becoming continuous with the periorbita and the inner ensheathing the nerve to the globe.

The ophthalmic artery supplying the retina and nerve exits the internal carotid at the superior part of its intracavernous course and travels deep to the nerve directly underneath it in its intracranial and proximal canalicular course. It then usually migrates to a more lateral position as it proceeds to the globe (11). The artery took a more medial course relative to the optic nerve within the optic canal in 16% of Lang's cases (8). The nerve itself is supplied along its course by numerous

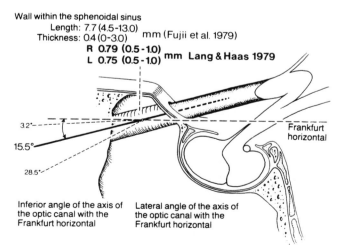

FIG. 4. Angle of optic nerve relative to Frankfort plane and bony thickness of sphenoid sinus aspect of optic canal. (From ref. 8, with permission.)

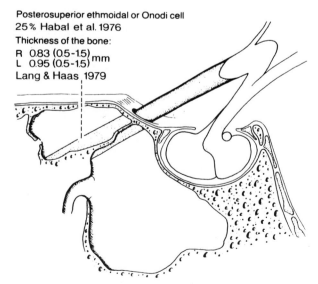

FIG. 6. Thickness of bony optic canal wall when optic nerve courses through a posterior superior ethmoid cell (cell of Onodi). (From ref. 8, with permission.)

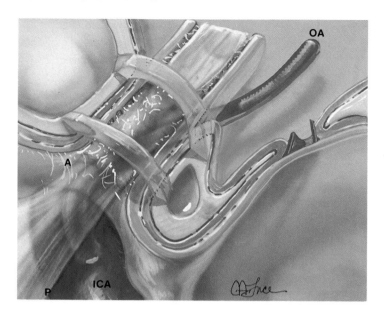

FIG. 7. Covering of optic nerve in intracranial, intracanalicular, and orbital parts. Also note relationship of ophthalmic artery. A, arachnoid; P, pia; ICA, internal carotid artery; OA, ophthalmic artery. (From ref. 11, with permission.)

vertically disposed perforating vessels by the investing pia mater.

The optic canal is surrounded anteriorly by the annulus tendineus (annulus of Zinn), which forms the origins of the four rectus muscles, as well as the levator palpebrae superioris. Besides the obvious risk of injury to the optic nerve and ophthalmic artery, fractures in this area can disrupt the function of these muscles as well.

In addition, the superior orbital fissure forms a passageway for the recurrent meningeal branch of the lacrimal artery, the superior and inferior ophthalmic veins, the oculomotor (III), the trochlear (IV), lacrimal, frontal, and nasal ciliary branches of the ophthal-

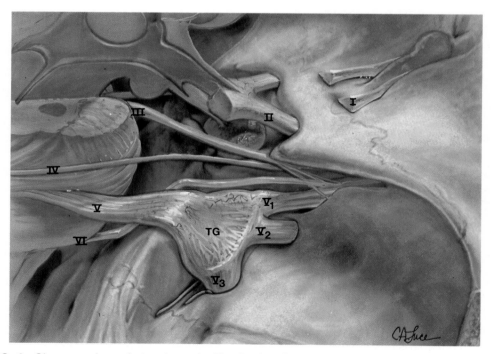

FIG. 8. Close-up view of structures in Fig. 3, showing cranial nerves I, II, III, IV, V, and VI. V₁, opthalmic; V₂, maxillary; V₃, mandibular.

mic (V Sub 1) and the abducens (VI) nerves, as well as the sympathetic supply to the globe (Fig. 8).

FRACTURE PATHOPHYSIOLOGY

Fractures of the sphenoid bone are relatively uncommon. In one review of 112 patients with skull base fractures, only 17 patients (15%) had radiologic evidence of sphenoid bone fractures (12). These sphenoid fractures themselves were most commonly associated with maxillary, zygomatic, ethmoid, frontal, and temporal bone fractures in descending order. The causes of these fractures are many but generally result from falls, sports injuries, blunt trauma, penetrating trauma, and motor vehicle accidents.

Orbital injury is a consequence of a high percentage of sphenoid fractures. Approximately 30% of patients in this group will have visual acuity loss from either direct ocular injury or from optic nerve damage. In one review of 63 cases of loss of vision following head injury all were noted to have sustained blunt trauma to the frontotemporal region (13). In one study, on cadaveric skulls, increasing frontotemporal compression yielded a fracture line somewhere in the floor of the anterior cranial fossa. Further increase in pressure merely deepened and extended the fracture line rather than producing additional ones (13). The fracture line developed as follows. Beginning in the frontal bone, the fracture spreads to the roof of the lateral orbit. A second fracture then forms on the medial floor of the anterior cranial fossa between the cribriform plate and the fovea ethmoidalis. These two fracture lines converge posteriorly on the roof of the orbit. The fracture line then continues posteriorly and inferiorly into the ethmoids and to the optic canal and sphenoid sinus. Further increase in pressure extends the fracture line across the optic canal to the petrous apex.

Damage to the optic nerve usually occurs within the optic canal from many different causes. In one study, the mechanisms of injury were classified as (a) mechanical impaction, (b) concussion, (c) hemorrhage, and (d) tear of the nerve (14). Damage may also occur from edema, necrosis, and infarction on a vascular basis. Ramsay (15) pointed out the potential importance of shearing forces, while Panje et al. (16) discussed the possibility of traction shearing and shock waves alone, or in combination, as additional potential causes of injury.

Concussion and traction with subsequent vascular injury are probably very significant causes of damage in optic canal injury. Edmund and Gadtfredsen (17) were able to identify an optic canal fracture in only 5 of 22 traumatically induced optic atrophy cases. Sofferman (18) postulates that shearing forces involving the peripheral microcirculation of the nerve may cause disruption of the nutrient vessels to the nerve, causing

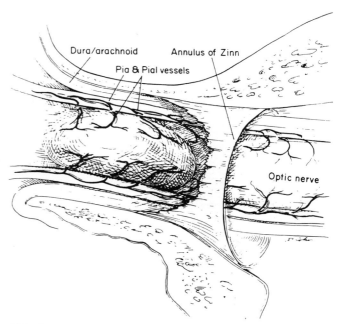

FIG. 9. Blood supply to nerve by perforating branches from the pia mater. (From ref. 21, with permission.)

infarction. Subsequent edema produces swelling of the nerve within the canal and compression, causing further injury. Edema alone may be enough even in the absence of hemorrhage to produce a mass effect within the canal, triggering a further compression–ischemia–edema process. Sofferman further postulates that most cases of post-traumatic atrophy result from a frontal blow. This may be a direct result of a stress concentration phenomenon brought about by the intrinsic nature of the bony configuration of the orbit

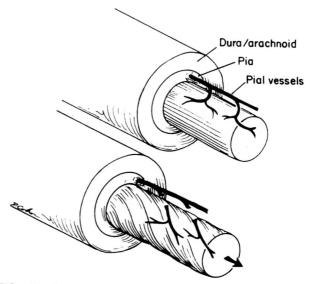

FIG. 10. Rotational force produces torsion of nerve, causing avulsion of nutrient vessels. (From ref. 21, with permission.)

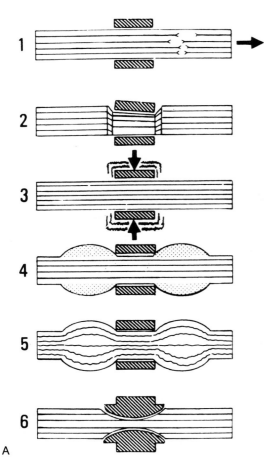

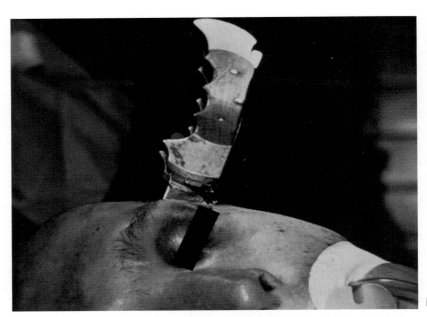

FIG. 11. A: Schematic representation of the various mechanisms of optic nerve injury. 1, stretching or torsion causing axonotmesis; 2, canal fracture; 3, shock waves; 4, hemorrhage; 5, edema; 6, callus formation. (From ref. 22, with permission.)**B:** Knife wound to orbital apex. No other significant injury occurred other than severance of the optic nerve.

and optic canal. Deduced from information derived from studies of holographic interferometry on dried human skulls (19), he concluded that force delivered to the brow will result in a stress concentration 5 to 8 mm from the optic canal (18).

Within the orbit itself, injuries, especially of the concussive type, are much less common. The nerve has a redundancy in length and has some room to stretch. Furthermore, there is a cushioning effect of the intraorbital fat and extraocular muscles. The final protective device is the stabilizing effect of the superior rectus muscle, which has a bony attachment outside the annulus of Zinn, directly on the sphenoid bone.

The optic nerve is most vulnerable to rotational force. Much of the nerve's blood supply in the optic canal comes from the small peripheral penetrating branches of the investing pia mater (Fig. 9). When the nerve undergoes torsion, these vessels are avulsed, producing neural ischemia (20,21) (Fig. 10). Another area of vulnerability outside the optic canal is the lamina cribrosa, where the nerve enters the globe. In the intraorbital course of the nerve, this is the most likely site of an avulsive, tearing injury.

The various mechanisms of injury are summarized in Fig. 11 (22).

CLINICAL PRESENTATION

Blindness following head injury can occur either early or late. Since any real chance of saving sight depends on the early identification of any degree of intact vision, the early establishment of this parameter is essential in the initial evaluation of the trauma patient. Unfortunately, in the flurry of activity surrounding the first assessment and resuscitation efforts, testing vision is often forgotten. The patient may also be unconscious, further hampering early testing.

The diagnosis of suspected optic nerve injury within the canal should be suggested by either immediate or progressive loss of vision. Slow loss of vision suggests increasing compression, while immediate blindness suggests severe injury or transection of the nerve (Fig. 11B). If a demonstrated fracture near or through the optic canal is coupled with loss of vision, it should be viewed as a definitive injury to the optic nerve or blood supply unless proved otherwise (23–25). If the optic nerve has been injured, a Marcus Gunn pupil would be expected (afferent pupillary defect). In this situation, the involved pupil reacts poorly, if at all, to light but reacts normally consensually. If there is a concomitant third nerve injury, a variable degree of pupillary dilatation will be seen. If there is a severe visual loss, but the retina is intact, visually evoked potentials will be markedly diminished or absent while the electroretinogram will be normal (26). Optic disc pallor and atrophy are delayed findings and will not be apparent on initial presentation.

In the awake patient, the early signs of optic nerve compromise include the reduced ability to discern red color discrimination, scotomata, and visual field constriction. Restriction of vision in the lower visual field is most commonly seen because of the narrowness of the superiormost aspect of the subarachnoid space in the optic canal (22). Frequent checks of these parameters of vision are essential in suspected injuries. Any deterioration should evoke a serious consideration of optic nerve decompression.

Spontaneous recovery of the visual acuity usually begins 2 to 4 days after the injury (25). Generally, the worse the vision, the less the potential for spontaneous recovery. However, even patients who are initially completely blind have been known to have made a spontaneous recovery (26). Maximal progression of recovery is usually seen at 4 weeks (25).

Fractures near or through the superior orbital fissure may cause injury to cranial nerves III, IV, and VI and the ophthalmic division of V (27). In this situation, the patient would have the classic superior orbital fissure syndrome, consisting of a dilated pupil, upper lid ptosis, and extraocular muscle dysfunction. When the optic nerve is injured in addition to the superior orbital fissure syndrome, it is more properly designated as an orbital apex syndrome.

IMAGING EVALUATION

While the diagnosis of optic nerve injury or superior orbital fissure syndrome can be made on clinical grounds, demonstration of the fracture or fractures themselves require various imaging studies. The fracture lines themselves are probably best visualized on computed tomography (CT) scan because of its far greater ability to show bony detail (Fig. 12). In one study, the CT scans of 490 blunt trauma victims were reviewed to establish the frequency of sphenoid fractures (28). Of these 490 patients, there were 111 with cranial facial fractures, 78 of whom had fractures of the sphenoid bone. Twenty-seven of the 78 had fractures involving primarily the skull base, while 51 had complex facial fractures in association. In this series of patients, optic nerve injury with total or partial loss of vision occurred in five, and extraocular muscle palsies occurred in six.

In another interesting study, it was noted that prior to 1980 and the routine use of computed tomography, the academic medical institution in question had made

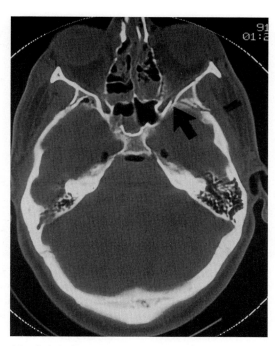

FIG. 12. Axial CT scan showing orbital apex fracture. *Arrow* points to fracture at apex.

the diagnosis of orbital apex fractures in only three patients. Beginning with the routine use of CT scans, in the subsequent 3 years, the diagnosis was made in 14 patients. The majority were caused by motor vehicle accidents, as one would expect. Optic nerve damage was demonstrated in three orbits, the superior orbital fissure in six, and the orbital apex syndrome in two. In the others, it was not possible to examine the orbit satisfactorily because of the severity of local soft tissue injury, globe rupture, or an altered level of consciousness (29). These studies and others show the superiority of CT scans in detecting fractures of the orbital apex. The standard projection is the axial one; in the multiple trauma patient by virtue of equipment design there is no additional risk imposed on the patient (Fig. 13) (12,13). Examination in the coronal projection may provide important additional information, but in some patients with multiple injuries, this may not be possible, particularly at their initial presentation (Fig. 14).

TREATMENT

The treatment of optic nerve injury from blunt trauma is as yet incompletely settled. Common wisdom is that optic nerve injury will either result in a diminution of visual acuity or immediate blindness. Should subsequent improvement in visual acuity occur, active intervention should be precluded. On the other hand, a gradually progressive decrease in visual acuity would suggest increasing compression of the nerve. At this

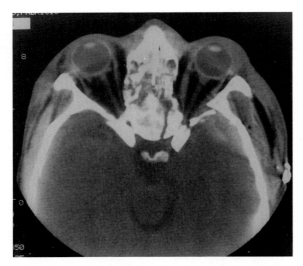

FIG. 13. Axial CT scan showing severe orbital apex fracture combined with nasoethmoid fracture.

juncture, a decision to treat medically or by operating intervention would have to be made.

With this in mind, it should be remembered that there is no universally accepted standard protocol for treating traumatic optic neuropathy. In cases of complete visual loss, some recommend surgery as soon as possible (30), while some believe surgery is not indicated if the blindness was instantaneous (31). Even when medical treatment is recommended, the dose of steroids advocated is quite variable. However, megadoses of steroids have been shown to produce a more marked reduction in cerebral edema than do conventional doses and therefore probably should be used (32).

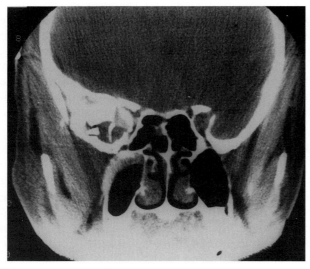

FIG. 14. Coronal CT scan showing superior orbital fissure fracture.

Very few trials have been conducted to establish the actual benefit of medical therapy. Panje et al. (16) proposed a scheme by which any patient with monocular trauma and diminished or absent vision on the basis of suspected canalicular trauma was given an initial bolus dose of 0.75 mg/kg of dexamethasone. This was followed by a dose of 0.33 mg/kg given every 6 hr for 12 hr. Nonresponse or failing vision after steroid taper was considered the primary indication for surgical decompression. This series unfortunately contained only seven patients. Most of the surgical patients did not recover useful vision; moreover, even the medical responders exhibited mediocre recovery at best.

Matsuzaki et al. (33) reported their results comparing medical and surgical decompression of optic canalicular injury with visual loss. The medical treatment consisted of prednisolone, mannitol, urokinase, and vitamin B_{12}. The decompressions were done at variable times after injury, even as long as 1 month later; this is one of the major analytic flaws in their series. Of the 22 patients managed medically, 59% were improved, while of the 11 patients that underwent decompression, 45% were improved.

Frenkel and Spoor (25) recommended an initial iv loading dose of 30 mg/kg of Solu Medrol and a second dose of 15 mg/kg two hours later. Treatment is continued at the 15-mg/kg dose every 6 hr for 48 to 72 hr. If there is no response, the medication is abruptly discontinued. If there is visual improvement, this therapy is maintained for 5 days and then rapidly tapered. If the patient is unconscious, he or she is followed by testing for an afferent pupillary defect. The dose is the same as for the awake patient. If there is no improvement in the afferent response, therapy is discontinued 24 to 48 hr later. If improvement is seen, the steroids are continued for an additional 3 to 5 days. If visual acuity deteriorates with withdrawal of steroid therapy, then it is reinstituted and a surgical decompression of the optic nerve is considered if a fracture is radiographically confirmed.

Several approaches have been recommended for optic canal decompression. The canal can be uncovered superiorly via a transcranial approach (34). Sewall (35) in 1926 described an external ethmosphenoidectomy for removal of part of the optic foramen and wall to relieve pressure on the optic nerve. Niho and colleagues (36) and Fukado (37) modified this technique and claimed excellent results in cases of traumatic neuropathy. This has been widely accepted as the approach of choice because it is less invasive and can be done under local anesthesia if necessary. Yet another approach is via a Caldwell–Luc incision in a transantral approach (38). In addition, a microsurgical endonasal technique can be used to decompress the optic canal extracranially (39). Optic canal decompression can also be performed using endoscopic sinus surgery instruments and techniques as described in the chapter, Endoscopic Sinus Surgery, by Rice.

In 1979, Sofferman (40) first described his sublabial transseptal sphenoidal approach to the optic canal. This avoids the dangers inherent in the transfrontal craniotomy and gives improved exposure over the more popularized transethmoidal sphenoidal approach.

In the Sofferman approach, the patient is placed in the slightly head-up position (about 20 to 30 degrees). Standard intranasal cocainization and local infiltration are administered as in a routine septoplasty. A hemi-transfixion incision is made in the membranous septum and superior septal and inferior premaxillary tunnels are made on the side *opposite* the nerve to be decompressed. On the side ipsilateral to the nerve in question, an incision along the entire nasal floor is made (Fig. 15). The inferior and superior tunnels are connected; the perpendicular plate of the ethmoid, vomer, and posterior cartilaginous septum is removed. The remaining cartilaginous septum is dislocated from the maxillary crest and displaced against the contralateral nasal wall (Fig. 16). This displacement is aided by the presence of the nasal floor incision.

A generous sublabial incision from canine to canine tooth is now made and the periosteum elevated to the pyriform rim. Removal of a small portion of bone of the pyriform rim and the sill of the nose is done with

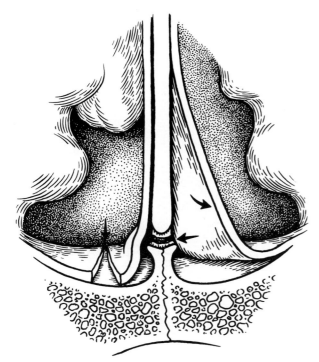

FIG. 15. Flap of mucoperiosteum and mucoperichondrium elevated over septum and floor of nose on side opposite nerve for decompression. Horizontal incision is made the length of the nasal floor on the opposite side. (From ref. 18, with permission.)

a cutting bur on the same side as the nerve. A limited excision of bone is required because of the septal dislocation (Fig. 16). The middle turbinate is removed and an ethmoidectomy performed with preservation of the lamina papyracea. Self-retaining nasal retractors of increasing length are employed so the dissection progresses deeper. Care is taken as the equator of the globe is passed and dissection proceeds posteriorly toward the orbital apex. Careful review of the computed axial tomography (CAT) scan is done preoperatively to establish the possible presence of an Onodi cell through which the optic nerve will run. As further progression to the orbital apex is made, the hard bone of the anterior aspect of the optic canal is encountered. The presence of fracture is diligently searched for as this dissection proceeds. The largest of the self-retaining retractors, the Cushing–Landau pituitary retractor, is inserted. The anterior face of the sphenoid sinus is exposed and the sphenoid sinus ostium is identified. The mucosa over the sphenoid is dissected free as much as possible and the bone of the sphenoid face is excised with pituitary and Kerrison rongeurs or the long pituitary drill. Suction irrigation greatly facilitates drilling in this area, keeping the drill bit clean and reducing generated heat. Attention is directed superolaterally to the point where the optic nerve traverses the superior wall of the sphenoidal sinus (Fig. 17). Using the pituitary drill and small pituitary rongeurs, the medial and inferior walls of the optic canal are removed. Visualization is aided by the operating microscope. Occasionally, the nerve does not make a noticeable bulge on the sphenoid sinus lateral wall. Sofferman (18) advises the use of the carotid bulge as a landmark to direct the surgeon to the optic canal. Beginning at the superiormost bulge of the carotid, a triangle of bone is removed between the bulge and the sphenoidal room (Fig. 18). Alternatively, the nerve can also be defined as it exits the posterior orbit. As the posterior limit of the lamina papyracea is reached, the posterior ethmoid foramen and artery are noted. Within millimeters, the bone immediately becomes much thicker as the sphenoidal–ethmoid articulation is passed and the optic foramen is reached. The periorbital sheath narrows and cones down as the foramen is approached. The nerve is then identified and followed posteriorly in its course in the superior aspect of the lateral sphenoidal sinus wall.

The nerve sheath is incised, taking great care to avoid the ophthalmic artery (Fig. 19). Fortunately, the artery is usually in an inferior course in most of the canal, then runs laterally within the orbit. However, the anomalous medial course previously alluded to may be encountered. Scant bleeding may be encountered by the lysis of small pial perforators but will be in marked contrast to damage to the ophthalmic artery if such a tragedy should ensue. Incision of the sheath

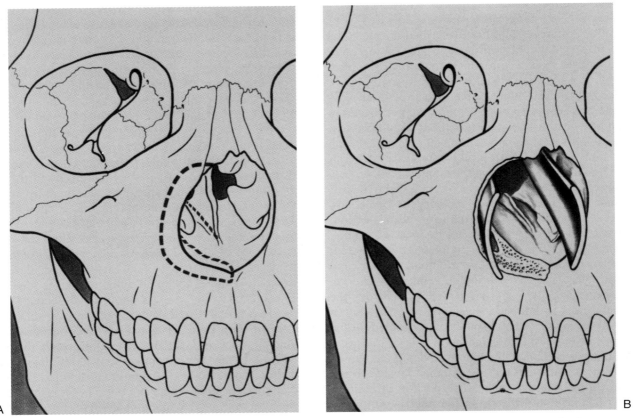

A

B

FIG. 16. Septal flap is displaced against the opposite nasal wall. Bone from the pyriform rim is removed to enhance exposure. **A:** Projected bone removal. **B:** Septum displaced and retractor in place. (From ref. 18, with permission.)

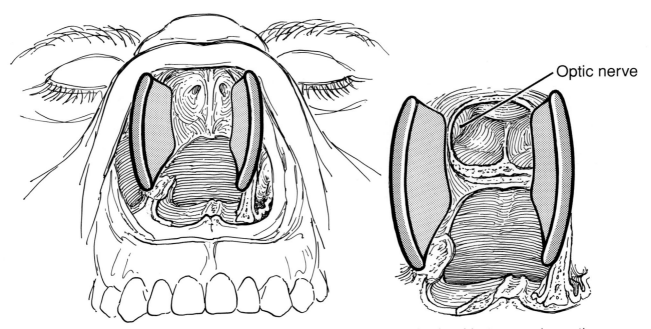

Optic nerve

FIG. 17. View through speculum after middle turbinate removal, ethmoidectomy, and resection of anterior wall of sphenoid are done, exposing optic nerve.

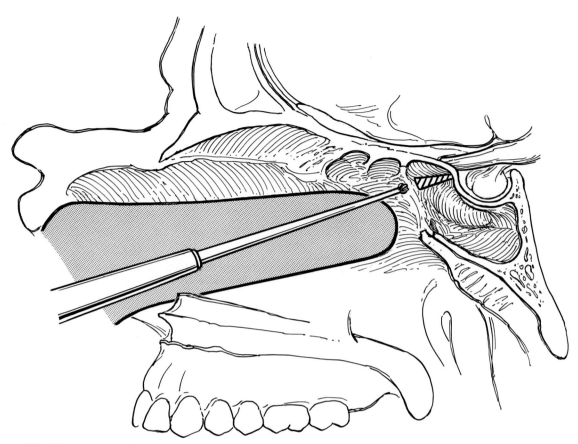

FIG. 18. Area of triangular bone removal from above carotid bulge in lateral sphenoidal sinus wall. (Adapted from ref. 18.)

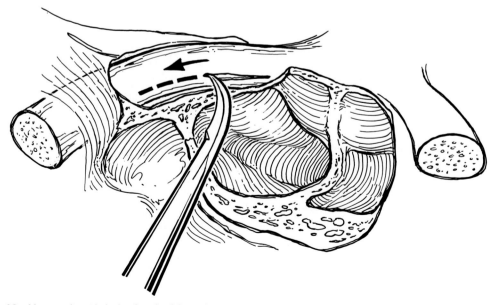

FIG. 19. Nerve sheath is incised with a sickle knife from the carotid through the annulus of Zinn.

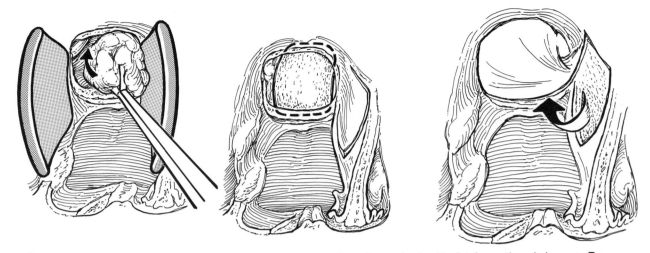

FIG. 20. Closure of the sphenoid sinus. **A:** The sinus is packed with fat from the abdomen. **B:** The anterior wall of sphenoid is plugged with a "cork" of septal bone. **C:** A posterior septal flap is swung over the sphenoid defect.

will be followed by a profuse flow of CSF. The sheath is split through to the annulus of Zinn and the annulus incised as well.

Once the decompression is completed, the sphenoidal sinus mucosa is completely stripped from the sinus cavity if not already done. An abdominal fat graft is placed within the sinus, replaced by a graft of septal bone (Fig. 20). A final seal is provided by a posterosuperiorly pedicled septal flap.

After the septum is returned to the midline and silastic splints are placed in the nose, the nose is packed with iodoform gauze. The packing is removed at 5 to 7 days and, in order to prevent synechiae formation, the splints are removed at 10 to 14 days.

The transethmoidal route can be used rather than the sublabial approach, but it gives a much less clear view of the field. It is a more direct approach as the removal of the lamina papyracea leads directly to the medial wall of the optic foramen. The major drawbacks are that it is a head-on view rather than a somewhat oblique view as provided by the sublabial approach, and the field is visually encumbered by a smaller incision and a restricted access.

Regardless of treatment, improvement is significantly related to extent of injury. In patients whose injuries result in no light perception, the improvement rate is 36% following medical treatment and 34% following surgical treatment. In contrast, patients with vision better than light perception had an improvement rate twice those with no light perception and the rate is 70% in both medical and surgical groups.

In addition, the prognosis seems dependent on the time interval between injury and the initiation of treatment. In general, the earlier the intervention the better the outcome; but most reported studies have a small

number of patients and the statistical significance is uncertain.

REFERENCES

1. Chadwick J, Mann WN. *The medical works of Hippocrates.* London: Blackwell Scientific, 1950.
2. Berlin R. Injuries to the optic nerve and ophthalmic artery from fracture of the optic canal. In: *Transactions of the 7th International Medical Congress, Vol 3.* London: Kolkmann, 1881.
3. Pringle HJ. Atrophy of the optic nerve following diffuse violence to the skull. *Br Med J* 1922;2:1156.
4. Hughes B. Indirect injury to the optic nerves and chiasma. *Bull Johns Hopkins Hosp* 1962;111:98.
5. Walsh FB. Pathological–clinical correlations. I. Indirect trauma to the optic nerve and chiasma. *Invest Ophthalmol* 1966;5:433.
6. Maisel H. Postnatal growth and anatomy of the face. In: Mathog RH, ed. *Maxillofacial trauma.* Baltimore: Williams & Wilkins, 1984.
7. Kattan KR, Potter GD. Lateral extension of sphenoid sinuses. *Med Radiogr Photogr* 1983;59:9–12.
8. Lang J. *Clinical anatomy of the nose, nasal cavity and paranasal sinuses.* New York: Thieme Medical Publishers, 1989;125–130.
9. Lang J, Oehmann G. Formentwicklung des Canals Opticus, Seine Masse und Einstellung Zu Der Schadelebenen. *Verh Anat Ges (Jena)* 1976;70:567–574.
10. Habal NG, Maniscalco JR, Lineweaver WC, Rhoton AL. Microsurgical anatomy of the optic canal. *Surg Forum* 1976;27:542–546.
11. Zide BM, Jelks GW. *Surgical anatomy of the orbit.* New York: Raven Press, 1985;53.
12. Ghobrial W, Amstutz S, Mathog RH. Fractures of the sphenoid bone. *Head Neck Surg* 1986;8:447–455.
13. Noyak AR, Kirtane MV, Ingle MV. Fracture line in post-head injury optic nerve damage. *J Laryngol Otol* 1991;105:203–204.
14. Walsh FB, Linderber R. *Die veranderungen des schnerven bei indirectetem trauma, n fortbildungskurs fur augenurzte.* Homberg: Erke Verlag, 1962.
15. Ramsay JH. Optic nerve injury and fractures of the canal. *Br J Ophthalmol* 1979;63:607–610.
16. Panje WR, Gross CE, Anderson RL. Sudden blindness following facial trauma. *Otolaryngol Head Neck Surg* 1981;89:941–948.
17. Edmund J Jr, Godtfredsen E. Unilateral optic atrophy following head injury. *Acta Ophthalmol (Copenh)* 1963;41:693.

18. Sofferman R. Transphenoethmoid decompression of the optic nerve. In: Johnson JT, Blitzer A, Ossoff R, Thomas JR (eds). *AAO instructional courses*, vol 1. St Louis: CV Mosby, 1988; 117–126.

19. DeKock JR, Hershkowitz N, Dross C, et al. Holographic interferometry applied to analysis of the human skull. *Opt Eng* 1979; 18(6):664.

20. Glaser JS. Clinical evaluation of optic nerve function. *Trans Ophthalmol Soc UK* 1976;96:359.

21. Wesley RE, Anderson SR, Weiss MR, Smith HP. Management of orbital–cranial trauma. In: Bosniak SL, Smith BC, (eds). *Advances in ophthalmic plastic and reconstructive surgery: orbital trauma*, vol 7, part 2. New York: Pergamon Press, 1988;16.

22. Osguthorpe DJ. Transethmoid decompression of the optic nerve. *Otolaryngol Clin North Am* 1985;18:125–137.

23. Manfredi SJ, Raji MR, Sprinkle PM, Weinstein GW, Minardi LM, Swamson TJ. Computerized tomographic scan findings in facial fractures associated with blindness. *J Plast Reconstr Surg* 1981;68:479–490.

24. Nickelson DH, Guzak SV. Visual loss complicating repair of orbital floor fractures. *Arch Ophthalmol* 1971;86:369–375.

25. Frenkel REP, Spoor TC. Traumatic optic neuropathies. In: Bosniak SL, Smith BC, eds. *Advances in opthalmic plastic and reconstructive surgery: orbital trauma*, vol 1, part 6. New York: Pergamon Press, 1981.

26. Hughes B. Indirect injury of the optic nerves and chiasm. *Bull Johns Hopkins Hosp* 1962;111:98–126.

27. Nesi F, LiVecchi J, Mathog RH. Orbital blow-out fractures. In: Mathog RH, ed. *Maxillofacial trauma*. Baltimore: Williams & Wilkins, 1984;21–38, 319–328.

28. Unger JM, Gentry LR, Grossman JE. Sphenoid fractures: prevalence, signs and significance. *Radiology* 1990;175:175–180.

29. Unger JM. Orbital apex fractures: the contribution of computed tomography. *Radiology* 1984;150:713–717.

30. Fujitani T, Inoue K, Takahashi T, Ikushima K, Asai T. Indirect traumatic optic neuropathy—visual outcome of operative and non-operative cases. *Jpn J Ophthalmol* 1986;30:125–134.

31. Kline LB, Morawetz RB, Swaid SN. Indirect injury of the optic nerve. *Neurosurgery* 1984;14:756–764.

32. Harrison MJG, Brownbill D, Lewis PD, Russell RWR. Cerebral edema following carotid artery ligation in the gerbil. *Arch Neurol* 1973;28:389–391.

33. Matsuzaki H, Kunita M, Kawai K. Optic nerve damage in head trauma: clinical and experimental studies. *Jpn J Ophthalmol* 1982;26:447.

34. Waga S, Kubo Y, Sakakura M. Transfrontal extradural microsurgical decompression for traumatic optic nerve injury. *Acta Neurochir* 1988;91:42–46.

35. Sewall EC. External operation on the ethmosphenoid–frontal group of sinuses under local anesthesia: technique for removal of part of optic foramen and wall for relief of pressure on optic nerve. *Arch Otolaryngol* 1926;4:377–411.

36. Niho S, Niho M, Niho K. Decompression of the optic canal by the transethmoidal root and decompression of the superior orbital fissure. *Can J Ophthalmol* 1970;5:22–40.

37. Fukado Y. Results in 400 cases of surgical decompression of the optic nerve. *Mod Prob Ophthalmol* 1975;14:474–481.

38. Kennerdell JS, Amsbaugh GA, Meyers EN. Transantral ethmoidal decompression of optic canal fracture. *Arch Ophthalmol* 1976;94:1040–1043.

39. Mann W, Rochels R, Bleier R. Mikrochirurgische endonasale dekompression des N. opticus. *Fortschr Ophthalmol* 1991;88: 176–177.

40. Sofferman RA. An extracranial microsurgical approach to the optic nerve. *J Microsurg* 1979;1(3):195–200.

CHAPTER 26

Frontal Sinus Fractures

Paul J. Donald

Frontal sinus fractures are uncommon and are the consequence of severe trauma. Because of its arch configuration and the thick bone of its anterior wall, the frontal sinus is highly resistant to fracture (see Fig. 26 in the chapter, Anatomy and Histology, by Donald). Motor vehicle wrecks, industrial accidents, and violent crime are the commonest causes. Occasionally, sporting accidents such as a fall from a horse, a kick such as in rugby, or a skate injury in hockey may result in such a fracture. Penetration by a bullet during criminal assault or self-inflicted gunshot wounds are unfortunately not uncommon. Suicide attempts using a shotgun placed under the chin almost invariably result in pellets penetrating the walls of the frontal sinus (Fig. 1).

PATHOPHYSIOLOGY OF FRONTAL SINUS MUCOSA

The mucosa lining the frontal sinus is unique in its behavior when compared to the other paranasal sinuses. When exposed to trauma, it tends to form cysts. These cysts secrete a mucus into the cyst lumen that thickens and becomes more proteinaceous, eventually assuming a brownish tinge with the passage of time. These cysts have the property of eroding bone, probably due to the pressure they exert against the sinus wall (1). Furthermore, a cyst may become infected, forming a mucopyocele, and can cause an osteomyelitis of the frontal bone and, worse, intracranial infection.

The experience of previously damaged frontal sinus mucosa by trauma producing a mucocele and secondary inflammatory complications is almost universal among practicing otolaryngologists. Often fracture fragments are depressed, entrapping mucosa between the pieces of broken bone. Some argue that most frontal sinus complications arise simply when fractures cross the frontonasal duct, resulting in duct stenosis and entrapment of secretions within the sinus. Although this is an important mechanism, it is not exclusively responsible for these complications. The experiments of Lotta and Schall (2), Schenck (3), and myself clearly show that injury to the mucosa alone is sufficient to produce pathological changes within.

Furthermore, the initial occult development of these pathological aberrations and their dire late consequences, coupled with the geographic mobility inherent in the facial fracture population, place the patient in extreme jeopardy. The patient in Fig. 2 was shot through the head 18 months prior to developing a near fatal bout of meningitis, which was the first sign of his frontal sinus mucocele that had extensive invasion of the anterior cranial fossa. An occult posterior wall fracture without frontonasal duct involvement was initially overlooked. The assault took place in Utah and his complication only manifested itself after he moved to California. The patient in Fig. 3 was in an automobile wreck 6 months prior to his admission. He suffered multiple trauma and, although comatose for a period, did not require intracranial intervention. His frontal sinus fracture went undiagnosed until he developed meningitis. The mucopyocele he developed as a result of this injury underwent drainage via trephination as his initial therapy. He subsequently underwent an osteoplastic flap procedure of the sinus that revealed evidence of extensive anterior fossa involvement (Fig. 3C).

Damaged frontal sinus mucosa tends to be markedly thickened and has extensive submucosal fibrosis with abundant inflammatory cells; also, the luminal cells lose their cilia (Fig. 4). There is often osteoneogenesis of the bone beneath the mucosa. The mucosa tends to form cysts (Fig. 5). When a mucocele or mucopyocele forms, the bone erosion at the interface of the cyst and the sinus wall may be due to the effect of pressure

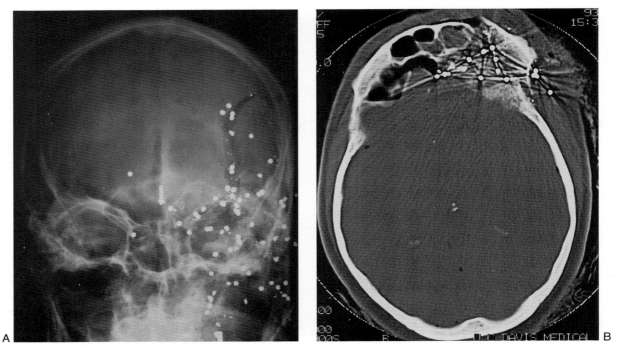

FIG. 1. Multiple shotgun pellets in frontal sinus following self-inflicted shotgun injury. **A:** Caldwell view. **B:** CAT scan.

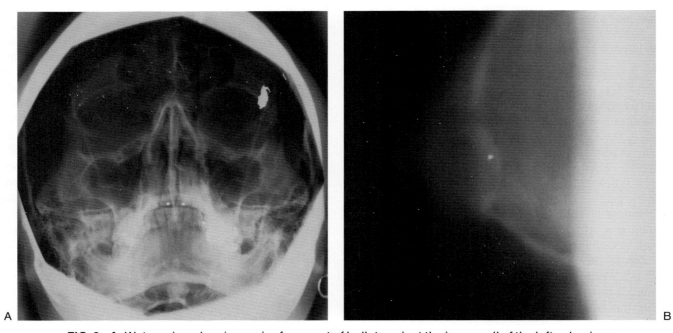

FIG. 2. A: Waters view showing major fragment of bullet against the inner wall of the left calvarium and opacification of right frontal sinus. **B:** Lateral tomographic view of frontal sinus showing posterior frontal sinus wall fracture and secondary mucocele to the gunshot wound.

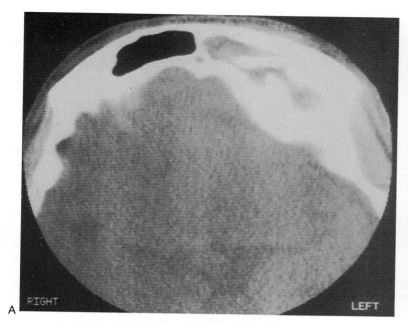

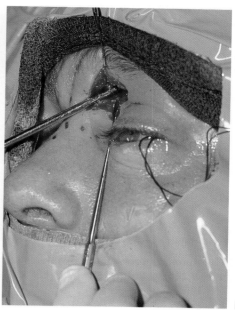

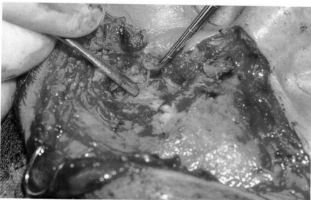

FIG. 3. A: Axial CT scan showing occult depressed posterior wall frontal sinus fracture. **B:** Trephination hole previously used to drain mucopyocele. **C:** Extensive intracranial invasion by mucopyocele. Suction tip is on the invading mucosa.

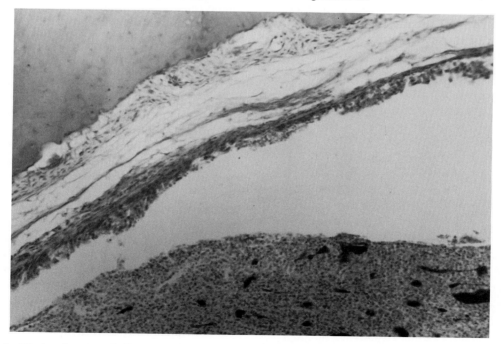

FIG. 4. Photomicrograph. The lining mucosa of a mucopyocele in a cat frontal sinus (H&E, ×100). (From ref. 5, with permission.)

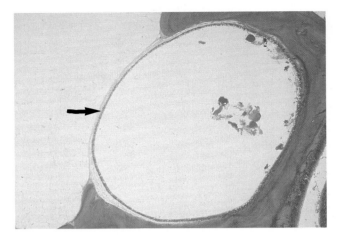

FIG. 5. Photomicrograph of cat frontal sinus that has been traumatized by currettage. Note the formation of a small cyst *(arrow)* (H&E, ×30). (From ref. 8, with permission.)

alone or the action of osteoclastic digestion (Fig. 6). Pressure studies done on experimentally induced mucoceles in cats were found to be statistically significantly elevated compared to pressures between the normal frontal sinus mucosa and underlying bone (Fig. 7). Osteoclastic digestion may arise as the result of a signal induced by pressure phenomena.

There are numerous vascular pits in the bone facing the sinus interior. These are foramina for the passage of veins from the subepithelium of the sinus mucosa to the subarachnoid space. Years ago, Mosher and Judd (4) made this discovery and theorized that these vessels were responsible for the spread of infection from the frontal sinus to the subarachnoid space. These so-called foramina of Breschet were noted by myself (5) to provide sites of imbrication of the frontal sinus mucosa. This fact has special relevance in the removal

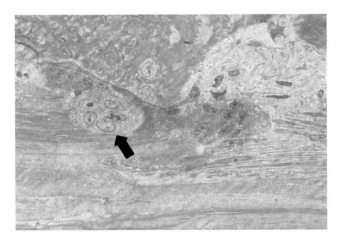

FIG. 6. Photomicrograph of a thin section of a mucocele and its interface with bone. Note osteoclast *(arrow)* (H&E, ×30). (From ref. 1, with permission.)

of mucosa required for frontal sinus obliteration and cranialization procedures.

CLINICAL PRESENTATION

Trauma is the obvious etiology in these fractures, with motor vehicle accidents leading the list. With the advent of the shoulder belt, the incidence of frontal sinus fractures in these accidents is much lower. Unrestrained occupants are at high risk for this fracture and make up the majority of cases. The bone is more resistant to fracture than any of the other facial bones. It takes approximately 550 to 900 foot pounds to fracture the mandible, but 800 to 1200 foot pounds to fracture the frontal sinus (Fig. 8) (6).

In a series of 72 frontal sinus fractures seen at the University of California, Davis Medical Center between 1974 and 1986 (7), the various causes of fracture are as listed in Table 1. To illustrate the severity of trauma, the frequencies of associated injuries are listed in Tables 2 and 3.

Many patients have a period of unconsciousness following the accident and often have amnesia for the event. The complaint of frontal headache is uncommon, but the problem of forehead numbness that often accompanies these fractures usually goes unnoticed. Nosebleed is a frequent complaint and careful inquiry regarding clear nasal drainage raising the suspicion of cerebrospinal fluid (CSF) rhinorrhea must be done. Anosmia is a symptom of anterior fossa floor fracture that may have a contiguous frontal sinus fracture and should raise suspicion. Massive hemorrhage is usually only seen in through-and-through fractures with brain injury and especially if the superior sagittal sinus is transected.

The initial deformity of a depressed anterior wall fracture may be effaced by overlying hematoma. A laceration in the forehead skin with the protrusion of underlying fractured bone or the exuding of CSF or brain is obvious. Oftentimes, there are no obvious signs save for frontal sinus tenderness, although this is of little help in the comatose patient and is often absent in isolated frontonasal duct, floor, or posterior wall fractures.

Being polytrauma victims, the patients commonly arrive in the emergency room and the usual attention to airway control, stemming of hemorrhage, and neurologic assessment take priority. The head injury victim has a computed tomography (CT) scan, as does the patient with obvious facial fractures. In the quick perusal of the head CT scan, the radiologist or neurological surgeon may overlook a frontal sinus fracture in the zeal to delineate any central injury. On the other hand, the facial CT scan will usually have the frontal injury included in the interpretation. It is important for the

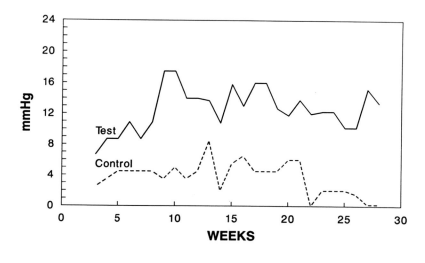

FIG. 7. Graph showing pressure exerted by the limiting membrane of a frontal sinus mucocele in one frontal sinus (test) compared to that produced by the frontal sinus mucosa of the normal mucosa on the sinus of the opposite side. (From ref. 1, with permission.)

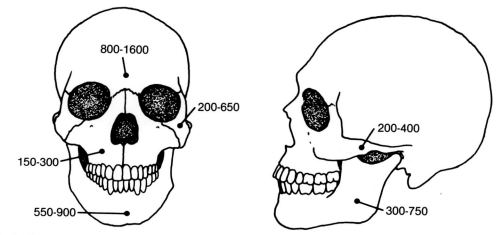

FIG. 8. Foot pounds of pressure necessary to fracture various elements of the facial skeleton. (From ref. 6, with permission.)

head and neck surgeon to personally review all the films to accurately assess the degree of injury. Fine cut CT scans at 1 or 2 mm intervals may be needed in order to better determine the extent and complexity of the fracture.

In the past, plane films of the facial skeleton and lateral laminography were the only means of radiographically demonstrating frontal sinus fractures. Cur-

TABLE 1. *Etiology of frontal sinus fractures*

Motor vehicle accident	51 (71%)
Assault	8 (10%)
Industrial accident	5 (7%)
Recreational accident	4 (4%)
Gunshot wound—self-inflicted	3 (4%)
—other	1 (2%)

From ref. 7, with permission.

TABLE 2. *Other craniofacial fractures: number per patient*

None	22 (31%)
One	27 (37%)
Two	12 (17%)
Three to seven	9 (12%)
Unknown	2 (3%)

From ref. 7, with permission.

TABLE 3. *Other craniofacial fractures by type*

Maxilla	27 (32%)
Zygoma	13 (16%)
Nasofrontoethmoidal	10 (12%)
Nasal	8 (10%)
Skull vault	8 (10%)
Skull base	8 (10%)
Mandible	8 (10%)
Total fractures	82 (100%)

From ref. 7, with permission.

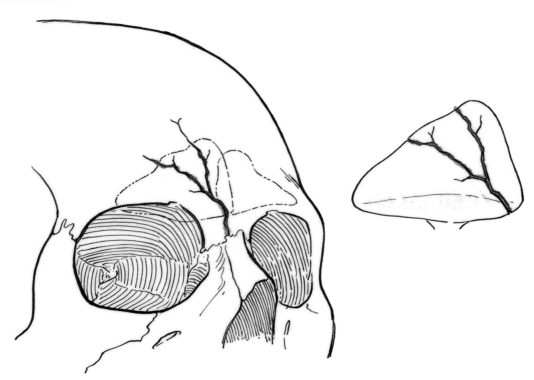

FIG. 9. Linear fracture, anterior wall of frontal sinus.

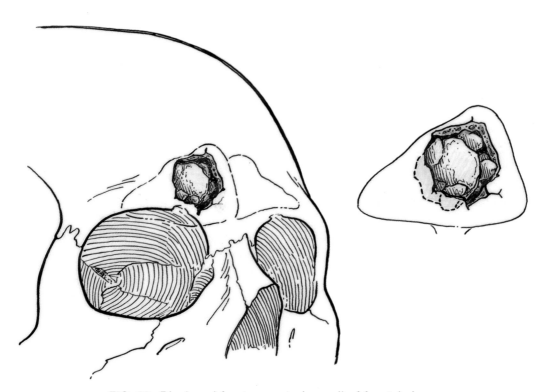

FIG. 10. Displaced fracture, anterior wall of frontal sinus.

rently, most hospitals have a CT scanner and the computer-assisted tomography (CAT) scan done in the axial plane gives the most definitive delineation of the injury (Fig. 3A). Magnetic resonance imaging (MRI), since it depicts only soft tissue injury, is of little value.

A classification system of frontal sinus fractures has been proposed on the basis of site and severity. Although it is uncommon for fractures to be limited to one specific site, treatment protocols often vary from one site to another, thus justifying this classification. Fractures are classified as follows:

Anterior wall
Posterior wall
Frontonasal duct
Floor
Corner
Through-and-through

Anterior wall fractures may be undisplaced or displaced, simple or compound, and with or without "missing bone." Undisplaced fractures are often linear and in continuity with an adjacent calvarial fracture (Fig. 9). In displaced fractures, fragments either prolapse into or project into the frontal sinus lumen (Fig. 10). Simple fractures occur beneath the cutaneous covering while compound fractures have an overlying laceration through which the fracture can be seen (Fig. 11). The concept of "missing bone" is in reality a misnomer. These fractures are usually comminuted and small fragments are lavaged or suctioned from the wound during its cleansing and debridement. Occasionally, small pieces of bone are so badly contaminated by road dirt or other materials that they cannot be saved.

Posterior wall fractures are either linear or displaced (Fig. 12). Linear fractures of this wall are uncommon in my experience. The displaced fracture may or may not have an associated CSF drainage.

The frontonasal duct is probably the most difficult

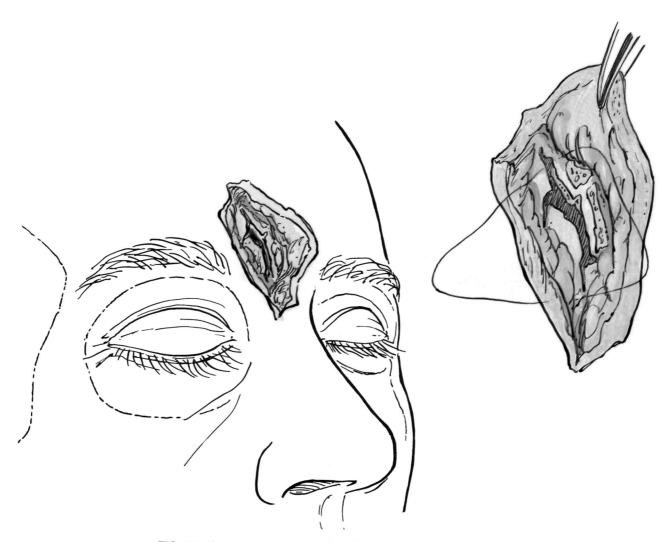

FIG. 11. Compound comminuted fracture of the anterior wall.

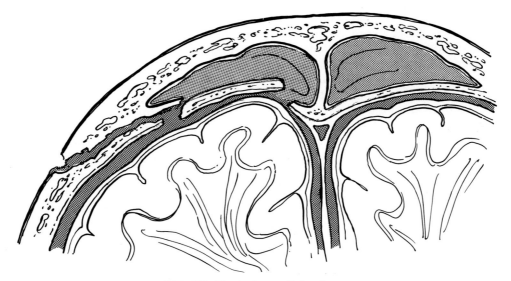

FIG. 12. Posterior wall fracture.

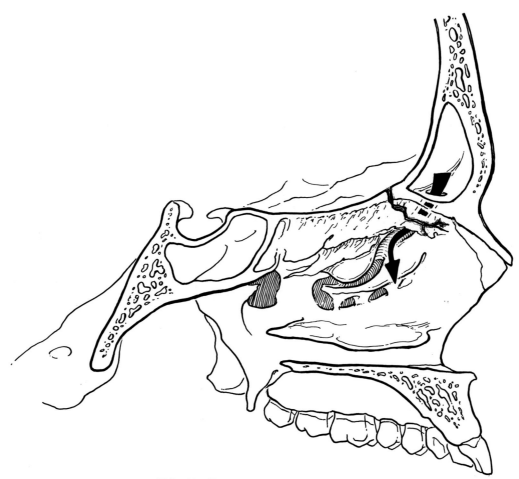

FIG. 13. Frontonasal duct fracture.

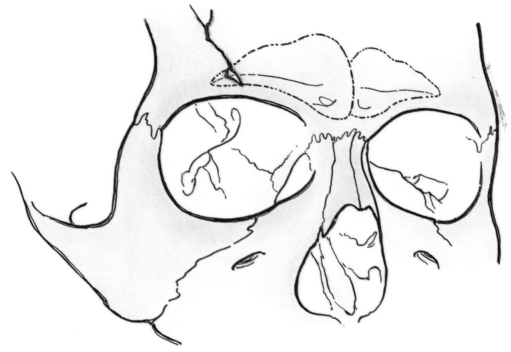

FIG. 14. Corner fracture.

fracture to demonstrate radiographically. It may or may not be in continuity with a frontal sinus floor fracture (Fig. 13). The floor fracture may be displaced or undisplaced into the sinus cavity itself, into the orbital ethmoids, or into the orbit.

The corner fracture is an innocuous fracture that nips the corner of the sinus, is undisplaced, and virtually always is in continuity with an adjacent calvarial fracture (Fig. 14).

The through-and-through injury is the most devastating fracture of all. The skin of the forehead is lacerated and both anterior and posterior walls of the sinus are fractured, usually always with displacement and comminution. The frontal lobe dura is torn and the frontal lobes of the brain are lacerated and contused (Fig. 15).

ANTERIOR WALL FRACTURES

Fractures of the anterior wall of the frontal sinus are the commonest. It is usually the first anatomical structure in the path of an oncoming traumatizing force and therefore obviously bears the brunt. Patients with anterior wall fractures tend to be less seriously injured than those with fractures of other sites within the sinus. They may not have an unconscious period. Those with linear fractures will complain of pain, have swelling over the forehead, but will not have a palpable step-off of the bone of the anterior sinus wall. One has to guard against the illusion of a step-off created by a

subgaleal hematoma. The edge of this lesion feels just like a fracture line. A careful check of the CT scan will show no evidence of displacement.

In displaced fractures, there will be obvious indentation in the forehead if the patient is observed soon after the accident. However, the space rapidly fills with hematoma, effacing the visual depression. Fortunately, the defect can commonly be palpated and will be confirmed on CT scan.

Compound fractures provide easy access for direct inspection of the fracture site and displacement or comminution, as well as for assessment of the degree of wound contamination (Fig. 16). It is important to conserve as many fragments of bone as possible and not discard them during any manipulations done in a preliminary attempt to assess the severity of the wound.

Linear fractures need no surgical intervention. The possibility of fractures of the other walls of the sinus must be investigated, but for purely linear fractures observation of the patient will suffice. The likelihood of a complication from linear nondisplaced frontal sinus fractures is distinctly remote.

Displaced fractures should be operated on. They present two separate problems: the almost inevitable development of a depression in the forehead and the possible formation of a mucocele. Although there is usually not much in the way of deformity in the early weeks following a depressed fracture, the inevitability of a significant cosmetic defect gradually becomes evi-

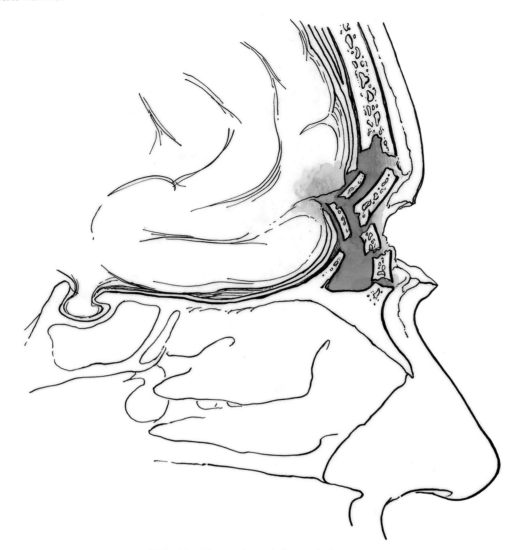

FIG. 15. Through-and-through fracture.

dent as hematoma resolves and fibrosis ensues (Fig. 17).

Entrapped mucosa between fracture fragments may lead to mucocele formation (Fig. 18). Plentiful research information is available to show that significant mucosal injury may lead to the formation of an abnormal mucosa that acquires the peculiar tendency to form cysts (3,8,9).

Access to repair a depressed fracture may be obtained through either a so-called butterfly incision or a coronal scalp incision (Fig. 19). If a forehead laceration is present over a compound fracture, extension of this incision into a natural forehead wrinkle will often provide excellent exposure of the fracture site (Fig. 20).

The fracture fragments are exposed, but great care is taken to preserve the maximal amount of periosteal attachments of the fragments. A skin hook or small stout bone hook is used to gently capture each fragment, preserving its periosteal pedicle (Fig. 21). The fragment is grasped and the margin of mucosa around the fracture line incised, cut, and stripped away (Fig. 22). A cutting bur is used to cut down a 1- to 2-mm thickness of bone at the site of mucosal removal (Fig. 23). The fragments are then replaced and fixed in site by wires and miniplates or microplates (Figs. 24 and 25). No packing is placed within the sinus. The frontonasal duct area is especially to be avoided in this regard. The rigid stabilization provided by the plating systems produces a stiffer fixation than the interosseous wires. The wound is sutured and the patient is advised to avoid sleeping in the prone position for 6 weeks and obviously to avoid the possible occasions of direct trauma.

When "missing bone" exists, significant gaps in the frontal sinus wall can be supplanted by split calvarial

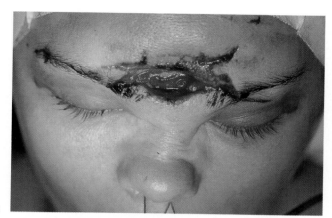

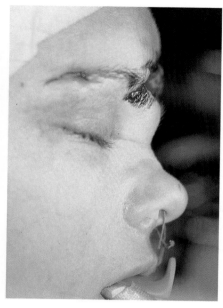

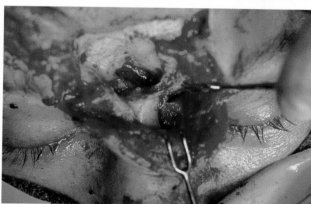

FIG. 16. Obvious compound anterior wall frontal sinus fracture seen through a forehead laceration. **A:** Frontal view. **B:** Lateral view. **C:** Intraoperative view.

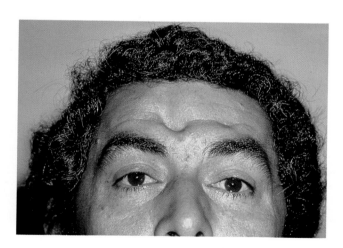

FIG. 17. Obvious deformity following nonintervention in a depressed frontal sinus fracture. (From ref. 10, with permission.)

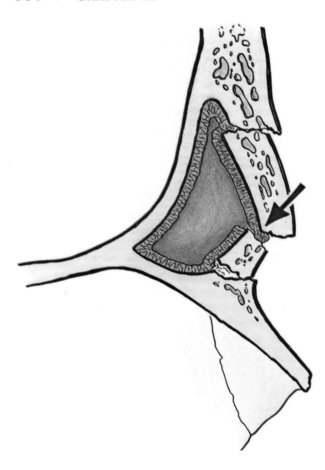

FIG. 18. Illustration of entrapped mucosa *(arrow)* between frontal sinus fracture fragments.

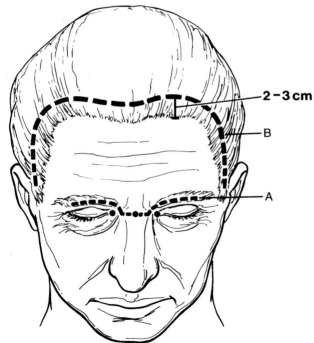

2–3 cm

B

A

FIG. 19. Incisions used for access for frontal sinus fracture repair. **A:** Butterfly incision. **B:** Coronal scalp incision.

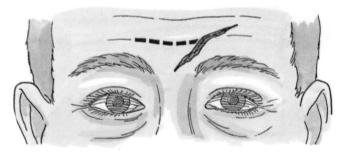

FIG. 20. Extension of laceration over compound frontal sinus fracture in a natural creaseline in forehead to gain exposure.

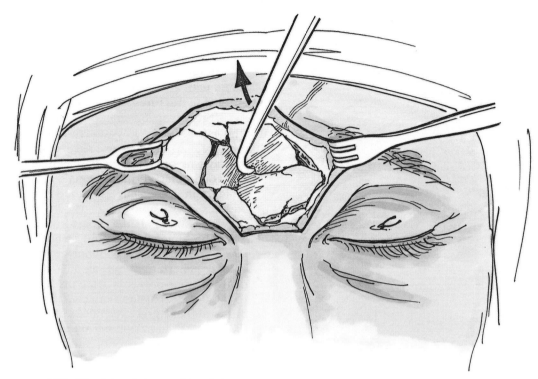

FIG. 21. A hook is used to disimpact the displaced anterior wall fragments.

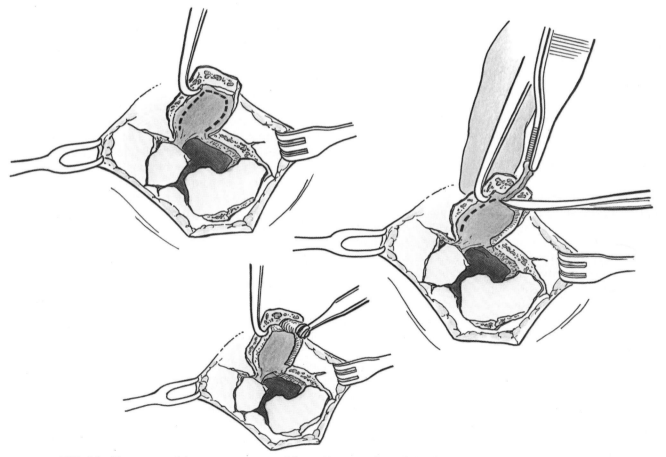

FIG. 22. Mucosa and bone are removed from the margins of the fracture fragments (see text).

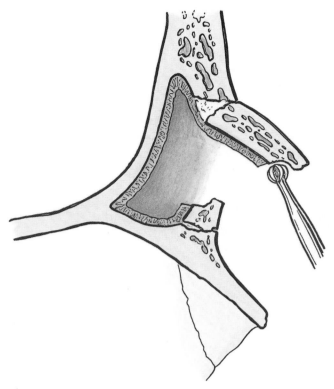

FIG. 23. One to two millimeters of bone are removed from the circumference of the fracture margin.

grafts. However, to take these grafts, the coronal scalp incision will be required for the initial exposure of the fracture. A vertical incision extending posteriorly from the middle of the coronal flap along the vertex of the skull may be required in order to provide exposure of the parasagittal aspect of the skull for harvesting this graft. This is fortunately usually unnecessary.

POSTERIOR WALL FRACTURES

The greatest degree of controversy in the management of frontal sinus fractures surrounds the issues in treatment of those of the posterior wall. The central problem is that of determining posterior wall displacement. Linear fractures would be safe to follow and observe if their linearity could be guaranteed. The problem arises in the differentiation on a radiographic basis between a linear and a displaced fracture. Even fine cut CT scanning cannot definitely distinguish linear fractures from minor degrees of displacement. The therapeutic choice between nonintervention and frequent close clinical observation, and immediate surgical treatment is an unresolved controversy. I recommend being conservative by being radical. The consequences of missing a displaced fracture with its attendant potential morbidity from intracranial mucocele or mucopyocele are dire. Brain abscess or meningitis may be the initial presenting feature of these com-

plications of frontal sinus fracture. Given the problems attendant to close follow-up inherent in the population that is victimized by maxillofacial trauma, an aggressive approach is advised.

With the exception of a posterior wall fracture associated with a "corner fracture," in my opinion, all posterior wall fractures should be operated on. The butterfly or brow incision should be limited to those patients who have a very low sinus. The coronal incision is preferred in most cases. An osteoplastic flap of the frontal sinus anterior wall is performed as described by Montgomery (9) and Donald (10). A 5-ft Caldwell radiograph of the sinuses is used as a template and the outlines of the sinus are marked with methylene blue. Care is taken to slant the perforating bur obliquely toward the lumen of the sinus when outlining its outer margins (Fig. 26). This not only avoids accidental intracranial penetration but creates an obliquely angled platform that prevents later prolapse of the flap into the sinus. Deep osteotomy cuts through the thick bony brows at the lateral extremities of the sinus and through the bone of the nasion permit easy greenstick fracture through the orbital roofs and avoid fragmentation of the anterior wall (Fig. 27). A broad flat osteotome through the intersinus septum is passed to the sinus floor. An upward prying in a firm but gentle fashion will again help to maintain the integrity of the anterior wall. Once the sinus is opened, the severity of the posterior wall fracture is assessed.

If a CSF leak is obvious, fracture fragments at its periphery are removed and the dural rent is identified. A dural suture is used to close the laceration in an interrupted fashion (Fig. 28). If a complex laceration exists or there is some concern regarding the watertight integrity of the closure, a graft of temporalis fascia or fascia lata is placed (Fig. 29). The graft is tucked under the edges of the posterior wall bone once a careful separation of the dura from the posterior sinus wall adjacent to the site of injury is done. All displaced fragments of bone are reduced anatomically. The interior of the sinus is divested of mucosa by blunt dissection. A cutting bur is used to drill away a 1- to 2-mm layer of the inner sinus wall bone to ensure total excision of all frontal sinus mucosal remnants. Loose unattached fragments of posterior wall bone are removed. If more than 25% of the posterior wall is missing, serious consideration of an alternative method of sinus obliteration or ablation should be entertained. Donald and Ettin (8) have shown that fat obliteration in frontal sinuses with a significant amount of missing bony walls will often result in reepithelialization, infection, and mucocele formation because of fat graft absorption. In sinuses with minimal bone loss, fat obliteration is the treatment of choice. However, obliteration, pedicled pericranium or cancellous bone chips from hip are also efficacious. In those patients with large dehiscences in the posterior wall, cranialization of the sinus is the most efficacious

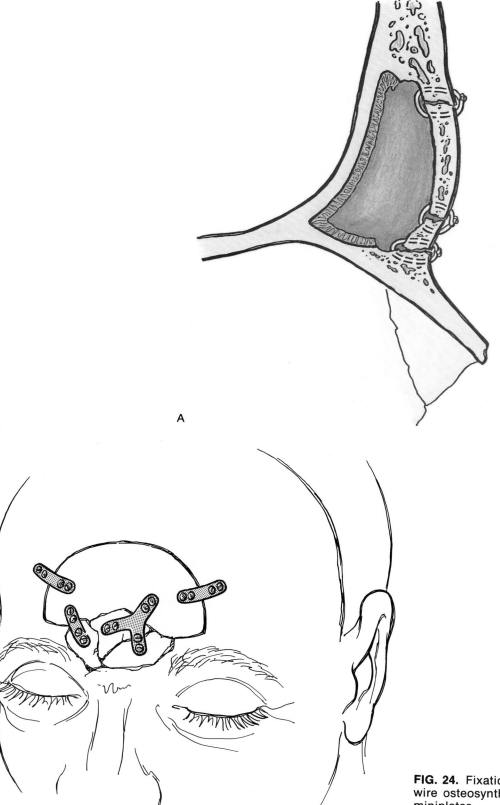

FIG. 24. Fixation of fragments done by **(A)** wire osteosynthesis and **(B)** application of miniplates.

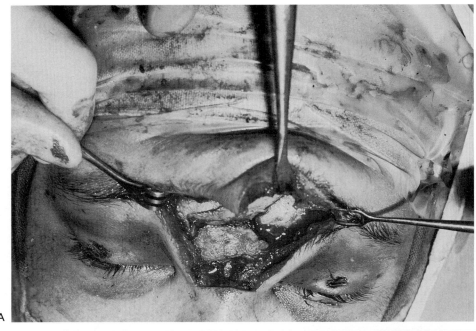

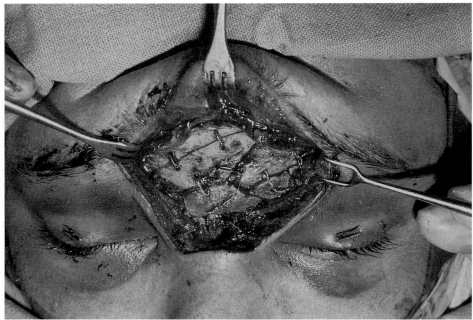

FIG. 25. Depressed anterior wall frontal sinus fracture. **A:** Fracture exposed through a butterfly incision. **B:** Fracture fragments are wired into position.

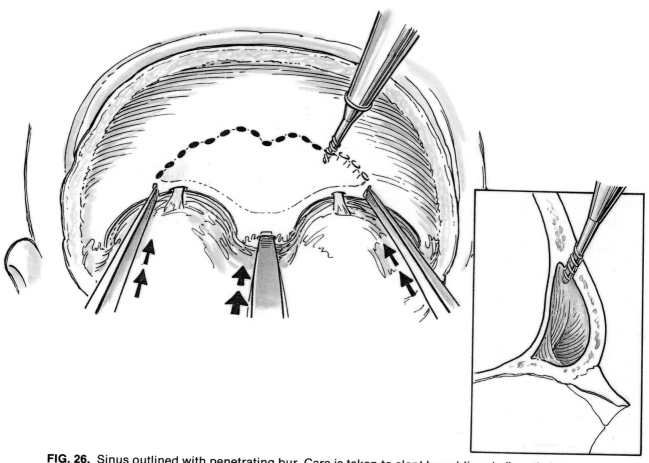

FIG. 26. Sinus outlined with penetrating bur. Care is taken to slant bur obliquely **(inset).** A sharp blow is delivered to the lateral brow areas and nasion to help mobilize the osteoplastic flap (see text).

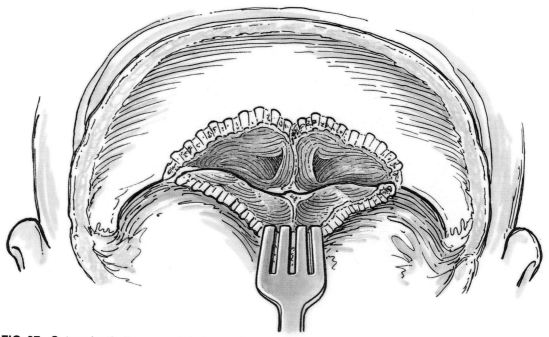

FIG. 27. Osteoplastic flap completed, anterior wall fractured across the orbital floors and pedicled on orbital periosteum.

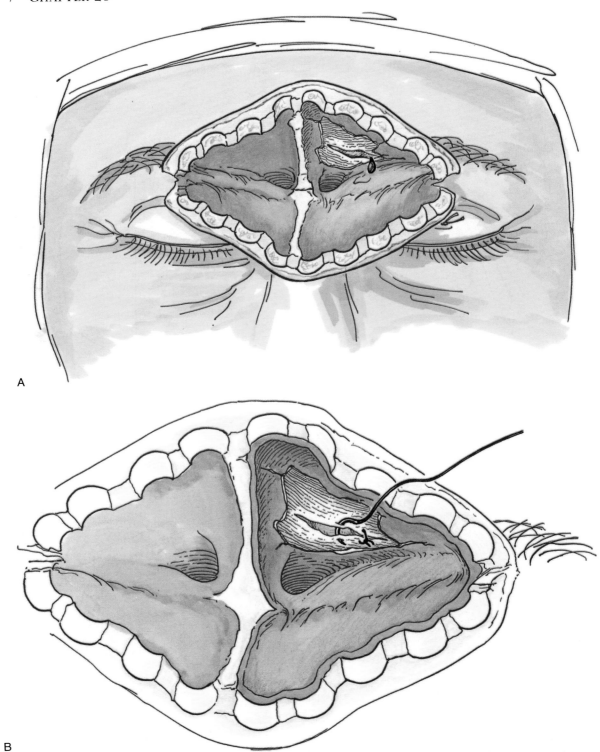

A

B

FIG. 28. Suture of dural laceration in posterior wall frontal sinus with CSF leakage. **A:** Dural laceration. **B:** Fracture bone debrided until limits of dural rent are apparent; tear is sutured with interrupted sutures.

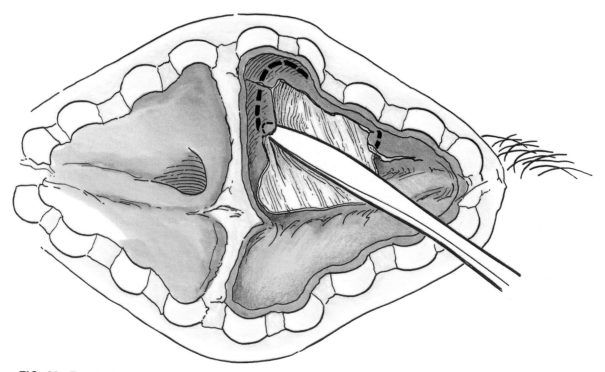

FIG. 29. Fascia graft being tucked into position to stem CSF leak in posterior wall fracture.

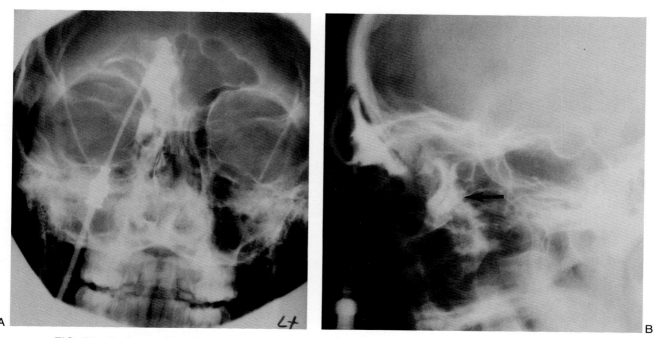

FIG. 30. Radiographic demonstration of nasofrontal duct patency in a suspected frontonasal duct fracture. **A:** Instillation of radio-opaque dye into frontal sinus cavity through a small trephination. **B:** Presence of dye in nose *(arrow)* demonstrates frontonasal duct patency.

alternative method (see upcoming section on through-and-through fractures).

FRONTONASAL DUCT FRACTURES

Of all the areas of the frontal sinus, the frontonasal duct is the most difficult area in which to diagnose an isolated fracture. An opacified sinus is often the only radiographic sign. Trephination of the sinus, lavage with warm saline, then instillation of cocaine or an epinephrine solution will clear the sinus and shrink the mucosa. Demonstration of ductal patency is done by installation of methylene blue into the sinus cavity and demonstrating its subsequent presence within the nose. Radiographic evidence of the passage of a radiopaque dye injected into the sinus into the nose also confirms patency and provides a permanent record (Fig. 30). Ductal fractures will almost always guarantee the future formation of mucocele if not effectively addressed (Fig. 31). An isolated frontonasal duct fracture can be managed by a slight enlargement of the trephination hole used for diagnosis and excision of the intersinus septum so that the sinus of the damaged side can drain through the duct of the untraumatized side. This technique can be done either through this trephination or through an osteoplastic flap (Fig. 32).

The more usual method of handling this fracture is by the osteoplastic flap and fat obliteration method. Since most frontal sinus fractures cut across both ducts, this technique is usually employed. Some authorities recommend a Lynch type resection of the frontal sinus floor and the use of the Sewell–Boyden flap (11) to reconstruct the duct area. This provides a mucosal covering and is said to prevent subsequent stenosis (see the chapter Surgical Management of Frontal Sinus Infections, by Donald).

THROUGH-AND-THROUGH FRACTURES

The through-and-through fracture is a devastating injury. It lacerates the forehead skin, produces a displaced, compound, comminuted fracture of both anterior and posterior frontal sinus walls, lacerates the underlying dura, and severely contuses the adjacent frontal lobes of the brain (Fig. 33). Fifty percent of victims die at the scene of the accident or in transit. Most are victims of polytrauma; and approximately 20% subsequently die of these multiple injuries or their cerebral contusions in the first weeks following the injury (Fig. 34). Management of these injuries in the past traditionally honored the basic tenets of neurosurgery and otolaryngology in the management of the head injury and the frontal sinus. Traditional neurosurgical thought dictated that compound penetrating injuries of

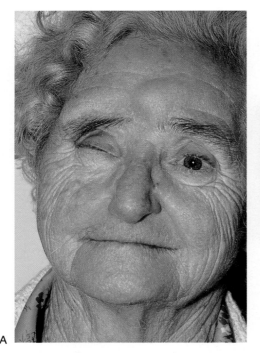

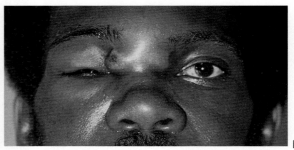

FIG. 31. A: Elderly woman with a frontonasal duct fracture sustained about 12 years previously and a history of some 10 trephinations for frontal sinus infection. Note the signs of mucopyocele. **B:** Young man who developed a massive mucopyocele 6 months following a Le Fort III fracture in which a nasofrontal duct fracture was missed.

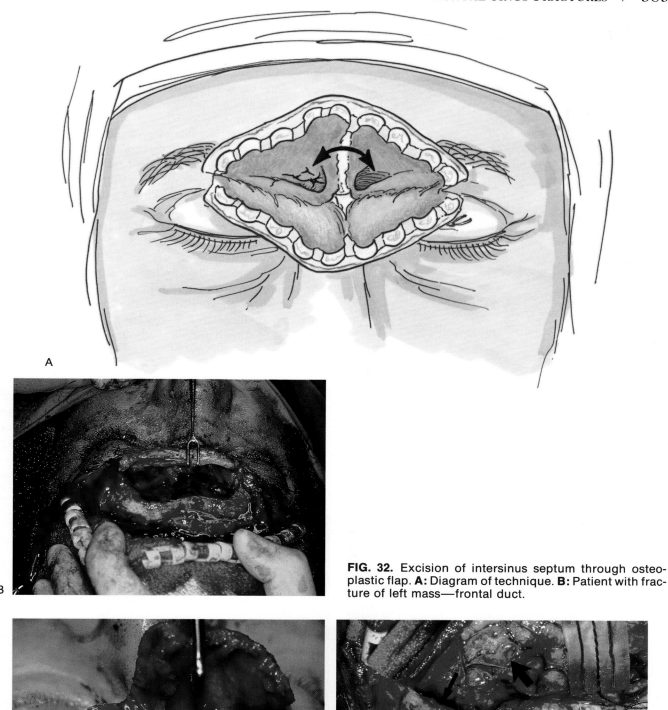

FIG. 32. Excision of intersinus septum through osteoplastic flap. **A:** Diagram of technique. **B:** Patient with fracture of left mass—frontal duct.

FIG. 33. Through-and-through fracture of frontal sinus. **A:** Penetrating injury to frontal skin, both frontal sinus walls, dura, and brain. **B:** Confusing appearance of injury in another patient. Note anterior frontal sinus wall *(open arrow)*, posterior frontal sinus wall *(closed arrow)*, brain frontal sinus wall *(arrow)*.

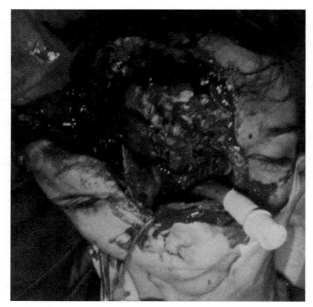

FIG. 34. Extensive frontal sinus fracture. (From ref. 12, with permission.)

the skull required control of the central injury but without return of the bone flap used for access or the pieces of fractured calvarium. On the other hand, basic otolaryngological practice was to totally eliminate the sinus for fear of risking infection or mucocele from possible retained mucosal remnants with its ready access to the anterior cranial fossa. Therefore sinus ablation by the

Riedel type was advised. The problems engendered by this approach in penetrating frontal sinus fractures into the anterior fossa are that the frontal lobes are rendered vulnerable to subsequent injury (13). The residual cosmetic defect is substantial (Fig. 35) and a second operation is required 8 to 14 months later to restore normal cranial contour.

The work of Nadell and Kline (14) clearly established, in compound skull fractures, the safety of returning the cleansed bone fragments involved in the compound fracture and the bone flap used for access after control of the central injury had been achieved. They found that in 124 consecutive cases of compound depressed skull fractures that they had no instance of brain abscess, meningitis, or osteomyelitis of the skull if they returned the bone fragments at the time of initial emergency surgery. Using this information, the technique of cranialization was developed (15).

Because of the severity of the intracranial injury, virtually all the patients have a frontal craniotomy (Fig. 36A,B). The neurosurgeon removes dead and necrotic brain, stops the central bleeding, and repairs the damaged frontal dura (Fig. 36C). This commonly requires a dural graft. Meanwhile, the calvarial bone fragments removed from the site of injury have been cleansed of road dirt and other contaminants. The bone from the anterior wall of the frontal sinus is divested of mucosa and the inner table burred. These fragments sit soaking in Betadine until the final phase of the operation.

The posterior wall of the sinus is completely re-

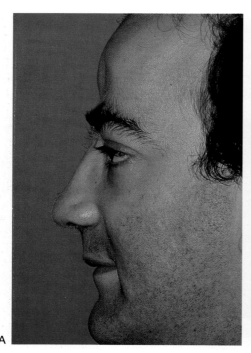
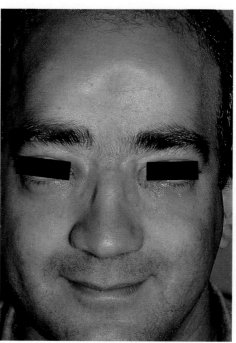

A   B

FIG. 35. Cosmetic defect left after the Riedel excision of the frontal sinus. **A:** Lateral view. **B:** Frontal view.

moved with a double actioned rongeur and the cutting bur (Fig. 36C,D). The posterior sinus wall is made flush with the anterior walls and floor of the anterior cranial fossa. All of the mucosal lining is carefully removed with the cutting bur. The very narrow recesses at the lateral and posterior extremities of the frontal sinuses are often difficult to visualize through standard frontal sinus surgical exposures. A view of these areas is greatly facilitated by the excellent exposure afforded by the anterior craniotomy. The frontonasal duct mucosa is inverted on itself and the funnel-shaped opening lightly abraded with the polishing bur. Grafts of temporalis muscle or fascia are forced into the ductal area (Fig. 36E). At this point, the bone fragments are washed in saline and the continuity of the anterior skull is restored. The bone is approximated by wire, plates, or both (Fig. 36F,G). The scalp is sutured in place.

Over the course of the ensuing days and weeks, the dura and dural grafts slowly expand into the newly expanded anterior cranial fossa. This is in part often initially very rapid because of the brain edema that is the consequence of the original injury.

Very often the head and neck surgeon's initial contact with the patient will be in the operating room after the neurosurgeon has completed the central repair. During the initial process of wound cleansing and debridement, it is not uncommon to wash away small fragments of "egg-shelled" bone. In addition, a few larger pieces may inadvertently be discarded during the procedure. Fragment of posterior wall (Fig. 37) may be used as free grafts to reconstruct the anterior wall. They are carefully divested of mucosa and fixed in place. Unfortunately, there is a discrepancy between the thickness of the anterior and posterior sinus walls. This produces a mild deformity with irregularity of the forehead contour. However, it still provides frontal lobe protection. A better choice is the use of split calvarial grafts.

Often there are concomitant facial fractures with disruption of the fovea ethmoidalis and cribriform plate. Although dural grafting is done to repair the resultant CSF leaks, reinforcement by a pericranial flap is often done to ensure a watertight closure and enhance healing by this introduction of fresh vascularized tissue.

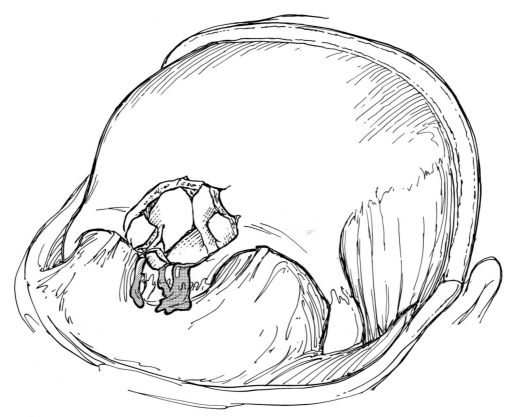

A

FIG. 36. Cranialization procedure. **A:** Through-and-through injury with CSF and brain oozing through the fracture. **B:** Anterior craniotomy done. Anterior wall fragments are cleansed and stored. Fracture of both sinus walls, dural rent, and damaged brain exposed. **C:** Brain debrided, dura patched, and posterior wall remnants removed with double actioned rongeur. **D:** Removal of remaining posterior wall of frontal sinus produces cranialization. **E:** The mucosa of the sinus is removed from the sinus lumen and the nasofrontal duct mucosa is inverted on itself and the frontonasal ducts are plugged with temporals muscle.

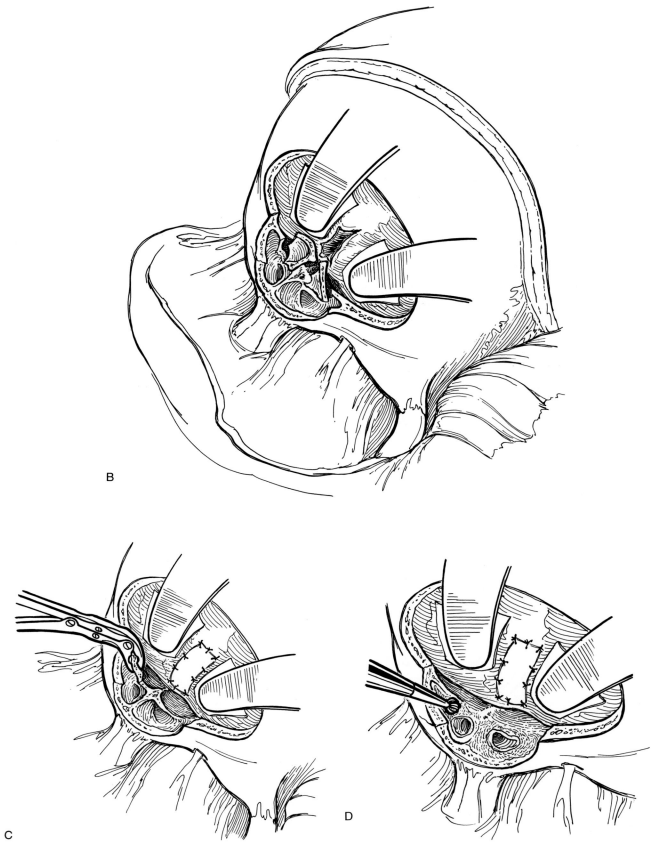

B

C

D

FIG. 36. *Continued.*

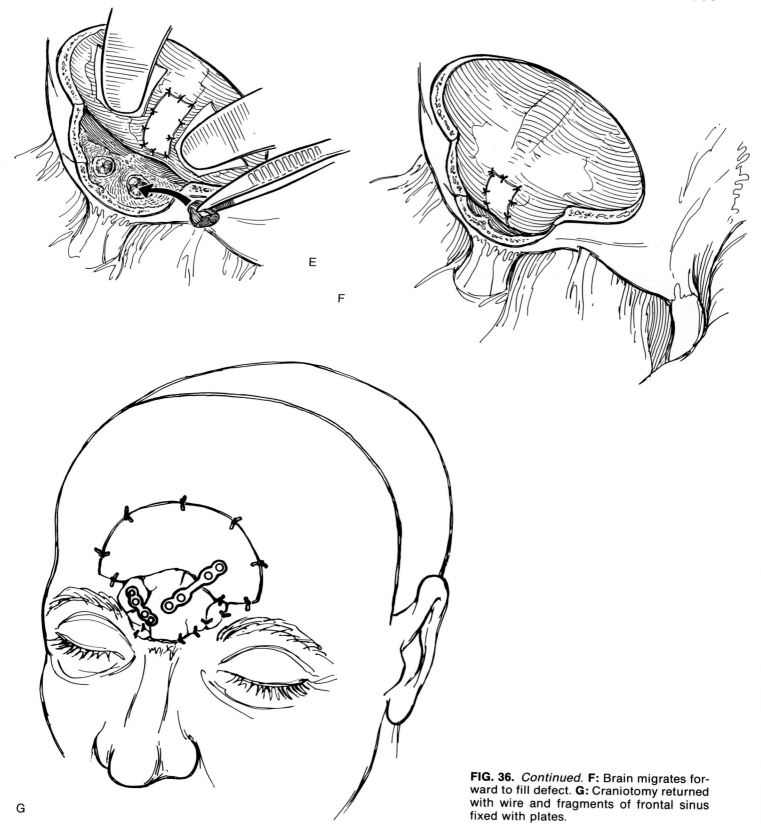

FIG. 36. *Continued.* **F:** Brain migrates forward to fill defect. **G:** Craniotomy returned with wire and fragments of frontal sinus fixed with plates.

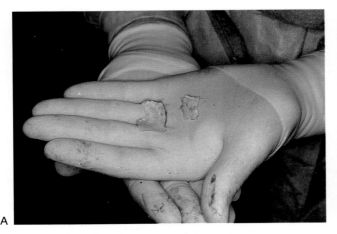

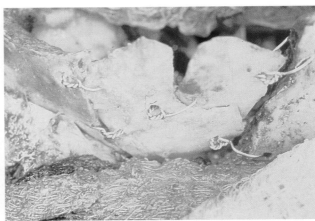

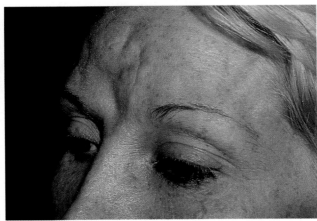

FIG. 37. A: Posterior wall fragments preserved to replace discarded anterior wall fragments. **B:** Fragments wired into place. **C:** Forehead deformity resulting from the discrepancy of the replaced fragments. (From ref. 10, with permission.)

Because of sometimes extensive tearing of pericranium in the fracture, the surgeon is challenged to develop inventive ways in which to design these flaps. A large redundant flap can be used, folded on itself to fill a flap left by frontal lobe excision necessitated by the injury. Dead space in the anterior fossa must be assiduously avoided at all costs. Extensive cerebral resection will mitigate against cranialization if such dead space cannot be filled. The employment of the pericranial flap in reconstruction will allow the use of intracranial free fat grafts to obliterate this space (Fig. 38). Without the pericranial flap, these grafts risk rapid absorption because of their placement between two other free grafts—the calvarial bone fragments and the dural patch grafts. Rapid absorption creates the potential for infection, especially in the face of a previously contaminated wound. The success of the pericranial flap in skull base surgery has been well established. Its use in the repair of frontal sinus fractures has recently been reported (16). The flap is tucked under the brain between the residual frontal lobes and the underlying calvarium. It may be fixed in place by sutures or stuck to the bone using fibrin glue. The fat grafts are then placed between the flap, which is created too long and

folded on itself like an accordion. The residual space is packed with fat grafts and the bone fragments are replaced.

In long-term follow-up (7), the cranialization technique has been found to be highly effective. A safe method of management, producing a normal frontal profile and frontal lobe protection, has been achieved. Complications are few, and no cases of meningitis, brain abscess or mucocele, or CSF leak from the sinus have occurred in the 18 years it has been performed (Fig. 39).

CONCLUSIONS

Frontal sinus fractures are uncommon and result from traumatic insults of considerable force. The most effective means of diagnosis is CT scanning. The therapeutic modality chosen is predicated on what walls are involved. Each injury is treated based on the aforementioned algorithm. Most fractures have multiple wall involvement and the exigencies of treatment are predicated on the requirements for treatment of each wall. For example, a linear fracture of the anterior wall cou-

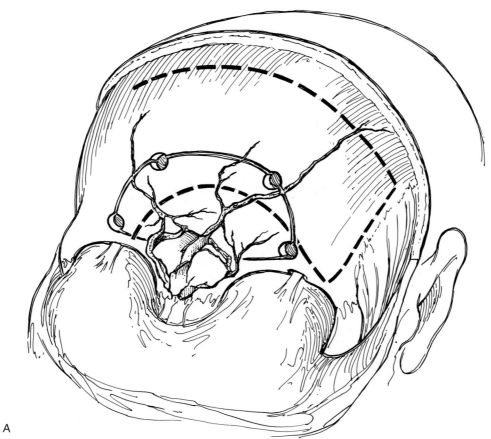

A

FIG. 38. Pericranial flap and free fat grafts used to obliterate dead space and reinforce areas of CSF leak. **A:** Pericranial flap designed and craniotomy flap cut.

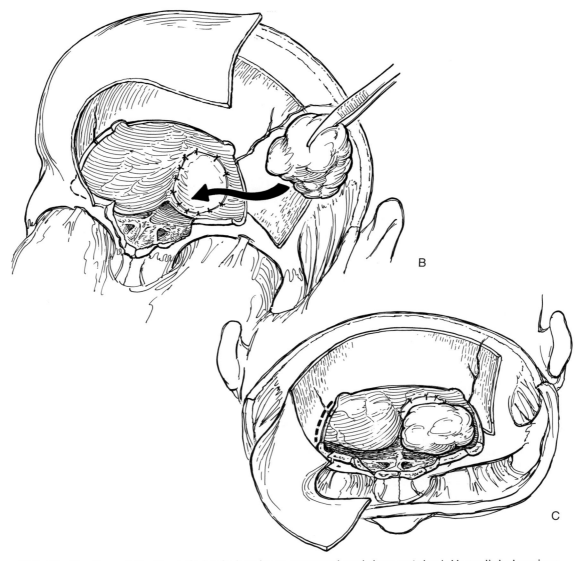

FIG. 38. *Continued.* **B:** Necrotic brain has been removed and dura patched. Unpedicled pericranial flap raised and fat graft to be inserted. **C:** Fat graft in place to obliterate dead space. Pericranial flap being rotated into position. Bony slot (see *dotted line*) cut out lateral to prevent pressure on flap once bone flap is replaced.

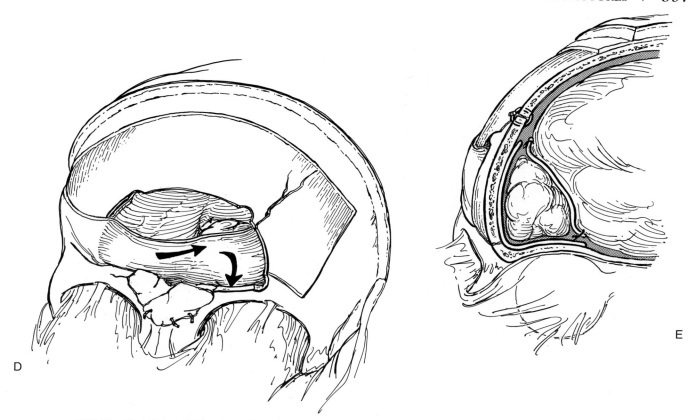

FIG. 38. *Continued.* **D:** Pericranial flap in place and anterior wall frontal sinus fragments returned. **E:** Craniotomy bone flap restored.

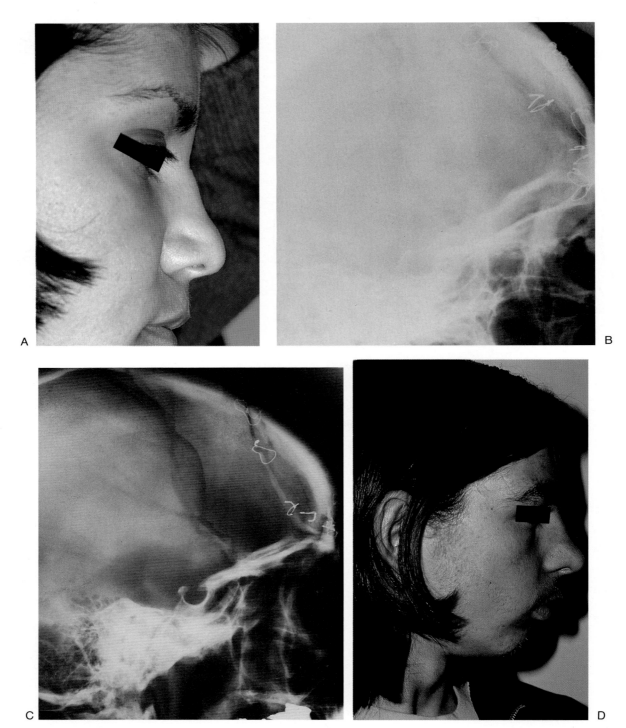

FIG. 39. A: Lateral view of patient following cranialization for through-and-through frontal sinus fracture 2 years postoperatively. **B:** Lateral skull film showing no bone absorption. (From ref. 10, with permission.) **C:** Typical lateral skull film, 5 years postcranialization. **D:** Profile view of patient, 4 years postcranialization, showing no bone resorption. (From ref. 17, with permission.)

pled with a frontonasal duct fracture cannot be managed by simple observation. The presence of the duct fracture mandates surgery.

This treatment protocol has been used by myself for over 20 years with a high degree of success.

REFERENCES

1. Fenton WH Jr, Donald PJ, Carlton W III. Pressure exerted by mucoceles in the frontal sinus. An experimental study in the cat. *Arch Otolaryngol Head Neck Surg* 1990;116(7):836–840.
2. Lotta JS, Schall RF. The histology of the epithelium of the paranasal sinuses under various conditions. *Ann Otol Rhinol Laryngol* 1934;43:945–971.
3. Schenck NL. Frontal sinus disease: III. Experimental and clinical factors in failure of the frontal osteoplastic operation. *Laryngoscope* 1975;85:76–92.
4. Mosher HP, Judd DK. An analysis of seven cases of osteomyelitis of frontal bone complicating frontal sinusitis. *Laryngoscope* 1933;43:153.
5. Donald PJ. The tenacity of the frontal sinus mucosa. *Otolaryngol Head Neck Surg* 1979;87:557–566.
6. Nahum AM. The biomechanics of maxillofacial trauma. *Clin Plast Surg* 1975;2:59.
7. Wallis A, Donald PJ. Frontal sinus fractures: a review of 72 cases. *Laryngoscope* 1988;98(6):593–598.
8. Donald PJ, Ettin M. The safety of frontal sinus fat obliteration when sinus walls are missing. *Laryngoscope* 1986;96(2):190–193.
9. Montgomery WW. *Surgery of the upper respiratory system.* Philadelphia: Lea & Febiger, 1971;126–135.
10. Donald PJ. Frontal sinus and nasofrontoethmoidal complex fractures. Self-instructional package #80400, American Academy of Otolaryngology–Head & Neck Surgery, Alexandria, Virginia, 1980.
11. Baron SH, Dedo HH, Henry CR. The mucoperiosteal flap in frontal sinus surgery (the Sewell–Boyden–McNaught operation). *Laryngoscope* 1973;83:1266–1280.
12. Schultz RC. *Facial injuries,* 2nd ed. Chicago: Year Book, 1977.
13. Neuman MJI, Travis LW. Frontal sinus fractures. *Laryngoscope* 1973;83:1281.
14. Nadell J, Kline DG. Primary reconstruction of depressed frontal skull fractures including those involving the sinus, orbit, and cribriform plate. *J Neurosurg* 1974;41:200–207.
15. Donald PJ, Bernstein L. Compound frontal sinus injuries with intracranial penetration. *Laryngoscope* 1978;88:225–232.
16. Thaller SR, Donald PJ. The use of pericranial flaps in frontal sinus fractures. *Ann Plast Surg* 1994;32(3):284–287.
17. Donald PJ. Frontal sinus ablation by cranialization: a report of 21 cases. *Arch Otolaryngol* 1982;108:142.

CHAPTER 27

Frontal and Ethmoid Complex Fractures

Paul J. Donald

Clearly the most difficult facial fracture injury in which to achieve a satisfactory cosmetic and functional result is the fracture of the nasofrontoethmoidal complex. These fractures are usually the consequence of severe trauma and produce disruption of a critical aesthetic and functional area. Signs and symptoms are pathognomonic and the diagnosis is clinically not difficult to make. Immediate surgery is much more successful than late, but a perfect result is difficult to obtain even in the early cases. Residua such as nasal depression, widened medial canthi, epiphora, and diplopia are not uncommonly seen.

ANATOMY

Osteology

The anatomy of the nasofrontoethmoidal complex, as the name implies, is complicated. The thin paired nasal bones articulate superiorly in a suture line with the nasal process of the frontal bone. In contrast with the somewhat flimsy nasal bones, this contribution from the frontal bone is extremely thick and strong. The nasal bones are inserted slightly under this process in the same way that the superior extent of the upper lateral cartilages underlie the nasal bones. The frontal sinus lies directly above the nasal process of the frontal bone and its aeration at this point is variable. In the midline, the nasal bones lie on a strong stout spine, extending anteroinferiorly from the frontal bone. The nasion and the glabella are important aesthetic features of this area. The nasion is the indented part of the nose as it flows into the contour of the forehead above. The glabella is the protuberant portion of the forehead just above the nasion (Fig. 1). Lang (1) states that the angle at the glabella should be around 115 degrees for males and 120 degrees for females. Powell and Humphries

(2) say the measurement should be 125 to 135 degrees (Fig. 2). Articulating with the nasal bones laterally as well as a part of the nasal process of the frontal bone superiorly is the frontal process of the maxilla. This thin bone is the most anterior projection of the maxilla and makes up a small portion of the lateral wall of the nasal dorsum. This process, however, rapidly thickens posteriorly as it becomes the anteromedial buttress of the face and that portion of the maxillary sinus. Superiorly, as one proceeds in a posterior direction into the medial wall of the orbit, the frontal process of the maxilla articulates with the lacrimal bone and the lamina papyracea of the ethmoid complex.

The lacrimal bone is the smallest bone in the facial skeleton and occupies the anteroinferior aspect of the medial wall of the orbit. It has rather stout anterior and posterior crests for the insertion of the medial canthal tendons but its central concave part has the thinness of onion skin paper. It articulates with the frontal process of the maxilla anteriorly, the frontal bone superiorly, and the lamina papyracea of the ethmoid posteriorly (Fig. 3). The lacrimal fossa measures about 16 mm high, 4 to 8 mm wide, and 2 mm deep (3). The nasal lacrimal duct leads from the inferior aspect of the lacrimal fossa, coursing through the maxilla in the anterior aspect of the lateral wall of the nose. It is approximately 12.5 mm long with a 5-mm extension in the inferior meatus. In its traverse, it is inclined in an anterior–posterior direction about 15 degrees. It runs a line roughly between the inner canthus of the eye and the first molar tooth. The duct bows slightly laterally in its course and is 4.5 mm wide. The termination at the inferior meatus of the nose under the inferior turbinate is about 7 mm from the bony nasal verge, its end being at about the level of the nasal ala (Fig. 4).

The lamina papyracea comprises most of the medial orbital wall. Attached to it, often at right angles, are the

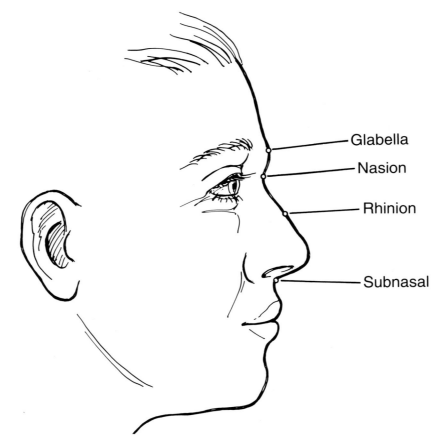

FIG. 1. Profile view of face with aesthetic landmarks.

Glabella

Nasion

Rhinion

Subnasal

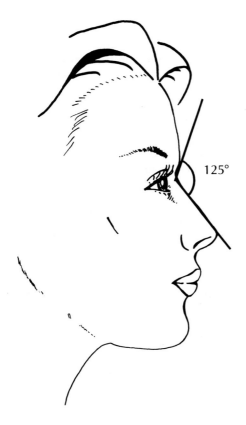

125°

FIG. 2. Ideal glabellar angle. (From ref. 2, with permission.)

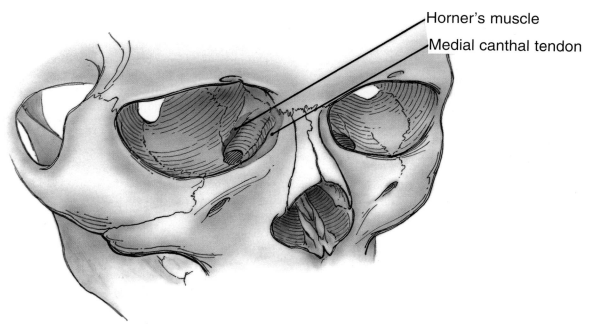

FIG. 3. Bony components of the region of the anteromedial wall of the orbit and points of insertion of Horner's muscle and medial canthal tendon.

septations between the numerous ethmoidal air cells, acting as a buffer against injury to brain and orbital contents. The lamina has a laterally facing concave surface and articulates with the sphenoid bone posteriorly, which thickens rapidly as it forms part of the medial wall of the optic canal. It articulates superiorly with the orbital process of the frontal bone and inferiorly with the orbital process of the maxilla—a bone of similar thinness, but without the support lent by the walls of the ethmoid cells. The lamina papyracea is penetrated by three foramina to permit the passage of the anterior, posterior, and middle ethmoid arteries.

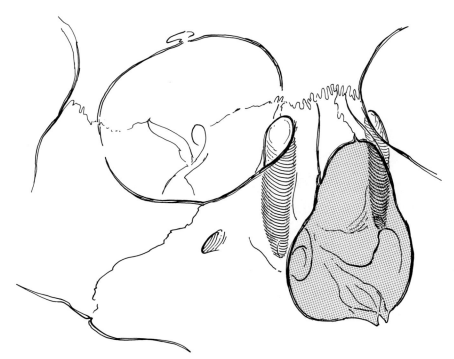

FIG. 4. Course of nasolacrimal duct.

Medial Canthal Tendon

We are greatly indebted to Lester Jones (4), whose definitive description of the medial canthal tendon has been little improved upon today. Much of our understanding of the anatomy and physiology comes from his extensive work.

The orbicularis oculi muscle is the main sphincter of the eyelids and its medial tendinous attachment makes up by far the largest portion of the medial canthal tendon. This structure is often referred to as the medial canthal "ligament" (5). The word ligament is a clear misnomer as this structure connects mainly muscle to bone, and not bone to bone, or bone to cartilage as the term "ligament" is defined (6).

The orbicularis oculi is made up of three portions: the orbital, pretarsal, and preseptal. Like the rest of the atavistic remnants of the panniculus carnosus, this muscle takes its origin on the hard tissues of the periorbital region and inserts into the skin of the eyelids and into itself at the lateral and medial raphes. The orbital part originates on the bone of the orbit, specifically the frontal bone and maxilla. It is the only portion of the orbicularis that does not contribute significantly to the formation of the medial canthal tendon. The preseptal part lies in front of the septum orbitale—that portion of the periorbital periosteum that connects the tarsal plates to the periorbital rims. The pretarsal segment lies on the anterior face of the tarsal plates. These latter two parts make up the bulk of the tendon (Fig. 5).

The next most important contribution to the medial canthal tendon is the suspensory ligament of Lockwood (Fig. 6). This structure lies under the globe and extends from the tendon's principal insertion at the frontal process of maxilla and anterior lacrimal crest, medially to its lateral insertion through Whitnall's tubercle on the medial aspect of the orbital process of the zygoma laterally.

Smaller contributions to the tendon are made by the check ligaments of the medial rectus muscle (7), the corrugator supercilii via the superciliaris muscle (4), a slip from the levator palpebra superioris, and the orbital septum (8) (Figs. 7 and 8).

The tendon has two separate insertions: anterior and posterior. The anterior insertion of the medial canthal tendon on the frontal process of the maxilla and the anterior lacrimal crest is by far the most substantial. However, both the preseptal and pretarsal muscles have smaller tendinous insertions to the posterior lacrimal crest. In this way, they straddle the lacrimal sac. The posterior portion is dubbed Horner's muscle and this sling comprises a sort of lacrimal pump so that when the orbicularis contracts, it aids in the passage of tears down the nasolacrimal duct (Fig. 9).

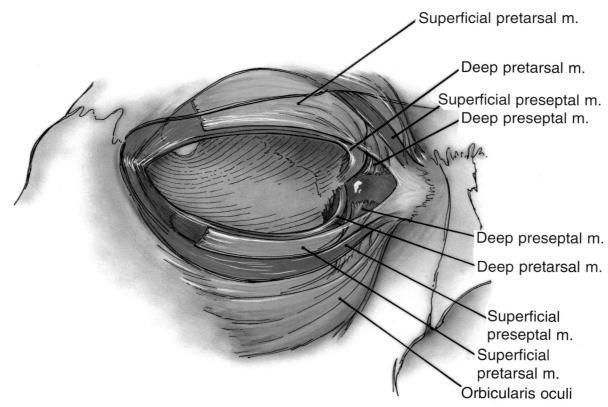

Superficial pretarsal m.

Deep pretarsal m.

Superficial preseptal m.
Deep preseptal m.

Deep preseptal m.

Deep pretarsal m.

Superficial preseptal m.

Superficial pretarsal m.

Orbicularis oculi

FIG. 5. Pretarsal and preseptal contributions to medial canthal tendon.

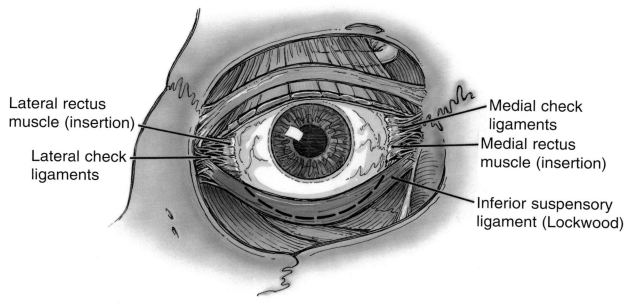

FIG. 6. Lockwood's suspensory ligament and its contribution to the medial canthal tendon.

The functions of the tendon appear to be (a) to tether the lids to the medial wall of the orbit, (b) to help in suspension of the globe within the orbit, (c) to act as a lacrimal pump, and (d) to assist in the function of the medial rectus muscle.

Some confusion exists between the terms telecanthus and hypertelorism. Hypertelorism is a condition usually caused by a congenital anomaly, such as an ethmoidal encephalocele, that produces an increased distance between the orbits. Tessier has established the criterion that if the distance between the lacrimal crests of each orbit exceeds the width of one bony orbit that hypertelorism exists (Fig. 10). Telecanthus is when the distance between the medial ends of the palpebral fissures of both eyes exceeds the distance measured between the medial and lateral canthi of an individual eye (Fig. 11). It is important to use calipers to measure this distance because the use of a flat ruler or paper tape has to negotiate the curve of the bridge of the nose, which will naturally increase the intercanthal

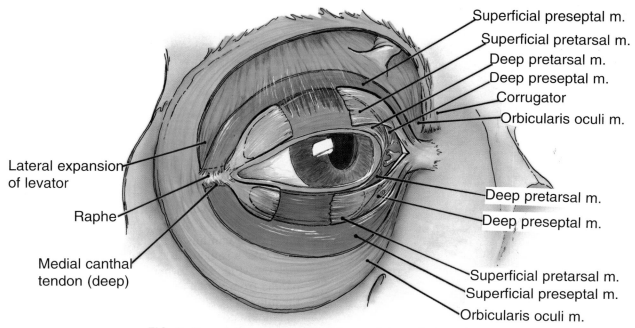

FIG. 7. Remaining contributions to medial canthal tendon.

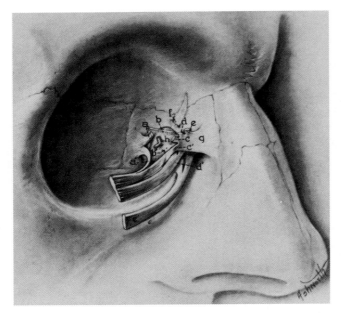

FIG. 8. All contributions to the medial canthal tendon. Shown are upper and lower deep heads of pretarsal muscles (a and a'); upper and lower deep insertions of preseptal muscles (b and b'); upper and lower insertions of superficial heads of pretarsal muscles (c and c'); upper and lower superficial parts of preseptal muscles (d and d'); orbital parts of orbicularis muscle (e and f); medial canthal tendon (g); and junction of canaliculi at lacrimal diaphragm (h). (From ref. 4, with permission.)

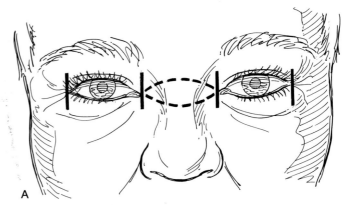

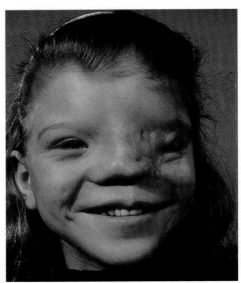

FIG. 10. A: Diagram showing measurement between orbits and orbit width showing parity. **B:** Patient with congenital hypertelorism.

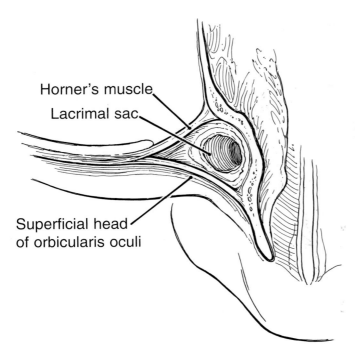

Horner's muscle

Lacrimal sac

Superficial head of orbicularis oculi

FIG. 9. Horner's muscle.

distance. "Eyeballing" along a flat ruler also has a great potential for error.

Lacrimal System

A detailed description of the lacrimal system is beyond the scope of this book. A cursory discussion is presented to enable understanding of disturbances in the system brought about by nasofrontoethmoidal complex trauma.

The lacrimal canaliculi each exit a punctum at the medial extremity of both upper and lower eyelids at the medial canthus just lateral to the caruncle. They each take a roughly L-shaped course to enter the lacrimal sac (Fig. 12), either separately or together. The papilla from which the canaliculi emerge is 8 mm from the inner canthus above and 10 mm for the lower. Each canaliculus has a 2-mm vertical course and then turns horizontally in the axis of the lid to empty into the sinus

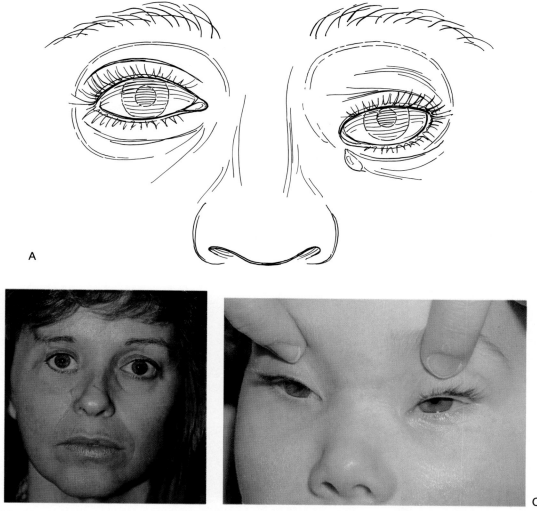

FIG. 11. A: Diagram showing telecanthus. **B:** Patient with unilateral telecanthus. **C:** Patient with bilateral telecanthus.

of Maier, which in turn empties into the lacrimal sac. The sac is 4 mm by 8 mm in size and several millimeters thick. Inferiorly, the lacrimal sac empties into a funnel-shaped lacrimal duct, which descends in the lacrimal canal into the inferior meatus of the nose at a 15-degree angle. The duct has five valves. They function to prevent dilation of the lacrimal sac on nose blowing. The closest valve to the sac is at the entrance of the sinus of Maier into the lacrimal sac. The furthest valve is the valve of Hausner located just adjacent to the opening of the duct in the inferior meatus of the nose. This opening is just opposite the nasal ala, approximately 7 mm from the bony nasal verge.

Trochlea

Another structure vulnerable to injury in nasofrontoethmoidal complex fractures is the trochlea. This fi-bro-osseous structure situated at the upper inner aspect of the orbit forms a pulley around which the superior oblique muscle takes a right-angled bend to insert on the globe. Although infrequently damaged in fractures even in extensive maxillofacial trauma, it is often dislodged during their repair. Injury or displacement of the tendon at the trochlea will produce diplopia, which usually resolves during the healing process when the trochlea reattaches to the medial orbit. (For more details on the trochlea, see the chapter, Surgical Management of Frontal Sinus Infections, by Donald.)

ETIOLOGY AND PATHOPHYSIOLOGY

Patients who sustain frontoethmoidal complex fractures are usually the victims of violent trauma. The blow is commonly received from a frontal direction, driving these contents of the central facial skeleton in

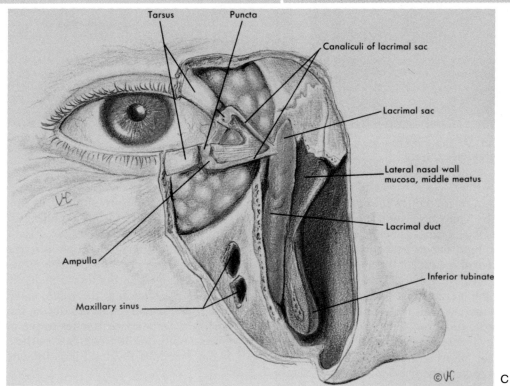

FIG. 12. Diagram of the lacrimal system. **A:** Schematic drawing of nasolacrimal excretory system to show valves. Valves represent central cells within developing epithelial cord that failed to degenerate. **B:** Approximate dimensions of nasolacrimal excretory system. In the adult the length of the system is about 35 mm; in the newborn the system measures about 25 mm. **C:** Nasolacrimal excretory system. (From ref. 9, with permission.)

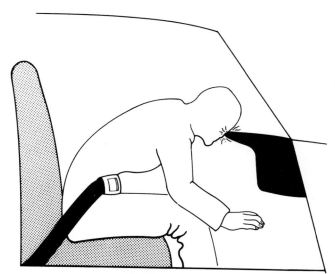

FIG. 13. Diagram of a head coming forward on dashboard indicating a common mechanism of injury producing frontoethmoidal complex fracture. (From ref. 10, with permission.)

a backward and upward direction. This was a more commonly encountered injury following motor vehicle accidents (Fig. 13) during the time prior to the extensive use of seat belts especially the shoulder type.

The blow fractures the nasal bones and they in turn prolapse into the ethmoid sinus complex. The nasal bones are pushed into the nasal cavity and lodge under the nasal process of the frontal bone. Sometimes the anterior wall of the frontal sinus is fractured also and is usually driven posteriorly. The fractures of the nasal bones are often carried through the ascending process of the maxilla as well. The lamina papyracea and the lacrimal bone often become fractured. This dislodges the medial canthal tendon. Because the tendon is the attachment of the orbicularis oculi muscle, the natural tone of the muscle will pull the medial canthus laterally (Fig. 11). The tendon may be lacerated or, more commonly, a piece of bone will be pulled laterally, attached to the tendon. An inferior displacement of the globe will result because of the loss of support of Lockwood's ligament.

The traumatic episode may also result in a laceration that cuts through the medial canthus, severing the lacrimal canaliculi. If more medial, the lacrimal sac may be disrupted or even the lacrimal duct transected. As the tension on the eye, placed by the tethering of the orbicularis oculi muscle, is released by the avulsion of the canthal tendon, the lacrimal punctum faces away from the lacus lacrimalis. This results in epiphora on blinking.

The possibility of fracture to the floor of the anterior cranial fossa exists, and careful observation for a cerebrospinal fluid (CSF) leak from the cribriform plate or

fovea ethmoidalis is essential. If the fracture extends into the orbital floor, the inferior oblique muscle and its check ligament may be injured, interfering with extraocular muscle function.

DIAGNOSIS

These patients often have a history of an unconscious period. They are frequently victims of multiple trauma including a head injury. The usual attention to emergency resuscitative measures and the ruling out of life-threatening injuries to the abdomen, thorax, or central nervous system are required. Skull computed tomography (CT) scans and cervical spine films precede any definitive attack on the facial fracture.

The patients usually complain of midfacial pain, epistaxis, nasal obstruction, and facial deformity. If there is an injury to the lacrimal drainage system, the patient will likely have epiphora and when there is avulsion of the medial canthal tendon, epiphora is almost invariable. If the inferior rectus or inferior oblique muscles are detached, the patient may have diplopia. Approximately 10% of patients with periorbital trauma have ocular injuries. Indeed, rupture of the globe, detached retina, vitreous hemorrhage, and dislocated lens may result from either direct trauma from the blow or injury from bone fragments.

The nose has a characteristic "pig snout" deformity (Fig. 14). This is produced by a loss of nasal tip and dorsal projection. The tip is abnormally tilted skyward and the nose appears shortened. The dorsum of the

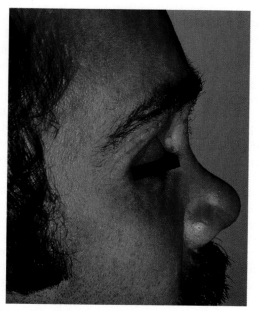

FIG. 14. "Pig snout" deformity characteristic of nasofrontoethmoidal complex fracture.

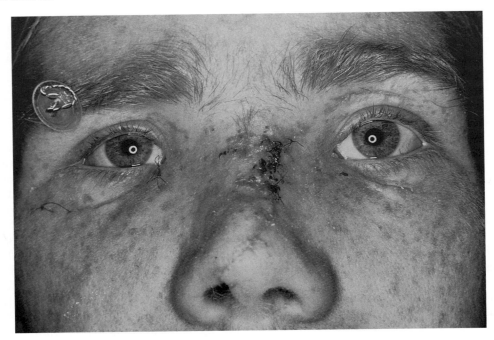

FIG. 15. "Wiped out" appearance between eyes.

nose is markedly reduced and usually flattened between the canthi. Even without telecanthus, the flattening between the eyes gives a "wiped out" appearance and mimics to some degree a splaying of the canthi (Fig. 15). There is often a marked indentation over the nasion. There may be epistaxis and it is important to test for the halo sign (see the chapter, Frontal Sinus Fractures, by Donald) to detect the presence of CSF.

When the medial canthal tendon is avulsed, the eye takes on a characteristic appearance (Fig. 11). The medial canthus is blunted, the lacrimal papilla is everted outward, and the lower lid is prolapsed downward. The lower lid margin is slightly everted away from the globe. The eye is slightly proptotic and the canthus is pointed downward as well as displaced laterally (Fig. 16). The mild proptosis comes about from the release of the backward tethering effect of the orbicularis oculi. The distance between the medial and lateral canthus of the affected eye is less than that of the normal eye. In addition, the distance between the eyes is greater than the width of the normal eye (Fig. 10). This was established by Günter (11) in 1933, to be from 25.5 to 37.5 mm in women and 26.5 to 38.7 mm in men. The average normal intraorbital distance in the adult is measured roentgenographically. It is the distance between the medial orbital walls and is 7 to 8 mm less than the intercanthal distance. If both canthal tendons are avulsed, the intraocular distance is far greater than the width of either eye. However, the distance rarely exceeds 1.5 times the width of the normal eye. The interorbital distance remains unchanged.

A common finding in medial canthal tears is absence of the "bowstring sign." When the patient looks laterally, the normal medial canthal tendon feels as tight as a bowstring. In medial canthal tears, palpation in the medial canthal area reveals no bowstring effect and feels soft.

Epiphora is common from both the dysfunction of the lacrimal lake and from the injury to either the lacrimal canalicular system or the lacrimal sac that is so common in these injuries. The eversion of the lacrimal punctum, coupled with the inefficiency of the disrupted lacrimal pump mechanism system resulting from the loss of fixation of Horner's muscle, causes the tears to overflow.

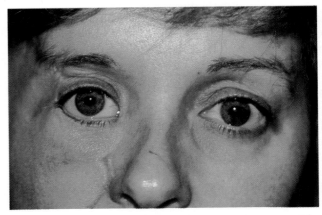

FIG. 16. Patient with characteristic downward and laterally displaced medial canthus from a medial canthal ligament avulsion (close-up of patient in Fig. 11B).

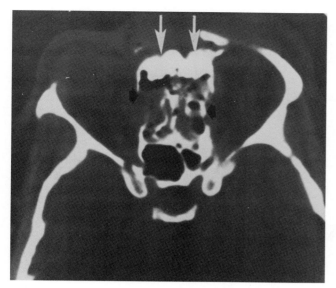

FIG. 17. Axial CAT scan of nasofrontoethmoidal complex fracture. (From ref. 12.)

An epicanthal web of soft tissue may form that obscures the caruncle and adds to the blunting of the inner palpebral angle. This excess skin from the nasojugal area forms as a result of the release of tension normally caused by the binding action of the medial canthal tendon.

Occasionally, fractures involving the medial or superior orbital wall (the lamina papyracea medially and the orbital process of the frontal bone superiorly) will result in ocular entrapment. This will cause diplopia on downward or outward gaze and restricted motion when the forced duction test is applied in these directions.

The diagnosis of nasofrontoethmoidal complex fractures is usually relatively easy to make on clinical grounds. There are sometimes associated soft tissue injuries, marked facial swelling, or associated maxillary fractures that tend to obscure these findings. The radiographic appearance best seen on the axial and coronal plane computer-assisted tomography (CAT) scan is characteristic. There is collapse and prolapse of the nasal bones. Telescoping of the ethmoid sinuses occurs as the nasal bones are pushed posteriorly (Fig. 17). Coronal scans will show splaying of the lacrimal crests and these are sometimes so badly shattered as to be unrecognizable. The nasal bones or a part of the nasal process of the frontal bone will be seen to be pushed into the ethmoid sinuses and be located directly adjacent to the globes (Fig. 18). The nasal bones often are blocked under the frontal bone from which they have been fractured. In some cases, the medial orbital wall may appear thicker by virtue of overlying bone fragments. The lamina papyracea is crushed, and the ethmoid block and usually frontal sinuses are opacified. Occasionally, there is intraorbital and even intracranial air (12).

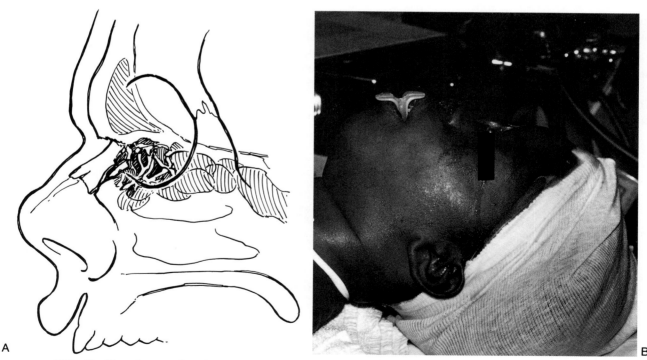

FIG. 18. Nasofrontoethmoidal complex fracture. **A:** Note nasal bones driven under the frontal. **B:** Patient with nasofrontoethmoidal complex fracture.

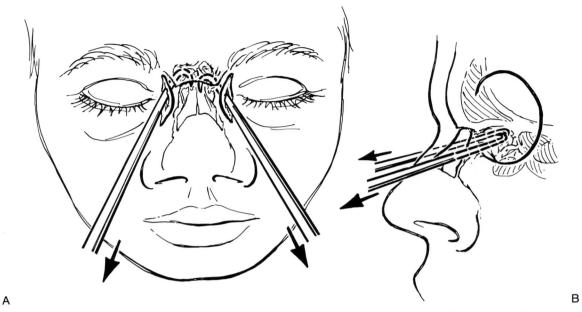

FIG. 19. Reduction of frontoethmoidal fracture. **A:** Stout bone hooks are placed through lamina papyracea into ethmoid fracture. **B:** Forward and downward traction is exerted until fracture is reduced.

TREATMENT

Early treatment is much more effective than late. This implies that the repair should be done as soon as possible after the injury. Once fibrosis sets in, it is extremely difficult to bring the canthus back to its normal anatomical position. Once the life-threatening problems are resolved, the patient should be operated on immediately.

Nose

The most difficult step is the actual reduction of the impacted nasal fracture. The depressed nasal dorsum

is not only difficult to disimpact, but it is equally hard to maintain in fixation. The depressed inferior fragment becomes locked under the frontal bone. The shattered, telescoped ethmoid sinuses do not afford an adequate foundation for stable reduction. The initial attempt at reduction using Walsham or Ashe forceps is met with only occasional success. Disimpaction usually requires placing stout hooks into the ethmoid labyrinth on each side. Access is achieved by using bilateral external ethmoidectomy incisions and, if necessary, a horizontal incision joining the two. The periorbitum is elevated to the level of the posterior ethmoid artery. Under direct vision, the hooks are placed into the fractured ethmoidal complex anterior to the posterior ethmoid arter-

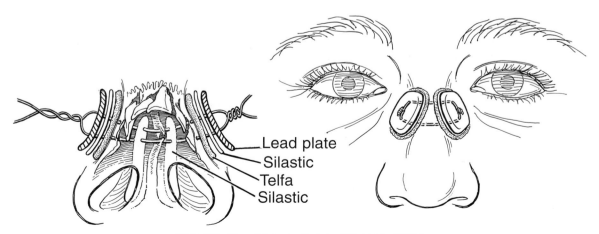

Lead plate
Silastic
Telfa
Silastic

FIG. 20. Nasal bones fixed with lead plates.

ies (Fig. 19). A downward–forward pull, often with considerable force, is required to achieve reduction. Some prying at the fracture site with an osteotome, coupled with the distraction force of the hooks, will usually disimpact the fracture.

The standard method of fixation is by the use of lead plates and suspension wires (Fig. 20). The wires are guided through the nasal and ethmoid fractures with a stout curved needle in a curvilinear manner. There are two wires passed one above and one below; and they go through one side of the nose and come out the other. The suspension wires are threaded through an ovoid piece of Telfa, then Silastic, and finally a thin lead plate. The two wires on each side are twisted down so as to be snug, but not tight. The lead plates serve as an anchor for the wires and not as a means of maintaining the fracture. Excessive tightening can produce sloughing of the underlying skin (Fig. 21).

Direct wiring or plating with microplates at the fracture site over the upper nasal dorsum is sometimes required to maintain the reduction. Small gauge wire can be used to approximate only the larger fragments of the shattered nasal dorsum. They may also be secured by microplates (Fig. 22). In the event that the bones are so severely comminuted that no discernible or predictably stable dorsum can be restored, a bone graft of split calvarial bone is placed over the dorsum and secured to the frontal bone with a microplate (Fig. 23).

An alternative method of fixation of the depressed dorsum is the use of a halo brace, such as that developed by Georgiade, and an external appliance. The frame is fitted to the outer table of the skull with bone screws. An outrigger is fixed to the frame and connected to wires hooked to the disimpacted fragments; it then is dropped from the frame in such a way that the wires are at a 90-degree angle to it. If disimpaction

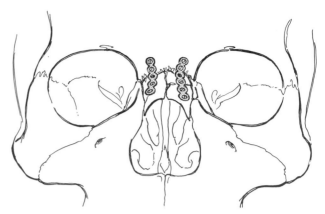

FIG. 22. Nasal dorsum restored with low-profile microplates.

of the fragments has been unsuccessful, then this system can be used for fracture reduction. Pieces of elastic interposed between the wire attached to the fragments and to the outrigger exert continuous traction that ultimately leads to reduction. To avoid overcorrection, care must be taken to substitute wire for the elastic once the nose has been satisfactorily reduced. With the advent of plating and more rigid fixation, this system has largely been abandoned.

Medial Canthal Tendon

The reduction of traumatic telecanthus is extremely difficult. It should be performed as soon after the injury as possible. The approach is through bilateral, external ethmoidectomy incisions. The displaced medial canthal tendon is often difficult to identify, and periodic traction on fibrous tissue that may resemble it is frequently the only means of localization. It is important to remember that the tendon is a subcutaneous structure and deep dissection is unnecessary to find it. Fortunately, there usually is a portion of lacrimal bone attached to the tendon that helps in identification and in reconstruction of its anatomic relationships.

The surgical goal is a slightly overcorrected reduction of the tendons. The principal impediment to permanently achieving this aim is the tearing of the wire through the tendon itself, and through the anchor site as well. Keeping this in mind, the surgeon must take maximum advantage of residual bone on the ligament and assure maximal security at the anchoring site.

A variety of techniques have been advanced to achieve fixation of the tendon. As is so often the case with multiple techniques, none is the most efficacious. The basic technique in all canthal fixation procedures is ligation of the tendon to a bony anchor somewhere between the ipsilateral medial orbital wall and that of the opposite orbit (Fig. 24). In the unilateral case, if

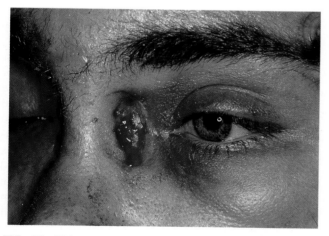

FIG. 21. Skin slough under excessively tightened lead plates.

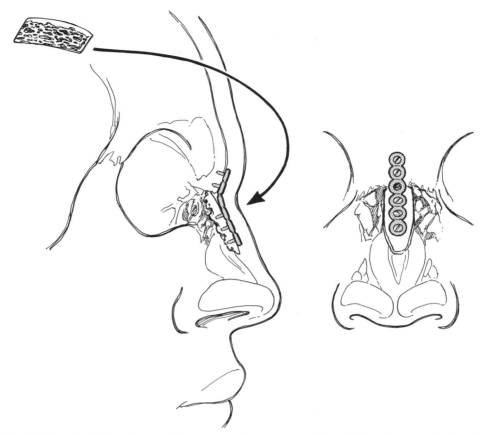

FIG. 23. Split calvarial graft, used to augment an irreversibly shattered nose, is fixed with a microplate.

no shattered bone exists in the medial orbital wall of the affected side, fixation can be achieved without crossing the nasal vault. Once the medial canthal tendon has been identified, two holes are made with a drill in the posterior lacrimal crest. Whenever possible, the drill holes should be placed behind the posterior lacrimal crest and above the lacrimal fossa. Unfortunately, this is not always feasible and the holes are made through the anterior crest. As big a gap as possible is made between holes in order to provide a firm anchor for the wire. Overcorrection produces better results. A 29- or 30-gauge wire is passed through the tendon. The wire is then passed through the holes in the lacrimal crest and twisted into place, thereby reducing the tendon. This is one of the first techniques described, but it has recently been modified by Duvall and Banovetz (13). Using an intranasal approach, they connected the medial canthal wire to a Silastic button via a pullout wire (Fig. 25). In this modification, the canthal wire is tightened, bringing the pullout wire with the button against the lateral wall of the nasal cavity. The pullout wire, when twisted up into the intranasal button, provides an excellent anchor for the wire. The pullout wire and button are removed in 14 days.

These two techniques are best suited to the delayed case, or to one in which the medial canthal tendon has been clearly avulsed, with minimal or absent fracturing of the medial orbital wall. In the nondelayed case, when the pullout button is not used, the probability of the wire spontaneously pulling through the small bony bridge around which it is anchored is extremely high. The intranasal button improves the results, but even the author of this innovation is less than completely enthusiastic about it.

Most commonly the medial wall of the orbit is shattered, eliminating the medial orbital wall as an anchor site for the medial canthal tendon. In these cases, the wire passed through the tendon and attached lacrimal bone must be secured to the lateral nasal wall of the opposite side. A Lynch incision is made in the nasojugal area of this opposing side and the frontal process of the maxilla on this side exposed to the tendon and above (Fig. 26A,B). Two drill holes are made in the bone above the tendon and the wire in the torn tendon is passed transnasally and brought through these drill holes with a curved or straight Keith needle (Fig. 26C). The wire is tightened and the tendon is reduced (Fig. 26D).

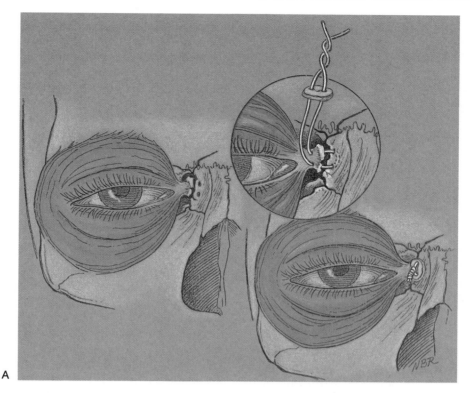

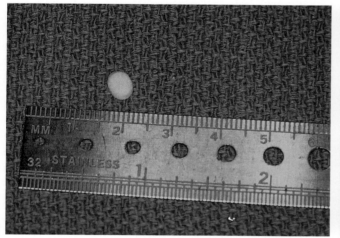

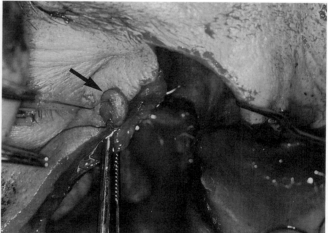

FIG. 24. Standard method of fixation of unilateral medial canthal tendon avulsion. **A:** Fixation to medial orbital wall with wire. **B:** Felt bolster. **C:** Wire is passed through a small Dacron felt bolster to prevent wire tearing through tendon. (*Arrow* points to felt bolster.)

In 1970, Converse and Hogan (14) described the "open sky" technique. This technique is especially good for the bilateral canthal avulsion. Bilateral external ethmoidectomy incisions are made and connected across the nasion (Fig. 26A). Once the fragments of nasal bone, nasal process of frontal bone, and frontal process of maxilla have been successfully wired or plated, two drill holes are created. The first goes from a point high on the anterior lacrimal crest on the fractured side to the same structure on the opposing side.

A second through-and-through hole is made through the posterior crest (Fig. 27). There may be such extensive fracturing that no drill holes can be made and subsequent wire passage is done by negotiating the needle with attached wire between fragments. Any substantial piece of bone, however, should be captured by the wire for stability. Passage of the wires through these holes constitutes one of the most difficult maneuvers of the entire operation. A curved Keith needle, or a large curved retention suture needle may be used to advance

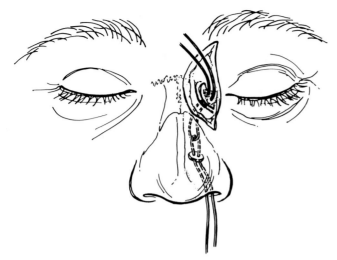

FIG. 25. Anchoring of medial canthal tendon wire using intranasal button technique as described by Duvall and Banovetz (13).

the wire through the holes (Fig. 26D). Another method of passing the wires is to drive a 16- or 18-gauge trochar through the holes, removing the stylet and using the trochar as a conduit. Great care must be exercised in placing and angulating the trochar to avoid penetrating the anterior cranial fossa. A careful check of the Caldwell radiograph, to ensure the relationship of the cribriform plate to the medial orbital wall, is essential prior to this maneuver. A horizontal line connecting the pupils usually marks the level of the cribriform plate. Once one wire is passed through, it is passed through each canthal tendon and clamped. The posterior wire is passed first and a second anterior wire next. The second wire is also passed through the tendon. Both wires are then twisted together to bring the medial canthal tendon into position.

A further modification of this technique is to use a Teflon or Dacron felt pad, or a bone or cartilage graft, as a bolster to secure the wire on the unfractured side in a unilateral case or on both sides for a bilateral case (Fig. 24). This prevents the wire from pulling through the anchor site. Kazanjian and Converse (15) added an additional modification to assist in redraping the soft tissue against the nasal bony framework. They recommended drilling an additional hole through the ascend-

ing processes of the maxilla, anterior to the holes for the canthal wires. A doubled-over wire is passed through the hole and punctured through the overlying skin. The wire is threaded through a Silastic button on either side of the nose. When the wires are tightened, the button will help to redrape the soft tissue, thereby effacing the epicanthal fold formed by the injury. The button on the opposite side will act simply as an anchoring bolster. If lead plates have been placed to reduce an unstable nasal fracture, they will accomplish the same objective. The epicanthal button also assists in maintaining the reduction of the canthal tendon. Care must be taken to avoid excessive tension on the plates as they may cause necrosis of underlying soft tissue (Fig. 21).

The goal one wishes to achieve by surgical management is slight overcorrection. The principal impediment in permanently achieving this aim is the tearing of the wire through the tendon. It is important to reemphasize that the wire has a tendency not only to tear through the tendon itself but to rip through the anchor site as well.

If the unilateral deformity is a problem to reduce, the bilateral deformity is even more difficult. The major obstacle centers around the fact that the canthal wire on each side acts as the anchor site for the opposing side. The risk of at least one wire pulling free is, of course, double that for the unilateral case. If one canthal tendon is anchored to its fellow, the cutting through of one wire will automatically release both sides, with relapse of the bilateral deformity.

The fixation of each canthal wire to a button or lead plate against the opposite side of the nose is probably the most effective means of fixation. However, the problem with this technique is that, in time, the wire needs to be pulled out. There is often a slow migration of the medial canthal tendon back to its original pathologic position. An anterior angulation in the direction of pull of the wire is also a drawback of this technique. The permanently placed wires obviate this problem and, despite their residence in the vault of the nose, cause little trouble.

Relaxation of the suspensory ligament via lateral canthotomy helps maintain the position of the repaired medial canthal tendon and probably should be performed routinely in bilateral cases. Some surgeons re-

FIG. 26. Repair of unilateral medial canthal tendon. **A:** Bilateral Lynch incisions are connected across nasal dorsum. **B:** Dissection of soft tissue demonstrates avulsed medial canthal tendon, medial orbital wall, and nasal dorsal fractures. **C:** Nasal fragments are approximated with low-profile microplates and avulsed tendon is fixed to opposite intact medial nasal wall by wires. **D:** Two wires are drilled in medial orbit, one high on the anterior lacrimal crest and one posteriorly and low on the posterior lacrimal crest. Large curved needle is used to pass wire between avulsed medial canthal tendons.

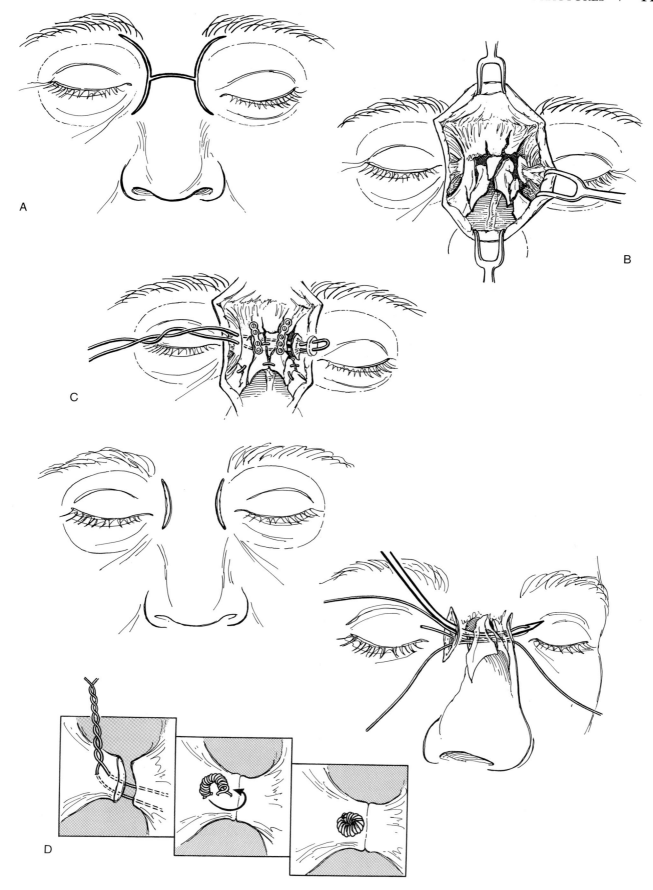

A

B

C

D

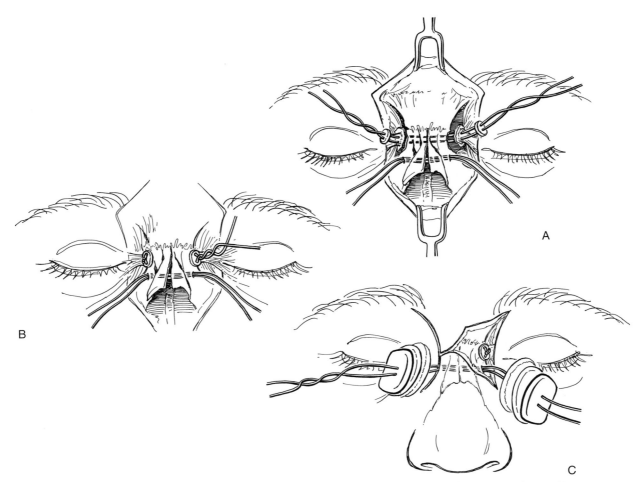

FIG. 27. Bilateral medial canthal tendon avulsion repaired using the Converse–Hogan "open sky" technique. **A:** Incisions opened. Two pairs of wires inserted—one through medial canthal tendons (above), the second through adjacent nasal bones (below). **B:** Wires are tightened, bringing canthal tendons into position. The wires are twisted together over each avulsed tendon, pulling the tendons together. **C:** Tendons supported and soft tissue splinted by Telfa pad-silastic-lead plate assembly (see Fig. 20).

lease the septum orbitale both above and below the medial canthus to the level of the superior and inferior orbital rims. However, this procedure usually is not necessary except in the delayed case.

Severe injuries to the medial canthus seldom occur without some damage to the lacrimal system. This is usually easiest to repair at the time of restoration of the medial canthus. Fixation of a large surgically created eventration in the lacrimal sac to the nasal mucosa, through a sufficiently large fenestration in the lacrimal fossa or just anterior to it, will bypass the nasolacrimal duct and ensure adequate drainage of tears. Prior to this, satisfactory drainage from the conjunctival sac should be ensured from its least one of the lacrimal canaliculi. If the lacrimal sac is unrecognizably damaged, then a Quickert tube is inserted through the lacrimal punctum into the nose, tied upon itself, and left in place for at least 3 weeks.

REFERENCES

1. Lang J. *Clinical anatomy of the nose, nasal cavity and paranasal sinuses.* New York: Thieme Medical Publishers, 1989:25.
2. Powell M, Humphries B. *Proportions of the aesthetic face.* Stuttgart: G Thieme, 1984;16.
3. Lemke BN. Lacrimal anatomy. In: Bosniak SL, Smith BC, eds. *Advances in ophthalmic plastic & reconstructive surgery,* vol 3. Elmsford, NY: Pergamon Press, 1984;11–23.
4. Jones LT, Raeeh MG, Wirtshafter JD. *Manual of ophthalmic anatomy.* Rochester, MN: American Academy of Ophthalmology & Otolaryngology, 1970.
5. Gross C. Pathophysiology and evaluation of frontoethmoid fractures. In: Mathog RN, ed. *Maxillofacial trauma.* Baltimore: Williams & Wilkins, 1984;280–287.
6. *Dorland's illustrated medical dictionary.* Philadelphia: Saunders, 1988.
7. Reeh MJ, Beyer CK, Shannon GM. *Practical ophthalmic plastic & reconstructive surgery.* Philadelphia: Lea & Febiger, 1976; 11.
8. Iliff CE, Iliff WJ, Iliff NT. *Oculoplastic surgery.* Philadelphia: Saunders, 1979;23.
9. Lemke BN. Anatomy of the ocular adnexa and orbit. In: Smith B, Della Rocca RC, Nesi FA, Lisman RD, eds. *Ophthalmic plas-*

tic & reconstructive surgery, vol 1. St Louis: CV Mosby, 1987; 23–24.

10. Beyer CK, Smith B. Naso-orbital fractures: their complications and treatment. In: Tessier P, Callahan A, Mustarde JC, Salyer KE, eds. Symposium on plastic surgery in the orbital region, vol 12. St Louis: CV Mosby, 1976;107.

11. Günter H. Konstitutionelle Anomalien des Augenabstandes und der Interorbitalbrilite. Virchows Arch A Pathol Anat 1933;290: 373.

12. Delbalso AM. Maxillofacial imaging. Philadelphia: Saunders, 1990;103.

13. Duvall AJ, Banovetz JD. Nasoethmoidal fractures. Otolaryngol Clin North Am 1976;9(2):507–514.

14. Converse JM, Hogan VM. Open-sky approach for reduction of naso-orbital fractures. Plast Reconstr Surg 1970;46:396.

15. Kazanjian VH, Converse JM. Surgical treatment of facial injuries, 3rd ed. Baltimore: Williams & Wilkins, 1974;698.

PART IV

Neoplastic Disease

CHAPTER 28

Tumors of the Nose and Paranasal Sinuses

Jack L. Gluckman

Tumors of the nose and paranasal sinuses are not common. The average head and neck surgeon will be exposed to only a limited number of benign, let alone malignant, tumors in an entire career and therefore it is difficult to attain a significant personal experience in managing these conditions. The differential diagnosis of tumors occurring in this area is considerable, ranging from tumors arising from dental structures and bone, to those arising from mucosa and the olfactory epithelium. They can be classified as per Table 1.

These tumors share common clinical features and radiologic findings with differences depending on the histologic type, the site of origin, and staging of the tumor at the time of presentation. Unfortunately, these tumors, whether benign or malignant, usually present at an advanced stage for the following reasons:

1. The nose and paranasal sinuses are air-filled cavities, which permit significant tumor growth before causing any symptoms or signs.
2. Many of the early symptoms caused by the tumors mimic those caused by rhinosinusitis (e.g., rhinorrhea, nasal obstruction, facial discomfort). These common symptoms can be misinterpreted and result in self-medication by the patient with significant *patient delay* before presenting to the physician.
3. Because of the rarity of these tumors and absence of objective signs early in the disease process, the clinician tends to have a low index of suspicion resulting in *physician delay* in diagnosis. In fact, the average delay from the onset of symptoms to diagnosis of maxillary sinus cancer is 8 months (1).

CLINICAL FEATURES

As already stated, the clinical features depend on the site of origin, the type of tumor, and the size and extent of tumor spread. These symptoms and signs can be categorized as follows.

1. *Nasal.* Unilateral nasal obstruction and rhinorrhea in an adult are a great source of concern. This discharge may be mucoid (due to mucosal irritation or secretion by the tumor), purulent (due to secondary obstructive sinusitis), sanguinous (which usually takes the form of blood-streaked rhinorrhea), or even clear cerebrospinal fluid (CSF) (indicative of intracranial extension). Frank epistaxis may signify a very vascular tumor or erosion of a blood vessel.

2. *Orbital.* Orbital symptoms depend on the degree of orbital involvement and whether the orbit is displaced or infiltrated. Diplopia and proptosis are invariably due to mass effect on the orbital contents, although in high-grade malignancy, they may be due to direct infiltration (Fig. 1). A focal periorbital swelling due to the mass itself may be seen in benign and malignant tumors. Diffuse periorbital edema may indicate regional lymphatic or venous obstruction. Pain and loss of visual acuity usually indicate malignant infiltration of the eye itself. Of course, ophthalmoplegia and decreasing visual acuity may indicate intracranial involvement of the cavernous sinus or the optic nerve. Sphenoid sinus involvement may present as unrelenting retro-ocular pain.

3. *Oral.* Distortion of the palate and alveolar ridge resulting in ill-fitting dentures and loose teeth can be early symptoms of a malignant tumor of the floor of the maxillary antrum. A persistent oroantral fistula after dental extraction is also suspicious. Tumor may overtly extend through the palate and fungate into the oral cavity (Fig. 2). Trismus is an ominous sign and may indicate malignant invasion of the pterygoid or masseter muscles. Referred dental pain may be an early symptom of paranasal sinus cancer and many of these patients may undergo dental extraction without relief of symptoms before the true diagnosis becomes established.

TABLE 1. *Tumors of the nose and paranasal sinuses*

Benign
  Epithelial
    Papilloma—fungiform
             —inverting
    Adenoma
    Nevus
    Mixed tumor
    Oncocytoma
  Mesenchymal
    Angiofibroma
    Hemangioma
    Lymphangioma
    Neurogenous—neurilemoma
                 —neurofibroma
    Fibroma
    Lipoma
    Chondroma
    Hamartoma
    Meningioma
  Osseous
    Osteoma
    Exostosis (torus palatinus)
    Osteoid osteoma
    Giant cell tumors—reparative granuloma
                 —giant cell tumor
                 —osteitis fibrosa cystica
                 —cherubism
    Ossifying fibroma
    Fibrous dysplasia
    Desmoplastic fibroma
    Chondromyxoid fibroma
  Odontogenic
    Ameloblastoma
    Pindborg tumor
    Adenoblastoma
    Myxoma
    Odontogenic fibroma
    Odontogenic fibromyxoma
    Cementifying fibroma
    Dentinoma
    Cementoma
    Mixed odontogenic tumors
Malignant
  Epithelial
    Squamous cell carcinoma
    Minor salivary gland cancers
    Adenocarcinoma
    Undifferentiated carcinoma
    Malignant melanoma
    Esthesioneuroblastoma
  Mesenchymal
    Sarcoma—chondrosarcoma
           —rhabdomyosarcoma
           —fibrosarcoma
           —angiosarcoma
           —neurofibrosarcoma
    Hemangiopericytoma
    Fibrous histiocytoma
    Lymphoreticular tumors—lymphoma
                     —plasmacytoma
  Osseous
    Osteogenic sarcoma
    Ewing's sarcoma
  Odontogenic
  Metastasis

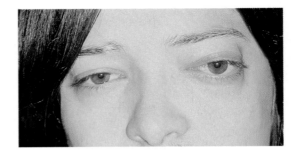

FIG. 1. Unilateral proptosis in a young man with an esthesioneuroblastoma extending into the ethmoid sinus.

4. *Facial.* Swelling and distortion of the nose and cheek may occur (Fig. 3). This may be diffuse and subtle or more localized. Facial pain, anesthesia, or paresthesia in the distribution of the branches of the trigeminal nerve may indicate an underlying malignancy. If confined to the distribution of the infraorbital nerve, this is indicative of involvement of the roof and/or the anterior wall of the maxillary sinus, but if the whole distribution of V_2 is involved, it suggests posterior base of skull extension.

5. *Intracranial.* Symptoms of intracranial extension include persistent intractable headache, ophthalmoplegia, and decreasing visual acuity if there is anterior cranial fossa or cavernous sinus involvement. CSF rhinorrhea is an uncommon, but obvious, sign of intracranial extension. Other cranial nerves may be involved if the middle cranial fossa is invaded.

6. *Base of Skull.* As the tumor extends posteriorly, trismus due to pterygoid muscle involvement, anesthesia and paresthesia in the distribution of the maxillary

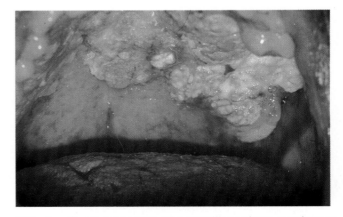

FIG. 2. Overt extension of a maxillary sinus carcinoma through the hard palate.

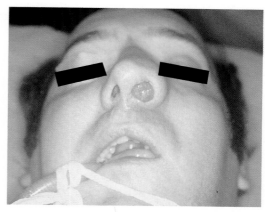

FIG. 4. Unilateral polypoid mass. Biopsy initially suggested chronic inflammation but on surgical exploration, inverting papilloma was noted.

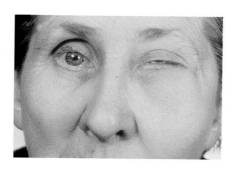

FIG. 3. Facial and orbital distortion due to carcinoma of the maxillary antrum extending through the anterior and superior walls.

and mandibular branches of the trigeminal nerve, and severe pain due to bone invasion may occur.

PATIENT EVALUATION

Clinical

In evaluating a patient with a suspected or overt nasal or paranasal sinus tumor, clinical examination is important in determining the site of origin of the tumor, the extent of spread, and even the tumor type. Unfortunately, even in large tumors, the findings may be minimal and the full extent of the tumor may only be apparent on imaging studies.

The head and neck examination should include palpation of the neck for cervical metastases although it should be appreciated that the first echelon drainage lymphatics for tumors of the posterior nasal cavity and sinuses is to the retropharyngeal nodes, which will only be apparent on imaging studies. Prior to examining the interior of the nose, the face should be examined for asymmetry or subtle distortion. If an overt mass is obvious, it is important to determine whether the overlying skin is infiltrated or free of tumor. If there is trismus, one should determine whether it is due to masseter or pterygoid muscle infiltration or even temporomandibular joint involvement.

The oral cavity should be examined for palatal distortion, loose teeth, overt tumor, and so on. It is important to evaluate the nasopharynx either by mirror examination or fiberoptic endoscopy as overt

involvement of the nasopharynx by tumor may signify a contraindication to surgery.

Nasal examination may reveal overt tumor or more subtle findings including unilateral mucosal thickening or benign looking polyps that may mask the presence of the underlying tumor. Unilateral findings should always be viewed with great suspicion (Fig. 4). Care should be taken to remove all crusts in the nose that may obscure the underlying pathology. Rigid nasal endoscopy has been suggested as improving the ability to detect early lesions (2).

The periorbita should be palpated for mass effect and the eyes examined for proptosis, ophthalmoplegia, and impaired visual acuity. If orbital exenteration is a consideration, an ophthalmologist should always be consulted to determine the status of the contralateral eye. A full cranial nerve examination is also necessary.

Imaging

While *plain sinus films* are not particularly helpful in diagnosing or delineating the extent of a tumor, they are frequently the initial radiograph obtained in evaluating a patient with sinus problems and may alert the physician to the presence of a sinus tumor.

Osteomas and fibrous dysplasia are readily apparent on plain radiographs with characteristic features and usually no further investigation is necessary to establish the diagnosis. Bowing of the posterior wall of the maxillary antrum is said to be diagnostic for angiofibroma. Bone erosion and a unilateral opaque antrum should always be viewed with great suspicion (Fig. 5). The real problem in evaluating plain films is to diagnose subtle changes and to differentiate inflammatory changes from tumor. Therefore, if a tumor is suspected, computed tomography (CT) and/or magnetic resonance imaging (MRI) should be obtained.

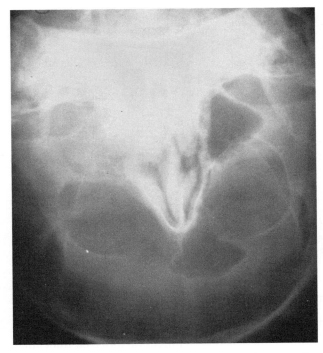

FIG. 5. Plain sinus radiograph demonstrating a unilateral opaque maxillary antrum with bone erosion (see *arrows*).

Computed tomography has revolutionized our ability to detect and delineate the extent of tumor. It is particularly useful in evaluating the extent of soft tissue changes and whether there is bone erosion. Behavior characteristics may be suggested, for example, bone destruction without remodeling is highly suggestive of an aggressive malignant tumor while necrosis with new bone deposition is more likely to be due to slow growing tumor (3) (Fig. 6). It is particularly useful in determining base of skull erosion. There are some drawbacks, however, and these include the scatter effect from dental amalgam, the relative difficulty in obtaining coronal images, and, of course, the problems of differentiating tumor from secondary inflammatory changes. The CT scan remains, however, an essential investigation for effective therapeutic planning.

Many of the problems associated with the CT scan have been solved by the introduction of *magnetic resonance imaging,* which permits multiplanar evaluation. While bone changes are not as well demonstrated as compared to the CT scan, the soft tissue imaging is better and inflammatory mucosal thickening and fluid can usually be differentiated from tumor (Fig. 7). It is therefore of great value to perform both a CT scan and MRI on all malignant tumors of the paranasal sinuses to aid in therapeutic planning.

Angiography is essential to establish the diagnosis and delineate the extent of vascular tumors (e.g., angiofibroma and hemangioma). In addition, if carotid

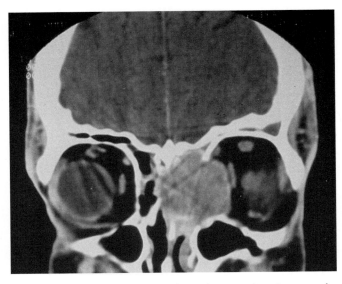

FIG. 6. CT scan demonstrating a low-grade adenocarcinoma of the ethmoid sinus causing bone erosion by ischemic necrosis.

resection is contemplated or if it is suspected that the cavernous sinus is involved and may need to be included in the resection, angiography is indicated. It is also important in identifying any feeder vessels that may require embolization and can be combined with a trial of carotid artery balloon occlusion before embarking on resection.

Biopsy

If tumor is easily accessible either intranasally or via the oral cavity, it should be biopsied directly. Occa-

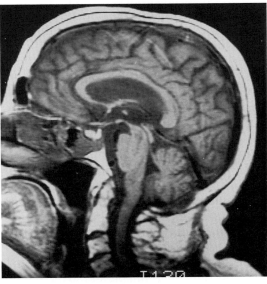

FIG. 7. Carcinoma of the sphenoid sinus with posterior erosion demonstrated by MRI.

sionally, it may be necessary to perform an open exploration of the sinus (e.g., via a Caldwell–Luc, external ethmoidectomy, or sphenoidotomy) to obtain tissue. The biopsy should be deep and include a substantial portion of the tumor as frequently overlying chronic inflammation or squamous metaplasia may obscure the true diagnosis. Some tumors may be very vascular and bleed significantly and it is therefore wise to have the facilities available to pack the nasal cavity after biopsy. If angiofibroma is suspected clinically, this, in my opinion, should *not* be biopsied even in the operating room, but rather the diagnosis established by angiography.

Antral lavage for a unilateral opaque maxillary antrum may yield nonpurulent necrotic material and, if thought to be suspicious, should be sent for cytology to rule out malignancy.

DIFFERENTIAL DIAGNOSIS

Patently, not all tumors that can occur in this area can be discussed in detail and the reader is encouraged to refer to the appropriate literature regarding the more unusual tumors. In addition, the chapter, Fibro-osseous Diseases by, Donald discusses the fibro-osseous diseases and these will therefore not be included in this chapter.

Benign Tumors

Papillomas

The mucosa of the nasal cavity and paranasal sinuses differs from that of the rest of the upper aerodigestive tract in that it is derived from ectoderm. Therefore papillomas arising from this mucosa have a unique behavior and appearance. These papillomas may be inverting or fungiform, although combinations of these have been described.

Fungiform papillomas usually arise on the nasal septum anteriorly, are localized, and have no propensity for malignant transformation. They are usually asymptomatic but may cause irritation or epistaxis. Treatment consists of excision and cautery of the base to prevent recurrence.

Inverting papillomas usually arise on the lateral wall of the nose but may develop *ab initio* in the paranasal sinuses, nasopharynx, and nasal septum (4). They are more common in men, occurring particularly in the fifth and sixth decades. These papillomas consist of epidermoid cells and occasionally columnar epithelium (5). The epithelial surface inverts into the underlying stroma, giving it its characteristic appearance. The basement membrane is intact. Clinically, they can be differentiated from allergic and inflammatory polyps by their gross appearance, which is more vascular,

firm, and nontranslucent, and their tendency to have a sessile base.

The etiology of inverting papillomas is unknown. Human papilloma virus (HPV) has been implicated, particularly HPV 6, 11, 16, and 18. It is possible that inverting papilloma that undergoes malignant transformation may be due to a HPV 16/18 hybrid (6).

Most present as a mass in the nasal cavity and, as they increase in size, extend into the paranasal sinuses. Bone destruction is due to pressure necrosis, although the bone may be invaded by aggressive disease with even intracranial extension.

The incidence of malignant transformation of inverting papilloma is as yet unresolved. The described incidence in the literature varies from virtually nonexistent (less than 2% of cases) (7) to as high as 50% (Fig. 8). Hyams (8) has noted a malignancy rate of 13% and this is approximately the generally accepted figure. A complicating and probably more common scenario is the presence of a coexistent malignancy (7), which may account for the discrepancy in the described incidence.

Diagnosis is made by deep biopsy with the tumor extent determined by CT scan.

Treatment of inverting papilloma consists of wide local excision and careful postoperative follow-up to ensure early diagnosis of any recurrence. In the case of lateral wall lesions, this usually necessitates a formal medial maxillectomy (8). In recent years, there has been a trend to more conservative resection even to the point of performing resection via the sinus endoscopes (9,10). This is possibly a satisfactory approach in expert hands for very limited lesions but should not be performed by the inexperienced occasional surgeon, as recurrence will inevitably occur. Large and recurrent tumors should undergo wide resection (i.e., medial maxillectomy), but extensive radical surgery (e.g., radical maxillectomy, craniofacial resection) is rarely necessary except in the rare aggressive tumors. Certainly if the tumor arises in the maxillary antrum, careful and

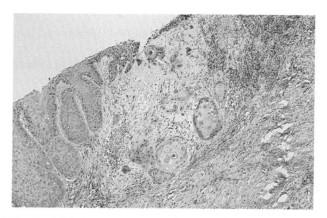

FIG. 8. Histology of an inverting papilloma undergoing malignant transformation with microinvasion.

meticulous mucosal stripping alone will suffice. Careful follow-up is essential, with most recurrences occurring within 2 years (11). Radiation is recommended for patients who are poor surgical risks, are unresectable, or have extremely aggressive disease (12). Some authors have suggested that malignant transformation may be induced by the radiation (13), while others have failed to confirm that this is a valid concern (12,14).

Minor Salivary Gland Tumors

Minor salivary glands (serous, mucous, or mixed) are present in the nose and paranasal sinuses. Tumors arising from these glands are uncommon, but when they do occur, approximately 50% are malignant (15). By far the most common of the benign tumors is the *pleomorphic adenoma,* which presents as a slow-growing mass filling the nose or paranasal sinus. Other benign tumors include *basal cell adenoma* and *oncocytoma.* These tumors may expand into the sinuses and achieve significant size before being detected. Treatment consists of wide local excision.

Juvenile Angiofibroma

Juvenile angiofibroma is a highly vascular benign tumor with a propensity for local extension. It is found exclusively in adolescent men.

Pathology

These tumors arise at the junction of the posterolateral wall and the roof of the nose at the superior margin of the sphenopalatine foramen, which embryologically represents the approximate location of the buccopharyngeal membrane (16). Previous studies had concluded that the site of origin was in the nasopharynx (17,18), hence the misnomer "nasopharyngeal angiofibroma."

This tumor presents as a lobulated submucosal mass, which is adherent to the surrounding structures at its site of origin but, as it extends laterally, is less adherent and has a fibrous pseudocapsule. While it may be quite firm to palpation, it is usually compressible and even sponge-like. The main arterial supply is the ipsilateral internal maxillary artery (19), but smaller contributions may arise from the dura and internal carotid or vertebral arteries.

Microscopically, this tumor consists of two components—the fibrous stroma and the vascular component—which consists of large channels lined by endothelial cells with no surrounding smooth muscle. These channels vary significantly in size. It is thought that

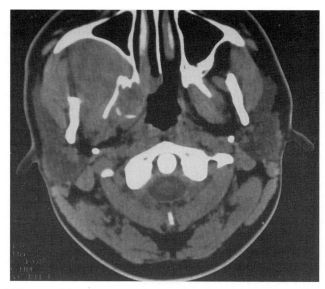

FIG. 9. CT scan demonstrating bowing of the posterior wall of the maxillary sinus by a juvenile angiofibroma extending into the pterygomaxillary fissure.

possibly the tumors become more fibrous and less vascular with time.

For some reason there is a dramatic surge in growth during the adolescent years, which is probably hormonally related. As the tumor enlarges, it fills the posterior choanae and the nasopharynx. It then extends laterally through the sphenopalatine foramen into the pterygomaxillary fissure, bowing the posterior wall of the maxillary sinus (Fig. 9). It then extends into the

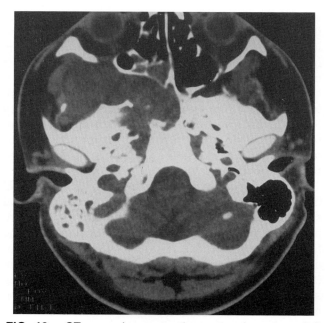

FIG. 10. CT scan demonstrating extension of angiofibroma through the inferior orbital fissure into the orbit.

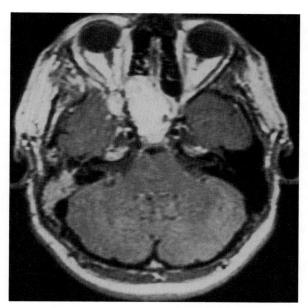

FIG. 11. MRI with contrast clearly demonstrating posterior extension of angiofibroma into the sphenoid sinus.

infratemporal fossa and around the lateral face of the maxilla, resulting in facial fullness. It may enter the orbit through the inferior orbital fissure (Fig. 10). The middle cranial fossa is entered via the infratemporal fossa or via the sphenoid sinus (Fig. 11). Intracranially, it can involve the optic chiasm and cavernous sinus; however, it usually just compresses the cavernous sinus. Intracranial extension only occurs in about 10% of patients (20,21).

Clinical Features

This condition is, for practical purposes, the exclusive domain of young adolescent men. The most common presenting symptom is *epistaxis,* with unilateral *nasal obstruction* and *unilateral rhinorrhea* also being common. Epistaxis can be particularly severe. Other symptoms and signs depend on the extent of the tumor; for example, if it extends into the nasopharynx, distortion of the soft palate occurs; if there is extension laterally into the infratemporal fossa, unilateral facial pain and swelling may result; if there is extension into the orbit, proptosis will be present; while intracranial extension may result in headache, impaired vision, and other cranial nerve palsies.

Diagnosis

Clinically, one should have a high level of suspicion in all adolescent men with recurrent epistaxis, unilateral nasal obstruction, and a submucosal posterior nasal or nasopharyngeal mass.

While *plain sinus films* are not necessary to establish the diagnosis, in over 90% of patients abnormalities can be detected consisting of opacity of one or multiple sinuses and bone displacement and/or erosion (22). In fact, the anterior bowing of the posterior wall of the maxillary sinus in young men has always been regarded as diagnostic for juvenile angiofibroma.

CT scan with contrast together with *MRI* provides the most detailed and accurate method of staging of angiofibroma with MRI being particularly useful in differentiating inflammation from tumor, as well as determining the presence and extent of intracranial extension.

Angiography is indicated to confirm the diagnosis in lieu of biopsy, to determine the extent of the tumor, to evaluate its blood supply, and to determine whether it is amenable to embolization preoperatively (21). While a number of complications secondary to angiography for angiofibromas have been described, including death (23), permanent transverse myelitis (24), transient hemiplegia (25), and retinal artery infarction (22), it is my opinion that the advantages to the clinician far outweigh the potential disadvantages. Others, however, believe that angiography is only indicated in unusual circumstances (16).

Examination under anesthesia and biopsy are recommended by some authors (16) and deemed unnecessary by most including this author. If a biopsy is to be taken, it should be performed with great caution in an operating room where facilities are available to control the inevitable hemorrhage.

Management

Over the years, innumerable therapies have been suggested and attempted. While surgery remains the most logical approach, it has its detractors because of the perceived morbidity that may result, particularly while excising the larger tumors. For this reason, radiotherapy has been embraced with great enthusiasm in some centers with apparently good results. Other proposed primary therapies, including hormone therapy, embolization, and even chemotherapy, have been discarded except in the most refractory of cases. Estrogens, particularly, have been used by a number of authors (either as definitive therapy or as preoperative treatment) but have never conclusively been shown to be of any real value (26,27).

The role of radiotherapy is controversial. In some centers, it is the definitive therapy of choice, while in others it is used only for advanced tumor with intracranial extension (28,29). Others, again, recommend it exclusively for recurrent inoperable tumors.

The most enthusiasm for radiotherapy as a primary modality is generated from the Princess Margaret Hospital in Toronto, with reported excellent results (30,31). In their large series, almost 80% were controlled by a single course of radiation and most of the refractory cases were controlled by a second course. Only a small percentage ultimately required salvage surgery. The dose of 30 Gy in 3 weeks induced thrombosis, fibrosis, and tumor regression, although it was acknowledged that it may take many years before the tumor completely disappeared.

Contraindications to radiation as a primary modality include the possibilities of radiation-induced malignant transformation of the angiofibroma (32,33), a sarcoma developing in the radiation field (34), or lesser sequelae of cataract formation, hearing loss, and eustachian tube dysfunction. An attempt was made by Cummings (35) to compare the risks of surgery and radiation and he concluded that the incidence of severe complications was the same for both these modalities.

In general, there is a trend toward surgical therapy as the primary modality of choice. Contraindications include those patients who are poor surgical risks, recurrent tumors that have proved refractory to previous excisions, and involvement of vital structures such as the carotid artery or optic chiasm.

If surgical resection is to be performed, preoperative embolization of the tumor is most useful, preferably the day prior to, or on, the day of surgery. It is certainly my opinion, with support from the literature, that this reduces intraoperative bleeding and makes the dissection easier (36–38).

The surgical approach has to be planned carefully and is dependent on the extent of the tumor.

If the lesion is confined to the posterior choana and nasopharynx, a transpalatal or medial maxillectomy approach can be used. The medial maxillectomy approach is more versatile, particularly if an extended lateral dissection needs to be performed. The transpalatal approach is really only of value for small tumors (39).

If there is significant lateral extension into the pterygomaxillary fissure, a medial maxillectomy via a lateral rhinotomy or degloving approach permits the best access. The posterior wall of the maxillary sinus is removed, the lateral extent of the tumor identified, and the internal maxillary artery isolated and divided before the tumor is removed.

If the tumor extends even further into the infratemporal fossa, a modified suprastructure maxillectomy will permit excellent exposure of the tumor. If necessary, even better exposure can be obtained via a mandibular osteotomy and swing. Control of the external carotid should always be obtained early in the operation for tumors with extensive infratemporal fossa involvement.

Intracranial extension will necessitate a craniotomy in combination with the above described procedures.

It has been our experience that the dura is rarely invaded and the cavernous sinus is usually compressed by the tumor, permitting a relatively easy dissection of the tumor off these structures.

Postoperative radiation is administered if inoperable residual tumor persists after resection. This usually consists of conventional cobalt therapy or even stereotactic radiosurgery if the residuum is localized.

The management of recurrent tumor is quite frustrating, with hormonal therapy, radiation, and even selective embolization alone being reported (40). Chemotherapy, consisting of doxorubicin or vincristine, dactinomycin, and cyclophosphamide combination, has been given with some limited success but should only be considered for refractory cases (41).

Results

An 80% success rate for extracranial tumor can be obtained with both radiation and surgery. Extensive tumors with intracranial extension have a higher recurrence rate (22,37) but can be treated surgically with satisfactory results.

Neurogenous Tumors

The most common of these tumors are the neurilemoma (schwannoma) and neurofibroma. *Neurilemomas* arise from the Schwann cells and present as encapsulated solitary tumors. They do not commonly occur in the nose and paranasal sinuses, constituting only 6% of all nerve sheath tumors in the head and neck (42). They may arise from any of the nerves in this area with the exception of the olfactory nerves. They most commonly arise in the nasoethmoid region. They rarely undergo malignant transformation (43).

Neurofibromas, on the other hand, are associated with von Recklinghausen's disease and present as multiple, nonencapsulated tumors, and sarcomatous degeneration is a distinct possibility.

These two tumors can easily be differentiated histologically. Neurilemomas are encapsulated with either palisading of nuclei (Antoni A) or loose stroma with no distinctive cell pattern (Antoni B). Cystic degeneration and necrosis are also noted in these tumors. Neurofibromas, on the other hand, are unencapsulated and incorporate the dendrites with a spindle cell pattern of growth. Neurons therefore do not traverse the body of neurilemomas but do in neurofibromas (44). Degenerative changes are not usually present. The malignant variant, neurofibrosarcomas, are associated with von Recklinghausen's disease in 6% to 16% of cases (45). These behave in a particularly aggressive manner.

Treatment of both neurilemomas and neurofibromas consists of wide local excision.

Meningiomas

Meningiomas most commonly present in the paranasal sinuses by direct extension from their intracranial origin. Rarely, they develop primarily in the nose and sinuses, originating from the arachnoid cells along the sheaths of cranial nerves (46). Their aggressiveness, like intracranial meningiomas, is variable. As expected, these tumors most commonly present in the frontal sinus, followed by maxillary and ethmoid sinuses. Essential to therapeutic planning is the determination whether there is intracranial involvement, which will necessitate a craniofacial as opposed to a purely facial approach.

Osteoma

This is the most common tumor arising in the nose and paranasal sinuses. Their true incidence is unknown, as most are asymptomatic, but they have been noted in under 1% of patients obtaining sinus radiographs (47). Their etiology is unclear. They tend to develop at the junction of membranous and endochondral bone and are most commonly noted in the frontoethmoid complex (Fig. 12) but may also rarely occur in the maxillary and sphenoid sinuses. They may continue to grow throughout life, but their growth is maximal during the period of skeletal development.

Grossly, they can easily be distinguished from the surrounding bone by their compact shiny appearance. Histologically, they can be subdivided into a *compact* variety with dense lamellar bone with no haversian system or marrow cavities; a *spongy* variety, which is predominantly cancellous with fatty marrow; and a *mixed* variety.

The vast majority are asymptomatic and may achieve considerable size before causing symptoms, which are due to distortion of surrounding structures (e.g., the orbit) or occlusion of a sinus ostium with a secondary mucocele or mucopyocele. Approximately 14% of patients with Gardener's syndrome have craniofacial osteomas, some of which can present in the paranasal sinuses (48).

Treatment is surgical. Basically, the tumor should only be removed if it is symptomatic. If the tumor is predominantly in the frontal sinus, the approach should be via an osteoplastic flap; however, if the tumor is in the ethmoids, an external frontoethmoidectomy approach is preferred. While occasionally they can be dissected out intact, this is usually technically difficult and the preferred approach is to drill out the tumor from within leaving an eggshell rim of tumor, which can be removed piecemeal.

Giant Cell Tumors

While there are a number of giant cell tumors that occur in this area, the giant cell reparative granuloma is the most common in the paranasal sinuses. These are usually diagnosed in young adults, predominantly involving the maxillary and sphenoid sinuses (49). These present as an expansile mass that is well demarcated from the surrounding structures. Treatment consists of curettage with a low local recurrence rate.

Malignant Tumors

Given the wide variety of tissues that comprise the paranasal sinuses and structures that surround them, it is apparent that a number of malignancies may arise from within the sinuses or from tissues that surround the sinuses and impinge on them.

Etiology

Unlike cancer elsewhere in the upper aerodigestive tract, cancer of the sinonasal area is apparently not related to tobacco products or alcohol. However, several occupations are hazardous for the development of these cancers, for example, nickel workers, woodworkers, leather workers, textile workers, petroleum refiners, isopropyl alcohol manufacturers, chrome pigment manufacturers, welders, and blast furnace operators (50). Nickel workers have a propensity for squamous cell cancers, which in one series was 28 times the expected incidence until the refining process was

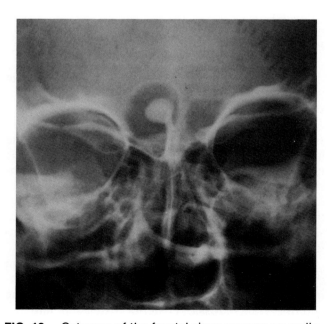

FIG. 12. Osteoma of the frontal sinus as seen on radiograph of the sinus.

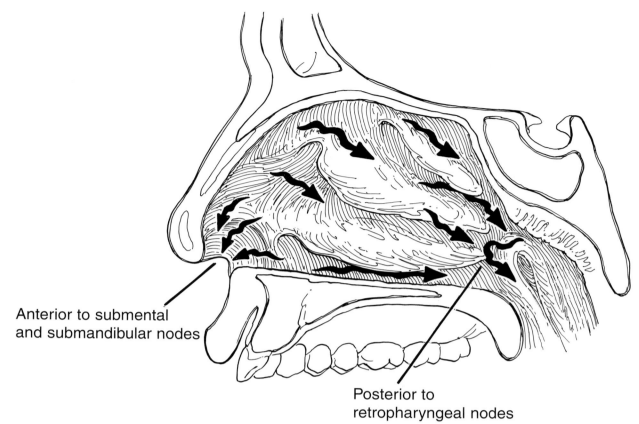

FIG. 13. The lymphatic pathway of the nose and paranasal sinuses.

modified (51). Woodworkers, on the other hand, are more likely to develop adenocarcinoma, with the specific carcinogens in woodwork and leather products being aldehydes, aflatoxin, and chromium (51). The described increase in risk in this group varies from 400 to 500 times as compared to the general population (52). Other activities associated with the development of these cancers include snuff users (particularly in Africa) and the injection of Thorotrast (thorium dioxide) into the sinus cavities.

Incidence

These cancers are rare, constituting 0.2% to 0.8% of all malignancies and 3% of all malignant tumors of the upper aerodigestive tract. The vast majority arise in the maxillary sinus (60%) followed by the ethmoids (15%) and nasal cavity (20%). Cancers of the nasal vestibule and frontal and sphenoid sinuses comprise the remaining 5%. Unfortunately, because most of these cancers present late, multiple sinuses may be involved by the time a patient first presents, making it difficult to determine the site of origin. Squamous cell carcinoma is the most common, comprising approximately

80% of all malignancies, while adenocarcinoma comprises 10% to 20% (53).

Pathology

Patterns of Tumor Spread

Local. Local tumor spread in this area is possible via natural ostia, by pressure necrosis, or direct invasion of bone (54).

Low-grade malignancies arising in the *maxillary sinus* may fill the sinus before spreading beyond the bony confines, but in high-grade malignancies, this rarely occurs and erosion of the bony walls and extension beyond the confines of the sinus develop early, for example, into the oral cavity, the cheek, the orbit, or nose depending on the site of origin. Posterior extension into the pterygomaxillary fissure and into the infratemporal fossa tends to occur late.

Ethmoid cancers tend to spread early into the antrum through the antroethmoid plate, through the thin lamina papyracea into the orbit, and superiorly into the anterior cranial fossa. Posterior extension into the sphenoid and nasopharynx tends to occur late and is not common and frontal sinus extension is rare. The cancer may spread into the nasal cavity to involve the septum and the opposite ethmoids (2). While the lamina papyracea is eroded easily, the orbital periosteum is relatively resistant to tumor invasion.

Frontal sinus tumors may spread posteriorly directly into the anterior cranial fossa or inferiorly into the ethmoids.

Sphenoid sinus tumors tend to spread laterally into the cavernous sinus and middle cranial fossa but may also present in the nasopharynx by anterior extension.

Tumors arising in the *nasal cavity,* per se, tend to fill the cavity before extending posteriorly into the nasopharynx or laterally into the paranasal sinuses.

Lymphatic. The direction of lymphatic spread depends on the site of origin of the tumor. Cancers of the nasal vestibule and anterior nose drain into the facial, parotid, submandibular, and submental nodes then to the upper deep cervical nodes. Tumors of the posterior nose and paranasal sinuses spread initially posteriorly to a plexus of lymphatics just anterior to the torus tubaris then to the retropharyngeal nodes and only then to the upper deep cervical nodes (Fig. 13). The true incidence of cervical metastases is difficult to determine because of the difficulty in evaluating involvement of the retropharyngeal nodes. The incidence at initial presentation is low, but 25% to 30% will eventually develop lymphatic metastases that may be bilateral (55,56).

Hematogenous. Although rare, spread to liver, lung, brain, and bones has been described in about 10% of cases with the incidence depending on the type of tumor (55,57).

Staging

The staging system used is recommended by the American Joint Committee on Cancer (1992) and applies to maxillary sinus cancers only (58). The anatomic descriptions are based on an imaginary line drawn from the medial canthus of the eye to the angle of the mandible, dividing the maxillary antrum into anteroinferior and posterosuperior areas (Ohngren's line). This was first described almost 60 years ago (59) (Table 2). The staging for nodal and distant metastases is identical to that used for other head and neck cancers. There is no similar staging system for cancers arising in the other sinuses, because they are relatively uncommon. Involvement of ethmoid and sphenoid sinuses by maxillary sinus cancer signifies advanced staging (60). Ohngren's concept that the anterior–medial tumors had a better prognosis than the posterolateral cancers based on the ability to surgically encompass the tumor still holds true in spite of advances in surgical technique. Other types of tumors may have their own unique stag-

TABLE 2. *Staging of maxillary sinus cancer*

T_{1s}	Carcinoma *in situ*
T_1	Tumor limited to the antral mucosa with no erosion or destruction of bone
T_2	Tumor with erosion or destruction of the infrastructure including the hard palate and/or the middle nasal meatus
T_3	Tumor invading skin of the cheek, posterior wall of the maxillary sinus, floor or medial wall of orbit, anterior ethmoid sinus
T_4	Tumor invades orbital contents and/or cribriform plate, posterior ethmoid or sphenoid sinuses, nasopharynx, soft palate, pterygomaxillary or temporal fossae or base of skull

From ref. 58, with permission.

ing system with close correlation with prognosis (e.g., esthesioneuroblastoma) (61) (Table 3).

Tumor Types

Squamous Cell Carcinoma

This is by far the most common cancer involving the sinonasal tract. It rarely arises in the nasal cavity *de novo,* but when it does, the majority arise from the turbinates (62). Involvement of the nasal septum, nasal floor, and nasal vestibule is most rare. Interestingly enough, tumors of the nasal vestibule appear to behave in a relatively nonaggressive manner (62). The maxillary sinus is the most common site of origin, but this tumor can arise *de novo* from any of the other sinuses. The poor prognosis associated with these lesions predominantly reflects late diagnosis and the advanced staging the tumor has achieved at the time of presentation. Histologic grading appears to be of no prognostic significance, although undifferentiated cancers do have a worse prognosis.

Minor Salivary Gland Cancers

Tumors of salivary gland origin account for 6% to 17% of all sinonasal cancers. Irrespective of the tumor type, they all appear to behave in a somewhat more aggressive manner than their counterparts elsewhere in the upper aerodigestive tract. Mucoepidermoid and

TABLE 3. *Staging for esthesioneuroblastoma*

Group A	Tumor confined to the nasal cavity
Group B	Tumor extending beyond nasal cavity into paranasal sinuses
Group C	Tumor spread beyond nasal cavities and paranasal sinuses

From ref. 61, with permission.

acinic cell cancers are rare with adenocarcinoma and adenoid cystic carcinoma being the most common (62). There is a propensity for extensive perineural spread, making wide local excision difficult. In addition, there is a tendency for distant metastases, particularly to bone and lung (63).

Adenocarcinoma of Mucosal Origin

These arise from the sinonasal mucosa itself (as opposed to the minor salivary glands) and occur predominantly in the ethmoids (64). These have been divided histologically into papillary, sessile, and alveolar-mucoid varieties by Batsakis et al. (62). The papillary form, which is most commonly associated with woodworkers, is the least aggressive, while the sessile group has the worst prognosis.

Malignant Melanoma

Malignant melanoma is extremely rare, comprising only 1% of all sinonasal cancers (65) and under 1% of all malignant melanomas (66). While it may present at any age, the vast majority of patients are older than 50 years. The most common site of origin is the septum followed by the lateral nasal wall of the nose (67). Over 75% are obviously pigmented, but amelanotic lesions may occur. Histologically, it may be difficult to differentiate from other small round cell tumors, but various immunohistochemical techniques facilitate this. The tumor tends to be more aggressive in its behavior than cutaneous melanoma with a worse prognosis (8% to 30% five-year survival) (67). Unfortunately, it has an unpredictable course with rapid progression or long periods of remission without any satisfactory explanation for this behavior. Staging techniques using tumor depth of invasion are invalid in mucosal melanomas. The best results have been reported with combination surgery and radiation (67).

Esthesioneuroblastoma

This is an aggressive malignancy of neural crest origin arising from the basal layer of the olfactory epithelium at the cribriform plate. It has always been regarded as rare but has been recognized with greater frequency in recent years predominantly because contemporary immunohistochemical techniques have enabled the pathologist to separate this tumor from the group of "small round cell tumors." It may present at any age but is commonly seen between the ages of 10 and 30 years. It is slightly more common in men.

It presents as a vascular, pinkish-grey polypoid mass arising from the cribriform plate. Histologically, it has a somewhat nondescript picture and is extremely difficult to differentiate from lymphoma, undifferentiated carcinoma, melanoma, sarcoma, and minor salivary gland cancers morphologically, but it can be diagnosed using immunohistochemical techniques (68). The classically described histologic feature is the presence of rosette formation, which has no prognostic significance (69).

The tumor is very aggressive in its behavior with a tendency for submucosal extension and nodal and distant metastases (69,70). In one series, metastases occurred in 62% of patients with some developing up to 10 years after the initial presentation (70). By far the most common sites of metastases are the cervical lymph nodes (17% to 48%) (71,72) and lung, although I have personally seen metastases to bone, skin, and liver. As the tumor increases in size, it may extend into the paranasal sinuses and intracranially with involvement of dura and even the frontal lobe.

The usual staging system used for this disease is that of Kadish, which has some correlation with survival (61,72) (Table 3) and is based on both clinical and radiologic evaluation.

Diagnosis and pretreatment evaluation should always include a metastatic workup to exclude distant metastases. Some authorities believe that routine CT screening of the neck is indicated to exclude occult metastases (72), but this has not been our routine.

Treatment consists of a combination of surgery and postoperative radiation for the primary tumor and elective neck dissection for overt neck metastases. A case can be made for prophylactic neck dissection, but we have not practiced this.

Resection of the primary tumor necessitates a craniofacial resection. Dura and even frontal lobe may be resected as indicated, but overt brain involvement is a poor prognostic sign (73).

Chemotherapy has been suggested as an adjunct particularly for advanced, recurrent tumors or tumor with evidence of metastases. Its exact value remains unclear, but recent series have shown an improved survival for stage C patients using a regimen of cyclophosphamide and/or vincristine (73,74).

Chondrosarcoma

These are uncommon tumors of the maxilla and predominantly are found in the anterior maxilla (75). A variant, *mesenchymal chondrosarcoma*, does, however, have a propensity for facial bones (76). It can be extremely difficult to differentiate histologically a benign chondroma from a low-grade chondrosarcoma. Tumor behavior can vary from relatively slow growing to a far more aggressive lesion.

The prognosis of these tumors depends on their aggressiveness and is usually characterized by multiple attempts at excision and local recurrence. There is approximately a 40% five year survival rate (77).

Rhabdomyosarcoma

The paranasal sinuses comprise a relatively common site of origin for this type of tumor in the head and neck following the orbit, temporal bones, upper aerodigestive tract, and neck (78). These are extremely aggressive lesions with their behavior depending on the histologic type (i.e., pleomorphic, alveolar, embryonal, and botryoid variants). Embryonal is the most common variety found in the head and neck while the alveolar form is the most aggressive. Regional lymphatic metastases are rare. Optimal treatment remains elusive and in a state of flux, with the mainstay consisting of chemotherapy and radiation, with surgery being reserved for salvage. Primary debulking of the tumor used to be the commonly employed technique but, while still used in some situations, is no longer the approach of choice. Of extremely ominous significance is the development of intracranial extension of the disease (79).

Fibrosarcoma

These uncommon tumors rarely involve the paranasal sinuses, but when they do occur, they are found in the maxillary and ethmoid sinuses. They are thought to arise from the periosteum of the paranasal sinus or occasionally from fibrous dysplasia that has been treated with radiation (80). They can be distinguished histologically into low-grade through high-grade with good clinical correlation. Low-grade lesions have an excellent 10-year survival but high-grade lesions have a dismal prognosis (45). They have a propensity for locally aggressive behavior with the incidence of regional and distant metastases seemingly related to histologic grade and the ability to adequately excise the tumor. There is some controversy as to whether aggressive fibromatosis (extra-abdominal desmoid) is in actual fact a low-grade sarcoma or a separate entity (81), but whatever the belief, the behavior pattern and prognosis are similar to low-grade sarcoma. Treatment consists of wide local excision and postoperative radiotherapy if possible to attempt to decrease the local recurrence rate.

Fibrous Histiocytoma

These are uncommon paranasal sinus tumors. The histologic picture varies from perfectly benign appearing to overt evidence of malignancy. Interestingly enough, the clinical behavior, which may vary from being slow growing and only locally aggressive to more aggressive local behavior with a 20% incidence of cervical metastases, bears no relationship to the histologic picture (82).

Hemangiopericytoma

From 15% to 25% of hemangiopericytomas arise in the head and neck, not uncommonly in the paranasal sinuses. They are most likely to occur in the nasal cavity, followed by the ethmoid sinus (83). These tumors have a variable histologic appearance with little correlation between clinical behavior and histology. They consist of thin-walled vascular spaces with the tumor cell (pericytes) surrounding these spaces. Mitoses, necrosis, tumor size, and site seem to have a slight correlation with malignant potential. Recurrence and metastases are characteristics of these tumors, but some feel that those arising in the head and neck have less of a propensity for this (83,84). Treatment consists of wide surgical resection.

Lymphoma

Lymphoma, particularly non-Hodgkin's lymphoma, is a fairly common tumor in the paranasal sinuses, comprising 8% of sinus malignancies in one series (85). These occur most commonly in the maxillary sinus but may arise in any of the sinuses. They may behave in an aggressive manner, presenting with all the manifestations of a high-grade malignancy, and it is important to differentiate these tumors from other small round cell cancers that occur in this area. Treatment consists of radiation and/or chemotherapy after the appropriate staging has been performed.

Plasmacytoma

Extramedullary plasmacytomas comprise 4% of all nonepithelial neoplasms of the nose and paranasal sinuses (86). They usually present as a submucosal mass that can be distinguished by its dark color. In 10% to 20% of cases, multiple lesions will be apparent and the possibility of systemic multiple myeloma needs to be excluded. The tumor may remain localized and relatively nonaggressive and can be controlled easily with radiation and/or surgery. It may, however, behave in a more aggressive manner with a local invasion and regional and distant metastases. The pattern of behavior cannot be predicted by the histology.

Osteogenic Sarcoma

After the mandible, the maxilla is the most common site of these tumors in the head and neck (87). Predisposing factors include Paget's disease and a history of radiation administered to this area. Histologically, they can be differentiated into osteoblastic, chondroblastic, and fibroblastic types. Their clinical course is characterized by local recurrences and distant metastases. The five-year survival of osteogenic sarcoma of the maxilla is 27% (75,88).

Odontogenic Tumors

Tumors of odontogenic origin should always be considered in the differential diagnosis of paranasal sinus tumors. It is beyond the scope of this chapter to discuss these; however, it should be noted that the most common tumor, and ameloblastoma, tends to be more aggressive in its behavior when it arises in the maxilla than in the mandible. It is therefore more difficult to treat and associated with a worse prognosis if not adequately excised (89).

Metastases

By far the most common source of distant metastasis to the paranasal sinuses is the kidney. Lung, breast, large bowel, and even prostate may also metastasize to this area. The clinician should always bear this entity in mind when evaluating any malignant paranasal sinus tumor and every attempt, both clinically and histologically, should be made to rule this out.

MANAGEMENT

As with tumors elsewhere in the upper aerodigestive tract, the factors that influence the decision-making process to determine the optimal therapy in any one given situation are multifactorial. These can be best categorized as follows.

1. *Type of Tumor.* Benign tumors are usually treated surgically unless they are inaccessible or are perceived as unlikely to cause the patient any harm (e.g., osteomas). Low-grade malignancies, on the other hand, always require treatment unless other patient factors mitigate. As surgery is usually successful and does not usually require radical excision, the approach recommended should balance adequate extirpation with the least amount of morbidity.

High-grade malignancies require more careful planning as wide field resection with or without craniotomy, orbital exenteration, and facial disfiguration may need to be performed. In addition, adjunct chemotherapy and radiation therapy may be needed and the timing for these will have to be considered.

2. *Stage of Tumor.* Unfortunately, most paranasal sinus cancers are diagnosed late and are therefore associated with a poor prognosis. The radical nature of the therapy required to effect cure needs therefore to be tempered by realistic expectations of survival and the impaired quality of life that the treatment may cause. This particularly applies to the extended surgical resections, but also to radical radiotherapy and chemotherapy, that may be used.

3. *General Physical and Emotional Status of Patient.* Once one has determined the optimal therapy for a particular *tumor,* it is then necessary to consider the ideal treatment for the *patient*. This necessitates careful evaluation as to whether the patient can physically withstand a prolonged and complex surgical procedure with its concomitant risks and whether the patient psychologically can tolerate the sequelae of the procedure (e.g., the loss of an eye, the need for prosthesis to replace the hard palate).

4. *Facilities Available.* While one can convincingly argue that ideally all these patients should be treated in a tertiary referral center where expertise in all therapeutic modalities is available, this is usually not possible and most patients will probably be treated in centers where facilities may vary in quality. The presence or absence of surgical expertise, sophisticated radiotherapy and chemotherapy, all will dictate the optimal treatment of the patient in any given situation.

5. *Philosophy and Experience of Oncologist.* In the final analysis, the oncologist in charge of managing the patient will need to make the final decision as to how best to manage the patient. While advice can be solicited from books, journals, and distant experts, the only individual who can really make the ultimate definitive decision is this individual, who knows the patient, the family, and the other intangible circumstances that need to be considered when making this decision.

Treatment Philosophy

In general, a combination of surgery and radiation offers the best chance of cure for most cancers of the paranasal sinuses (90,91), provided this is technically feasible. Adjunct chemotherapy may be of value in certain cancers (e.g., esthesioneuroblastoma), but its true role in managing squamous cell cancers has not yet been defined. Radiation alone is rarely possible as a curative entity except in rare tumors (e.g., lymphoma). Surgery alone will usually suffice for low-grade malignancies but in some situations will be very technically difficult (e.g., sphenoid sinus tumors).

Radiation

Radiation therapy plays an important role in the treatment of cancer of the paranasal sinuses. It may occasionally be used as definitive curative therapy (e.g., lymphoma) but usually is used as an adjunct to surgery or for palliation in advanced incurable cancer.

Curative Radiation

Certain tumors (e.g., lymphoma, plasmacytoma, and even juvenile angiofibroma) have been treated successfully with radiation as the definitive modality. Occasionally, radiation is recommended by default because the area to be treated is not amenable to surgical ablation or the patient is not deemed fit enough to withstand surgery.

The exact dosage would depend on the type, stage, and site of the tumor, but in general, 50 to 55 Gy over 5 to 6 weeks should be administered and, if well tolerated, a booster dose of 15 to 20 Gy given. Unlike the mandible, the bone of the paranasal sinuses tolerates radiation quite well with very little danger of osteoradionecrosis. Every attempt should be made to protect the orbit unless cancer cure will be sacrificed. If the orbit is included in the field, loss of vision in that eye is to be expected (92).

If it is thought that there is a significant possibility for retropharyngeal or cervical metastases (e.g., posterior sinus tumors or cheek skin involvement), these should prophylactically be included in the radiation fields.

Adjunct Radiation

In general, the same guidelines that have already been described for definitive radiation apply to adjunct radiation. The major debate is whether the treatment should be given preoperatively or postoperatively.

Preoperative radiotherapy shrinks the cancer and occasionally the resected specimen will demonstrate no evidence of microscopic residua (93), but it is unclear whether this has any bearing on improving cure rates (94). Preoperative radiation does, however, have a significantly adverse effect on the operative complication rate (94).

Postoperative radiotherapy is probably equally effective with the greatest advantage being that after surgery the exact site of potential residual cancer is known, and the radiation fields are tailored to encompass these.

In general, we tend to use postoperative radiation as the approach of choice.

Palliative Radiation

This is usually given when the tumor is too advanced for curative surgical therapy or if there has been recurrence after surgical resection. In these situations, the radiation may be augmented by hyperthermia and implants or intracavitary irradiation via mold applications.

Chemotherapy

The exact role of chemotherapy in managing paranasal sinus cancers is controversial. While its role in some tumors (e.g., lymphomas and rhabdomyosarcoma) is quite obvious, its role in others (e.g., esthesioneuroblastoma) is less clear and, of course, in squamous cell cancers, it is even more vague. Groups from Japan and Holland have reported impressive results using chemotherapy and radiation together with tumor debulking (95,96); however, this has not been the accepted approach in the United States. Only time and greater experience will determine the validity of these results.

The use of adjunct chemotherapy together with radiation for inoperable advanced cancer for the sole purpose of palliation has its proponents and is worth considering.

Surgery

The cornerstone for the management of benign, low-grade, and most malignant tumors involving the nose and paranasal sinuses is surgery. There exists a bewildering array of surgical approaches and techniques designed to resect any portion of the midface that is affected. No attempt will be made to describe in detail the technical aspects of these procedures; the appropriate surgical atlases should be consulted for this information. In addition, the topic of craniofacial resection is presented elsewhere in this book.

The basic surgical procedures can be categorized as follows and, in general, usually consist of some form of maxillectomy for exposure or resection:

1. Medial maxillectomy.
2. Suprastructure maxillectomy.
3. Infrastructure maxillectomy.
4. Radical maxillectomy.

These dissections may be extended to include:

± Orbital exenteration.
± Infratemporal fossa dissection.
± Craniotomy (craniofacial resection).
± Contralateral maxillectomy.

Surgical Approaches

In order to perform these procedures, three transfacial approaches have been designed:

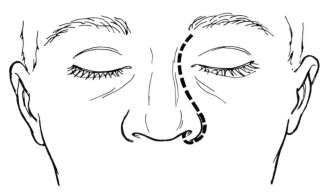

FIG. 14. Incision for the lateral rhinotomy approach.

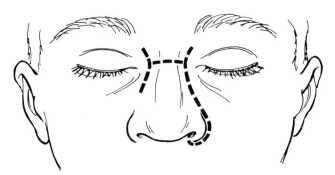

FIG. 16. Incision used to perform a total rhinotomy.

1. *Lateral Rhinotomy* (Fig. 14). This incision provides an excellent exposure to permit a medial maxillectomy or improved intranasal exposure. It can be extended into a lip-splitting incision (Weber–Ferguson incision) (Fig. 15) to permit access to a radical maxillectomy. The key to obtaining a good cosmetic result is to carefully follow the nasolabial crease. By elevating the nasal alar off the underlying bone forming the pyriform aperture, an excellent exposure of the nasal cavity and lateral wall of the nose can be obtained.

2. *Total Rhinotomy* (Fig. 16). A total rhinotomy is of value if the tumor is midline and exposure is required of the cribriform plate and ethmoids bilaterally. It frequently is combined with a craniotomy to provide access for a craniofacial resection. It essentially consists of performing a lateral rhinotomy on one side and connecting the incision with a Lynch incision on the contralateral side. After the cartilaginous septum is divided, an osteotomy through the frontal process of the maxilla is performed bilaterally and the nasal skeleton swung laterally based on the contralateral facial artery. This provides outstanding access to the anterior base of the skull. At the termination of the procedure, the nasal bones are plated into position.

3. *Midface Degloving Incision* (Fig. 17). The advantage of this technique is that it avoids any facial incisions. It consists of making a gingivobuccal incision extending from maxillary tuberosity to tuberosity and communicating this with columella transfixion and intercartilaginous incisions between the upper and lower nasal cartilages. This does provide excellent visualization for unilateral or bilateral infrastructure maxillectomy although access to the roof of the ethmoids is sometimes difficult.

Medial Maxillectomy

This technique is most commonly used for benign and low-grade malignancies involving the lateral wall of the nose, but it can also be used for high-grade cancers. It can easily be combined with a craniofacial re-

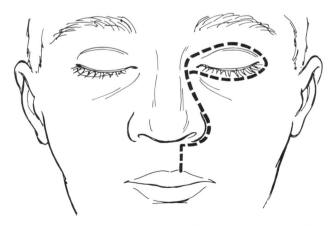

FIG. 15. Weber–Ferguson incision to permit a radical maxillectomy.

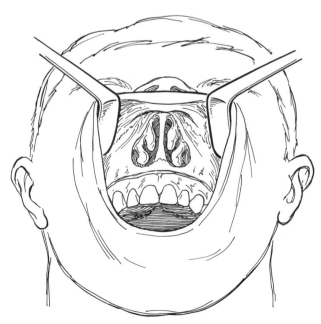

FIG. 17. Midface degloving approach to the paranasal sinuses.

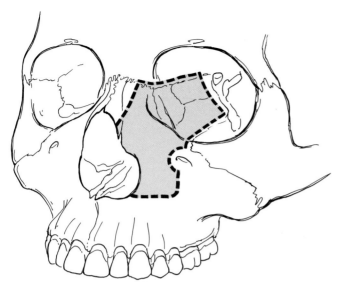

FIG. 18. Area resected via medial maxillectomy.

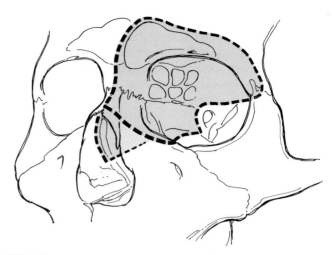

FIG. 20. Area to be resected via suprastructure maxillectomy with craniotomy.

section, suprastructure maxillectomy with or without orbital exenteration, or resection of the contralateral side. The customary incisions used for this procedure are the lateral rhinotomy or midface degloving approaches. The area resected via the classical technique is demonstrated in Fig. 18.

Variants of this procedure include an inferior medial maxillectomy (where the superior extent is the middle meatus) and a superior limited medial maxillectomy where the nasolacrimal system is not disrupted (97) (Fig. 19). These techniques are commonly used for benign or low-grade malignancies (e.g., inverting papilloma). A medial maxillectomy may also be performed, not as the definitive ablative procedure but rather to

obtain access to a posteriorly placed benign tumor (e.g., angiofibroma).

Complications are minimal following medial maxillectomy. Crusting can be treated with meticulous nasal toilette and usually spontaneously resolves with time. Nasolacrimal duct stenosis is rarely a problem but can easily be managed by a dacryocystorhinostomy if necessary.

Suprastructure Maxillectomy

A suprastructure maxillectomy (Fig. 20) is indicated for ethmoid cancers that have extended laterally to involve the orbit and the upper half of the maxillary sinus

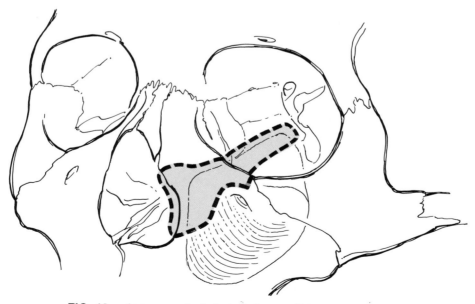

FIG. 19. Area resected via inferior medial maxillectomy.

and usually has extended intracranially. It therefore is frequently combined with a craniotomy to permit a craniofacial resection. The approach is usually via a lateral rhinotomy incision with lateral infraorbital extension to incorporate the orbital exenteration. The floor of the orbit, orbital contents, and ethmoid complex are removed en bloc, together with the superior half of the maxillary sinus.

Infrastructure Maxillectomy

This procedure (Fig. 21) is performed for tumors confined to the floor of the maxillary antrum, hard palate, or superior alveolar ridge. The entire procedure can be performed via an intraoral approach after diagnostic antrotomy through the anterior face of the maxillary has been performed to ensure that the tumor is resectable by this approach. As the hard palate has been removed, the defect is closed by an obturator placed at the time or surgery, or a pack of iodoform gauze held in place with a hammock created by O-silk sutures.

Radical Maxillectomy

A radical maxillectomy (Fig. 22) is the therapeutic procedure of choice for advanced cancer of the maxillary sinus. It consists of en bloc removal of the maxilla and the lower half of the ethmoid sinus and may be extended posteriorly to include the pterygoid plates

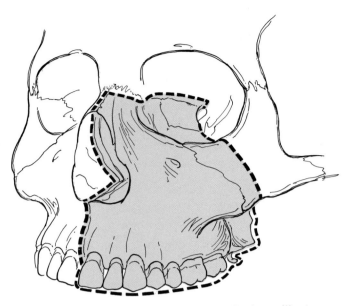

FIG. 22. Area to be resected by a radical maxillectomy.

and pterygoid muscles and superiorly to include the orbital contents. If combined with a craniotomy, the whole ethmoid complex and anterior skull base can be incorporated in the resected specimen. It is most effective when the tumor is confined to the cavity of the maxillary antrum.

Contraindications include:

1. Involvement of the sphenoid.
2. Involvement of the nasopharynx.

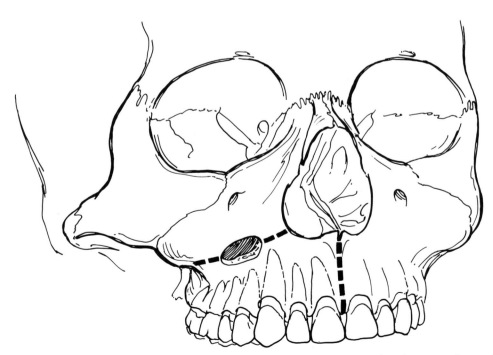

FIG. 21. Infrastructure maxillectomy after diagnostic antrotomy has been performed.

3. Middle cranial fossa extension.
4. Extensive infratemporal fossa involvement.
5. The presence of bilateral cervical metastases. This is somewhat controversial, but multiple series have reported dismal survival regardless of the therapeutic regimen in this situation (98–100). On the other hand, other authors believe that some of these cases can be salvaged by performed neck dissections and radiation to the retropharyngeal nodes (101). In the final analysis, as long as realistic expectations are present, it is not unreasonable to make an aggressive attempt at cure.
6. Distant metastases. Obviously the presence of distant metastases should preclude the use of radical local therapy. The only possible exception would be in slow-growing adenoid cystic carcinoma, where the patient is able to live for many years in symbiosis with the tumor even with extensive distant metastases. A case can therefore be made to resect the primary tumor in this situation.

A wide-field radical maxillectomy necessitates a Weber–Ferguson incision with lateral infraorbital extension to permit the lateral dissection. Once the tumor has been resected, the cavity is skin grafted to prevent contracture and a temporalis muscle flap is used to support the orbital contents if exenteration has not been performed. The cavity is then packed or a temporary prosthesis is placed.

Orbital Exenteration

Indications for orbital exenteration remain controversial, particularly because of the emotions involved in "removing the eye." In spite of newer sophisticated imaging techniques, the need for orbital exenteration can usually only be made definitively at the time of surgery.

If the orbital contents are grossly involved, the eye needs to be removed. If only the periosteum is involved with no extension into the underlying periorbital fat and muscles, then the periosteum alone can be removed and replaced with a skin graft.

A confusing situation exists if preoperative radiation has been administered, making evaluation of the periorbita both clinically and by frozen section difficult. Other factors including subtle intraoperative findings and the preradiotherapy imaging studies all help in deciding whether to remove the eye. In general, if the disease is extremely extensive, and it is felt that residual cancer has been potentially left in multiple sites after resection, it is better *not* to sacrifice the eye. In addition, if the other eye has no serviceable vision or both eyes need to be sacrificed, I tend not to sacrifice the eye or for that matter, not to operate at all. Total blindness, in my opinion, is not compatible with a satisfactory quality of life, particularly if the chances of cure are minimal.

Infratemporal Fossa Dissection

The infratemporal fossa may occasionally need to be accessed for overt tumor extension. This can be achieved by a lateral dissection, removing the zygomatic arch and dissecting the mandibular condylar head out of the glenoid fossa, or performing an anterior mandibular osteotomy and "mandibular swing," exposing this area from below. While one may argue against performing this dissection in high-grade cancers, it certainly is valuable in managing low-grade and benign tumors.

Reconstruction

Reconstruction is dependent on the type of surgical procedure performed. No formal reconstructive procedure is necessary after the medial maxillectomy. Reconstruction after a simple radical maxillectomy essentially consists of lining the intracavitary soft tissue with a skin graft to prevent contracture. If the floor of the orbit has been removed and the orbital contents remain, a sling should be fashioned to support this structure consisting of pedicled temporalis muscle or a free fascia lata graft, which diminishes the entropion that inevitably results.

If a craniofacial resection is performed, a far more elaborate approach to reconstruction is necessary to prevent the development of intracranial infection, cerebrospinal fluid leak, and pneumocephalus. The closure for the most part depends on the size and type of defect but usually consists of repair of the dura, reinforced with fascia lata if needed, a muscle flap (e.g., pericranial flap or temporalis muscle graft), and a skin graft (102). Palatal defects are best closed using an obturator and while multiple creative flaps have been designed to close these defects, in my opinion, they have never been particularly satisfactory.

Rehabilitation

Rehabilitation of the patient is a team approach necessitating the skills of the prosthodontist, speech therapist, social worker, nurse, and psychologist, as well as the surgeon acting as a coordinator. The ultimate goal should always be to restore the patient back into the previous role in society.

The prosthodontist's role is key. Without an adequate palatal prosthesis, the patient will not be able to eat or speak properly (Fig. 23). A skilled prosthodontist can perform miracles and without this expertise being

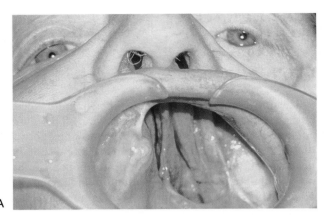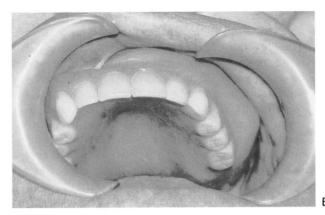

A

B

FIG. 23. **A:** Palatal defect after radical maxillectomy. **B:** Defect closed by prosthesis.

available, one wonders whether this surgery should be performed at all! Usually, multiple steps are needed over the course of weeks and months before the final prosthesis can be placed. In order to facilitate this process, the surgeon should adhere to the following rules:

1. Place a skin graft at the time of surgery to prevent contracture.
2. Preserve as much anterior maxilla as possible.
3. Preserve as many teeth as possible.
4. Remove any redundant bony projections that may interfere with placement of the obturator (e.g., nasal septum).

The soft palate defect can easily be corrected by posterior extension of the prosthesis. Replacement of the eye, nose, and even cheek skin is possible using a prosthesis, but commitment and patience by both the prosthodontist and patient alike are essential.

Prognosis

The late diagnosis and the aggressive nature of many of these malignancies, and the difficulty in effectively treating the primary tumor and the retropharyngeal nodes, all contribute to the extremely poor prognosis for cancers of the nose and paranasal sinuses. An overall 30% five-year survival for squamous cell cancer has been our experience and is similar to that reported in the literature. Local recurrence is the most common cause of failure with regional and distant metastases being less common.

Obviously the earlier the diagnosis, the better the chance to surgically and radiotherapeutically encompass the tumor. Efforts therefore need to be directed to raising the index of suspicion and improving our imaging studies in order to diagnose these lesions earlier.

While sporadic reports have supported the potential role of adjunct chemotherapy in improving prognosis and minimizing the need for less radical surgery, this has still not been clarified and will require further investigation.

REFERENCES

1. Gullane RP, Conley J. Carcinoma of the maxillary sinus. *J Otolaryngol* 1983;12:141–145.
2. Sisson G, Toriumi D, Atiyah RA. Paranasal sinus malignancy: a comprehensive update. *Laryngoscope* 1989;99:143–150.
3. Som PM, Shugar JM. The significance of bone expansion associated with the diagnosis of malignant tumors of the paranasal sinuses. *Radiology* 1980;136:97–100.
4. Astor FC, Donegan JO, Gluckman JL. Unusual anatomic presentations of inverting papilloma. *Head Neck Surg* 1985;7:243–254.
5. Batsakis JG. The pathology of head and neck tumors. Nasal cavity and paranasal sinuses. *Head Neck Surg* 1980;2:410–419.
6. Brandwein M. Human papilloma virus 6/11 and 16/18 in schneiderian inverted papillomas: in situ hybridization with human papilloma virus RNA probes. *Cancer* 1989;63:1708–1713.
7. Batsakis JG. Nasal (schneiderian) papillomas. *Ann Otol Rhinol Laryngol* 1980;90:190–196.
8. Hyams VJ. Papillomas of the nasal cavity and paranasal sinuses: a clinico pathologic study of 315 cases. *Ann Otol Rhinol Laryngol* 1971;80:192–206.
9. Waitz G, Wigand ME. Results of endoscopic sinus surgery for the treatment of inverted papillomas. *Laryngoscope* 1992;102:917–922.
10. Dolgin SR, Zaveri VD, Casiano R, Maniglia AJ. Different options for treatment of inverting papilloma of the nose and paranasal sinuses. A report of 41 cases. *Laryngoscope* 1992;102:231–236.
11. Vrabec DP. Inverted schneiderian papillomas: a clinical and pathological study. *Laryngoscope* 1975;85:186–220.
12. Weissler MC, Montgomery W, Turner P. Inverted papilloma. *Ann Otol Rhinol Laryngol* 1986;95:215–221.
13. Maybery TE, Devine KD, Harrison EG. The problem of malignant transformation in a nasal papilloma. *Arch Otol* 1965;82:296–300.
14. Mendenhall WM, Million R, Cassisi NJ. Biologically aggressive papillomas of the nasal cavity. The role of radiation therapy. *Laryngoscope* 1985;95:344–347.
15. Gluckman JL, Barrord J. Nonsquamous cell tumors of the minor salivary glands. *Otolaryngol Clin North Am* 1986;19:497–505.
16. Neel HB. Juvenile angiofibroma. In: Blitzer A, Lawson W, Friedman W, eds. *Surgery at the paranasal sinuses*. Philadelphia: Saunders, 1991.

17. Brunner H. Nasopharyngeal fibroma. *Ann Otol Rhinol Laryngol* 1942;51:29–65.
18. Holman CB, Miller WE. Juvenile nasopharyngeal fibroma, roentgenologic characteristics. *Am J Roentgenol* 1965;94:292–298.
19. Rosen L, Hanafee W, Nahum A. Nasopharyngeal angiofibroma, an angiographic evaluation. *Radiology* 1966;86:103–107.
20. Sarpa JR, Novelly NJ. Extra nasopharyngeal angiofibroma. *Otolaryngol Head Neck Surg* 1989;101:693–697.
21. Jones GC, DeSanto LW, Bremer JW, Neel HB. Juvenile angiofibromas: behavior and treatment of extensive and recurrent tumors. *Arch Otolaryngol Head Neck Surg* 1986;112:1191–1194.
22. Bremer JW, Neel HB, DeSanto LW, Jones GC. Angiofibromas: treatment trends in 150 patients during 40 years. *Laryngoscope* 1986;96:1321–1329.
23. Fitzpatrick PT. The nasopharyngeal angiofibroma. *Can J Surg* 1970;13:228–235.
24. Wilson GH, Hanafee WN. Angiographic findings in 16 patients with juvenile nasopharyngeal angiofibroma. *Radiology* 1969;92:279–284.
25. Thomas ML, Mowat RD. Angiography in juvenile nasopharyngeal hemangiofibroma. *Clin Radiol* 1970;21:403–406.
26. Johnsen S, Kloster JH, Schiff M. The actions of hormones on juvenile nasopharyngeal angiofibroma: a case report. *Acta Otolaryngol* 1966;61:153–160.
27. Brentani MM, Butugan O, Oshima CT. Multiple steroid receptors in nasopharyngeal angiofibromas. *Laryngoscope* 1989;99:398–401.
28. McGahan CA, Durrance FY, Parke RB. The treatment of advanced juvenile nasopharyngeal angiofibroma. *Int J Radiat Oncol Biol Phys* 1989;17:1067–1072.
29. Enconomou TS, Abemayor E, Ward PH. Juvenile nasopharyngeal angiofibroma: an update of the UCLA experience 1960–1985. *Laryngoscope* 1988;98:170–175.
30. Fitzpatrick PJ, Briant TDR, Berman JM. The nasopharyngeal angiofibroma. *Arch Otol* 1980;106:234–236.
31. Cummings BJ, Blend R, Keane T. Primary radiation therapy for juvenile nasopharyngeal angiofibroma. *Laryngoscope* 1984;94:1599–1605.
32. Haughey BH. Malignant angiofibromas. *Otolaryngol Head Neck Surg* 1988;99:607.
33. Makek MS, Andrews JC, Fisch U. Malignant transformation of a nasopharyngeal angiofibroma. *Laryngoscope* 1989;99:1088–1092.
34. Spangnolo DV, Papadimitriou J, Archer M. Post irradiation malignant fibrous histiocytoma arising in juvenile nasopharyngeal angiofibroma and producing alpha-1-antitrypsin. *Histopathology* 1984;8:339–352.
35. Cummings BJ. Relative risk factors in the treatment of juvenile nasopharyngeal angiofibroma. *Head Neck Surg* 1980;3:21–26.
36. Wilms G, Reene P, Baert AL. Pre-operative embolization of juvenile nasopharyngeal angiofibroma. *J Belge Radiol* 1989;72:465–470.
37. Roberts JK, Korones GK, Levine H. Results of surgical management of nasopharyngeal angiofibroma: the Cleveland Clinic experience 1977–1986. *Cleve Clin J Med* 1989;56:529–534.
38. Robertson GH, Biller H, Sessions DE, Ogura JH. Presurgical internal maxillary artery embolization in juvenile angiofibroma. *Laryngoscope* 1972;82:1524–1532.
39. Cocke EW. Transpalatine surgical approach to the nasopharynx and posterior nasal cavity. *Am J Surg* 1964;108:517–525.
40. Robertson GH, Price AC, Davis JM. Therapeutic embolization of juvenile angiofibroma. *Am J Radiol* 1979;133:657–663.
41. Goepfert H, Cangir A, Lee Y-Y. Chemotherapy for aggressive juvenile nasopharyngeal angiofibroma. *Arch Otol* 1985;111:285–289.
42. Hillstrom RP, Zarbo RJ, Jacobs JR. Nerve sheath tumors of the paranasal sinuses, electron microscopy and histopathologic diagnosis. *Otolaryngol Head Neck Surg* 1990;102:257–263.
43. Toriumi DM, Atiyah R, Murad T, et al. Extracranial neurogenic tumors of the head and neck. *Otolaryngol Clin North Am* 1986;19:609–619.
44. Leakos M, Brown DH. Schwannomas of the nasal cavity. *J Otolaryngol* 1993;22(2):106–107.
45. Enterline HT. Histopathology of sarcomas. *Semin Oncol* 1981;8:133–155.
46. Granich MS, Pilch BL, Goodman ML. Meningiomas presenting in the paranasal sinuses and temporal bone. *Head Neck Surg* 1983;5:319–328.
47. Atallah N, Jay MM. Oteomas of the paranasal sinuses. *J Laryngol Otol* 1981;95:291–304.
48. Huvos AG. *Bone tumors. Diagnosis, treatment and prognosis.* Philadelphia, Saunders, 1979.
49. Waldon CA, Shafer WG. The central giant cell reparative granuloma of the jaws: an analysis of 38 cases. *Am J Clin Pathol* 1968;45:437–447.
50. Voss R, Stenersen T, Oppedel BR. Sinonasal cancer and exposure to soft wood. *Acta Otolaryngol* 1985;99:172–178.
51. Roush GC. Epidemiology of cancer of the nose and paranasal sinuses. *Curr Concepts Head Neck Surg* 1979;2:3–8.
52. Nunez F, Suarez C, Alvarez I. Sinonasal adenocarcinoma. Epidemiological and clinicopathological study of 34 cases. *J Otolaryngol* 1993;22(2):86–90.
53. Barnes L. Intestinal-type adenocarcinoma of the nasal cavity and paranasal sinuses. *Am J Surg Pathol* 1986;10:192–202.
54. Batsakis JG, Sciubba JJ. Pathology. In: Blitzer A, Lawson W, Friedman W, eds. *Surgery of the paranasal sinuses.* Philadelphia: Saunders, 1991.
55. Krespi YP, Levine TM. Tumors of the nose and paranasal sinuses. *Otolaryngology* 1991;3(10):1935–1958.
56. Rice D, Stanley R. Surgical therapy of nasal cavity, ethmoid sinus and maxillary sinus tumors. In: Thawley S, Panje W, Batsakis J, Lindberg R, eds. *Comprehensive management of head and neck tumors*, vol. 19. Philadelphia: Saunders, 1987;368–390.
57. Kraus DH, Sterman BM, Levine HL, et al. Factors influencing survival in ethmoid sinus cancer. *Arch Otolaryngol Head Neck Surg* 1992;118:367–372.
58. Beahrs OH, Henson DE, Kennedy BJ, eds. *American Joint Committee on Cancer. Manual for staging of cancer*, 4th ed. Philadelphia: Lippincott, 1992.
59. Ohngren LG. Malignant tumors of the maxillo-ethmoidal region—a clinical study with special reference to the treatment with electrocautery and irradiation. *Acta Otorhinollaryngol Belg* 1933;19(1):476–482.
60. Har-EL G, Hader T, Krespi YP. An analysis of staging systems of carcinoma of the maxillary sinus. *Ear Nose Throat J* 1988;67:511–524.
61. Kadish S, Goodman M, Wang CC. Olfactory neuroblastoma: a clinical analysis of 17 cases. *Cancer* 1976;37:1571–1576.
62. Batsakis JG, Rice DH, Solomon AR. The pathology of head and neck tumors. Squamous and mucous gland carcinomas of the nasal cavity, paranasal sinuses, and larynx. *Head Neck Surg* 1980;2:497–508.
63. Regine WF, Mendenhall WM, Parsons JJ. Radiotherapy for adenoid cystic carcinoma of the palate. *Head Neck* 1993;15:241–244.
64. Knegt PP, De Jong PC, Van Andel JG. Carcinoma of the paranasal sinuses: results of a prospective pilot study. *Cancer* 1985;56:57–62.
65. Snow GM, VanderEsch EP, VanSlooten EA. Mucosal melanomas of the head and neck. *Head Neck Surg* 1978;1:24–30.
66. Moore ES, Martin H. Melanoma of the upper respiratory tract and oral cavity. *Cancer* 1955;8:1167–1176.
67. Lund VJ. Malignant melanoma of the nasal cavity and paranasal sinuses. *Ear Nose Throat J* 1993;72:285–290.
68. Frierson HF, Mills SE, Fechner RE, Taxy JR, Levine P. Sinonasal undifferentiated carcinoma. *Am J Surg Pathol* 1986;10:771–779.
69. Djalilian M, Zuko RO, Weiland LH. Olfactory neuroblastoma. *Surg Clin North Am* 1977;57:751–762.
70. Olsen KD, DeSanto LW. Olfactory neuroblastoma, biologic and clinical behavior. *Arch Otolaryngol Head Neck Surg* 1983;109:767–802.
71. Beitler J, Fass D, Brenner H. Esthesioneuroblastoma: is there a role for elective neck treatment? *Head Neck* 1991;4:321–326.

72. Davis RE, Weissler MC. Esthesioneuroblastoma and neck metastasis. *Head Neck* 1992;14:477–482.
73. Zappia JO, Carroll W, Wolf G. Olfactory neuroblastoma: the results of modern treatment approaches at the University of Michigan. *Head Neck* 1993;15:190–196.
74. Spaulding CA, Kranyak MS, Constable WC, et al. Esthesioneuroblastoma. A comparison of two treatment eras. *Int J Radiat Oncol* 1988;15:581–590.
75. Batsakis JG, Solomon AR, Rice DH. The pathology of head and neck tumors: neoplasms of cartilage, bone and the notochord. *Head Neck Surg* 1980;3:43–57.
76. Block DM, Bragoli AJ, Collins D, et al. Mesenchymal chondrosarcomas of the head and neck. *J Laryngol Otol* 1979;93:405–412.
77. Kragh LV, Dahlin DC, Erich JB. Cartilaginous tumors of the jaws and facial regions. *Am J Surg* 1960;99:852–856.
78. Dito WR, Batsakis JG. Rhabdomyosarcoma of the head and neck. An appraisal of the biologic behavior in 170 cases. *Arch Surg* 1962;84:582–588.
79. Berry MP, Jenkin RDT. Parameningeal rhabdomyosarcoma in the young. *Cancer* 1981;48:281–288.
80. Farr WH. Soft part sarcomas of the head and neck. *Semin Oncol* 1981;8:185–189.
81. Fu Y-S, Perzin K. Non-epithelial tumors of the nasal cavity, paranasal sinuses and nasopharynx. A clinicopathologic study. Fibrous tissue tumors. *Cancer* 1976;37:364–376.
82. Blitzer A, Lawson W, Biller HF. Malignant fibrous histiocytoma of the head and neck. *Laryngoscope* 1977;87:1479–1499.
83. Batsakis JG, Rice DH. The pathology of head and neck tumors. Vasoformative tumors. *Head Neck Surg* 1981;3:326–339.
84. Eichorn JH, Dickersin G, Bhan AK. Sinonasal hemangiopericytoma: a reassessment with electron microscopy, immunohistochemistry and long term follow-up. *Am J Surg Pathol* 1990;14:856–868.
85. Sofferman RA, Cummings CW. Malignant lymphoma of the paranasal sinuses. *Arch Otolaryngol* 1975;101:287–292.
86. Batsakis JG, Fries GT, Goldman RT. Upper respiratory tract plasmacytoma. *Arch Otolaryngol* 1964;79:613–618.
87. Batsakis JG. Osteogenic and chondrogenic sarcomas of the jaws. *Ann Otol Rhinol Laryngol* 1987;96:474–475.
88. Caron AS, Hajdu SI, Strong E. Osteogenic sarcoma of the facial and cranial bones. A review of 43 cases. *Am J Surg* 1971;122:719–725.
89. Sehdev M, Huvos G, Strong EW. Ameloblastoma of maxilla and mandible. *Cancer* 1974;33:324–333.
90. Lavertu P, Roberts JK, Kraus D, et al. Squamous cell carcinoma of the paranasal sinuses: the Cleveland Clinic experience 1977–1986. *Laryngoscope* 1989;99:1130–1136.
91. Flores AD, Anderson DW, Doyle PJ. Paranasal sinus malignancy: a retrospective analysis of treatment methods. *J Otolaryngol* 1984;13:141–146.
92. Ellingwood KE, Million RR. Cancer of the nasal cavity and ethmoid/sphenoid sinuses. *Cancer* 1979;43:1517–1526.
93. Shidnia H. The role of radiation therapy in the treatment of malignant tumors of the paranasal sinuses. *Laryngoscope* 1984;94:102–105.
94. Jesse RH. Preoperative versus postoperative radiation in the treatment of squamous cell carcinoma of paranasal sinuses. *Am J Surg* 1965;110:552–556.
95. Sakai S. Multidisciplinary treatment of maxillary sinus carcinoma. *Cancer* 1983;52:1360–1364.
96. Kneght P, de Jong PC, VanAnder JG. Carcinoma of the paranasal sinuses. Proceedings of the International Conference on Head and Neck Cancer, 1984.
97. Sessions RB, Larson DL. En bloc ethmoidectomy and medial maxillectomy. *Arch Otol* 1977;103:195–202.
98. Stell RM. The management of cervical lymph nodes in head and neck cancer. *Proc R Soc Med* 1975;68(2):83–85.
99. Schechter GL, Ogura JH. Maxillary sinus malignancy. *Laryngoscope* 1972;82:796–806.
100. Weymuller EA, Reardon EJ, Nash D. A comparison of treatment modalities in carcinoma of the maxillary antrum. *Arch Otol* 1980;106:625–629.
101. Som ML. Surgical management of carcinoma of the maxilla. *Arch Otol* 1974;99:270–273.
102. Freije JE, Gluckman JL, VanLoveren H, et al. Reconstruction of the anterior skull base after craniofacial resection. *Skull Base Surg* 1992;2(1):17–21.

CHAPTER 29

Skull Base Surgery for Sinus Neoplasms

Paul J. Donald

One of the greatest advances in head and neck surgery in the past two decades, and especially in the last 10 years, has been the development of skull base surgery. This approach embodies the concept of a surgical team comprised principally of a head and neck surgeon and a neurological surgeon who together, in a planned, co-ordinated way, can resect neoplasms that encroach upon or penetrate through the bones at the base of the skull. The surgical team may also include a neuro-ophthalmologist, vascular surgeon, or plastic surgeon. The latter is especially important if a free flap will be needed for reconstruction. Other members of the team obviously will include the diagnostic and interventional radiologist during the patient's preoperative workup, the nurse clinician, dietitian, and social worker, as well as the maxillofacial prosthodontist. The nurse clinician deserves special notice because of the important input in the management of the family, reassuring the patient, and providing valuable information in preparation for the patient's impending surgical ordeal.

A sense of collegiality and cooperation, as well as an attitude of mutual respect and understanding, are critical elements to the smooth functioning of the team. The neurosurgeon and the head and neck surgeon require a clear understanding of the anatomy, physiology, and surgical requirements and exigencies in one another's areas of expertise. The emergence of formalized skull base teams at major institutions throughout the world, as well as the establishment of societies and study groups dedicated to study and research in skull base surgery, has led to rapid advances in this challenging field.

HISTORY

Skull base surgery first began with attempts to resect extensive primary sinus neoplasms, and thereby extending intracranially, or as a means to solve an intra-cranial problem by using an extracranial approach, such as was done with pituitary adenoma surgery.

The advances experienced in modern otolaryngology–head and neck surgery, neurosurgery, and plastic surgery have been little short of amazing. However, until relatively recently, tumor unresectability had been established at artificial boundaries, in essence created by the lack of understanding of the anatomy and physiology of the areas of interface between traditional head and neck surgery and neurological surgery. Moreover, the concern regarding the potential problem of reconstructing the resected area limited the aggressiveness of the ablative surgeon.

In the preantibiotic era, pioneering neurosurgeons such as Schloffer (1), Cushing (2), and Hirsch (3) were the first to enter the cranial vault through the structures of the face. This was in the form of the transnasal approach to the pituitary fossa. The mortality rate was only 5%, and mostly due to meningitis. This was the preferred route for Cushing and his colleagues for the next 10 to 20 years. They then, for reasons that remain unclear but presumably due to the problem of infection, elected to resume the transcranial approach. Osker Hirsch, however, continued to use the transnasal route and, in 1952 (4), reported on 425 such procedures he had done.

The history of modern craniofacial surgery probably began in 1941 when Dandy (5), while removing an orbital tumor with an approach through the anterior cranial fossa, extended his resection through the ethmoids. Rae and McLean (6) in 1943 reported a combined transorbital, transcranial excision of a retinoblastoma. However, the landmark article in skull base surgery was in 1954, when Klopp teamed up with Smith and Williams (7) to do what is recorded as probably the first craniofacial resection in that area, performed through separate transcranial and transfacial incisions. The tumor was described as a cancer of the frontal sinuses. It is ironic to note that it was said that it "gained little acceptance at the time," an experience not unfamiliar to many of us in our early attempts to do skull base surgery for tumors. Malecki (8) in 1959 reported a craniofacial resection for ethmoid carcinoma and described a resection of the cribriform plate. However, it was not until 1963 that Ketcham (9) and his colleagues reported the first group of patients who had undergone skull base surgery for malignancy. They described 19 patients with malignant tumors, mostly originating in the paranasal sinuses, that had undergone anterior craniofacial resections. Ketcham followed this up with a paper on complications (10) and finally a report in 1974 (11) of a 14-year experience with 48 patients who had a 53% determinate 5-year survival rate.

The development of the binocular operating microscope by Holmgren (12) in 1922 revolutionized the surgical treatment of deafness. In 1961, Dr. William House (13) pioneered the subspecialty of neurotology by removing an acoustic neuroma for the first time through the middle fossa approach. He combined with a neurosurgeon, John B. Doyle, to form one of the first skull base teams. In the years since, the subspecialty of neurotology has flourished with the development of many new and innovative procedures. However, for more extensive tumors, the cooperative efforts of the neurological surgeon became obviously indispensable.

The next major breakthrough was made by Dr. Ugo Fisch (14) when he described in 1977 his approach to glomus jugulare tumors through the infratemporal fossa. In the same year, Gardner and Cocke (15) described their unique approach to glomus tumors through the transcervicomastoid approach. Schramm (16) and Sekhar (17), using an adaptation of Fisch's infratemporal approach, developed an attack on benign and malignant tumors of this region. Using a craniotomy flap that includes part of the middle fossa floor produced excellent access to the petrous carotid, cavernous sinus, and nasopharynx. Further work by Sekhar (18), Parkinson (19), Dolenc (20), and Al-Mefty (21) has revealed the intimate anatomy of the cavernous sinus, as well as providing a number of safe approaches to resections of tumors contained therein. This frightening area was always considered surgically inviolable until these surgeons showed us that surgery was not only possible, but safe and effective.

With the development of microvascular surgery in 1960 by Jacobson and Suarez (22) and then Nakayama (23), the transplantation of free flaps was born. This has become an essential adjunct to the reconstruction of the extensive defects left by cranial base exenteration. Although free grafts and regional flaps are important elements in the resurfacing and reconstruction of these areas, often a free flap will give the only real insurance of a clear separation of the intracranial cavity and the upper aerodigestive tract.

Although the surgical management of these cases is the central focus, a revolution in the accuracy of preoperative evaluation of precise tumor extent has been made possible by the introduction of the computer-assisted tomography (CAT) scan and magnetic resonance imaging (MRI). The development of gadolinium as a tumor enhancing agent has greatly improved this precision. This has been improved even further by the advent of fat suppression software. Balloon occlusion arteriography, especially when combined with radioactive xenon cerebral blood flow scanning, helps in predicting the integrity of contralateral internal carotid artery blood flow to the brain. This renders much more predictable the safety of internal carotid artery sacrifice.

PATHOPHYSIOLOGY

The majority of patients who require skull base surgery involving entrance into the anterior cranial fossa suffer from malignancies of the paranasal sinuses. The maxillary and ethmoids are most commonly the source, with the maxillary cancers having the highest incidence. Maxillary tumors spread to the anterior fossae via the ethmoids or orbit or both. The usual area of penetration of maxillary sinus tumors is either through the narrow common wall it shares with the ethmoid at the medial roof of the maxillary sinus or through the superior aspect of the medial wall of the maxillary ascent into the bulla ethmoidalis. Further extension superiorly will take the tumor to the ethmoidal fovea. Extension of maxillary tumors medially brings them into the nasal cavity, while further growth in a rostral direction results in encroachment on the cribriform plate (Fig. 1).

In days gone by, malignancies behind Ohngren's line were thought to carry a virtually hopeless prognosis. This was because of their rapid spread to the orbit and orbital apex with access to both the anterior and middle cranial fossae. The access to the middle fossa is by virtue of the proximity of the lateral wall of the optic canal, as well as the posterolateral orbital wall, to the anteriormost extension of the temporal lobe (Fig. 2). It is important to realize that the beginning of the canal is approximately 1 cm posterior to the posterior wall of the maxillary sinus.

Posteriorly, tumor spread will be through the thin posterior sinus wall into the pterygomaxillary space or laterally beyond to the infratemporal fossa. Spread to the former permits access to the foramen rotundum and the vidian canal. The bone at this particular portion of the skull base near where the pterygoid plates subtend from the body of the sphenoid is extremely thick

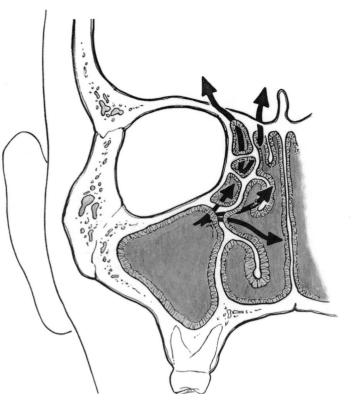

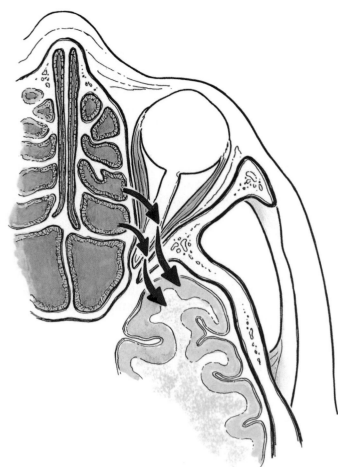

FIG. 1. Routes of spread of tumor from the maxillary sinus to ethmoids to anterior cranial fossa.

FIG. 2. Spread of tumor from the posterior ethmoids and sphenoidal sinus to the middle cranial fossa.

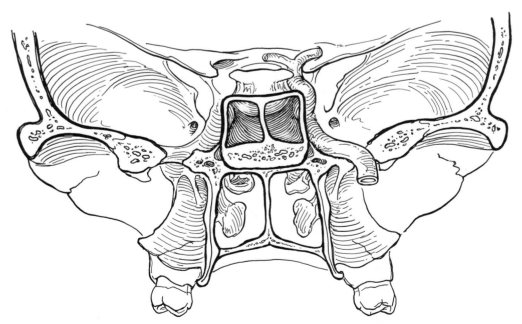

FIG. 3. Coronal cut through the sphenoid bone demonstrating the thickness of the sphenoid body near the level of the origin of the pterygoid plates.

(Fig. 3). Erosion into the middle fossa at this site takes a substantial amount of time. Extension of tumor into the deep aspects of the infratemporal fossa provide an intracranial route of spread through the foramen ovale. Further progress posteriorly provides access to the undersurface of the temporal bone, the stylomastoid foramen, carotid canal, and jugular foramen. Sinus tumors rarely ever extend this far except in the most advanced cases.

Inferior spread through the palate and alveolar ridge, penetration into the soft tissues of the cheek anteriorly, and extension into the nose with presentation at the nares are more common modes of tumor presentation (Fig. 4).

The next commonest of the sinuses to be afflicted by tumor are the ethmoids. Their commonest route of spread is medially into the orbit. They can extend inferiorly into the maxillary sinus, but most remain confined to the superior half of the maxilla. Superior extension will breach the fovea ethmoidalis and the cribriform plate. Progress posteriorly encroaches on the sphenoid sinus. Extension to the sphenoid sinus from an ethmoid or maxillary sinus carcinoma is far more common than sphenoidal primaries themselves. Anterior tumor growth will result in involvement of the lacrimal sac and duct. The eyelids may be invaded (Fig. 5) and even the nasal dorsum itself.

The sphenoid sinus rarely has tumors beginning there *de novo*. Wylie et al. (24) in 1973 reported only six primary sphenoid malignancies seen at the Mayo Clinic. There were two squamous cell carcinomas, two lymphoepitheliomas, one adenocarcinoma, and one of undifferentiated type. Alexander (25) reported a variety of tumors including malignant melanoma, basal cell carcinoma, and reticulum cell, osteoblastic, and transitional cell sarcoma. The most common presentation is an extension from another site. The roof of the sphenoid sinus, the planum sphenoidale, has an intimate relationship to the optic chiasm (Fig. 6). This provides in some patients a therapeutic dilemma in that resec-

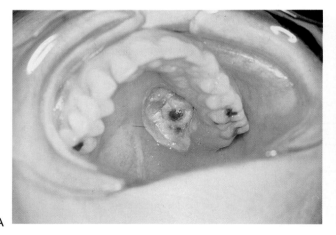

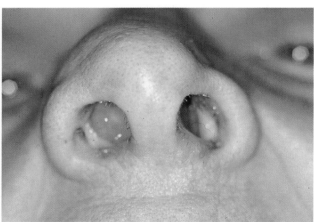

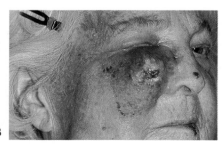

FIG. 4. Routes of spread of maxillary carcinoma. **A:** Through the palate. **B:** Through the soft tissues of the cheek. **C:** As a soft tissue mass in the nose.

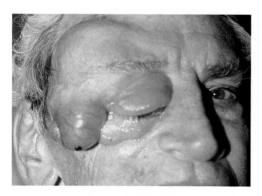

FIG. 5. Invasion of the periorbital tissues and eyelids by an adenoid cystic carcinoma of the maxillary and ethmoid sinuses.

tion at this site may lead to complete amaurosis. Invaginating the sphenoid sinus is the sella turcica, which contains the pituitary gland. Surrounding the pituitary stalk in the region of the diaphragma sella is the circular sinus that connects one cavernous sinus to its fellow on the opposing side. Often, there are extensions of the circular sinus into the dura encasing the pituitary.

The posterior wall of the sphenoidal sinus is the basal portion of the sphenoid bone into which the sinus is merely an invagination. The basisphenoid articulates through a synostosis with the occipital bone to form the clivus. The floor of the sinus is the roof of the nasopharynx. The roof of the nasopharynx is characterized by numerous short spike-like protrusions called the pharyngeal tubercles, to which are attached the pharyngobasilar fascia and origin of the superior constrictor. The floor of the sinus is 3 to 5 mm thick.

The most important anatomical relationships of the sphenoid sinus are related to its lateral walls. The cavernous sinus, a dura-encased network of veins, venous sinusoids, and vascular spaces, is intimately related to the lateral aspect of the sinus (Fig. 7). The dura lining the cavernous sinus is relatively tough, especially on the lateral side. Contained within the sinus are the internal carotid artery, cranial nerves III, IV, and VI, and two branches of the trigeminal nerve, V_{II} (maxillary branch) and V_{III} (mandibular branch) (Fig. 8). The

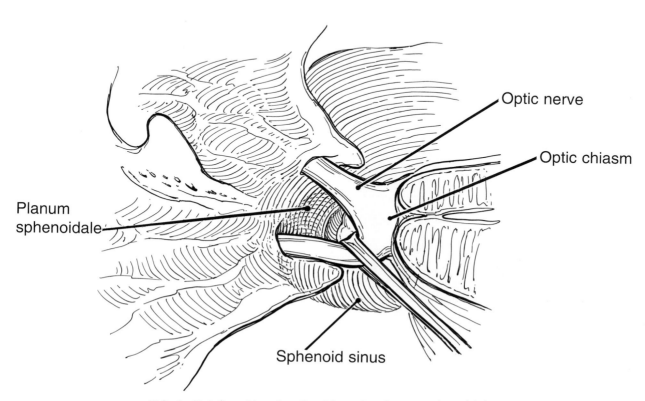

FIG. 6. Relationship of optic chiasm to planum sphenoidale.

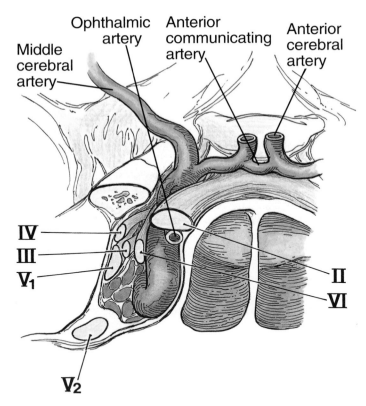

FIG. 7. Cavernous sinus.

carotid artery often indents the inferolateral wall of the sphenoid sinus. Some of the aforementioned cranial nerves will often produce prominences as well (Fig. 9). The cavernous sinus begins anteriorly as the ophthalmic vein and receives a host of venous connections from other regions of the face as well as many dural sinuses. Small projections of the sinus occur along the sheaths of V_{II} and V_{III}, occasionally extending slightly extracranial through their exiting foramina. Tumor invading the cavernous sinus tends to compress it and

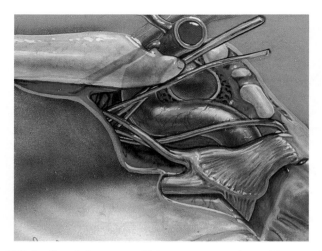

FIG. 8. Cranial nerves within cavernous sinus. (From ref. 49, with permission.)

even results in thrombosis. Usually the thrombosis is asymptomatic.

The cranial nerve most commonly afflicted in cavernous involvement is VI. In the initial one-third of its course in the sinus, this nerve lies in the adventitia of the lateral surface of the internal carotid (see Fig. 5 in the chapter by Rice, Ethmoid, Maxillary, Frontal, and Sphenoid Sinusitis). The III and especially the IV nerves are plastered against the dural wall on the lateral side of the sinus or may be enclosed in two sheaths of dura. The third division of the trigeminal nerve has a very short course in the sinus prior to diving into the foramen ovale, whereas the second division courses all the way through the floor of the cavernous sinus.

The sphenoid sinus often has more than one septation and may even have a transverse one. The sphenoid may have within itself a very large posterior ethmoid or sphenoethmoid cell called an Onodi cell (26).

The frontal sinus is rarely afflicted by malignant tumors. Tumor spread from the ethmoids, orbit, or nasal cavity is commonest. So-called benign tumors of the meninges, such as meningioma, can invade the sinus as well. Most meningiomas affecting the frontal sinus are primary within the dura of the anterior fossa and extend into the sinus. Of the 36 so-called primary meningiomas of the paranasal sinuses, most have arisen within the frontal sinus (27,28). They have a variable degree of invasive potential and are histologically usually of either the meningoendothelial or psammomatous type (29). There are about 100 cases of carcinoma of the frontal sinuses in the literature, usually invading the ethmoid sinuses (30). They often present like a frontal sinus mucocele, commonly with bone erosion (Fig. 10).

Much of the floor of the frontal sinus makes up a good part of the orbital roof. However, in many instances, a portion of this floor is displaced by the intrusion of an orbital ethmoid cell. In coronal section this gives a three-tiered appearance with the roof of the orbit the bottom tier, the roof of the orbital ethmoid cell the middle tier, and the floor of the frontal sinus the top tier (see Fig. 24 in the chapter by Donald, Anatomy and Histology). The paired frontonasal ducts will allow egress of primary frontal sinus tumors into the nose or provide conversely a pathway for maxillary and ethmoid tumors into the frontal. The posterior wall of the sinus makes up the anterior wall and part of the anterior floor of the anterior cranial fossa. It is very thin and tumor transgression is relatively easy. A dural sinus lies directly against the frontal crest, which runs in the midline of the posterior sinus wall. This is the superior sagittal sinus, which begins in the foramen cecum anterior to the crista galli and extends superiorly along the frontal crest over the vertex of the skull. This sinus starts as a dorsal nasal vein and slowly enlarges in size as it proceeds to the level of the coronal suture.

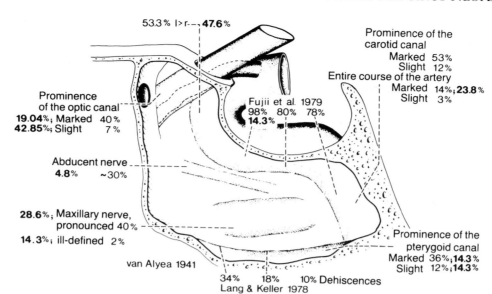

FIG. 9. Prominences produced on the lateral wall of the sphenoidal sinus. (From ref. 26, with permission.)

In its situation behind the frontal sinus, it has a rather small caliber.

The intracranial contents of direct concern for lesions encroaching on the anterior fossa are not too complex. The dura lining the anterior wall of this fossa tends to be somewhat brittle in the elderly and will tear easily during craniotomy. At the region of the cribriform plate, which is on the average 20.8 mm long (31), the dura encases the olfactory filaments as they pass through the olfactory foramina. The plates are roughly elliptical in shape and are penetrated by an average of 43 fila per side. The level of the cribriform plate is at about the interpupillary line, but this is somewhat variable.

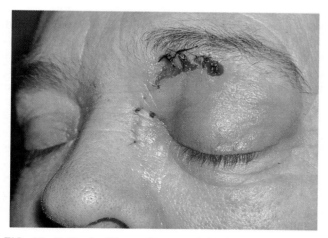

FIG. 10. Patient with carcinoma of the frontal sinus presenting with proptosis and inflammation of the upper eyelid.

The frontal lobes and the underlying olfactory bulbs lie directly over the floor of the anterior fossa. The medial aspect of the floor is composed of the roof of the frontal sinus, as well as the roofs of the ethmoids anteriorly, and some of the sphenoid sinus posteriorly. The orbital roofs make up the remainder.

The superior sagittal sinus, already alluded to, is roughly triangular and is contained within the dura of the falx cerebri. It expands in volume from inferior to superior and is usually not a problem during low anterior craniotomy.

The middle cranial fossa is shaped somewhat like a bow tie with the sella turcica being like the central knot. Much more vital anatomy lies adjacent to the middle fossa floor than the anterior fossa. Laterally, the temporal lobes overlie the floor. Anteriorly, they invaginate under the lesser wing of the sphenoid to lie lateral to the apical portion of the lateral orbital wall. Medially lies the midbrain and the circle of Willis. Just anterior to the anterior clinoids is the optic chiasm lying directly above the sphenoid sinus on the planum sphenoidale. The internal carotids emerge from the cavernous sinus to course directly lateral to the chiasm.

In addition to the internal carotid artery, there are two additional vascular structures of importance in the middle fossa—the middle meningeal artery and the vein of Labbé. Of least importance is the middle meningeal artery. It ascends through the foramen spinosum just medial to the sphenoid spine and traverses the floor of the middle fossa. The artery is almost always controlled subcranially in the various skull base approaches. The vein of Labbé (Fig. 11) is a more vitally

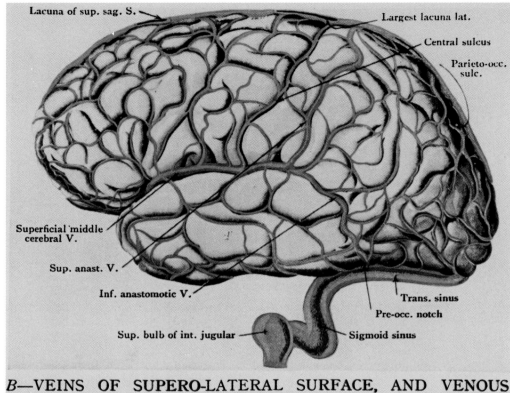

Lacuna of sup. sag. S.

Largest lacuna lat.

Central sulcus

Parieto-occ. sulc.

Superficial middle cerebral V.

Sup. anast. V.

Inf. anastomotic V.

Trans. sinus

Pre-occ. notch

Sup. bulb of int. jugular

Sigmoid sinus

B—VEINS OF SUPERO-LATERAL SURFACE, AND VENOUS SINUSES

FIG. 11. The vein of Labbé or inferior anastomotic cerebral vein. (From ref. 50, with permission.)

important structure. It is more correctly called the inferior anastomotic cerebral vein. Beginning in the Sylvian fissure, it usually empties into the lateral sinus. In some patients, its termination will be more anteriorly, located just posterior to the sigmoid sinus. Its critical importance stems from the occasions when it is the principal vein of drainage of that cerebral hemisphere. In this situation, if the vessel is compromised, cerebral infarction will eventuate.

In head and neck surgery in which principally soft tissues of the upper aerodigestive system are resected, surgeons are accustomed to taking 2-cm margins. This especially pertains to resection width in pharyngeal tumors, and tongue width and thickness in lingual carcinoma. This rule of thumb is considered by many to be inviolable; but there are many instances in common practice when this dictum is not followed. In the larynx, a 1-mm margin is acceptable for adequate resection on the vocal cord. Posterior pharyngeal wall cancers of considerable extent can be resected with a narrow margin between the deep surface of the tumor and the prevertebral fascia. On the other hand, skin penetration or hypopharyngeal extension of tumors need wider margins for safe resection.

What constitutes an adequately safe resection margin in skull base surgery is still as yet unestablished.

It is clear that certain anatomical structures have a resistance to tumor penetration. Just as the prevertebral fascia and the carotid arterial adventitia offer stout barriers to tumor penetration (although they indeed can be penetrated), certain tissues in the skull base offer this same resistance. Dura has the property to contain tumor penetration for consideration periods of time. Sisson (32) presents a case of ethmoid carcinoma that remained stuck to dura, without penetration, for 12 years. Actual cerebral invasion of malignancies even as aggressive as squamous cell carcinoma is an uncommon occurrence (Fig. 12). The periosteum of the carotid canal also offers a strong barrier to tumor penetration. It is my experience that resections of very extensive cancers can safely be limited to millimeters at dura and at the carotid, obviating the necessity of cerebral or carotid artery resection. Cerebral tissue, however, offers very little resistance to tumor penetration once invaded, and whether patients with gross cerebral involvement can successfully be salvaged by excision is unclear. There are some anecdotal cases where successful resection has been achieved.

The biology of sinus tumors of certain histologies requiring skull base surgery often determines the extent of resection. If a basal cell carcinoma has invaded the cranial base, as it might from an origin in the skin

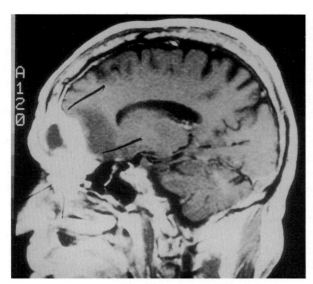

FIG. 12. Sagittal view MRI scan with gadolinium contrast showing poorly differentiated carcinoma invading the frontal lobe of the brain. Note area of edema adjacent to tumor as isolated by the *two grease pencil marks.*

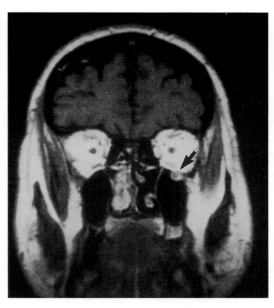

FIG. 14. Coronal CAT scan showing perineural spread of a squamous cell carcinoma of the skin along the infraorbital nerve. (*Arrow* points to tumor.)

of the periorbital region, resection margins do not often need to be as wide as with, for instance, squamous cell carcinoma. Although basal cell carcinoma never takes its origin within a paranasal sinus cavity, the sinus may be invaded by direct extension from nasal skin or the periorbital region (Fig. 13). Since basal cell carcinomas in general, except for the morphea type, have more of a pushing margin rather than a creeping infiltrative one, resection margins are often easier to manage. This is in contrast to squamous cell carcinoma, which, as a rule, is much more infiltrative and aggressive. Certain tumors possess a peculiar propensity to travel along perineural sheaths. The most notorious among these is adenoid cystic carcinoma, which is infamous for its

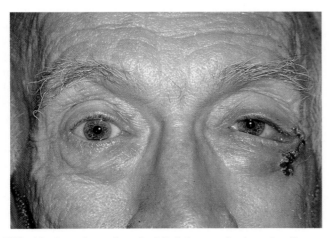

FIG. 13. Invasion of periorbital tissues by basal cell carcinoma.

ability to extend along perineural spaces for considerable distances from the primary tumor. In some instances, squamous cell carcinoma may also acquire this property (Fig. 14). Melanomas, and rarely adenocarcinoma and acinic cell carcinoma, may do this as well. The characteristic of neuroblastoma to pass freely along nerves may be the result of polysialic acid containing epitopes called neuronal cell adhesion molecules (NCAMs) (29). They may act like a biochemical passport for perineural spread. Perhaps a similar enzyme may also be possessed by these neurotropic epithelial neoplasms. Preliminary study of this phenomenon suggests that NCAMs may be involved in this process. The relevance in surgical resection is that in those neoplasms that invade the skull base, consideration must always be given to their potential for perineural spread. This is especially true for those lesions presenting with cranial nerve dysfunction.

Lymphatic metastases to regional lymphatics from sinus carcinomas are uncommon. Neck dissection is advisable only in those individuals with manifest metastatic disease. Considerable discussion occurs in the literature describing the route of metastases of tumors from the maxillary sinus posterior to Ohngren's line and from the posterior ethmoids. These channels are said to interconnect with the peritubal lymphatics of the eustachian tube and thence to the posterior pharyngeal nodes or directly to the middle group of internal jugular nodes (33,34). This pattern of lymphatic spread has been quoted as being one of the major reasons for the poor prognosis for tumors at these sites. The incidence of cervical lymph nodal metastases from squamous cell carcinoma of the sinuses is quoted to be between 16% and 25% (35,36). Sisson and Goldstein (37) state that a palpable retropharyngeal node was found in only 3% of their patients. In my own experience, direct extension of tumor to peritubal tissues is by far a more common occurrence, and lymphatic spread of cancer here has not yet been seen. Thanks to the modern techniques of cranial base surgery, direct spread can often be safely resected. Retropharyngeal lymphatic tissue does occur without doubt, but it is scant; and, in my own experience, lymph nodal metastases to this area from sinus tumors are decidedly rare.

DIAGNOSIS

The diagnosis of cranial base extension of sinus tumors frequently cannot be made on the basis of presenting signs and symptoms. Most of these tumors present in the same way any sinus carcinoma presents, as described by Gluckman in Tumors of the Nose and Paranasal Sinuses. Unfortunately, the subtle symptoms of epistaxis (Fig. 15), nasal obstruction (see Fig. 4C), ill-fitting dentures (see Fig. 4A), and sinusitis are often misconstrued by the primary care physicians as conditions of more benign character.

Symptoms and signs suggesting extension to the skull base most commonly include ocular dysfunction and cranial nerve abnormalities. Proptosis, especially with visual loss, is an important sign and symptom. Ptosis, ophthalmoplegia (Fig. 16) with diplopia, or, worse still, ocular fixation suggests orbital apex invasion with impairment of the first division of the trigeminal nerve. Anesthesia over the infraorbital, infratrochlear, or external nasal nerves or of the upper teeth on the affected side suggests second division trigeminal invasion.

Trismus is symptomatic of posterior or posterolateral wall invasion with extension to the masticatory muscles, especially the pterygoids and masseter. Careful testing of the third division of the trigeminal nerve is mandatory because of the possibility of extension of tumor along the undersurface of the sphenoid bone to the foramen ovale. Involvement of cranial nerve VII suggests extremely far posterior extension and is seen only very rarely. Involvement of cranial nerves X, IX, and XI with symptoms of hoarseness, dysphagia, aspiration, and shoulder weakness are more suggestive of metastasis than direct extension to the jugular foramen. The so-called node of Rouviere (33), the highest lateral pharyngeal node, located deep to the neck of the mandible, may be affected by metastatic disease. Because of its proximity to the jugular foramen, it may bring about the symptoms of a jugular foramen syndrome. In addition, further extension to nerve XII as it emerges close by may produce slurred speech, oral dysphagia, and unilateral lingual atrophy.

Visualization of tumor by indirect nasopharyngoscopy further suggests skull base invasion. Unilateral otitis media with effusion is symptomatic of eustachian tube involvement.

RADIOGRAPHIC EXAMINATION

For sinus tumors, as well as any tumors that invade the skull base, CAT scanning and MRI examination are absolutely essential to determine preoperative extension of tumor. The two studies complement one another in that the CAT scan shows bony detail whereas soft tissue involvement can be more accurately determined by MRI.

When ordering the CAT scans, it is essential to obtain coronal cuts as well as the standard axial views. The reconstructed view derived data, obtained from 5-mm thick axial cuts, are of very limited value. At sites of vital concern, the cuts should be narrowed to 1-mm thickness (Fig. 17). Bone and soft tissue contrast settings are important for more accurate determination of bony and soft tissue extension (Fig. 18). The critical element of cranial base erosion can be determined when it is gross but subtle degrees are less amenable to discernment.

MRI scanning often provides outstanding contrast between tumor and surrounding soft tissues in previously unoperated and unirradiated individuals. Axial, coronal, and sagittal views are all important in assessing tumor extent and creating a mental three-dimensional construction of tumor extent. Distinction between tumor and adjacent soft tissue can best be done when comparing T1 to T2 weighted images. In the T2

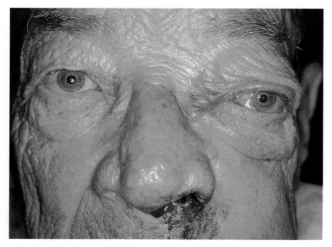

FIG. 15. Patient with extensive carcinoma of ethmoid sinuses presenting as an epistaxis. Note marked lateral displacement of globe.

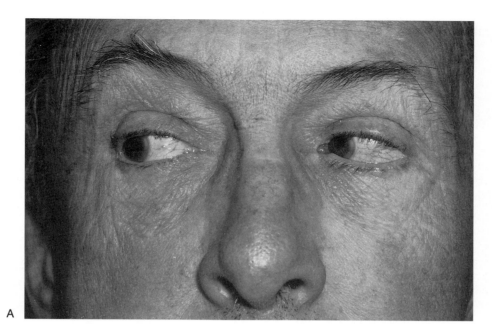

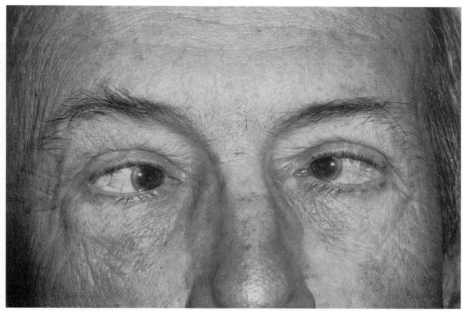

FIG. 16. Patient with carcinoma of the sphenoid sinus presenting with an abducens nerve palsy. **A:** Right lateral gaze. **B:** Left lateral gaze showing paralysis of left abducens nerve.

image, the tumor shows up much brighter than the surrounding soft tissue (Fig. 19). The advent of gadolinium as a contrast material, which has preferential uptake by tumor, has greatly enhanced the ability to diagnose tumor extension and to differentiate tumor from surrounding tissues (Fig. 20). Unfortunately, edema, fibrous tissue, and highly vascularized tissues and fat pick up the contrast as well (38). The use of fat suppression programs helps greatly in eliminating the image of fat, which obscures the signal produced by tumor. The

swelling of nerves in their foramina is highly suggestive of perineural invasion. This is especially important in the superior orbital fissure and foramen rotundum in sinus tumors. Any widening of nerves V1 or V2 as they traverse their respective foramina must be presumed to be evidence of tumor invasion. Dural displacement and direct invasion can be seen with MRI. Furthermore, direct cerebral invasion can be presumed by MRI with gadolinium contrast (Fig. 21). The patient in Fig. 21 had no symptoms of cerebellar or cerebral

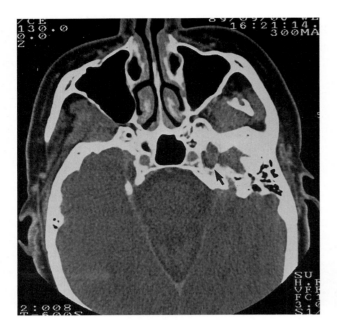

FIG. 17. CAT scan of middle-aged woman in axial projection showing widening of V3 in the foramen ovale resulting from recurrent acinic cell carcinoma of the deep lobe of the parotid. *Black arrow* points to enlarged foramen.

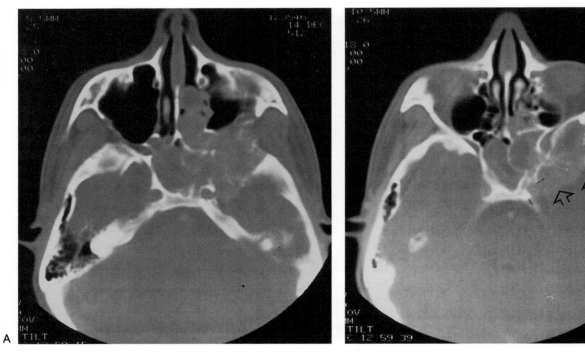

A

B

FIG. 18. CAT scan of 14-year-old boy with a highly invasive juvenile angiofibroma extending into the middle fossa. **A:** Bone windows showing extensive erosion of the floor of the left middle fossa. **B:** Soft tissue window illustrating extension into orbital apex and middle cranial fossa. *Open arrows* point to middle fossa invasion.

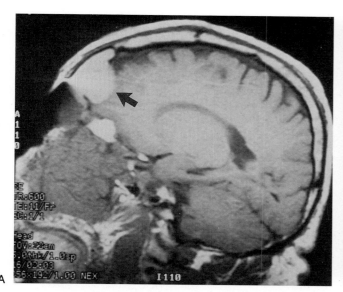
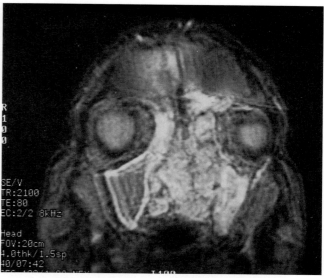

FIG. 19. Middle-aged man with a massive esthesioneuroblastoma with intracranial invasion. **A:** T1 weighted image in sagittal plane showing massive tumor density in nose and ethmoid sinuses at a similar density to surrounding soft tissue *(solid arrow).* Note fluid-filled frontal sinus mucocele, which gives a very bright signal. **B:** T2 weighted image showing much brighter signal from tumor than surrounding soft tissue.

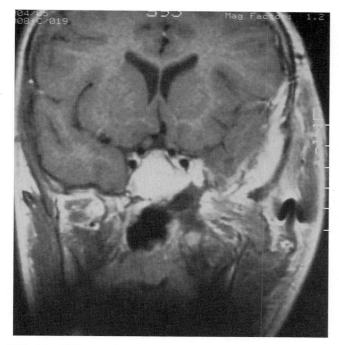

FIG. 20. MRI scan in coronal plane in patient with recurrent nasopharyngeal angiofibroma of the sphenoidal sinus. Gadolinium contrast creates a bright signal on T1 image.

involvement but had strong evidence of invasion of these structures with MRI that discouraged me from operating on him. However, often cerebral findings are equivocal and the only definitive reliable finding thus far has been the presence of brain edema adjacent to the area of invasion (Fig. 22).

The cavernous sinus is one of the most difficult areas to assess by any means. Coronal CAT scans and MRI scans are studied carefully in an attempt to assess symmetry, carotid displacement, dural displacements, irregularity of outline, or changes in sinus density. Extension from the sphenoid sinus with a homogeneous opacity, especially when it contrasts with adjacent cavernous tissues, is helpful (Fig. 23).

CAROTID ASSESSMENT

With very extensive tumors of the sinuses that have marked posterior and posterosuperior extension, the internal carotid artery may be in jeopardy. This is especially true of tumors beginning in the posterior ethmoids and sphenoid sinuses. Very extensive maxillary tumors spreading to these aforementioned areas are, however, the most common to spread in this fashion. By this mode of spread they are in the substance of the bone that makes the major contribution to the floor of the middle cranial fossa: the temporal bone.

The intracranial portion of the internal carotid artery begins at its entry into the undersurface of the anterior aspect of the temporal bone at the entrance to the carotid canal. It is encased at this point in a ring of fibrous

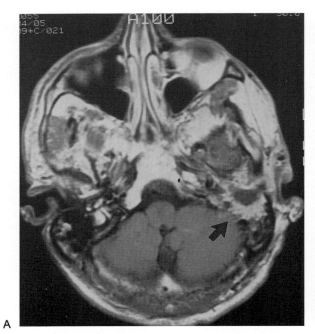
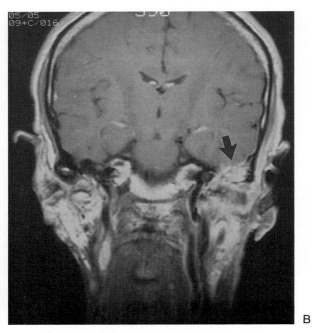

FIG. 21. MRI scan of young man with temporal bone carcinoma and central extension. **A:** Axial view shows evidence of extension into the cerebellum *(solid arrow)*. **B:** Coronal view demonstrates tumor extension into the temporal lobe *(solid arrow)*.

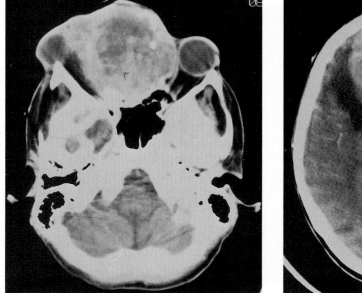
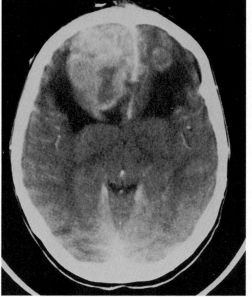

FIG. 22. Nineteen-year-old woman with a massive esthesioneuroblastoma with extensive brain invasion. **A:** Axial scan showing gross displacement of left eye by tumor. **B:** CAT scan shows a considerable rim of edema around the tumor pathognomonic of brain invasion.

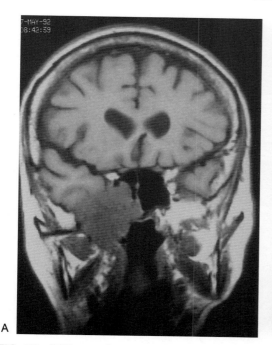
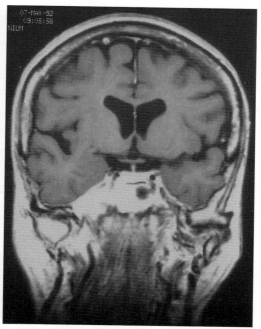

FIG. 23. CAT scan in coronal plane showing involvement of the left cavernous sinus extending from the left nasopharynx. **A:** T1 image. **B:** T1 image with gadolinium contrast.

tissue. The carotid ascends in a vertical direction in the temporal bone medial to the bony eustachian tube (Fig. 24). It is separated from the tube by a thin plate of bone and in some instances there are areas of dehiscence. Just under the floor of the middle fossa, the artery makes a right angle bend and courses horizontally in the axis of the temporal bone into the petrous apex. During the lateral portion of the artery's horizontal traverse of the temporal bone, the artery is intimately related to the medial bony and lateral aspect of the cartilaginous eustachian tube. An intimate understanding of this important relationship is vital to the safe dissection of this vessel during infratemporal fossa surgery. On its way to the foramen lacerum at the petrous tip, the artery is separated from the middle fossa contents by a 1- to 3-mm thin bony plate that, in some individuals, is partially dehiscent. As it travels under Meckel's cave, the vessel is overlain by the gasserian ganglion and the three branches of the trigeminal nerve (Fig. 25). The carotid ascends into the cavernous sinus through the upper one-half of the foramen lacerum. The artery is separated from the nasopharynx at this point by a cartilaginous plug (Fig. 24). Once in the cavernous sinus the artery takes an S-shaped bend, becoming closely related in the top of its course to the lateral aspect of the optic chiasm (Fig. 7). Just below this point, it gives off the ophthalmic artery, which travels into the optic foramen just below the optic nerve. The carotid then ascends to enter the cerebral circulation at the circle of Willis.

One of the prime dilemmas posed by surgery on tumors that encroach on the middle fossa floor or cavernous sinus is the management of the internal carotid artery. The burning question is whether or not the artery can safely be sacrificed. When the tumor is close, neither MRI nor CAT scan can determine if the carotid artery has been invaded. Tumor proximity is not synonymous with carotid invasion. If arterial involvement is extensive and the artery is already occluded, this may be demonstrable on MRI as absence of carotid flow void. Prior to any skull base surgery procedure when the internal carotid artery is in jeopardy, it is essential to establish preoperatively whether or not there is adequate collateral cerebral circulation. It is incumbent then to ascertain as clearly as possible if the contralateral cerebral circulation can maintain an adequate blood supply to the cerebrum of the operated side if the internal carotid is taken.

In the past, numerous studies such as ophthalmodynamometry, the Matas test, and arterial back pressure studies were done in an attempt to make this determination. Unfortunately, most of these lack adequate predictive value. More recently, balloon occlusion arteriography (39) has come to the fore as a more accurate method of determining adequacy of arterial crossfill. In the angiography suite, with the patient sedated, a small inflatable intra-arterial balloon on a long arteriography catheter is run up into the internal carotid artery on the test side. The balloon is inflated for 15 to 20 min and the patient carefully monitored for any change in neurological status. If any change such as dysarthria, muscle weakness, or alteration in cognitive

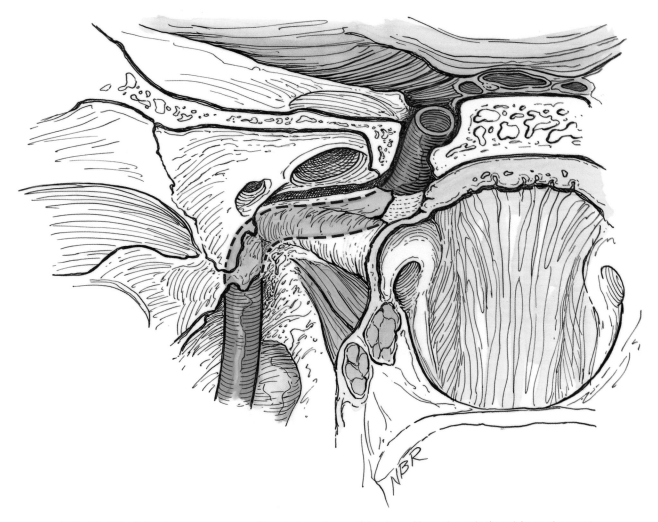

FIG. 24. The intrapetrous course of the internal carotid artery. Note the relationship to the eustachian tube. Also note the cartilaginous plug in the inferior aspect of the foramen lacerum. (From ref. 51, with permission.)

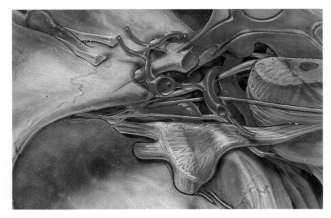

FIG. 25. Gasserian ganglion overlying the terminal portion of the petrous portion of the internal carotid artery.

functioning occurs then the test is considered to be a failure. The patient is thereby established to be at risk for stroke in the event of subsequent carotid sacrifice. If no neurological changes ensue, then the patient is adjudged to be at low risk for stroke. To further refine this test, some individuals have deliberately induced hypotension to determine whether the patient might fall into that small percentage of balloon occlusion successes who fail carotid sacrifice. Others have attempted to enhance the validity of the test by incorporating an ongoing electroencephalogram (EEG) that will monitor brain wave functioning during the occlusive episode.

The most helpful refinement of the balloon occlusion test was the introduction of radioactive xenon cerebral blood flow studies. It is unfortunately a highly technique-intensive study and requires substantial training

TABLE 1. *Xenon cerebral blood flow rates versus risk of stroke*

Blood flow rate (cc/100 gm/min)	Stroke risk
>40	Low
30–40	Moderate
<30	High

of ancillary personnel for its successful performance. A carefully measured amount of radioactive xenon gas of a precisely determined concentration is inhaled by the patient. A CAT scan of the head is done while the intra-arterial balloon is inflated. Either derivations of information recorded on the scan or, using a scintillation counter, a precise calculation of blood flow to the arterially occluded hemisphere from the contralateral side can be made. With certain refinements in software, maps of the hemisphere can be created, showing areas of high and low flow. Table 1 shows the relative risk of stroke compared to blood flow rates as determined by xenon gas inhalation reported by Sekhar and Janecka (40). If flow is greater than 40 ml of blood per 100 g of brain tissue per minute, then the risk of stroke is extremely low.

The newest form of blood flow determination technology to enter the arena is the single photon emission computed tomography (SPECT) scan. This is a much less invasive study, which hopefully will supplant the highly technical xenon flow study. A cerebral map is made after the infusion of radiolabeled D-glucose and the artery balloon occluded. Areas of poor perfusion will show up as regions of poor isotope uptake.

SURGICAL TECHNIQUE

Preparation

Prior to the extensive workup so far described, the patient's general health, cardiovascular fitness, and status of any intercurrent disease must be clearly established. The absence of distant metastases must be ruled out, usually by chest radiograph but occasionally supplemented by CAT scanning if adequate suspicion of a malignancy arises. Bone, liver, and spleen scans are done only if biochemical abnormalities appear in the blood but especially if signs or symptoms of dysfunction of these organs appear. Control of diabetes, heart disease, and chronic obstructive ·pulmonary disease (COPD) are commonly done "fine-tuning" procedures necessary in this patient population.

Preoperative visitations by the nurse clinician, psychiatric social worker, dietitian, and dentist are done, as well as consultations with other members of the skull base surgical team. The nurse clinician counsels

the patient and holds meetings with the family, setting a solid framework of understanding of the rigors and functional consequences of the impending surgery. Although the surgeon is responsible for providing as much information to the patient as possible and obtaining an informed consent, the nurse converses with the patients, often on a more simplistic basis, so that they more easily comprehend the innumerable details that may not have been made clear to them and their family. The nurse clinician helps in the education of the intensive care unit (ICU) personnel and floor nurses in the care of these complex patients and is the essential person in discharge planning and aftercare. Training of the family in wound care, tracheostomy care (if necessary), and nasogastric feeding is particularly helpful.

Many patients after radical sinus surgery require maxillofacial prosthetic rehabilitation. The preoperative assessment by the prosthodontist establishes the premorbid physiognomy of the patient and the dental status. Dental impressions can be taken and a facial moulage if indicated. An intraoperative splint is of great value in the functional rehabilitation of the patient. Being able to take oral sustenance and having clearly understandable speech give the patient a significant psychological boost in the early postoperative period (41).

The informed consent process is difficult. It is very hard to try to transmit to the patient an appreciation of the functional and aesthetic compromise that may be experienced. Most patients appear to readily accept the disability described to them if they know they have a reasonable chance at life. Most therapeutic options have been exhausted, and they are in the court of last resort trying to make a life or death decision concerning their surgery. A substantial time period must be set aside to educate the patients and family, giving them adequate time to ask all their questions so that they will feel fully aware of the surgery about to be done. Care must be taken not to make the procedure and the prognosis sound too rosy; but on the other hand, one must not be overly pessimistic or excessively graphic in detail during this dialogue. Drawing the line between adequate informed consent and minimizing fears and apprehension are difficult tasks.

Anterior Resection

The earliest craniofacial or skull base procedures done were anterior resections (42–44). These were performed usually for ethmoidal or maxillary tumors with ethmoidal extension. Anterior resection should be done for any nasal, orbital, or ethmoid malignancy that abuts against or penetrates through the anterior fossa floor.

Formerly, an oral endotracheal anesthetic was

given. Because of problems with pulmonary toilet, with occasionally even some time on a mechanical respirator, a tracheostomy is done. Tracheostomy also prevents the early development of tension pneumocephalus. If any threat to the internal carotid artery is anticipated, then EEG leads are sewn into the scalp preoperatively so that cerebral electrical activity can be monitored. Usually the carotid is at risk only if additional excursions into the middle fossa are needed. An arterial line, and occasionally cerebrovascular profile (CVP) lines, are established. If there is a cardiac problem, a Swan–Ganz catheter is placed.

Temporary tarsorrhaphy stitches are placed to close the eyelids; the face, scalp, and neck are surgically scrubbed. Corneal shields are avoided because of the prolonged nature of the case with the potential for damage to the eye. The scalp may be shaved according to the surgeon's bias. Graft donor sites are prepped if grafts such as fat, bone, fascia, or free tissue transfer are anticipated.

There are a host of different approaches to lesions at the anterior site. It is beyond the purpose of this chapter to describe them all in detail. What is described are my favored approaches. For lesions confined to the anterior ethmoid, and possibly the upper portion of the maxilla and nasal cavity, the preferred approach is through a lateral rhinotomy that is extended into the upper brow (Fig. 26).

During the incision, care is taken to ensure hemosta-

sis of the nasolabial and angular vessels. The periosteum is cut throughout the course of the incision. The sill is cut through in order to enhance exposure. A curved osteotome is placed along the frontal process of the maxilla low down near the maxillary face in a similar manner to a low osteotomy done for rhinoplasty (Fig. 27). The osteotome is driven medially toward the nasal dorsum near the articulation of the nasal process of the frontal bone and the nasal bones. The nasal skeleton of the operated side is outfractured in greenstick fashion at the midline dorsum (Fig. 27). At this point, the orbital periosteum is elevated from the lamina papyracea and a determination is made as to whether the eye should be sacrificed or not. Although controversy exists concerning how much periorbital bone or orbital tissue involvement mandates orbital exenteration (45,46), I sacrifice the eye in most cases in which a malignancy invades the periorbita. The justification for this is that I have had no periorbital recurrences to this point following resections in which this rule was followed but have had to revise many cases in which this principle was violated by others. In limited lesions, the eye can be preserved. The ethmoid is resected sufficiently to visualize tumor and its degree of encroachment on the floor of the anterior fossa. An extended Denker procedure is done to assess the degree of maxillary involvement (Fig. 28).

During the ethmoidectomy and the Denker procedure, it is necessary to excise some of the tumor in a

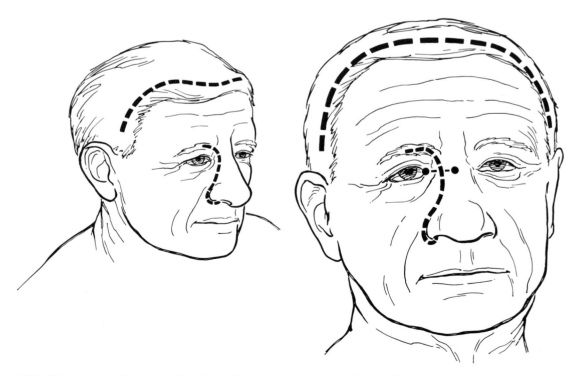

FIG. 26. Lateral rhinotomy incision. Note coronal scalp flap incision for anterior craniotomy approach.

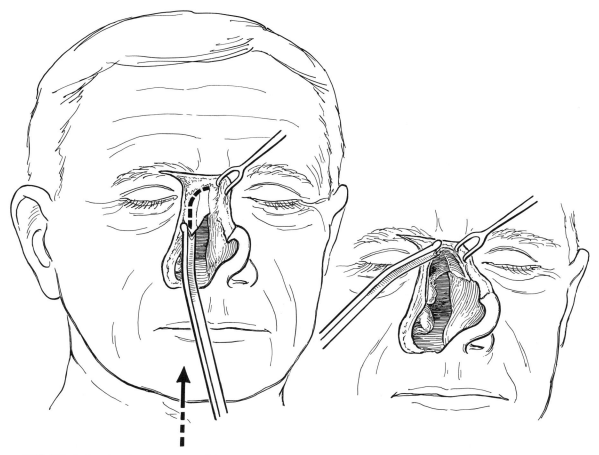

FIG. 27. Lateral osteotomy cut with a rhinoplasty-type osteotome. Lateral nasal skeleton is green-stick-fractured out laterally.

piecemeal fashion. This violates a basic principle of cancer excision, namely, that of en bloc resection. There is much controversy over the safety of piecemeal resection. However, I have used this technique for 20 years with a level of local recurrence and incidence of distant metastasis that is comparable to published results of leading authorities. The drawback to the slavish commitment to en bloc resection is the frequent unnecessary sacrifice of noninvolved tissues beyond what would be a safe resection margin. Once the initial incisions are made, there is a serious problem of inadequate visualization of the margins of resection by the presence of tumor in the line of sight. Partial piecemeal resection then permits a clear appreciation of tumor extent, the margins can be established, and the bulk of the tumor removed en bloc. Strict reliance on MRI and CAT evidence of degree of tumor extent is frequently disappointing as under- and overestimation of tumor size are not uncommon.

Once fovea and cribriform involvement is established, a craniotomy is done to expose the intracranial extent of tumor and protect the dura and brain. Usually a bicoronal incision is done in the scalp (Fig. 26), not

so much for exposure for the craniotomy, but in order to raise the pericranial flap for later reconstruction. The bicoronal flap is elevated without cutting the calvarial periosteum (pericranium). The scalp flap is elevated to just over the brows, taking care when possible to preserve the supraorbital and supratrochlear neurovascular bundles. The pericranium is elevated as a separate layer, taking great care not to put any holes in it (Fig. 29).

Intracranial exposure is done through a low craniotomy that includes the frontal sinus in the bone flap. There are two basic approaches used, based on eliminating the hazard posed by the frontal sinus. One is to remove a bone flap containing the frontal sinus, either leaving the brow and orbital roofs behind or removing these structures with the flap (Fig. 30). The second approach is to create an osteoplastic flap of the frontal sinus that will later be cranialized to eliminate any chance of remucosalization and infection (Fig. 31). The posterior wall of the sinus is removed to provide the anterior fossa exposure. This can be used if the frontal sinus is capacious enough.

The tumor is now visualized from below and all mar-

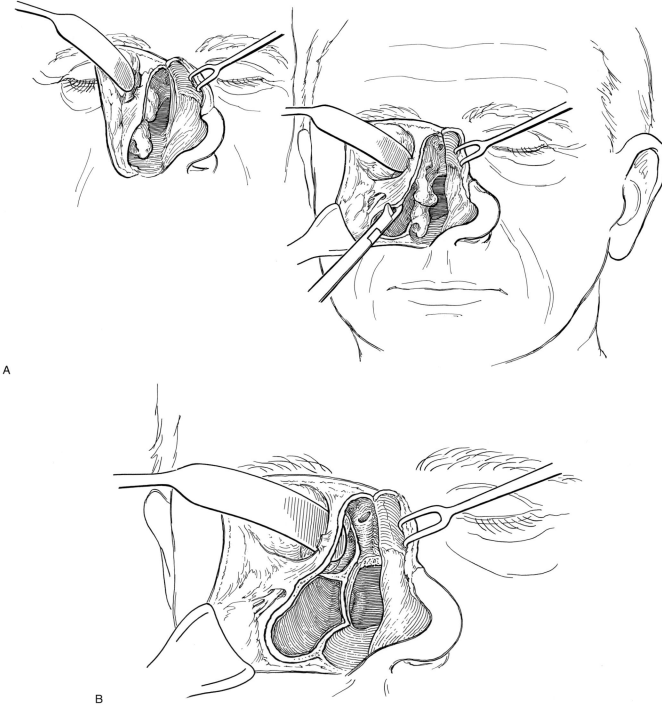

A

B

FIG. 28. A: Denker procedure done by excision of junction between the anterior and medial walls of the maxillary sinus. **B:** Denker procedure finished along with medial maxillectomy and complete ethmoidectomy. **C:** Denker procedure, ethmoidectomy, and sphenoidotomy completed. Residual tumor in lateral wall of sphenoid is still apparent.

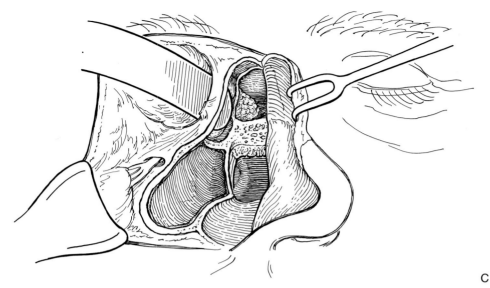

C

FIG. 28. *Continued.*

gins of the anterior fossa floor involved with tumor are outlined (Fig. 32). The dura is elevated from the projected area of resection and the cerebral contents are protected with a Teflon-coated retractor and telfa strips (Fig. 33). Dural elevation over the cribriform plate will by necessity cause amputation across the fila olfactoria; this produces a number of small CSF leaks. These will require repair, usually accomplished by merely placing a number of individual dural sutures at the closure phase of the procedure. Further elevation will reveal areas of tumor involvement. If dura is in-

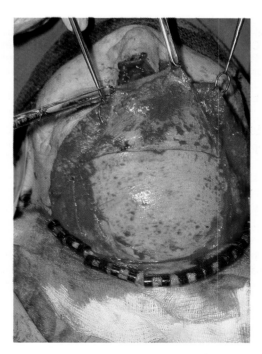

FIG. 29. Pericranial flap.

volved, it should be resected with a 3- to 5-mm margin unless the tumor appears to have a more infiltrating character on gross examination. Frozen sections are taken to ensure adequate resection. If cerebral tissue is involved, a wide margin is necessary but how wide is not yet clear. In my own experience, narrow resections of brain result in local recurrence. Fortunately, the frontal lobes are mainly "silent" areas, and resection usually has only minor sequellae. A margin of about 1 cm is preferred.

Excision of the tumor is made with the appropriate bony margin from below with a small osteotome. The dura and brain are protected with a Teflon-coated retractor from above by the neurosurgeon. The bloc is delivered through the face with the suction tip (Fig. 34).

Most tumors require more extensive resections and the lateral rhinotomy approach is not adequate for exposure. A modified Weber–Fergusson incision is used to enable a radical maxillectomy (Fig. 35). If orbital exenteration is required, a determination as to whether the lids should be preserved or not should be made. If there is tumor invasion of the lids, then a wide field resection is required (Fig. 36). Some advocate a lid excision in any orbital exenteration because of the difficulty in prosthetic rehabilitation of the exenteration cavity. It is much simpler then to place an onlay prosthesis. Without some bony or soft tissue support for the cavity, there is no support for the residual lids if they are preserved. In addition, the mucosa of the eye socket tends to exude mucus. Oral exenteration with lid resection is much simpler because the incision goes directly through skin, the orbital portion of the orbicularis oculi, and the orbital periosteum. The dissection to the orbital apex is fast. With lid preservation, a

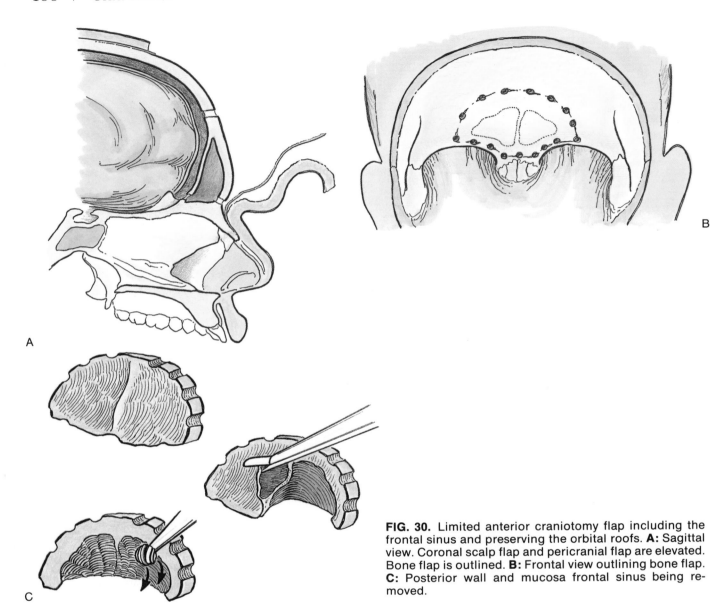

FIG. 30. Limited anterior craniotomy flap including the frontal sinus and preserving the orbital roofs. **A:** Sagittal view. Coronal scalp flap and pericranial flap are elevated. Bone flap is outlined. **B:** Frontal view outlining bone flap. **C:** Posterior wall and mucosa frontal sinus being removed.

transconjunctival incision takes the surgeon through the septum orbitale and the orbital fat. This makes the dissection tedious and messy as dissection to the periorbita is finally reached. Complete subperiosteal dissection around the superior pole of the globe to the orbital apex is done. If tumor penetration through the orbital roof is seen, it is noted and skirted if possible. However, if access to the orbital apex is prohibited by tumor, piecemeal resection is done until visualization and control of the ophthalmic artery and nerve can be accomplished. A short right-angled clamp is used to secure the neurovascular bundle, and it is clamped, cut, and tied with a nonabsorbable suture.

Delineation of tumor is carried posteriorly from below to establish the posterior margin. As the planum sphenoidale is reached and the posterior limits of the anterior fossa floor are approached, the optic chiasm is jeopardized. Careful dissection and exposure from above by the neurosurgeon simultaneously with inferior establishment of tumor limits are required in order to maximally protect the chiasm.

Any frontal sinus involvement is managed by excision. If the anterior wall is involved with tumor, then it is excised full thickness and removed with a dental burr, preserving the outer cortex at those sites for areas of lesser involvement. Bone excision must be extensive enough to result in complete and safe resection of tumor. Invasion posteriorly into the body of the sphenoid bone will be handled similarly with excision using the cutting burr.

Once all tumor has been removed and this has been confirmed with frozen sections, the wound is thor-

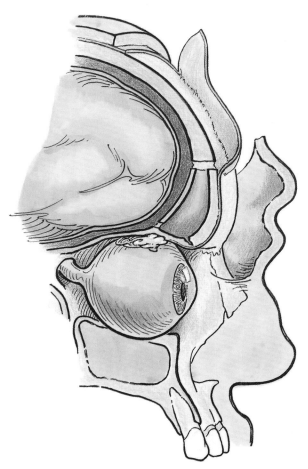

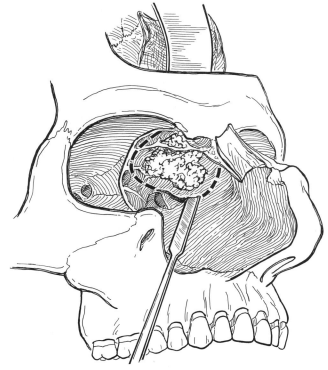

FIG. 32. Tumor invading anterior cranial fossa floor is outlined from below. (From ref. 51, with permission.)

FIG. 31. Osteoplastic flap is used in a capacious frontal sinus giving limited but adequate anterior cranial fossa extension.

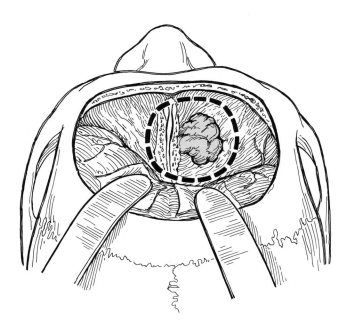

FIG. 33. Brain is protected through anterior craniotomy. Teflon-coated retractor retracts brain and margins of bone and/or dura are outlined. (From ref. 51, with permission.)

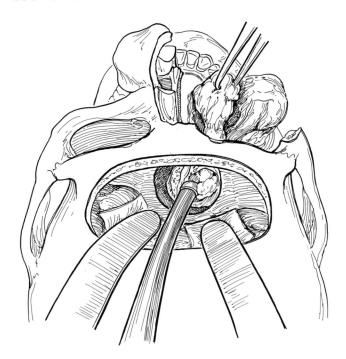

FIG. 34. Tumor bloc delivered from above through the facial wound. (From ref. 51, with permission.)

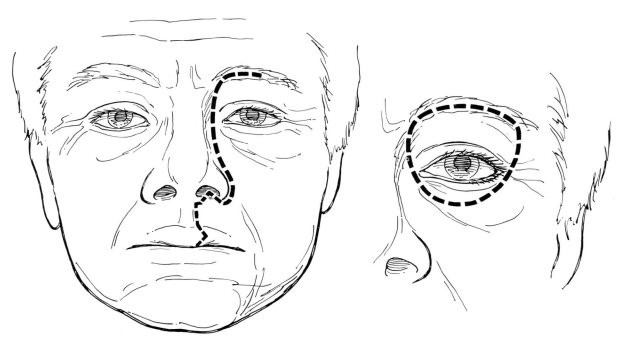

FIG. 35. Modified Weber–Fergusson incision. Note dart in sill of nose and around sucking tubercle of upper lip to prevent scar contracture. Incision courses down a philtral ridge in attempt to camouflage scar.

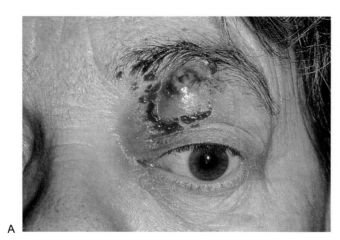

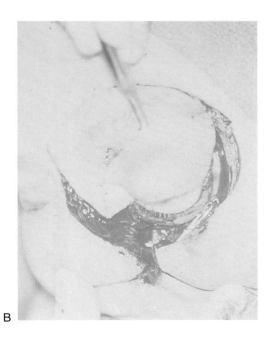

FIG. 36. A: Large squamous cell carcinoma of the frontal and ethmoid sinuses invading eye and upper eyelid. **B:** Surgical resection of lid margins outlined.

oughly irrigated with sterile water. The closure is now begun. The first exigency is to establish a watertight closure of the dura. Fascia lata, temporalis fascia, or lyophilized dura is used and sutured in place and fixed with tissue glue if available. An especially difficult area of closure is posteriorly near the optic chiasm. Tissue glue is especially helpful at this site as suturing varies from tenuous to impossible.

One of the greatest advances in maintaining support of the intracranial contents is the advent of the pericranial flap. This highly vascularized tissue provides not only a tough viable support for the dural graft and overlying brain but a bed that will nourish a split thickness skin graft. The flap is either tucked over the superior aspect of the osteoplastic flap and run along the anterior fossa floor (Fig. 37) or, if a frontal bone flap is to be replaced, tucked between the flap and the bone of the brow (Fig. 38). The cavity and cheek flap are covered with split thickness skin and the wounds closed.

Case 1

Patient M, an 80-year-old healthy woman, was admitted with a 2-month history of progressive nasal obstruction and epistaxis. Over the preceding 3 weeks,

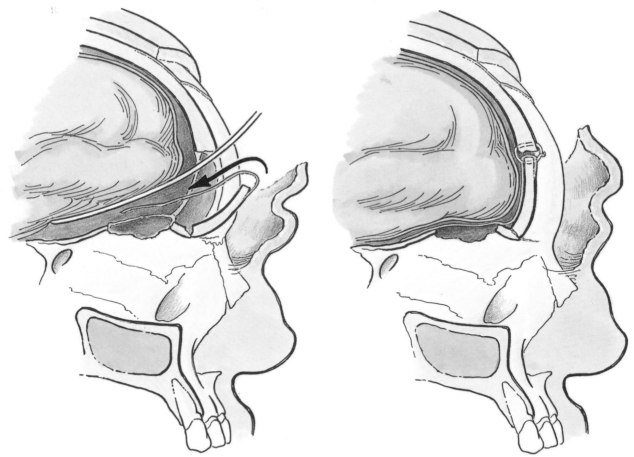

A   B

FIG. 37. A: Pericranial flap tucked over the superior rim of the osteoplastic flap. **B:** Bone flap anchored in place with stainless steel wire.

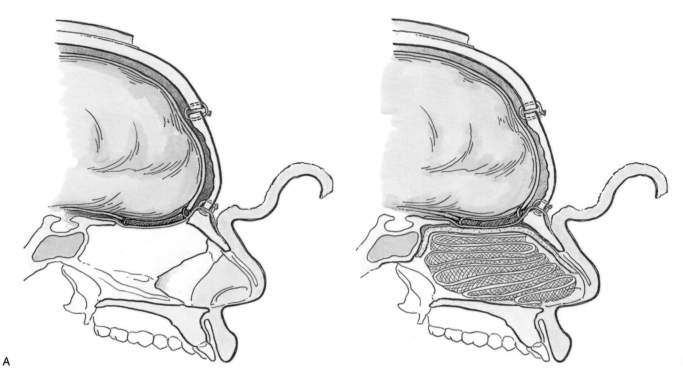

A   B

FIG. 38. A: Pericranial flap tucked under the inferior edge of low frontal craniotomy flap. **B:** Cavity lined with split thickness skin graft and packed with iodoform gauze.

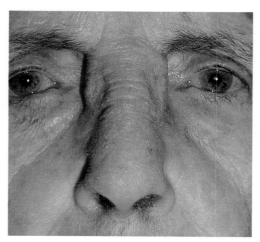

FIG. 39. Case 1. Eighty-year-old woman with a carcinoma of the nasal cavity invading the nasal bones.

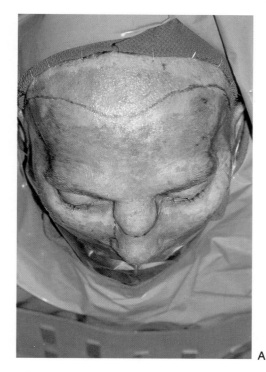

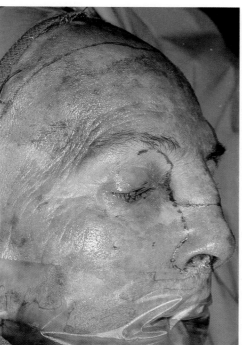

FIG. 40. Case 1: incisions. **A:** Bicoronal scalp flap with modified nasal flap. **B:** Modified nasal flap incision and lateral rhinotomy.

she noticed a gradual swelling and widening of her nasal dorsum (Fig. 39). Physical examination revealed an alert, healthy, very active, elderly woman with an intranasal mass and swelling of the nasal dorsum with dissolution of the nasal bones. Biopsy showed a mixed cellular picture comprised of both esthesioneuroblastoma and squamous cell carcinoma. CAT scan and MRI showed tumor in the anterior ethmoid sinuses, through the floor of the frontal sinus, and in the nasal cavities, eroding the nasal bones and septum.

A bicoronal scalp flap was combined with a separate bilateral brow incision that extended down one side of the nose in a lateral rhinotomy (Fig. 40). A skin flap over the nasal dorsum was dissected over the tumor mass, which was then circumscribed by a wide margin of nasal septum. The lamina papyracea of both ethmoids was intact, and ethmoidectomies were done bilaterally. Tumor was seen to be entering the frontal sinus in the midline and was adherent to the cribriform plate.

An anterior craniotomy was done through a frontal sinus osteoplastic flap with removal of the posterior wall as well as the frontal sinus floor to which tumor was attached (Fig. 41). A large pericranial flap was elevated. En bloc removal was then performed after amputation of some anteriorly located fila olfactoria was done in order to obtain a margin on the cribriform plate. These CSF leaks were sealed with dural sutures.

Closure was obtained by turning the pericranial flap

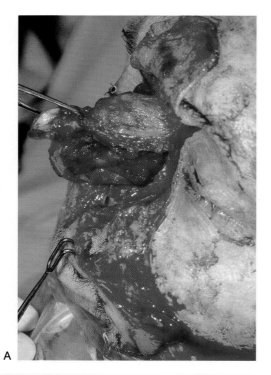

A

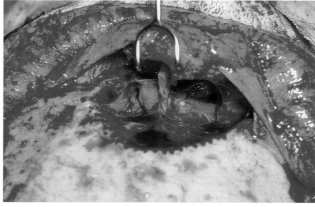

B

FIG. 41. Case 1: resection. **A:** Tumor including septal and nasal bones. **B:** Osteoplastic flap exposing superior tumor extent. **C:** Tumor bloc ready for excision.

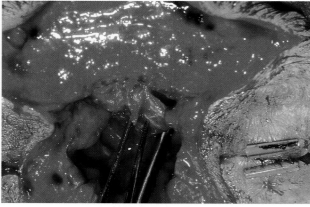

C

over the top of the osteoplastic flap and laying it across the anterior fossa floor to cover the defect left by the cribriform resection. The flap of skin over the nasal dorsum was used to cover the nasal side of the craniotomy defect and the wound closed.

The patient was discharged on the ninth postoperative day and received a full course of radiation therapy. Patient is alive and well without disease 4 years postoperatively. She is presently wearing a prosthesis and awaiting reconstruction (Fig. 42).

Case 2

Patient EW, a 53-year-old man, presented with a history of nasal obstruction. Physical examination revealed a mass in the right nasal cavity. CAT scan demonstrated a mass in the right ethmoid sinus invading

the right orbit and maxilla (Fig. 43). Biopsy of the nasal mass showed adenoid cystic carcinoma.

A modified Weber–Fergusson incision and coronal scalp flap were done for exposure. A maxillectomy, ethmoidectomy, and orbital exenteration were necessary to encompass the subcranial portion of the tumor. As dissection proceeded posteriorly, the tumor was revealed to have traveled along the optic nerve almost to the chiasm. Tumor excision from below went posteriorly through the planum sphenoidale.

The craniotomy needed to be low enough to allow a view as far as the sphenoid ridge (Fig. 44). Tumor was removed with the optic nerve just at the chiasm. Tumor was also dissected away from the internal carotid artery. A large defect in the anterior fossa floor resulted (Fig. 45). This was closed with lyophilized dura and a pericranial flap. The cavity was skin grafted.

Postoperatively, the patient received a full course of

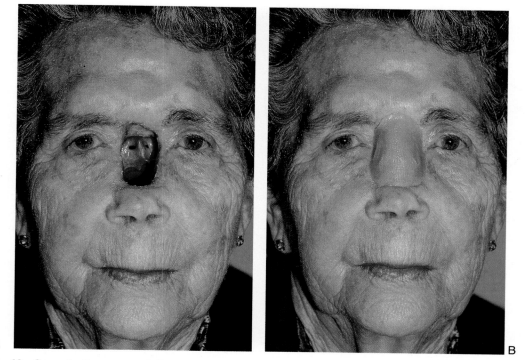

FIG. 42. Case 1: three-year follow-up. **A:** Frontal view of patient without prosthesis. **B:** With prosthesis.

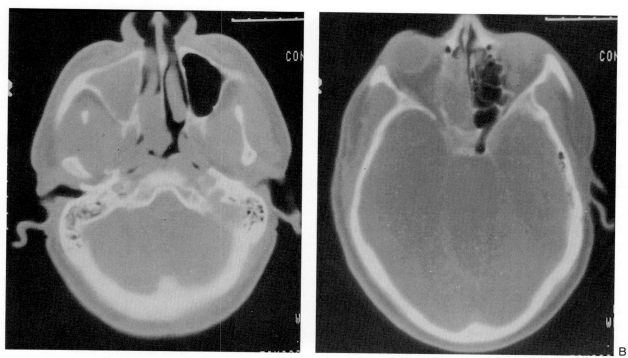

FIG. 43. Case 2. **A:** CAT scan in axial plane shows tumor of the ethmoids invading the maxillary sinus. **B:** CAT scan in axial plane shows tumor of the ethmoids invading the orbit, sphenoid sinus, and cavernous sinus.

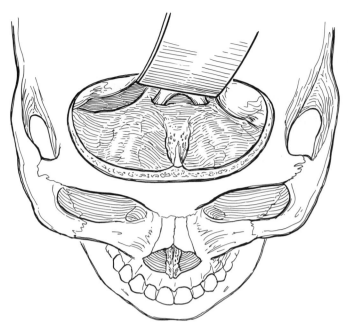

FIG. 44. Case 2. Anterior fossa floor dissection is carried back to the lesser sphenoid ridge exposing optic chiasm. (From ref. 51, with permission.)

radiation therapy. He is now alive and well without disease 9 years postoperatively.

Case 3

Patient VC is a 64-year-old woman who 3 years prior to presentation had an orbital exenteration, partial maxillectomy, and partial rhinectomy for an aggressive basal cell carcinoma of the facial skin. A large local flap was used for reconstruction, which precluded a clear view of her resection site. Thus a local recurrence of tumor was effaced until it attained a substantial size (Fig. 46). Extensive disease was obscured by the facial flap with erosion throughout the internal aspect of the nose and cheek flap.

A frontal craniotomy and facial excision were outlined (Fig. 47). A much wider resection of facial skin was required once the extent of tumor was determined when the facial flap was developed. Widespread invasion of frontal lobe dural and frontal bone required excision of much of the anterior cranial fossa dura and wide frontal craniectomy (Fig. 48). Split calvarium, lyophilized dura, and a wide pericranial flap pedicled on the uninvolved side were needed (Fig. 49) to close the defect.

Patient is alive and well 1.5 years status postresection and in the process of prosthetic reconstruction (Fig. 50).

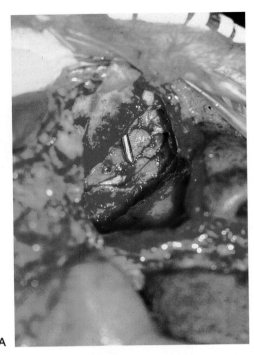

A

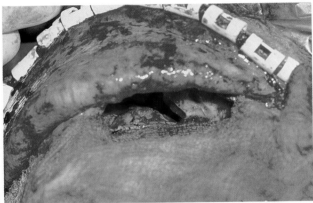

B

FIG. 45. Case 2. **A:** Large defect in the anterior cranial fossa floor as seen from below through maxillectomy and orbital exenteration site. **B:** View from above through frontal craniotomy.

Sphenoid Sinus Resection

The sphenoid sinus has for a long time been considered to be a site that, when invaded by malignancy, was unresectable. This was due, in part, to the fact that most of its walls are exceedingly thin and vitally important anatomical structures are in their near proximity. Carcinomas primary to the sphenoid sinus are rare. However, invasion from an adjacent sinus or the nasal cavity is not uncommon. If the tumor is represented by just its protuberance into the sinus cavity proper, this does not constitute a real problem. Difficulty in resection results when there are erosion of sinus walls and extension of tumor into adjacent tissue.

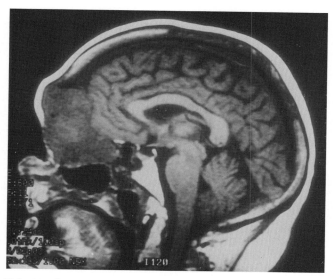

FIG. 46. Case 3. MRI scan in sagittal plane showing massive intracranial extension of locally recurrent aggressive basal cell carcinoma.

An anterior transfacial approach is the most efficacious as long as there is not direct tumor involvement along the petrous carotid for any appreciable distance, erosion into the middle cranial fossa, or too much infratemporal fossa extension. A factor that greatly enhances the ability to resect sphenoid sinus tumors is the ability to cut away all diseased bone with a cutting

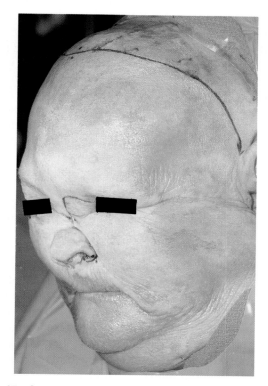

FIG. 47. Case 3. Patient with frontal craniotomy and facial excision outlined.

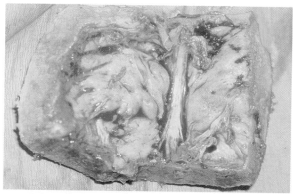

FIG. 48. Case 3. Wide-field craniectomy and dural excision were required by extensive tumor invasion. Brain was uninvolved.

bur, avoiding an en bloc resection that would seriously endanger optic nerves, internal carotid arteries, and brain.

Perhaps the best way to illustrate the resection is to show how I serendipitously came to realize that such resections were possible when an occasion arose in which this became the only viable option.

Case 4

Patient JJ, a 38-year-old woman, presented with the rapid onset of facial swelling and pain, proptosis, and a mass under the skin of the nasal dorsum. The only significant feature in her past history is that she had been treated as an adolescent with low-dose irradiation to the face for acne. Physical examination revealed a mass in the nasal cavity, mild proptosis, a small mass under the skin of the nasal dorsum, and a slight swelling of the cheek. A CAT scan revealed a mass in the maxil-

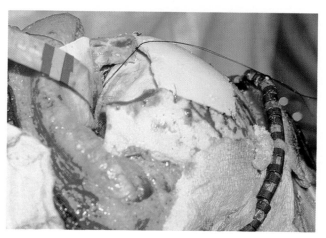

FIG. 49. Case 3. Split calvarium was used to replace the resected calvarium. Lyophilized dura was used to repair the excised dura.

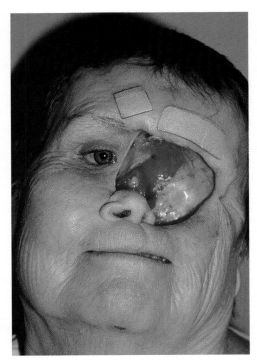

FIG. 50. Case 3. Patient at 1 year following resection with a healed cavity and no evidence of disease.

lary sinus extending to the ethmoid sinus and orbit on that side. The sphenoid sinus was opacified, but densiometric readings interpreted this finding as fluid rather than tumor.

A modified Weber–Fergusson incision was done to include excision of an area that encompassed the nasal skin involvement (Fig. 51). A radical maxillectomy, orbital exenteration, and ethmoidectomy were done. As dissection proceeded posteriorly, it became obvious

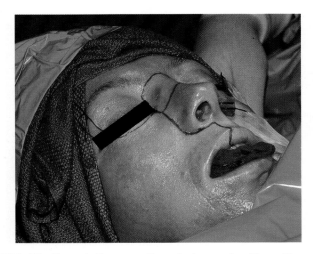

FIG. 51. Case 4. Preoperative photograph with outline of Weber–Fergusson incision and skin excision for tumor invading dorsum of nose.

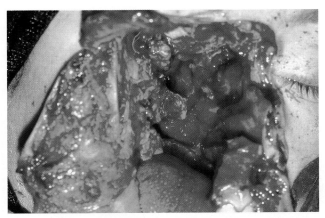

FIG. 52. Case 4. Cavity after maxilloethmosphenoidectomy with resection of medial cavernous sinus wall.

that tumor, not fluid, was present in the sphenoid sinus. Tumor was excised from the sinus cavity, and the walls were excised with a dental cutting burr. The area of the body of the sphenoid from which the pterygoid plates subtend was completely removed. The lateral wall of the affected sinus was removed, exposing the dura of the cavernous sinus. The posterior wall was cut back to the marrow of the sphenoid body and the sinus floor was completely removed (Fig. 52). There was no encroachment on the roof, so the planum sphenoidale and pituitary fossa were left undisturbed.

Because of frozen section positive margins on the nasal skin, a subtotal rhinectomy was necessary. Split thickness skin grafts were placed in the cavity. The wound was closed. An obturator was placed and fixed to the remaining teeth. Postoperatively, there was a wound dehiscence at the medial end of the periorbital incisions (Fig. 53A). The patient underwent a full course of postoperative irradiation. Electing not to undergo reconstruction, she wears a maxillofacial prosthesis. She is alive and well nine years postoperatively (Fig. 53B).

It became apparent with this case that sphenoid tumors can be excised with safe margins, in that all bony walls can be adequately excised with the cutting burr. The only limitation of soft tissue resection outside these confines is superiorly beyond the pituitary gland. Careful preoperative scrutiny of the CAT scan in the lateral projection is essential to assess bony thickness of the posterior wall of the sphenoid sinus to protect against transgression of the clival cortex on the brain stem side. The burr can be used to excise bone down to and including parts of the cervicobasilar junction, taking care laterally to avoid the vertebral arteries.

Table 2 lists the patients and their tumor types that have had sphenoid sinus excision because of tumor originating there or having spread from the ethmoids. It also includes three cases of inverting papilloma that

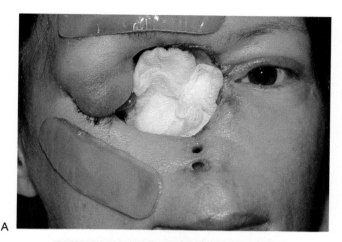

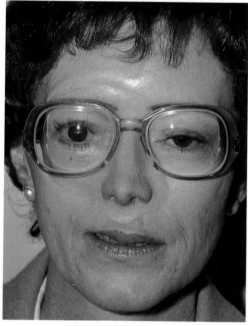

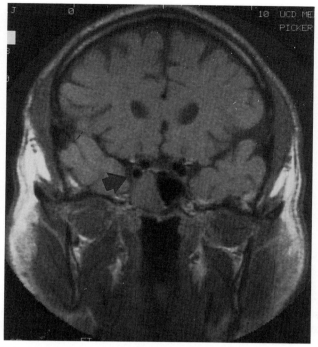

FIG. 54. MRI scan showing inverting papilloma of sphenoid sinus adjacent to cavernous sinus and internal carotid artery *(solid arrow).*

FIG. 53. Case 4. **A:** Immediately postoperatively. **B:** Nine years postoperatively patient is alive and well without disease and wearing a prosthesis.

TABLE 2. *Survival of patients with malignancy and inverting papilloma of the sphenoid sinus following complete excision*

1. Inverting papilloma, 3 cases no recurrence at 3–7 years
2. Small cell carcinoma, 2 cases no recurrence at 4 years
3. Mucoepidermoid carcinoma, 1 case recurrence anteriorly at 18 months, alive with disease at 3.5 years
4. Squamous cell carcinoma, 5 cases
   (1) No recurrence at 7 years
   (1) No recurrence at 1 year
   (1) Postop death of stroke
   (1) DOD at 6 months
   (1) DOD at 7 months
5. Adenoid cystic, 1 case no recurrence at 5 years

(From ref. 53, with permission.)

took origin in the sphenoid sinus. These tumors are not frank malignancies but are very aggressive locally and have heretofore not been considered amenable to excision when adherent to the walls of the sphenoid sinus. The patient whose MRI scan is illustrated in Fig. 54 had inverting papilloma of the sphenoid sinus with erosion of the lateral sinus wall and invasion of the cavernous sinus. Complete resection was attained by the lateral rhinotomy approach coupled with a Denker procedure on the maxilla. The patient is now 5 years status postresection with no recurrence (Fig. 55). None of the patients with inverting papilloma have had a recurrence, with follow-up from 3 to 6 years. The squamous cell carcinomas have had the poorest prognosis, with two of five cases surviving better than 2 years and one case at only 6 months follow-up.

Infratemporal Fossa Approach

In very extensive sinus neoplasms that have breached the posterolateral wall of the maxillary sinus and have invaded the pterygomaxillary space, infratemporal fossa, and nasopharynx, the infratemporal fossa approach is the most efficacious means to attain complete excision. This is actually a combined middle cranial fossa/infratemporal fossa approach. If no transgression of the skull base has occurred, then the craniotomy portion of the procedure can be eliminated.

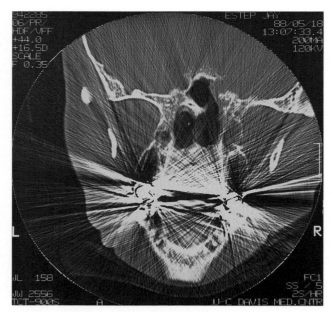

FIG. 55. CAT scan showing absence of tumor in sphenoid sinus 1 year postoperatively. Patient is now 5 years free of disease.

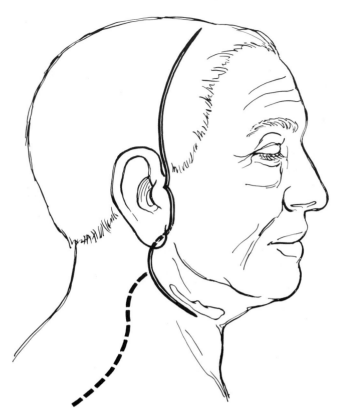

FIG. 56. Incision for infratemporal fossa approach. For sinus tumors the preauricular incision is preferred. The *dotted line* represents an extension if a radical neck dissection is required.

Occasionally, it is very difficult to detect on the preoperative radiographs whether there is extension into the fossa that cannot be resected from the anterior approach or if there is invasion of either the foramen rotundum or foramen ovale by tumor. During the performance of the maxillectomy, whenever the posterior or posterolateral walls of the sinus have been penetrated by neoplasm, I always drill out the foramen rotundum and the vidian canal, then sample the nerve stumps flush with the dura at these sites to look for tumor invasion on frozen section. If the section is positive, then a middle fossa approach will be necessary. When the infratemporal fossa is invaded, then a similar procedure is done for V3. If this is positive, then a middle fossa approach is definitely indicated.

The procedure is done with the patient supine and the head turned laterally on a Mayfield horseshoe head rest. An incision is made from the vertex of the scalp and continued in a preauricular crease, then carried into the neck similar to a modified Blair incision (Fig. 56). The flap is elevated in the subcutaneous plane lateral to the submucosal aponeurotic system (SMAS) fascia. The elevation extends from the angle of the mandible to the lateral orbital rim to the calvarial vertex. At a level halfway along the zygomatic arch, a small semicircular flap of temporalis fascia is elevated in order to protect the frontal branch of the facial nerve (Fig. 57).

An incision in the pericranium is made 2 cm wide of the temporalis muscle, and the muscle is elevated from the infratemporal fossa (Fig. 58). Careful protection of

the muscle is essential to preserve it from damage or infarction. The blood supply comes from two branches of the internal maxillary artery just posterior and just anterior to the foramen spinosum through which the middle meningeal artery traverses. The muscle is dissected into the deep aspects of the infratemporal fossa toward its insertion on the coronoid process (Fig. 59). At this point, the surgeon may encounter tumor. If so, the temporalis muscle or its blood supply may need to be sacrificed. When this muscle is resected with tumor, alternative methods of reconstruction, such as myocutaneous flaps or a free flap, may need to be invoked. Further dissection into the infratemporal fossa anteriorly brings the surgeon into the territory of the pterygoid venous plexus. Hemostasis is best handled with the bipolar cautery.

The next step in the procedure is the zygomatic ostectomy (Fig. 60). A subperiosteal dissection of the zygoma is done with a narrow periosteal elevator. The body of the zygoma is approached through a stab incision over the malar eminence into the same plane as the zygomatic branch of the facial nerve. The power saw is used to incise the arch just in front of the articular eminence. The next osteotomy is through the lateral

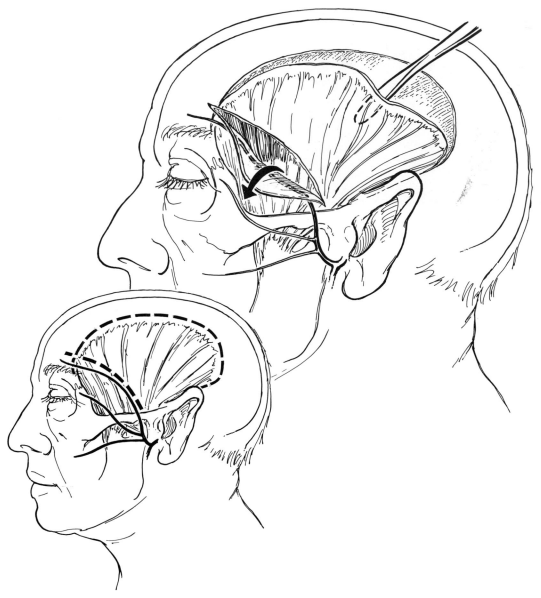

FIG. 57. Small flap of deep temporalis fascia is elevated to preserve the temporal branch of the facial nerve.

orbital rim and carried through the lateral orbital wall inferiorly to the inferior orbital fissure. The final osteotomy is made through the stab incision in the malar eminence. As little of the malar portion as possible is included in the ostectomy. The osteotomy saw is run up to the inferior orbital fissure. A final bit of periosteal stripping and soft tissue dissection is often necessary and finally the zygoma is delivered (Fig. 61). The bone is wrapped in a saline-soaked sponge until the end of the case.

To further enhance infratemporal fossa exposure, the mandibular condyle is removed. An incision in the temporomandibular joint capsule is followed by exci-

sion of the meniscus and osteotomy of the mandibular neck (Fig. 62). A malleable retractor is placed deep to the mandibular neck and condyle to preserve the internal maxillary artery. Once the condyle has been removed, further dissection will reveal the medial termination of the glenoid fossa, at the anteromedial end of which is located the foramen spinosum. Just anterior to the foramen spinosum is the foramen ovale, through which travels V3. If a middle fossa craniotomy is planned, this area will be its medial boundary. If all tumor can be excised at this point and there is no tumor in the foramen ovale, the procedure can be terminated.

If a middle fossa craniotomy is needed, soft tissues

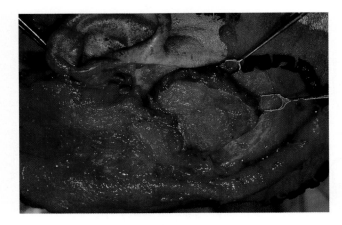

FIG. 58. Temporalis muscle is elevated from the infratemporal fossa with a 2-cm cuff of pericranium.

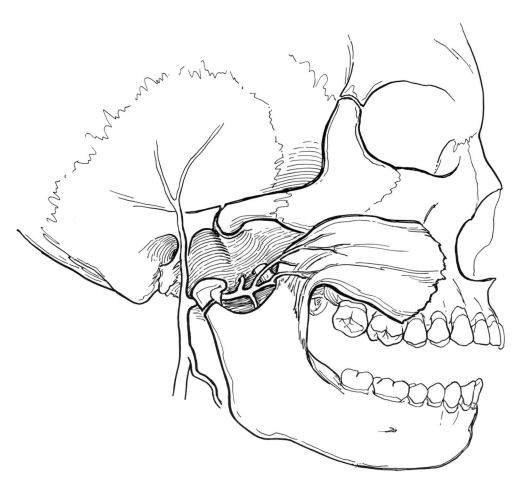

FIG. 59. The temporalis muscle is dissected inferiorly to its point of insertion on the coronoid process.

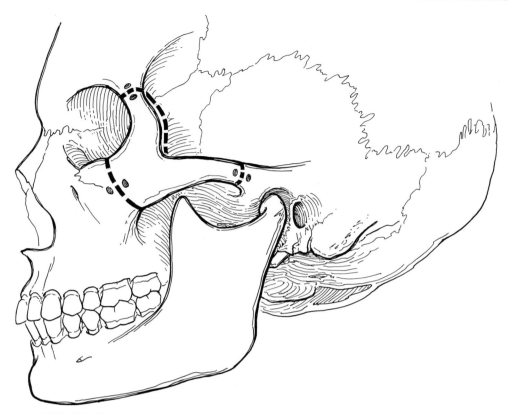

FIG. 60. Zygomatic ostectomy incisions. (From ref. 52, with permission.)

are completely dissected from the medial end of the glenoid fossa to the foramen spinosum, where the middle meningeal artery is controlled by ligature. Just anterior is the foramen ovale, and dissection proceeds thence to the base of the lateral pterygoid plate. The craniotomy is carried from these points (Fig. 63), which in fact are osteotomized last, superiorly through the lateral orbital wall arching over the greater wing of the sphenoid through the pterion, and curving down the squamous temporal bone into the external auditory

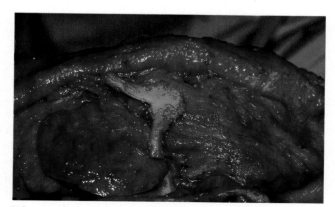

FIG. 61. Zygoma is removed and stored in a saline-soaked sponge.

canal at 12 o'clock. Obviously when the craniotomy is elected, the external auditory canal must be transected at the bony cartilaginous junction and the pinna and cartilaginous canal retracted posteriorly. Prior to canal transection, a flap of anterior canal wall skin is elevated pedicled laterally on the concha. The skin incision is made at 12 and 6 o'clock and down medially as close to the annulus as possible (Fig. 64). The tympanic annulus is elevated from its sulcus from the anterior edge of the notch of Rivinus to about 6 o'clock. The craniotomy goes through the external auditory canal at about 10 o'clock and enters the protympanum (Fig. 64). This is done with a small cutting bur. The inferior cut through the inferior aspect of the eustachian tube orifice is made with the drill carried through the annulus and out the external auditory canal at about 5 o'clock (Fig. 65). The anterior cut goes almost completely through the bone of the glenoid fossa and is carried medially and forward to the foramen spinosum.

The craniotomy is done with a cutting bur or a craniotome. The otologic portion of the incision and the inferior cuts through the foramen spinosum and ovale, then up to the base of the pterygoid plate, are made with the otologic drill and a small cutting bur. The dura is carefully elevated from the bone flap and the flap removed, then wrapped in a saline-soaked sponge (Fig. 66). It will be noted that the craniotomy flap actu-

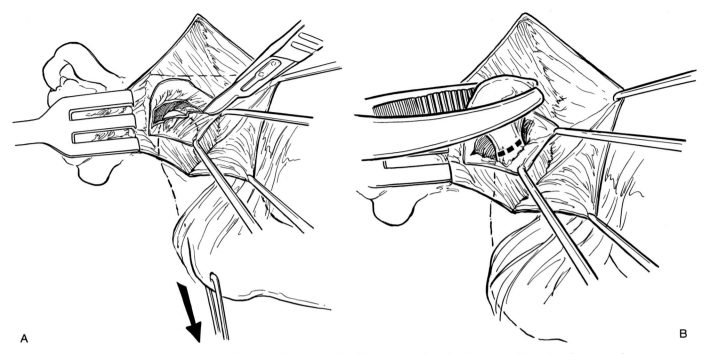

FIG. 62. Condylectomy. **A:** Temporal mandibular joint incised while downward traction is exerted at mandibular angle. **B:** Condyle grasped and excised. (From ref. 51, with permission.)

ally has vertical and horizontal components. The horizontal part is, in fact, part of the middle fossa floor. Sufficient CSF is removed via the lumbar drain to allow the brain to relax such that little or no retraction of the temporal lobe is required for exposure. The craniotomy will have fractured along the longitudinal axis of the eustachian tube and connected foramen spinosum to foramen ovale. The third branch of the trigeminal nerve is easily seen (Fig. 67). The fracture across the bony eustachian tube is the key maneuver in terms of identifying and dissecting the internal carotid artery.

The next step is to dissect out the infratemporal part of the internal carotid artery. The artery is identified in the neck through the cervical portion of the incision and is controlled with a loosely applied tie tape, as is the internal jugular vein. The artery is dissected up until the point that it disappears into the carotid foramen in the temporal bone. This is the point where it is protected by the fibrous ring. The bony eustachian tube has been exposed by the craniotomy. Using loupes or the dissecting microscope, an otologic cutting burr is used to drill the tube away. The posterior wall of the eustachian tube is the common wall of the carotid. Careful removal of the bony wall of the artery is done, keeping the internal carotid canal periosteum intact. This is not too difficult as this is a tough anatomical layer. Dissection of the vessel is done in an anteromedial and inferior direction. As soon as there is no tumor left, the dissection can stop. Otherwise, the dissection proceeds and the course of the eustachian

tube will be seen to diverge somewhat from that of the artery. Very soon V3 will be seen to cross the artery and in most instances will need to be cut across in order to give adequate exposure. On the undersurface of the temporal bone, the palatal musculature is taking its origin. This soft tissue will be removed if involved with tumor or dissected to the side if not, unless it is found to interfere with exposure.

Deeper dissection of the carotid will reveal the gasserian ganglion with V1 and V2 overlying it (see Fig. 25). On occasion, the ganglion can be retracted and tumor in the proximity removed. More medial progression toward the nasopharynx and cavernous sinus will necessitate sacrifice of the ganglion. At this point, the carotid ascends into the cavernous sinus through the foramen lacerum.

If tumor is in the cavernous sinus, it is dissected in slow, careful, piecemeal fashion. Most of the sinus that is invaded by tumor will be compressed and the venous sinusoids will be collapsed and some even thrombosed. Once the limit of tumor extent is reached, however, hemorrhage is brisk. Hemostasis is ensured by slow progression, microscopic control, compression with Gelfoam soaked in thrombin with overlying cottonoids, and finally generous use of the bipolar cautery. The CO_2 laser can be used in those cases in which the vessel size is small and flow is not too great. Great care is taken to preserve the oculomotor nerves when possible. The trochlear nerve is plastered to the supe-

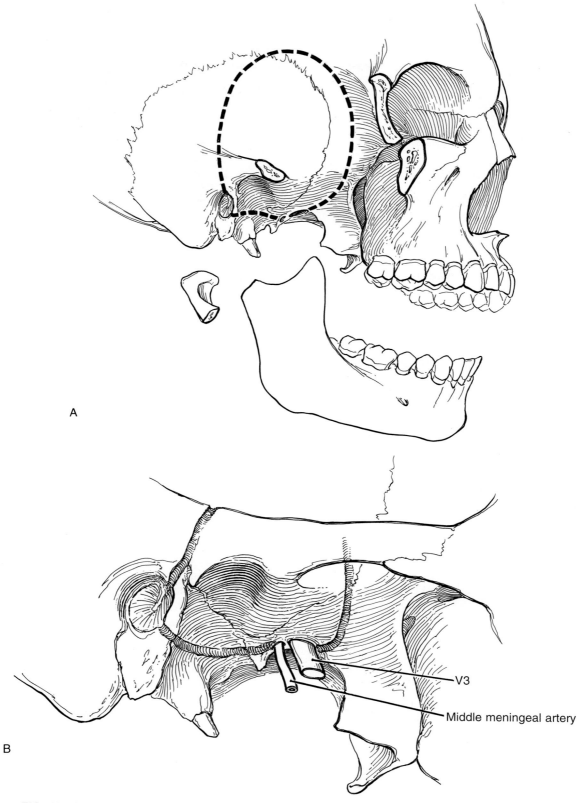

FIG. 63. Craniotomy. **A:** J-shaped craniotomy performed over wing of sphenoid and squamous temporal bone. **B:** Close-up view of inferior aspect of cut through the external auditory canal, glenoid fossa, and connecting foramen spinosum to foramen ovale.

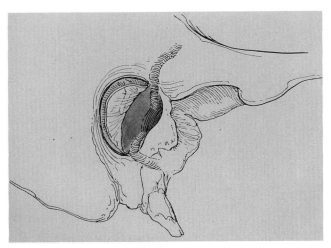

FIG. 64. A tympanomeatal flap is elevated and the anterior external auditory canal cuts are made into the superior and inferior part of the protympanum.

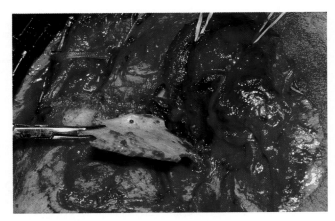

FIG. 66. Craniotomy flap is separated from dura.

rior aspect of the lateral dura of the sinus and is most likely to be injured first.

If tumor is invading the carotid, the decision whether to sacrifice the artery or to graft it has to be made. If the balloon occlusion was negative and the SPECT scan or xenon scan shows good collateral flow, the chances of stroke following carotid sacrifice are low but significant. When at all possible, the safest course is to preserve the internal carotid. If the vessel wall is directly

invaded by tumor, then grafting with a saphenous vein graft is performed. Although there is a significant complication rate when the graft is done, it is an acceptable risk in an otherwise fatal disease. If all the preoperative tests of collateral vascular integrity show excellent cross-fill, an additional assurance of collateral flow is obtained by cross-clamping the internal carotid artery with heparinization and watching the EEG for any spectral drift that is an indicator of cerebral hypoxia. If the EEG remains unchanged, and a decision is made to sacrifice the artery, it is taken as close to the posterior communicating artery as possible. This is to prevent thrombus formation in the distal stump and possible late embolization. The ophthalmic artery is obviously taken in this instance. In the rare circumstance in which the eye is preserved, the ophthalmic artery may be spared and the artery taken distally to it. However, later embolization is a risk and perhaps low-dose heparin beginning at 48 to 60 hr postoperatively may be justified. This has been done on patients in whom the internal carotid artery has been sacrificed in the neck without problems to date of late bleeding or stroke.

Following management of the carotid artery and the cavernous sinus, resection can proceed into the sphenoid sinus, if not yet done, or into the nasopharynx (Fig. 68). Resections of the clivus and portions of the body of C1 are done as necessary, avoiding damage to the basilar arteries. Tumor excision can be extended to the opposite torus tubarius. If the tumor extends further to the opposite side, then a staged procedure through the opposite infratemporal fossa will be necessary.

Nerve root extension along the branches of the trigeminal can be followed toward the brain stem. Obviously, involvement at brain stem level denotes incurability. What margin of resection is required at the nerve root level is uncertain. Presently, frozen section evidence of tumor absence 2 to 4 mm along a nerve is

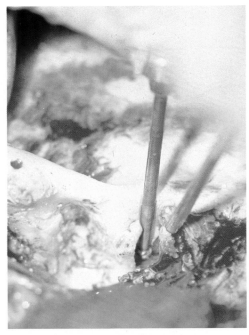

FIG. 65. A cutting bur is used to cut the superior and inferior aspects of the external auditory canal as far as the superior and inferior limits of the protympanum. Bur is cutting inferior canal wall.

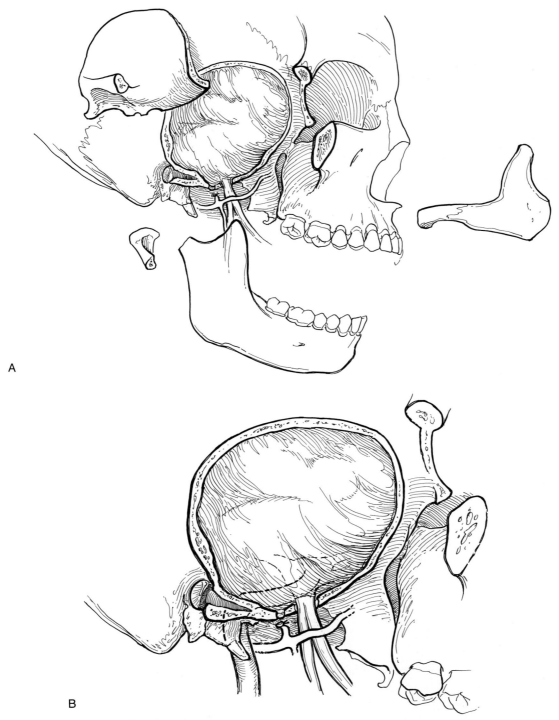

A

B

FIG. 67. Diagram summarizing the steps in the infratemporal fossa–middle fossa approach to the skull base. **A:** Zygomatic ostectomy, mandibular condylectomy, and middle fossa craniectomy done. Note V3 emanating from the foramen ovale. **B:** Note how the craniotomy fractures across the bony eustachian tube. **C:** Patient after craniotomy. *Arrow* points to mandibular branch of V5.

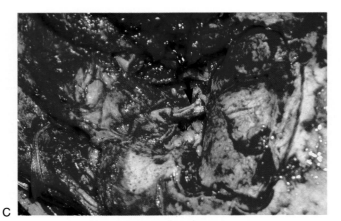

C

FIG. 67. *Continued.*

considered adequate, especially if followed by a full course of irradiation.

The next step is to do the reconstruction and closure. When complete, tumor clearance has been assured, and all margins have been checked, the wound is copiously irrigated with sterile water. The closure begins with establishing a watertight seal of the dura. Dural grafts of fascia or lyophilized material are used. When some additional support is required to further aid in preventing or stopping dural leaks, a fat graft is sutured into place.

Support for the undersurface of the temporal lobe of the brain, coverage of the internal carotid artery, and support for the dural seal are essential. This goal and separation of these vital central structures from the upper aerodigestive tract can be done with the temporalis muscle flap, developed at the beginning of the case, a free flap transfer with microvascular anastomosis, or occasionally a musculocutaneous flap. The temporalis muscle flap is the most commonly used technique. The flap is turned into the defect and the pericranial cuff on the muscle is sutured to the pharyngobasilar fascia

on the opposite side of the nasopharynx (Fig. 69A). If the temporalis has been resected or is unusable, the most commonly used free flap is the rectus abdominis. Its vessels are usually anastomosed to the superficial temporal or external carotid arteries and the superior temporal vein or in an end-to-side fashion to the internal jugular vein. The two musculocutaneous flaps most often utilized are the posterior trapezius flap (47) and the pectoralis major musculocutaneous flap. These flaps are especially good if there is a necessity for an epithelial lining facing the upper aerodigestive stream or if a cutaneous resection has been required.

The cranial bone flap is fixed in place with wires, with the muscular flap turned beneath it. Dural anchoring sutures are placed as well. The zygoma is replaced either with miniplates or wire fixation (Fig. 69B).

Because the eustachian tube has been eliminated, the middle ear must be aerated with a tube. The canal skin is restored, and the external auditory canal is dressed with a thin Silastic sheet and a gauze pack.

The infratemporal fossa defect is a problematic area to reconstruct. If a free flap or musculocutaneous flap is used for reconstruction, then little defect exists, at least until flap atrophy takes place. The defect can be filled with irradiated cartilage grafts or a free fat graft and the skin closed. More and more often the defect is filled by the free flap, thus precluding any further procedure. Hemovac drainage may be used, but this often necessitates the addition of a large pressure dressing.

Case 5

Patient S, a 28-year-old Navy serviceman, first presented with right facial pain and purulent nasal drainage. He was treated initially for maxillary sinusitis (Fig. 70). Because he was refractory to conservative medical treatment and had sinus opacification that had re-

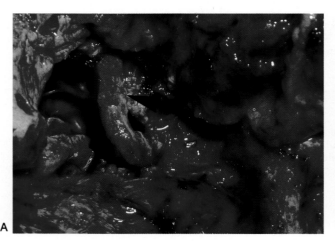

A

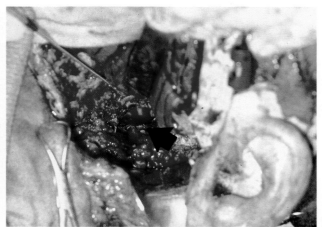

B

FIG. 68. **A:** Petrous carotid *(arrow)* dissected to the foramen lacerum. **B:** Exposure of the nasopharynx *(arrow)* via infratemporal fossa–middle fossa exposure.

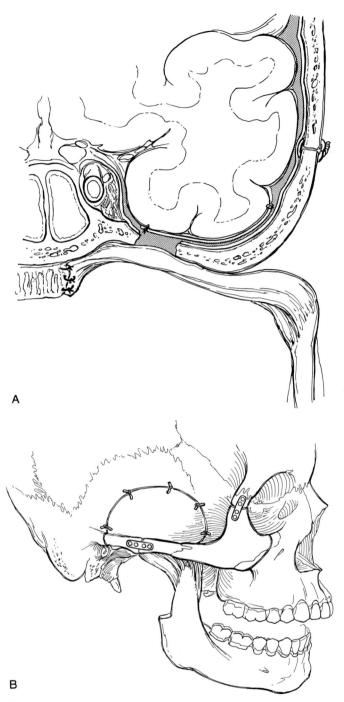

FIG. 69. A: Temporalis muscle sutured across the skull base defect and the craniotomy flap returned. **B:** Zygoma is replaced and secured by osteosynthesis plates.

mained unchanged, a Caldwell–Luc procedure was done. Tumor was seen to fill the maxillary antrum. Biopsy showed adenoid cystic carcinoma. Subsequent CAT scans demonstrated an extensive tumor eroding the walls of the maxillary sinus into the infratemporal fossa (Fig. 71).

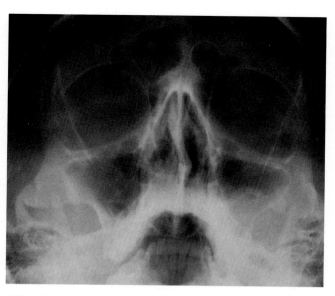

FIG. 70. Case 5. Water's view radiograph of a mass in floor of left maxillary sinus mimicking a maxillary sinusitis.

Because there was doubt of foramen rotundum invasion, an anterior approach was used. The modified Weber–Fergusson incision was followed by a total maxilloethmoidectomy and orbital exenteration. The anterior fossa was not encroached upon, so anterior craniotomy was unnecessary. The sphenoid was unaffected except the anterior wall, which was removed. The limited infratemporal fossa extension was excised and the foramen rotundum exposed once the pterygoid plates had been removed. The cutting bur was used to remove approximately 5 mm of bone from the foramen. Tumor invasion of V2 was found at the level of the dura on frozen section. A staged infratemporal fossa resection was planned.

Through the standard vertical preauricular cervical incision, the temporalis muscle was elevated, the zygoma removed, and the mandibular condylectomy performed (Fig. 72). The craniotomy was done and V3 was unaffected and preserved. The maxillary branch was identified and traced intradurally (Fig. 71). A tumor-free margin was obtained next to the Gasserian Ganglion. The wound was closed.

Postoperatively, the patient developed a CSF leak and meningitis. The meningitis was controlled with antibiotic medication, and the CSF leak repaired through a portion of the original incision. He subsequently underwent a full course of irradiation and is now 5 years free of disease.

Case 6

Patient FG, a 14-year-old boy, presented with a 6-month history of gradually progressive left nasal ob-

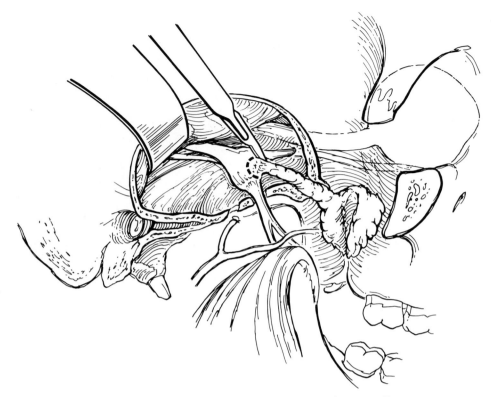

FIG. 71. Case 5. Diagram of resection of V2 within the gasserian ganglion.

struction and two bouts of vigorous epistaxis that had occurred in the 3 weeks prior to presentation. On physical examination, he was breathing through an open mouth and the only other physical finding was a mass occluding the left nares and the left nasopharynx. CAT scans showed a massive tumor filling the left ethmoid and sphenoid sinuses, the nasopharynx, the infratemporal fossa, the cavernous sinus, the left orbital apex,

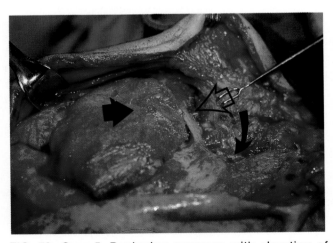

FIG. 72. Case 5. Beginning exposure with elevation of temporalis muscle *(solid arrow)*. Zygomatic ostectomy *(open arrow)* and mandibular condylectomy done *(curved arrow)*.

and eroding the floor of the left middle cranial fossa (see Fig. 18A). Soft tissue contrast suggested dural penetration (see Fig. 18B). Biopsy under general anesthesia confirmed the suspicion of a diagnosis of nasopharyngeal angiofibroma. Arteriography demonstrated a highly vascularized tumor and the patient successfully passed the balloon occlusion test.

Under general anesthesia with a tracheostomy in place, a combined transpalatal, Calwell–Luc, and infratemporal fossa–middle fossa approach were used for extirpation because of the concern of intracranial presentation. The transpalatal approach allowed for mobilization and, in the end, partial removal of tumor from below, whereas the infratemporal fossa approach permitted access to the intracranial part.

An Owen's incision was made in the palatal mucoperiosteum (Fig. 73). The palate and septum were drilled away in the vicinity of the lesion and the tumor exposed from below. A vertical preauricular cervical incision was made (Fig. 74), the skin flap was elevated, the temporalis muscle was reflected, and the zygoma and condyle were removed (Fig. 75). At craniotomy, the tumor could be seen wrapped around V3 (Fig. 76). This was dissected away and tumor was seen to pass through a hole in the dura and to be fixed to the temporal lobe of the brain (Fig. 77). The connection to cerebral tissue was dissected away with the bipolar cautery. Removal of tumor from the cavernous sinus

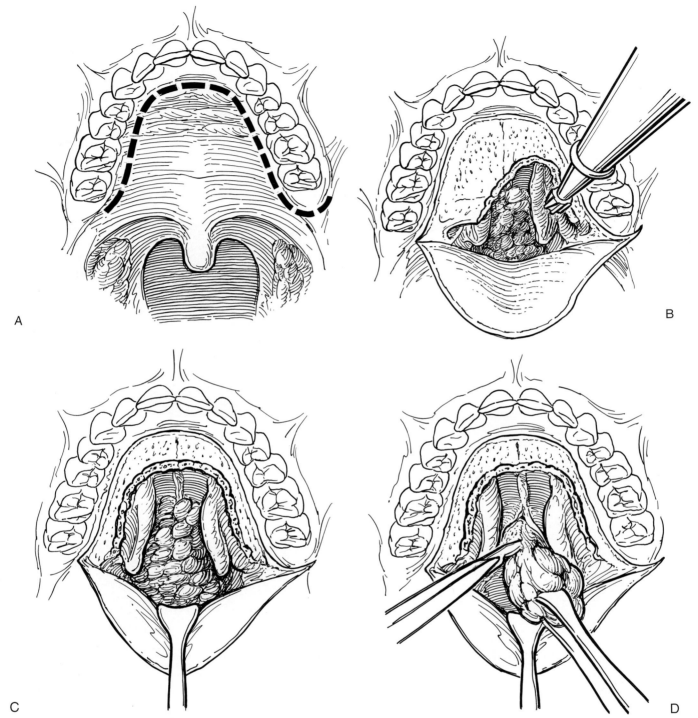

FIG. 73. Case 6. **A:** Owen's incision marked out in hard palate. **B:** Hard palate being drilled away and soft palate split in the paramedian plane. **C:** Exposure of the large nasopharyngeal and postnasal space tumor that filled the sphenoid and ethmoidal sinuses. **D:** Tumor being removed. **E:** Area of tumor origin in basisphenoid being drilled away.

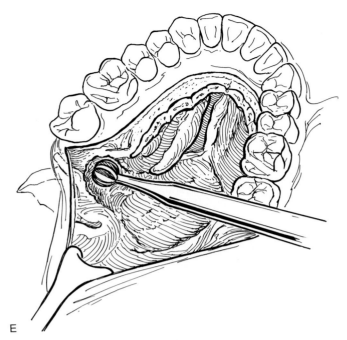

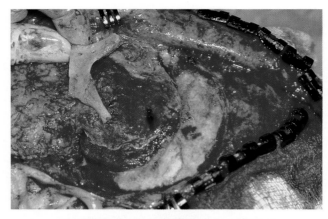

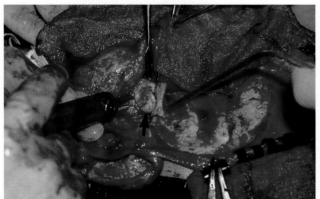

FIG. 73. *Continued.*

FIG. 75. Case 6. **A:** Zygomatic ostectomy. **B:** Condylectomy (*arrow* points to condyle).

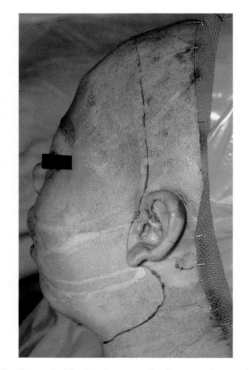

FIG. 74. Case 6. Vertical preauricular craniocervical incision.

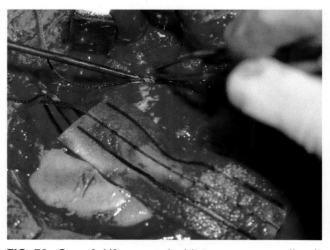

FIG. 76. Case 6. V3 exposed with tumor surrounding it.

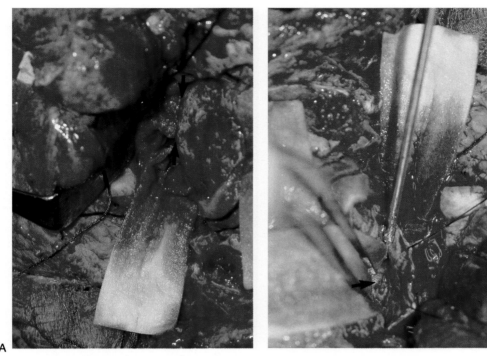

FIG. 77. Case 6. **A:** Tumor growing through hole in dura *(arrow)*. **B:** Dura opened. Tumor adherent to temporal lobe of brain *(arrow)*.

and orbital apex was done, occasionally aided by the CO_2 laser (Fig. 78).

The bulk of the tumor was pushed from above down and out through the transpalatal incision, whereas the remainder was removed piecemeal from the infratemporal fossa dissection. The large defect in the skull base and subcranial area was filled in with a rectus abdominis free flap.

The patient had a smooth recovery but was found to have residual tumor in the sphenoid sinus on follow-up MRI. This was removed with a sinus endoscope approximately 6 weeks following his skull base proce-

dure. The patient is alive at 2 years, without evidence of intracranial disease and with minimal residual problems (Fig. 79). He has required two additional local excisions into the nasopharynx for recurrence.

CONCLUSION

The skull base approach to sinus neoplasms is a great advance in the salvage of previously inoperable and incurable patients. The problems of actual salvage rates are uncertain at this time but appear to be around

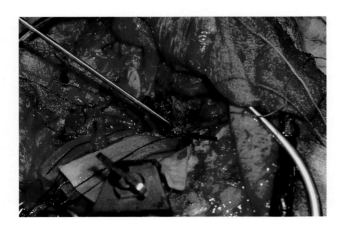

FIG. 78. Case 6. Tumor reduction in cavernous sinus done with CO_2 laser. Suction points to tumor. *White spot* corresponds to laser spot *(arrow)*.

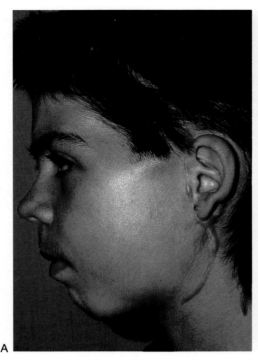 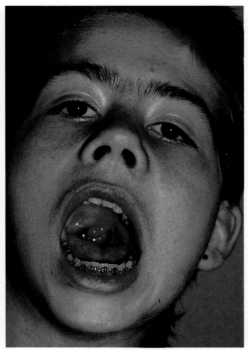

A   B

FIG. 79. Case 6. **A:** Patient 2 years following resection (is a hypertrophic scar former). **B:** Patient with mouth open, illustrating excellent temporomandibular joint function despite condylectomy.

50% (48). Controversial issues such as the width of safe resection margins, the curability of patients with frank intracerebral spread, and the management of carotid involvement as yet remain unresolved.

REFERENCES

1. Schloffer H. Zur frae der operation en an der hypophyse. *Beitr Klin Chir* 1906;50:767.
2. Cushing H. Partial hypophysectomy for acromegaly: with remarks on the function of the hypophysis. *Ann Surg* 1909;50:1002.
3. Hirsch O. Demonstration eines nach eines neuen method operiten hypophysentumors. *Verh Dtsch Ges Chir* 1910;39:51.
4. Hirsch O. Symptoms and treatment of pituitary tumors. *Arch Otolaryngol* 1952;55:268.
5. Dandy WE. *Ortibal tumor. results following the transcranial operative attack.* New York: Oskar Piest; 1941;168.
6. Rae BS, McLean JM. Combined intracranial and orbital operation for retinoblastoma. *Arch Ophthalmol* 1943;30:437.
7. Smith RR, Klopp CT, Williams JM. Surgical treatment of cancer of the frontal sinus and adjacent areas. *Cancer* 1954;7:991–994.
8. Malecki J. New trends in frontal sinus surgery. *Acta Otolaryngol (Stockh)* 1959;50:137.
9. Ketcham AS, Wilkins RH, Van Buren JM, Smith RR: A combined intracranial facial approach to the paranasal sinuses. *Am J Surg* 1963;106:698–703.
10. Ketcham AS, Hoyle RC, VanBuren JM, Johnson RH, Smith RR. Complications of intracranial facial resection for tumors of the paranasal sinuses. *Am J Surg* 1966;112:591–596.
11. Ketcham AS, Chretien PB, Schour L, et al. Surgical treatment of patients with advanced cancer of the paranasal sinuses. In: Ketcham AS, Chretien PB, Schour L, et al. eds. *Neoplasia of the head and neck.* Chicago: Year Book; 1974;187–209.
12. Shambaugh GE, Glasscock ME III. *Surgery of the ear,* 3rd ed. Philadelphia: Saunders; 1980;426.
13. House WF. Surgical exposure of the internal auditory canal and its contents through the middle cranial fossa. *Laryngoscope* 1961;71:1363–1385.
14. Fisch U. Infratemporal fossa approach for extensive tumors of the temporal bone and the base of the skull. In: Silverstein H, Norrell H eds. *Neurological surgery of the ear.* Birmingham, Alabama: Aesculapiul; 1977;34–53.
15. Gardner G, Cocke EW, Robertson JT, et al. Combined approach surgery for removal of glomus jugulare tumors. *Laryngoscope* 1977;87:665–688.
16. Schramm VL. Infratemporal fossa surgery. In: Schramm VL, Sekhar LN eds. *Tumors of the cranial base.* New York: Futura; 1987;421–437.
17. Sekhar LN. Operative management of tumors involving the cavernous sinus. In: Schramm VL, Sekhar LN eds. *Tumors of the cranial base.* New York: Futura; 1987;393–419.
18. Sekhar LN, Burgess J, Akin O. Anatomical study of the cavernous sinus emphasizing operative approaches and related vascular and neural reconstruction. *Neurosurgery* 1987;21:806–816.
19. Parkinson D. A surgical approach to the cavernous portion of the carotid artery: Anatomical studies and case report. *J Neurosurg* 1965;23:474–483.
20. Dolenc V. Direct microsurgical repair of intracavernous vascular lesions. *J Neurosurg* 1983;58:824–831.
21. Al-Mefty O, Smith RR. Surgery of tumors invading the cavernous sinus. *Surg Neurol* 1988;30:307–381.
22. Jacobson JH, Suarez EL. Microsurgery in anastomosis of small vessels. *Surg Forum* 1960;11:243.
23. Nakayama K, Tamiya T, Yamamoto K, Akimoto S. A simple new apparatus for small vessel anastomosis. *Surgery* 1962;52:9118.
24. Wylie JW, Kern EB, Djalilian M. Isolated sphenoid lesions. *Laryngoscope* 1973;83:1252.
25. Alexander FW. Primary tumors at the sphenoid sinus. *Laryngoscope* 1963;73:537.
26. Lang J. *Clinical anatomy of the nose, nasal cavity and paranasal sinuses.* New York: Thieme Medical Publishers, 1989;85–98.

27. Atherino CCT, Carcia R, Lopez LJ. Ectopic meningioma of the nose and paranasal sinuses (report of a case). *J Laryngol Otol* 1985;99:1161–1166.
28. Perzin KR, Pushparaj N. Nonepithelial tumors of the nasal cavity, paranasal sinuses, and nasopharynx: a clinicopathologic study XIII meningiomas. *Cancer* 1984;54:1860–1869.
29. Blitzer A, Lawson W, Friedman WH, eds. *Surgery of the paranasal sinuses*, 2nd ed. Philadelphia: Saunders; 1991;119–159.
30. Rice D, Stanley RB. Surgical therapy of nasal cavity, ethmoid sinus and maxillary sinus tumors. In: Thawley SE, Panje WR, eds. *Comprehensive management of head and neck tumors, vol I.* Philadelphia: Saunders; 1987;380.
31. Lang J. *Clinical anatomy of the nose, nasal cavity and paranasal sinuses.* New York: Thieme Medical Publishers, 1989;121.
32. Sisson G. Personal communication, 1988.
33. Rouviere H. *Anatomie des Lymphatiques de l'Homme.* Paris: Masson, 1932;132.
34. Goss CM. *Gray's anatomy of the human body,* 29th ed. Philadelphia: Lea & Febiger, 1975;741.
35. Chung CT, Rabuzzi DD, Sagerman RN, et al. Radiotherapy for carcinoma of the nasal cavity. *Arch Otol* 1980;106:763–766.
36. Adams GL. Malignant tumors of the paranasal sinuses and nasal cavity. In: McQuarrie DG, Adams GL, Shows AR, Browne GA, eds. *Head and neck cancer: clinical decisions and management principles.* Chicago: Year Book Publishers, 1986;326–327.
37. Sisson GA, Goldstein JC. Tumors of the nose, paranasal sinuses and nasopharynx. In: Paparella MM, Shumrick DA, eds. *Otolaryngology,* vol III N&N. Philadelphia: Saunders; 1973;123.
38. Jackler R, Parker DR. Radiographic differential diagnosis of petrous apex lesions. *Am J Otol* 1992;13:561–574.
39. Vories de EJ, Sekhar LN, Horton JA, Eibling DE, Janecka IP, Schramm VL, Yonas H. A new method to predict safe resection of the internal carotid artery. *Laryngoscope* 1990;100:85–88.
40. Sekhar L, Janecka IP. Extracranial extension of cranial base tumors and combined resection: the neurosurgical perspective. In: Jackson CG, ed. *Surgery of the skull base tumors.* New York: Churchill Livingstone, 1991;211–250.
41. Gillis RE. Psychological implications of patient care. In: Laney WR, ed. *Postgraduate dental handbook series.* Littleton: PSG Publishing, 1979;21.
42. Malecki J. New trends in frontal sinus surgery. *Acta Otolaryngol (Stockh)* 1959;50:137–140.
43. Smith RR, Klopp CT, Williams JM. Surgical treatment of cancer of the frontal sinus and adjacent areas. *Cancer* 1954;7:991–994.
44. Ketcham AS, Wilkins RH, Van Buren JM, Smith RR. A combined intracranial facial approach to the paranasal sinuses. *Am J Surg* 1963;106:698–703.
45. Perry C, Levine PA, Williamson BR, Cantrell RW. Preservation of the eye in paranasal sinus cancer surgery. *Arch Otolaryngol Head Neck Surg* 1988;114:632–634.
46. Mann W, Rareshide E, Schildwächter A. Nasennebenhöhlentumor nit orbitaler Beteiligung. *Laryngorhinootologie* 1989;68:667–670.
47. Netterville J, Wood DE. The lower trapezius flap: vascular anatomy and surgical technique. *Arch Otolaryngol* 1991;117:73–76.
48. Donald PJ. Skull base surgery: combined results of treatment of malignant disesae. *Skull Base Surg* 1992;2:76–79.
49. Zide BM, Jelks GW. *Surgical anatomy of the orbit.* New York: Raven Press, 1985;59–60.
50. Jamieson EB. *Illustration of regional anatomy,* 8th ed. Edinburgh: Livingstone, 1956;8.
51. Donald PJ. *Head and neck cancer: management of the difficult case.* Philadelphia: Saunders, 1986.
52. Donald PJ. Cranial facial surgery for head and neck cancer. In: Johnson JT, ed. *American Academy of Otolaryngology–Head & Neck Surgery: instruction course,* vol 2. St. Louis: CV Mosby, 1989.
53. Donald PJ, Boggan JE. Sphenoidal and cavernous sinus resection for tumor. *J Otolaryngol* 1990;19(2):127.

CHAPTER 30

Restoration of Palatal, Nasal, and Orbital Defects

John Beumer, Russell Nishimura, and Eleni Roumanas

Resection of tumors involving the sinuses and nasal cavities may require removal of portions of the hard and soft palate and occasionally these resections can result in removal of facial structures such as the orbital contents, nose, and cheek. The surgical resection can cause facial disfigurement and severe functional disabilities. Many of these defects are best restored prosthetically and it is the purpose of this chapter to describe how this is best accomplished.

The care of patients with nasal and paranasal sinus neoplasms does not cease with elimination of the tumor. Rehabilitation, an essential phase of cancer care, should be considered from the time of diagnosis. Surgical resections often create large defects accompanied by dysfunction and disfigurement. Speech, swallowing, control of saliva, and mastication can be affected adversely. If these cosmetic and functional impairments are not corrected or minimized, the patient may be unable to resume a normal working and social life.

TREATMENT OBJECTIVES

The primary objective of rehabilitation is the restoration of appearance and function. How successfully this is accomplished depends on the judgment and skill of the therapist and the post-treatment anatomic, physiologic, and psychological makeup of the patient. In the rehabilitation of these patients, certain basic considerations apply:

1. The process of rehabilitation begins at the time of diagnosis. For example, if surgery is to be employed, the configuration of the surgical defect can have great impact on the design and effectiveness of the prosthetic restoration. These issues should be discussed before surgery if the level of rehabilitation is to be maximized.

2. When surgical resections involve the hard and/or soft palate, the teeth should be preserved if possible. Teeth that might be considered inadequate for conventional prosthodontic purposes may prove valuable in patients with large palatal defects.

3. Treatment plans should be developed carefully using basic prosthodontic principles with the aid of mounted diagnostic casts and appropriate radiographs. The prostheses are designed to be as simple and lightweight as possible.

4. Further surgery to improve existing anatomic configurations may be required. The successful use of a prosthesis may depend directly on secondary surgical procedures—lining a defect with skin, creation of soft tissue undercuts, placement of osseointegrated implants, and so on.

5. Ideally, comprehensive care of the cancer patient recognizes that this disease has both physical and psychological components and demands teamwork by health care professionals with expertise in these areas. Surgeons, prosthodontists, and others may be able to resolve the physical defects associated with cancer care, but psychological intervention in some patients may be equally important if recovery is to be as complete as possible. After primary treatment, many patients with cancer of the head and neck fail to return to work, become socially isolated, and experience feelings of shame, worthlessness, and dejection—even when they have been rehabilitated by prosthetic and/or surgical means. Therefore a support system should be initiated at the patient's entry into the health care system and should continue throughout the course of treatment. A physically restored patient who withdraws from a usual pattern of social interaction represents a failure of the health care team (1).

THE TEAM APPROACH TO REHABILITATION

Rehabilitation of head and neck cancer patients requires the team approach, often employing specialists outside the medical and dental professions who are available at a large medical center complex. An important member of a maxillofacial rehabilitation team is the clinical social worker. Since severe emotional distress may accompany the diagnosis and treatment of head and neck cancer, the patient's emotional resources can be strained, sometimes beyond endurance. The patient's family, which is called upon to provide support and comfort, often does not know just how to help. The clinical social worker sees the patient at the time of diagnosis (whenever possible), during primary cancer treatment, and during the long period of rehabilitation. The primary function of this team member is to help the patient understand the process of treatment and to mobilize his or her resources to cope with the situation. The social worker also serves as the patient's advocate in the large medical center and with government agencies, as well as dealing with the myriad of other problems that patients and their families must face. When specific problems arise in the patient's relationship with his or her work, a vocational rehabilitation counselor can also be of great assistance.

Other professionals who may contribute to the care and rehabilitation of the head and neck cancer patient are nurses, dietitians, occupational therapists, physical therapists, speech pathologists, and dental hygienists. Nurses can provide support and comfort for the patient, give instruction on the care of the surgical defect or tracheostomy, and arrange for a visiting nurse support when the patient returns home. The dietitian advises the patient on his or her changing dietary requirements. Occupational and physical therapists help retrain altered muscular systems, and the speech pathologist can help the patient to adapt the speech mechanism to a new prosthesis or to altered physiology. The dental hygienist is an important member of the team because maintenance of dentition is a vital factor in successful maxillofacial rehabilitation. A thorough prophylaxis and instruction in plaque control before and periodically after cancer therapy are essential to avoid severe dental disease. The services of these clinicians broaden a maxillofacial rehabilitation program so that the entire scope of problems faced by these handicapped patients can be treated.

MAXILLARY DEFECTS

Most tumors requiring maxillary resection arise either from paranasal sinus or palatal epithelium or from the minor salivary glands present in the submucosa. Resection of many of these tumors requires either a partial or a radical maxillectomy. A radical maxillectomy entails resection of the entire maxilla to the midline, usually with exposure gained by reflection of a lip and cheek flap (Weber–Fergusson incision). A partial maxillectomy is less encompassing and may be performed transorally. The amount of soft palate included in these resections is variable and depends on the need to obtain tumor-free margins.

Disabilities

Defects of the hard or soft palate produce a variety of problems. Hypernasality makes speech unintelligible; mastication is difficult, particularly for the edentulous patient, because dental structures or denture-bearing tissue surfaces are lost; swallowing is awkward since food and liquids may be forced up into the nasal cavity and out of the nose; the nasal mucous membranes become desiccated by abnormal exposure to the oral environment; nasal and sinus secretions collect in the defect area and may be difficult to control; and facial disfigurement can result from lack of midface bony support or resection of a branch of the facial nerve. In some cases, tumor invasion requires exenteration of the orbital contents or the cheek.

Rehabilitation after resection of the hard or soft palate is best accomplished prosthodontically. Customarily, a temporary prosthesis, known as an immediate surgical obturator, is placed at the time of surgery. During the healing period, this prosthesis is relined periodically with temporary denture reliners to compensate for tissue changes secondary to organization and contracture of the wound. When the defect becomes well healed and dimensionally stable (usually 3 to 4 months after surgery), the definitive prosthesis is made.

Compromised retention, stability, and support are the main problems encountered when the patient attempts to use an obturator prosthesis. The remaining teeth therefore become extremely valuable in providing support, retention, and stability for these restorations. Unilateral prostheses are particularly difficult because movement of the prosthesis may accelerate resorption of alveolar bone and subject abutment teeth to excessive lateral stress. The purpose of these prostheses is to restore the physical separation between the oral and nasal cavities, thereby restoring speech and swallowing to normal and providing support for the lip and cheek.

Alterations at Surgery Improving Prosthetic Prognosis

It is essential that the prosthodontist examine and consult with the patient before surgery. The sequence of treatment should be explained to the patient, and diagnostic casts and appropriate radiographs should be obtained. With this information, the prosthodontist is ready to consult with the surgeon about the design and fabrication of the surgical obturator. Modifications in the surgical plan that may improve the prosthetic prognosis without adversely affecting tumor removal should be discussed at this time.

The surgeon can improve the prosthetic prognosis by considering the following modifications (2).

Hard Palate. An attempt should be made to retain as much of the hard palate as possible, consistent with adequate tumor-free margins. Today presurgical radiographic studies enable the surgeon to outline the extent of the tumor with some accuracy. Therefore significant portions of the hard palate, particularly the premaxillary segment, can often be identified as being free of disease. Retention of the premaxillary segment in partially edentulous patients significantly improves the support, stability, and retention of the future prosthesis under function, thereby enhancing speech, swallowing, and mastication (Fig. 1). Retention of this segment is particularly helpful for the edentulous patient because the remaining palatal surface area provides more support for the obturator prosthesis. Enhanced support for the prosthesis leads directly to improved chewing efficiency for the patient.

Transalveolar Resections. In dentulous patients, transalveolar bony cuts should be made as distant as possible from the tooth that will be adjacent to the palatal defect. The abutment tooth adjacent to the defect is subject to significant occlusal forces and must be well anchored in bone. It is highly advisable that bony cuts should not be made interproximally (between adjacent teeth) since this results in the loss of bone on the defect side, thereby compromising the tooth's periodontal support and predisposing it to premature loss (Fig. 2). When possible, the next adjacent tooth should be extracted and the transalveolar cut made through the defect side of the extraction socket. This approach will result in a sufficient amount of bone on the defect side of the remaining tooth and thus make it a more suitable abutment for the support, stability, and retention of the obturator prosthesis. Additionally, retention of key teeth, particularly the cuspid, may be quite valuable because of its longer root and superior bony support as compared to its immediate neighbors.

Palatal Mucosa. In many instances, the surgeon can save some of the palatal mucosa normally included in the resection and use this keratinized mucosa to cover the margins of the cut palatal bone (Fig. 3). If this tissue is tumor free, it can be reflected prior to the medial bony cut made through the palatal vault. If the exposed bony surface is allowed to granulate and epithelialize spontaneously, it usually becomes lined with respiratory mucosa or poorly keratinized squamous epithelium and provides a decidedly inferior denture-bearing surface. The palatal margin of the defect, particularly in the edentulous patient, serves as the fulcrum around which the prosthesis rotates during function. A keratinized surface in this region will enhance patient comfort and improve the stability of the obtura-

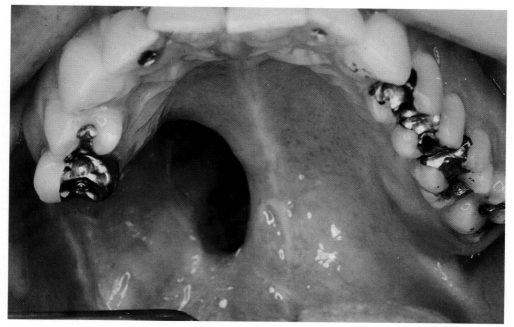

FIG. 1. Retention of the premaxillary segment improves the support and stability of the future obturator prosthesis.

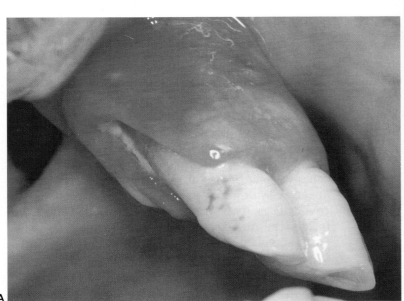
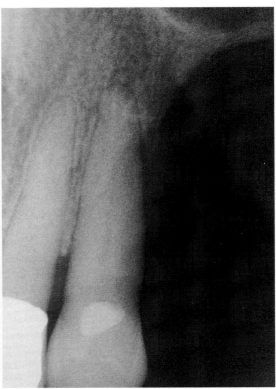

A   B

FIG. 2. Note the gingival and bone recession associated with the root of the tooth adjacent to the surgical defect.

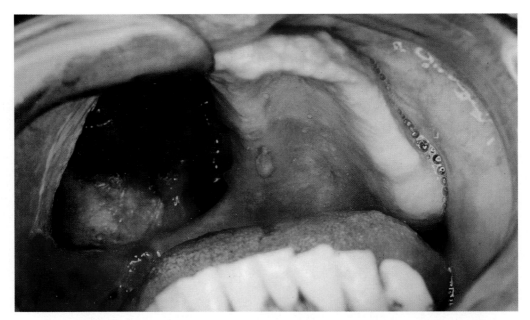

FIG. 3. The palatal margin of this defect has been lined with a palatal mucosa.

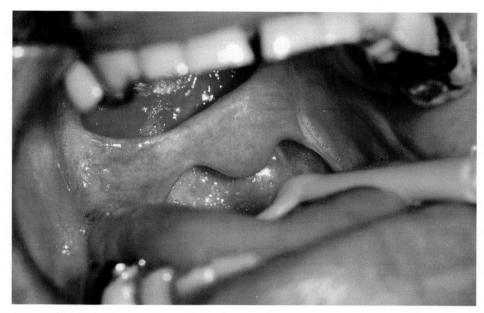

FIG. 4. This soft palate remnant is nonfunctional and must be removed if an effective obturator prosthesis is to be made.

tor prosthesis by providing resistance to lateral displacement during mastication and swallowing.

Soft Palate. In a maxillectomy or palatectomy that involves a significant portion of the soft palate or in resection of tumors primarily confined to the soft palate, the remaining portion of the velopharyngeal mechanism must be accessible to the prosthesis if proper velopharyngeal closure is to be achieved during speech and swallowing. If the resection includes the anterior and middle third of the soft palate, a posterior narrow

nonfunctional band of intact soft palate may remain postsurgically (Fig. 4). This remnant may lack innervation and/or the capacity for normal elevation. These bands of soft palate contract superiorly, thus preventing proper positioning of an obturator prosthesis designed to interface with the residual velopharyngeal musculature. Resultant speech will be hypernasal and leakage of fluids into the nose will occur during swallowing. Therefore, on the resected side if less than one-third of the posterior aspect of the soft palate is to

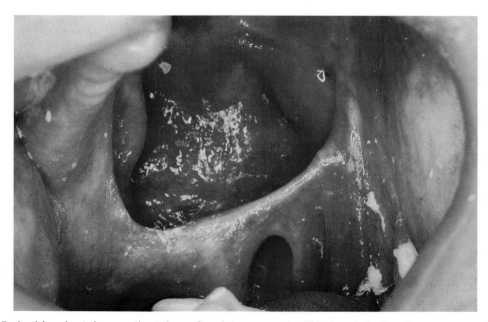

FIG. 5. In this edentulous patient the soft palate remnant will help retain the obturator prosthesis.

remain postsurgically, the entire soft palate should be removed. An exception should be made for an edentulous patient undergoing a radical maxillectomy. Retention of the obturator prosthesis is always difficult in such situations and a distal extension of obturator prosthesis onto the nasal side of the soft palate is an advantage that outweighs the possible speech and leakage problems previously mentioned (Fig. 5). In such patients, osseointegrated implants can also be placed in the residual premaxillary segment, thereby providing retention for the anterior portion of the obturator prosthesis (Fig. 6).

Skin Grafts. The surgeon can improve the tolerance and retention of the obturator prosthesis dramatically if the reflected cheek flap and other adjacent raw tissue surfaces are lined with a split-thickness skin graft (Fig. 7). Keratinized stratified squamous epithelium is more resistant to the abrasion caused by the obturator prosthesis than is respiratory epithelium or nonkeratinized stratified squamous epithelium. The latter epithelium will line the defect if it is allowed to granulate and epithelialize spontaneously. Placement of the skin graft also limits scarring and increases the flexibility of the cheek area. This flexibility enables the prosthodontist to more effectively support and reproduce midfacial contours with the obturator prosthesis. In addition, a longitudinal scar band is formed at the junction of the skin graft and the oral mucosa, which creates a retentive pocket above and a support area below the band. Engaging the scar band superiorly and inferiorly with the obturator prosthesis enhances its stability, support, and retention. At surgery the amount of the skin graft survival and defect coverage is improved by the use

of an immediate surgical obturator. This device supports a bolus placed into the defect, usually gauze packing, and keeps the graft in place and properly adapted to the raw tissue surface of the cheek. Thermoplastic material like black gutta percha attached to the obturator and molded to the limits of the defect can also be used for this purpose.

Access to the Defect. The surgeon should provide access to the superior and lateral aspects of the defect for the prosthodontist. Extending the obturator up the lateral walls of the defect provides retention and stability for the prosthesis. Engaging the lateral nasal side of the orbital floor provides vertical support for the obturator prosthesis. Such structures as the turbinates and bands of oral mucosa may prevent the prosthesis from engaging key areas of the defect, dramatically compromising its function (Fig. 8). If the postsurgical defect is large, these structures provide little benefit to the patient if oral integrity is not maintained and severely limit the ability of the prosthodontist to seal the defect and provide proper obturation. Furthermore, the turbinates can enlarge secondary to changes in normal nasal environment and from irritation from food and liquids leaking into the nasal cavity. These edematous turbinates may extend below the normal palatal plane, distorting the contour of the palatal portion of the prosthesis, impairing tongue space, and thereby disrupting speech and swallowing. Consequently, these structures should be considered for inclusion in the resection. This suggestion may not apply to small midline defects of the hard–soft palate junction.

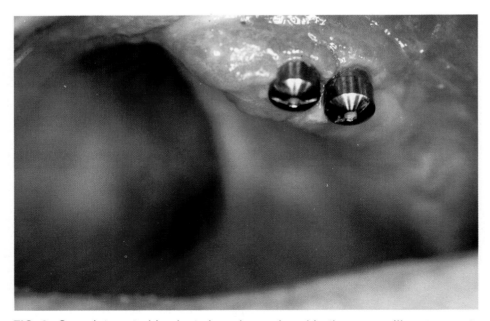

FIG. 6. Osseointegrated implants have been placed in the premaxillary segment.

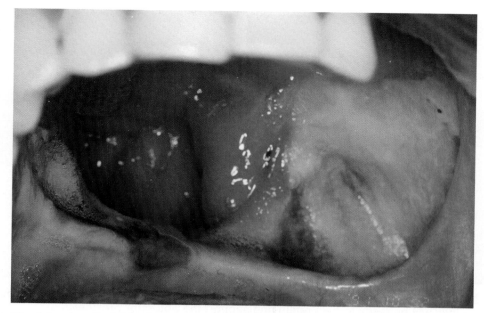

FIG. 7. The lateral wall of this defect is lined with skin, facilitating the stability and retention of the obturator prosthesis.

Osseointegrated Implants. In edentulous patients or when the prognosis for remaining dentition is poor, placement of osseointegrated implants at the time of tumor resection should be considered (Fig. 9) (3). These implants can be placed immediately upon tumor removal and require little additional operating time. The most suitable sites for implant placement are the remaining premaxillary segment and the maxillary tuberosity. In some edentulous patients, there may be sufficient bone remaining in the alveolar process below the maxillary sinus. The use of bone sites within the defect should be discouraged except in extraordinary circumstances. Compromised oral hygiene access makes it difficult to maintain healthy peri-implant soft tissues around implants positioned in the surgical defect. The prospect of pre- or postoperative radiation

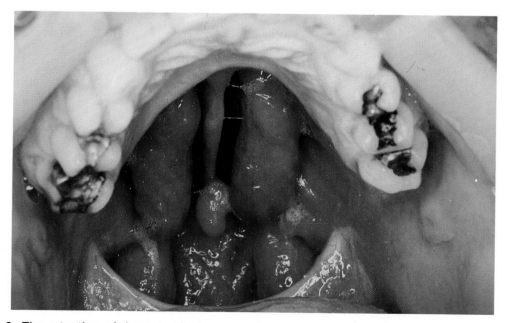

FIG. 8. The retention of these turbinates prevents proper extension of the obturator into the defect.

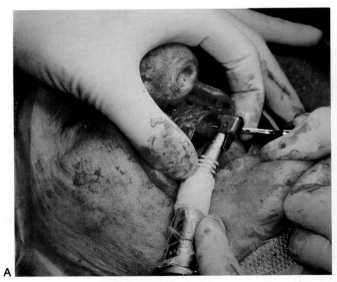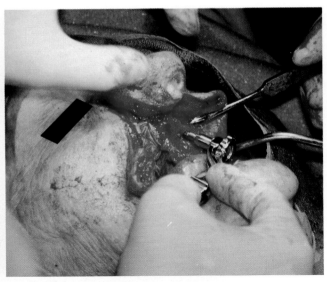

A

B

FIG. 9. These implants are being positioned immediately following resection of the tumor. In 6 months they will be ready to help retain and support the obturator prosthesis.

does not appear to preclude the use of osseointegrated implants in these patients.

Surgical Reconstruction of Palatal Defects

Attempts should not be made to close large defects of the hard palate by surgical means (Fig. 10). Such surgical closures disrupt normal contours and eliminate tongue space, resulting in difficulty in speech articulation and swallowing. These flaps also make it difficult, if not impossible, for the patient to wear a prosthesis and may also delay detection of recurrent tumor. An exception would be of defects of 2 cm or less of the palate. Surgical closure of such defects generally does not distort palatal contours.

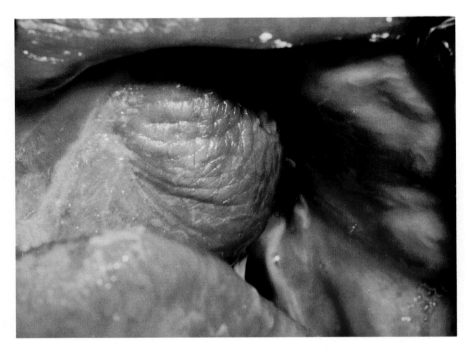

FIG. 10. This defect has been covered with a myocutaneous flap. Consequently, palatal contours are distorted. The flap must be reduced or removed if a dental prosthesis is to be fabricated.

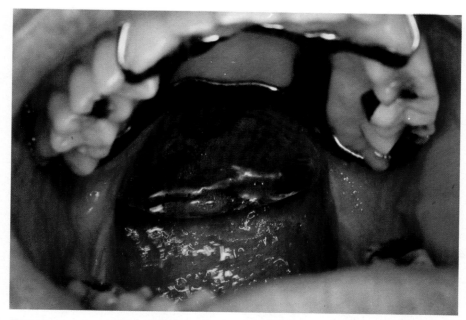

FIG. 11. The musculature of the residual velopharyngeal complex will interact with this obturator, enabling the patient to achieve velopharyngeal closure. Normal speech and swallowing are the result.

Likewise, soft palate defects should not be reconstructed by surgical means. Surgical reconstruction of these defects may result in nonfunctional denervated tissues, which are incapable of functioning in a coordinated fashion with the residual velopharyngeal musculature. If the remaining velopharyngeal structures retain the capacity for some movement, a properly contoured speech prosthesis will restore normal speech and eliminate almost all nasal leakage of food and liquids. The obturator prosthesis consists of a platform of acrylic resin positioned in the nasopharynx around which the surrounding velopharyngeal musculature functions in a coordinated manner (Fig. 11). If the peripheral musculature retains capacity for contraction, the patient is able to control the magnitude of nasal airflow, allowing for normal speech and swallowing. Therefore surgical closures that impair the function of the residual velopharyngeal musculature should be discouraged. For example, tethering a tongue flap to the residual soft palate may limit palatal elevation and make difficult the proper positioning of the obturator prosthesis, leading to hypernasal speech and nasal leakage of bolus.

Immediate Surgical Obturators

Immediate or early coverage of a palatal defect with an obturator prosthesis will greatly facilitate the patient's postoperative course (4). The obturator pro-vides a matrix on which the surgical packing can be placed, minimizes contamination of the wound in the immediate postoperative period, and enables the patient to speak and swallow effectively immediately after surgery. The immediate surgical obturator is useful in both dentulous and edentulous patients.

Making the prosthesis is simple for the prosthodontist. An impression is obtained of the maxillary arch and the anterior portion of the soft palate, and a cast is retrieved. The obturator's size is determined by the surgical boundaries of the resection, as indicated by the surgeon. In the dentulous patient, teeth in the path of the surgical resection are removed from the cast (Fig. 12). Care should be taken to extend the surgical obturator posteriorly past the proposed posterior soft palatal resection line to effectively seal off the defect. These prostheses are processed in autopolymerizing methylmethacrylate. They can be altered at surgery by trimming or by adding a temporary denture reliner. The prosthesis is wired to remaining teeth, alveolar ridge, or other available structures (e.g., zygomatic arch, anterior nasal spine) (Fig. 13).

After the surgical packing is removed (6 to 10 days after surgery), the prosthesis is relined with a temporary denture reliner. As healing progresses, the obturator is periodically relined and extended further into the defect and adaptation is improved. Three to five months after surgery, and after initial wound contracture is essentially complete, the definitive prosthesis is begun. Edentulous patients with maxillary de-

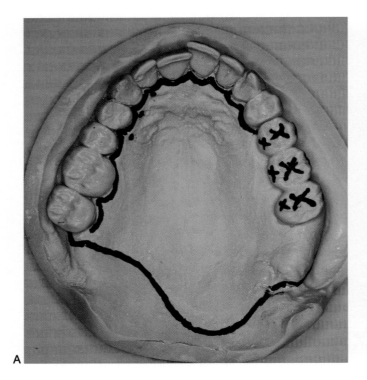

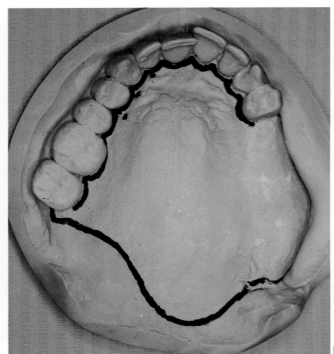

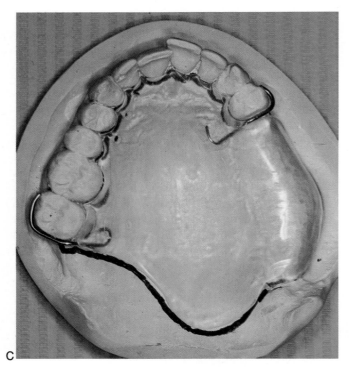

FIG. 12. A cast of the maxilla is made **(A)**. Teeth in the path of the resection are removed **(B)** and the immediate surgical obturator is fabricated **(C)**.

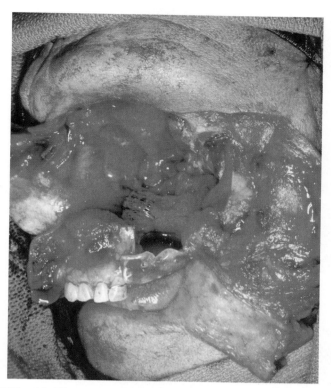

FIG. 13. The immediate surgical obturator has been wired to the remaining dentition.

fects often require a longer period of healing because the defect must be engaged more aggressively so as to maximize stability, support, and retention.

Definitive Obturator Prostheses

Defects of the hard palate are restored effectively with a prosthesis. If teeth are present, they greatly improve obturator retention and stability. Speech, swallowing, mastication, and facial contour can be restored with proper extensions and obturation. The obturator should extend maximally along the lateral wall of the defect (Fig. 14). This high lateral extension improves retention and lateral stability and provides support for the lip and cheek. The movement of the coronoid process into the distolateral area of the defect must be accounted for during border molding and final impression procedures. The extension superiorly along the medial margin of the defect should not exceed the level of the repositioned palatal mucosa. If it does, little mechanical benefit results and unnecessary and painful ulceration of the respiratory mucosa lining the nasal septum may result. In some patients, extension across the nasal surface of the soft palate or into the nasal aperture may be necessary to facilitate obturator retention (5). When the prosthesis is completed, speech and swallowing are restored to normal limits and appearance is greatly improved.

Fabrication of an obturator prosthesis for an edentulous patient will challenge the ability of the most skilled clinician. In the presence of a sizable palatal defect, air leakage, compromised stability, and reduced bearing surface will compromise adhesion, cohesion, and peripheral seal of the prosthesis. However, the use of osseointegrated implants can resolve many of these difficulties. The contours of the obturator prosthesis, however, must still be used to maximize the retention, stability, and support for the obturator prosthesis. On the defect side, engaging the skin-lined lateral wall and extending a lip onto the nasal side of the soft palate will facilitate retention. Support for the prosthesis on the defect side can be obtained by extending the prosthesis superiorly to contact the lateral portion of the orbital floor. On the unresected side, the restoration obtains its retention from the retentive mechanism attached to the implants. Support is provided by engaging the residual palatal structures in the usual manner. The implant secured overdenture retention mechanism must take into account the axis of rotation of the prosthesis when occlusal loads are applied (Fig. 15). In most patients it is advisable to first fabricate a trial denture with an accompanying dental index, thereby establishing the most ideal position of denture teeth, before the retentive mechanism is fabricated. In some patients the retentive apparatus can be a useful aid in making altered cast impressions or centric relation records. These records are then transferred to an articulator in the usual fashion. For most edentulous patients nonanatomic posterior teeth are preferred. Processing the prosthesis must take into account the special needs related to the retentive devices. The resulting prosthesis can be gratifying to the patient as well as the clinician. In large defects dramatic improvements in function can be effected as a result of the improved retention and increased support and stability provided for the prosthesis by osseointegrated implants.

Definitive Soft Palate Prostheses

Defects of the soft palate require different and more complex prosthetic treatment. Velopharyngeal closure normally occurs when the soft palate elevates and contacts the contracting lateral and posterior pharyngeal walls of the nasopharynx. When a portion of the soft palate is excised or when the soft palate is perforated, scarred, or neurologically impaired, complete velopharyngeal closure cannot occur. Speech becomes hypernasal, and normal swallowing is not possible. With a pharyngeal obturator the patient may be able to reestablish velopharyngeal closure if the residual portion of the velopharyngeal mechanism still exhibits reasonable

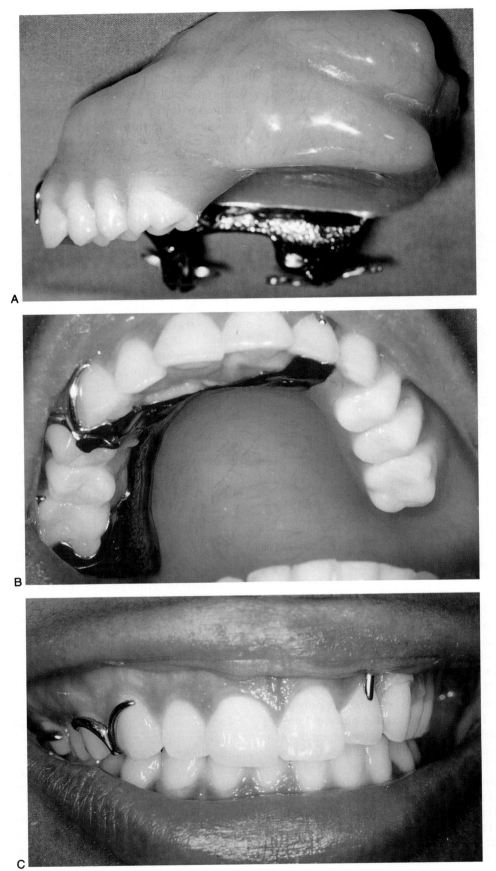

FIG. 14. The obturator prosthesis extends up the full height of the lateral wall of the defect and restores the partition between the oral and nasal cavities in this patient.

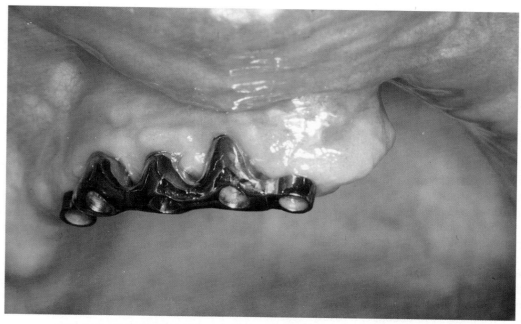

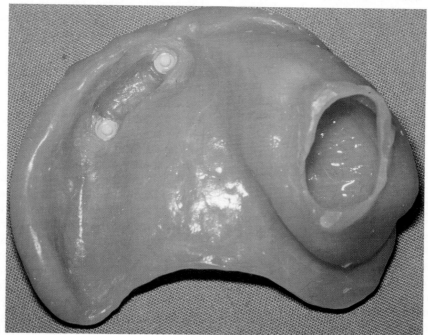

B

FIG. 15. The implant secured retention mechanism shown here allows for several axes of rotation upon application of occlusal loads.

movement (see Fig. 11). Properly designed and fabricated, the obturator will not interfere with breathing, impinge on soft tissues during postural movements, or hamper the tongue during swallowing and speech (6).

The soft palate obturator remains in a fixed position in the nasopharynx and does not attempt to duplicate normal movements of the soft palate. The inferior surface of the obturator remains level with the hard palate contour, which in most patients is approximately the level of the anterior tubercle of the atlas. The inferior margin of the posterior surface of the obturator contacts Passavant's pad, if present, and extends approximately 10 mm superiorly into the nasopharynx. During breathing and the production of nasal speech sounds, the space around the obturator reflects the potential for muscular contraction. During swallowing and the production of other speech sounds, this sphincteric muscular network moves into contact with the stationary acrylic resin obturator, establishing velopharyngeal closure. A correctly constructed obturator will result in the return of normal speech and swallowing for patients with acquired soft palate defects.

NASAL AND ORBITAL DEFECTS

General Comments

Restoration of facial defects is a difficult challenge for both the surgeon and the prosthodontist. Surgical reconstruction and prosthodontic restoration both have distinct limitations. The surgeon is limited by the availability of tissue, the damage to the local vascular bed in tumor patients, the need for periodic visual inspection of an oncologic defect, and the physical condition of the patient. The prosthodontist is limited by the materials available for facial restoration, the movable tissue beds, the difficulty in retaining large prostheses, and the patient's willingness to accept the result. The difficulty encountered in retaining a large facial prosthesis has largely been overcome by the use of osseointegrated implants. Whatever the mode of rehabilitation, the patient should be informed about these choices and should participate in the decision-making process. A well-informed patient with realistic expectations is the objective to be achieved before surgical resection of tumors requiring nasal resection or orbital exenteration.

Surgical Reconstruction Versus Prosthetic Restoration

The choice between surgical reconstruction versus prosthetic restoration of large facial defects is difficult and complex and depends on the size and etiology of the defect as well as the wishes of the patient. Surgical reconstruction of small facial defects is possible and in most cases is preferable. Many patients prefer masking a small defect with their own tissue rather than with a prosthetic restoration. It is safe to say, however, that it is difficult, if not impossible, for the surgeon to fabricate a facial part that is as effective in appearance as a well made prosthesis. However, not everyone will accept an artificial part, and many would rather have a permanent, even if less esthetic, partial nose or ear. In general, younger patients prefer to have a permanent reconstructed facial part rather than an artificial one. The application of osseointegrated implants in facial defects has, in part, changed patient perceptions about facial prostheses because of the effectiveness of retention achieved.

A variety of circumstances may dictate prosthetic restoration of rhinectomy–orbital defects.

1. When a large resection is necessary and reoccurrence of tumor is likely, it is advantageous to be able to monitor the surgical site closely. A prosthesis permits such observation, whereas primary surgical reconstruction may make it more difficult.

2. Surgical restoration of large defects is technically difficult and requires multiple procedures and hospitalizations. Patients confronted with this type of defect are usually older and less able or willing to tolerate the multiple procedures required for surgical reconstruction.

3. Increasing numbers of these types of tumors are being treated with radiation therapy. Reduced vascularity, increased fibrosis, and scarring of the tissues bordering the defect increase the risk of complications associated with reconstruction. In many patients, full-course radiation therapy precludes successful surgical reconstruction.

Even when surgical reconstruction is deemed possible, significant delay may be necessary to ensure control of the tumor. Most surgeons prefer to wait at least 1 year after a large resection before beginning surgical reconstruction of a facial defect resulting from removal of a malignant tumor.

Alteration at Surgical Resection to Enhance the Prosthetic Prognosis

Nasal Defects

When a total rhinectomy is contemplated, the nasal bones should be removed, even though these structures may not be infiltrated with tumor (Fig. 16). If the nasal bones remain, the prosthesis must either terminate just above the superior surgical margin, disrupting concealment of the prosthetic margin, or extend superiorly over the nasal bridge. Extension of the prosthesis over the nasal bones results in proper margin placement but creates a thin, overcontoured prosthesis in this area. In addition, these areas of the prosthesis are subject to tearing. Additionally, retained nasal bones will dictate the prosthetic contours of the nasal tip. The resultant nasal prosthesis may then appear larger than normal, leading to an unesthetic result (Fig. 16).

Whenever possible, care should be taken to avoid surgical displacement and/or distortion of the upper lip during resection and closure. If the lip is retracted posteriorly or displaced vertically to accomplish closure, it is not possible to fabricate a nasal prosthesis that can faithfully reproduce presurgical facial contours, particularly from the lateral perspectives (Fig. 17). A retracted upper lip immediately draws attention to the patient's midface defect and compromises the concealment of the prosthetic margins.

During surgical resection of the tumor, care should also be taken to avoid undue distortion of the cheeks

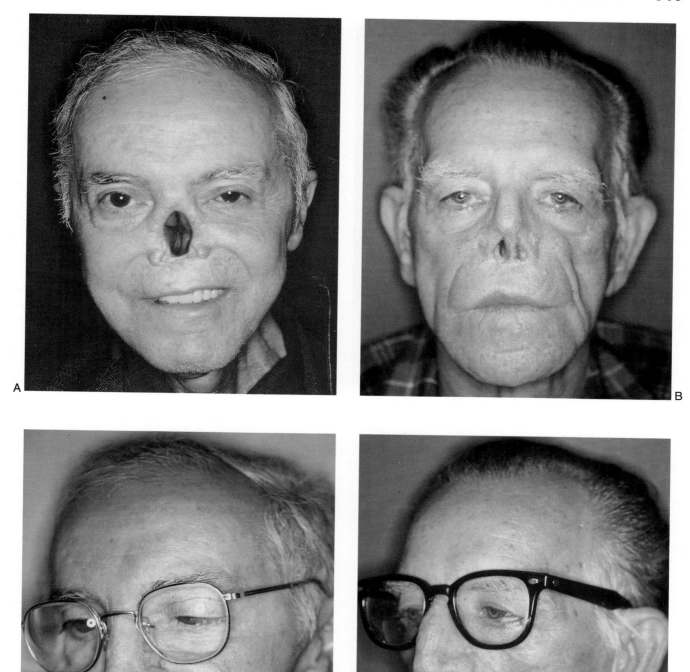

FIG. 16. In one patient **(A)** the nasal bones have not been removed, while in another **(B)** the bones have been removed. Note the difference in the esthetic results **(C,D).**

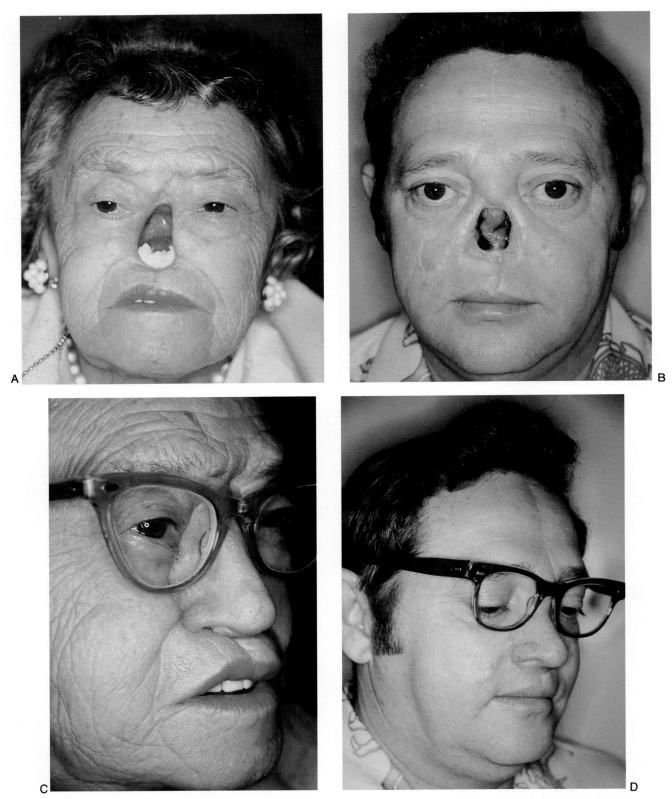

FIG. 17. In one view **(A)** the lip is retracted posteriorly and superiorly; in another view **(B)** they are not. Note the difference in the esthetic results **(C,D).**

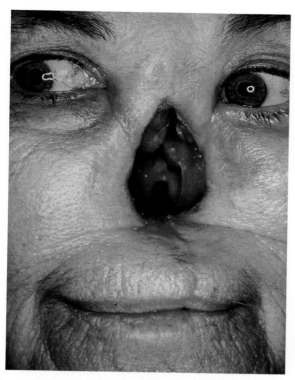

FIG. 18. Note the distortion of the tissues adjacent to the defect area. It will be difficult to fabricate an esthetic facial prosthesis.

and nasolabial folds. Obliteration or displacement of the nasolabial folds adversely affects the contour and position of the nostril and columella portion of the prosthesis. During surgical resection, the nasal bones, alae, columella, and the anterior portion of the nasal septum should be removed without distortion of adjacent facial contours. The osseous and soft tissue margins of the surgical defect should be smooth and covered with skin grafts. Primary closure of such defects should be avoided because of the possibility of distorting midfacial contours (Fig. 18). In selected patients, osseointegrated implants can be placed immediately following tumor resection. The preferred site is the maxilla on the floor of the nose. In dentulous patients care must be taken to avoid the roots of teeth during implant placement (Fig. 19) (7).

Orbital Defects

Resections confined to removal of orbital contents are prosthetically easier to restore than those extending beyond the orbit. As surgical margins extend beyond the orbital confines, the prosthesis becomes less esthetic because of the inability to camouflage lines of juncture between skin and prosthesis. Additionally, as the prosthesis extends beyond the orbit, movable tis-

sue margins are encountered. This results in further exposure of the lines of juncture and compromises retention of the prosthesis.

As with rhinectomies, the surgeon should avoid procedures that lead to distortion of adjacent facial structures. In particular, slight discrepancies in the position of the globe or eyebrow are noticed by even the most casual observer. Orbital defects should be lined with split-thickness skin grafts (Fig. 20). Pedicle flaps intended to fill the orbital cavity are discouraged since access to the defect and sufficient depth of defect are essential in order to fabricate an esthetic orbital prosthesis. When the orbital contents are resected, the eyelids should also be removed since retaining them only hinders access to the defect and often prevents the clinician from placing the globe in proper position (7).

Midfacial Defects

These defects usually result from resection of advanced nasal or nasal cavity tumors and may lead to resection of the nose, upper lip, and orbital contents with extension into the oral cavity. The prosthetic prognosis is primarily dependent on the presence and condition of the teeth, the amount and contour of the remaining hard palate, the functional status of the lower lip, and the motivation and adaptability of the patient. The presence of small amounts of upper lip is usually of little value and in most defects it is not advisable to reconstruct the upper lip surgically. The reconstructed upper lip is often improperly positioned and immobile and access to the oral cavity is compromised as a result. In addition, the reconstructed lip can prevent normal lip valving during speech. Furthermore, the poor esthetics of the reconstructed upper lip often focuses more attention on the defect and the midfacial prosthesis. Usually, the reconstructed upper lip must be overlaid and covered with the prosthesis to restore speech and esthetics. The small oral opening and impaired flexibility of the reconstructed oral stoma make it difficult for the prosthodontist to fabricate any necessary oral prostheses and make their insertion/removal difficult for the patient. In addition, oral hygiene procedures will invariably be compromised by the impaired oral opening (Fig. 21).

Surgical modifications at tumor resection that may be indicated include retention of key teeth that can be used to support and retain the combined facial and intraoral prosthesis; preparation of the soft tissue bed with the intent of creating retentive pouches; and placement of skin grafts to minimize distortion and contraction of the tissue bed (Fig. 22). If soft tissue undercuts are created surgically, they should be lined with split-thickness skin grafts. Failure to do so results in excessive contracture and, in some cases, loss of the

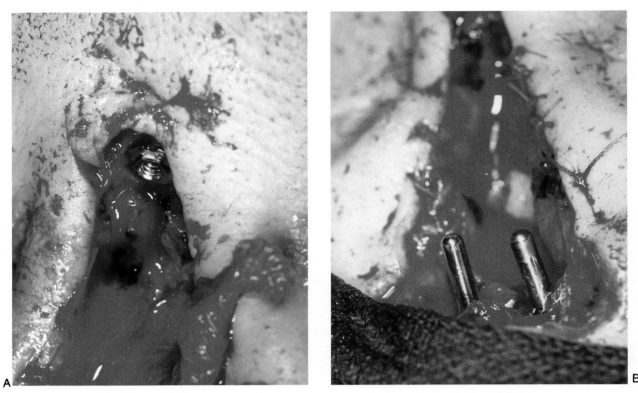

FIG. 19. These implants have been placed immediately upon resection of the tumor.

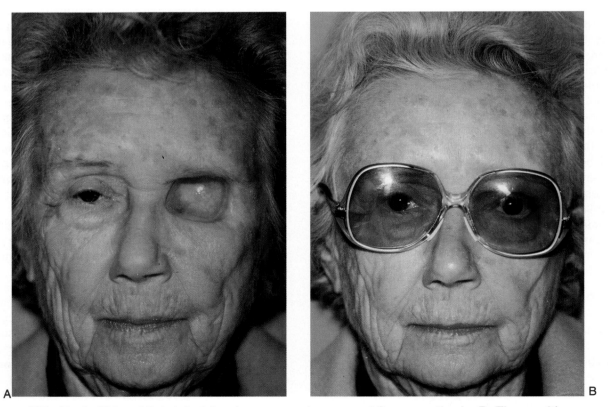

FIG. 20. A: This orbital defect has been properly prepared for a prosthesis. **B:** The resulting prosthesis is quite esthetic.

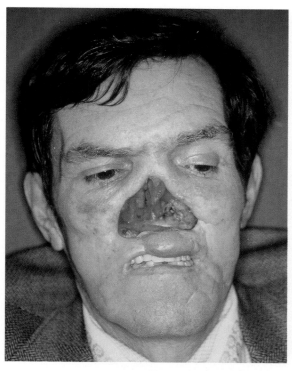

FIG. 21. The upper lip has been reconstructed. The size of the oral stoma is minimal and insertion of the obturator prosthesis is made very difficult.

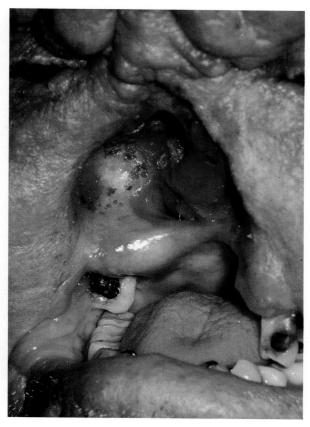

FIG. 22. Teeth have been retained and undercuts have been lined with skin in this large midfacial defect.

created undercut. Additionally, these undercut areas usually become epithelialized with nonkeratinized squamous epithelium or respiratory mucosa, thereby limiting their usefulness as a prosthesis-bearing surface. A keratinized tissue at the anterior palatal margin will also improve patient comfort. In addition, if the nasal floor of the residual hard palate is skin grafted, this surface may be used to retain the maxillary and nasal prosthesis (8).

Placement of osseointegrated implants has had a dramatic impact on the function of these large and heretofore difficult to retain midfacial prostheses. Possible sites include the orbital rim, the floor of the nose, residual malar or zygoma segments, and the glabella. With implants in position, these large facial prostheses can be retained effectively (Fig. 23). When possible, the implants should be placed at the time of the tumor resection.

Prosthetic Restorations

The challenge to the prosthodontist is to fabricate an esthetically pleasing restoration. A conspicuous prosthesis may produce more anxiety and permit less social readjustment than a simple facial bandage or eye patch. Since successful use of the restoration may depend on the patient's psychological acceptance of it, it

is beneficial to have the patient seen by a social worker during the rehabilitation period. The most critical period is the first 2 to 3 days after delivery of the prosthesis. The conflicting emotional responses of the patient should be anticipated and discussed before delivery. In some cases, a patient will not wear a facial prosthesis because of unrealistic expectations. Since all facial restorations are detectable under close scrutiny, the patient must understand that the prosthesis has two different roles. For family, close friends, or business associates, it can only cosmetically replace the tissues excised. For the public at large, however, it generally provides enough concealment to render the reconstructed defect inconspicuous.

Materials Used for Facial Prostheses

A number of materials have been used for facial prostheses. These include wax, metals, and, recently, polymers. Current materials exhibit some excellent properties, but also some frustrating deficiencies, and all possess some undesirable characteristics. The materials most often used today are the silicone elastomers. The newest silicone elastomers have been shown

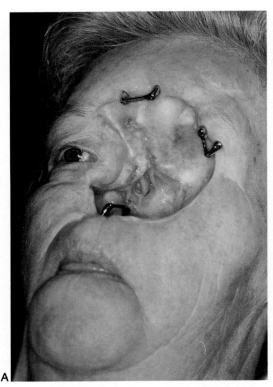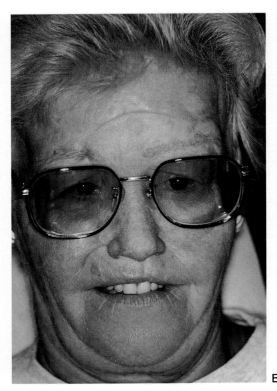

FIG. 23. Implants are very useful in retaining this large midfacial prosthesis.

to be the most clinically acceptable material and have achieved wide acceptance.

Retention and Osseointegrated Implants

A major development in recent years has been the use of osseointegrated implants for retention (9). In eligible patients with sufficient bone at the desired sites, the result is an extremely well-retained prosthesis, allowing for vigorous physical activities. The tissue-adhesive systems used during the last 40 years are rapidly being discarded in favor of these new implant systems.

The use of osseointegrated implants is having a dramatic impact on restoration of facial defects. The retention and support derived from these implants eliminate some of the primary limitations of adhesive-retained facial restorations. Benefits derived from implant-retained prostheses include (a) improved retention and stability of the prosthesis, (b) elimination of the occasional skin reaction to the adhesives, (c) ease and enhanced accuracy of prosthesis placement (particularly important in orbital prosthesis), (d) improved skin hygiene and patient comfort, (e) decreased daily maintenance associated with removal and reapplication of skin adhesives, (f) increased life span of the facial restoration, and (g) enhanced lines of juncture between

the prosthesis and skin. When skin adhesives are used for retention, they must be removed and reapplied each day, leading to loss of colorants at the margin of the prosthesis, eventually rendering the prosthesis unacceptable. When an implant prosthesis is fabricated, its margins can be made thinner and positive pressure developed with the prosthesis. These two factors can be especially useful when a facial prosthesis extends into movable tissue beds.

When implants are to be placed, the clinician is best advised to develop a wax sculpting of the facial part to be replaced. From this sculpting a surgical template can be fabricated and used at surgery to identify appropriate implant positions (Fig. 24). In rhinectomy defects, two implants placed into the floor of the nose positioned so as not to distort the contours of the future nasal prosthesis are sufficient for retention and support. More implants are needed to support an orbital prosthesis, not for retention but because of the higher rate of implant loss at this site (10,11).

Surgical Placement

The craniofacial implants are fabricated of commercially pure titanium. They are available in lengths of either 3 or 4 mm and have a 5-mm diameter flange (Fig. 25). The short lengths are designed to allow placement

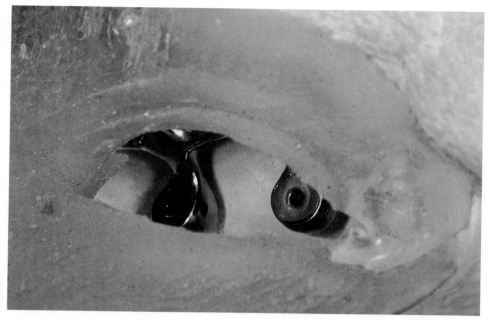

FIG. 24. This surgical template was used to help position implants during surgery.

in limited bone beds. The flange facilitates initial immobilization of the implant and prevents undue penetration into interior compartments.

A two-stage surgical procedure, basically the same as used in the intraoral application, is employed. Surgical placement can be conducted with local anesthesia but sterile conditions must be observed. A full-thickness flap is reflected and potential implant sites evaluated with the help of a surgical stent. The implant sites are prepared and tapped in the usual manner (12). A titanium cover screw is placed into the implant to prevent ingrowth of bone and soft tissue during the 4 to 6-month healing period.

In the orbital area the supraorbital rim is usually the preferred site for the fixtures since the bone thickness is adequate in this area. A skin incision just below the eyebrow is made, the periosteal flap is reflected inferiorly, and, if the bone thickness allows, 4-mm long fix-

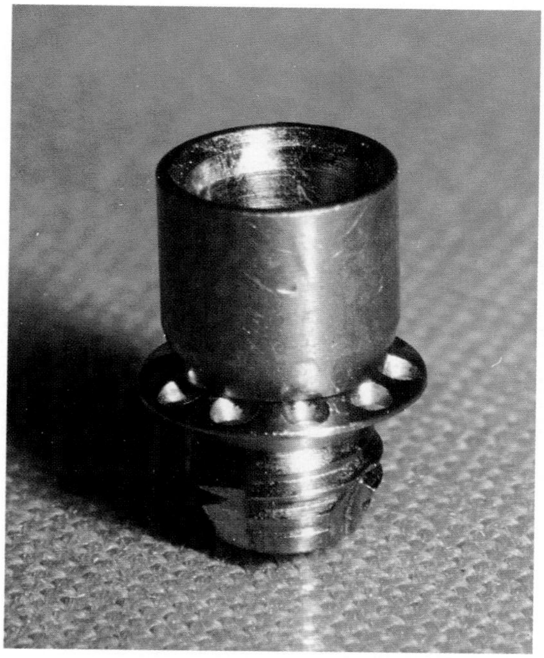

FIG. 25. An osseointegrated implant designed for use in the nasal, orbital, or auricular area.

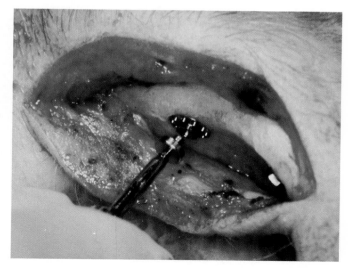

FIG. 26. Implant fixtures are being placed in the orbital rim.

tures are used. Two to three fixtures are sufficient to retain an orbital prosthesis (Fig. 26).

In the nasal area, there are three possible sites for the installation of the fixtures. If the patient is edentulous in the anterior maxillary area, two fixtures can be placed in the anterior nasal floor. When roots of teeth are present, the lateral wall of the periform aperture can be used as an implant fixture site bilaterally. Sufficient bone volume does not always exist in this area, however, and if not, the superior nasal area is another option. At this site one 4- to 7-mm fixture can be placed in what remains of the nasal bones or into the anterior wall of the frontal sinus. The nasolabial fold area should be avoided. Mobility of the tissues in this area

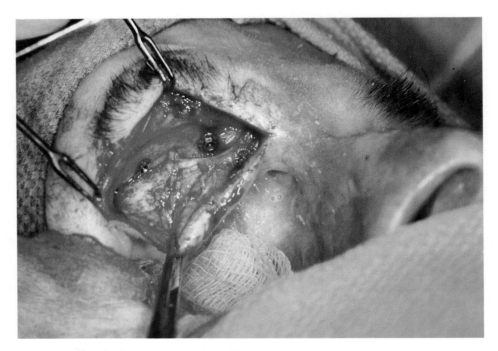

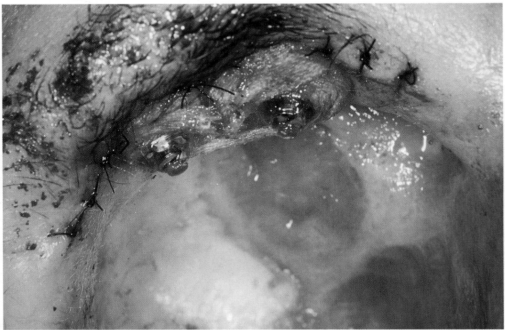

FIG. 27. At the second stage the implants are exposed, abutments are connected **(A)**, and a compression dressing is placed **(B)**.

from lip movement results in frictional irritation of the soft tissues around the implants, leading to inflammation and proliferation of granulation tissue.

At the second stage a transcutaneous abutment cylinder is attached. Special care must be directed toward thinning the tissue flap over the implant sites prior to placement of the abutments. This procedure will lead to the formation of epithelial cuffs around the abut-

ments and facilitate the maintenance of healthy peri-implant soft tissues.

The second surgical exposure of implants and the placement of the transepithelial abutments are generally performed 4 to 6 months after the first stage. In cases where the total length of the fixture was not seated within the cortical bone at the time of installation or the fixture was seated in loose cancellous bone,

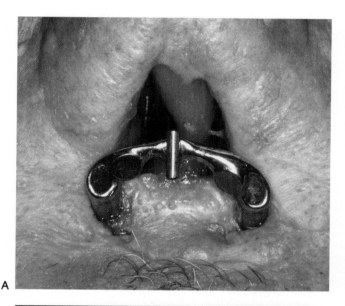

A

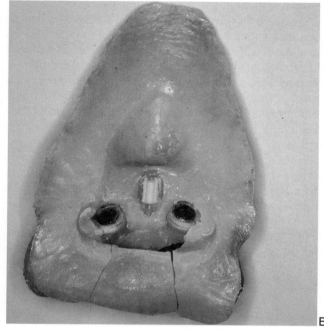

B

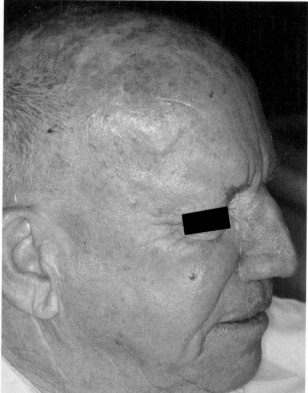

C

FIG. 28. The retentive mechanism has been designed so as not to distort the contours of the prosthesis.

a healing time of 6 months is preferred. The second-stage surgical procedure can be performed with local anesthesia and, when necessary, conscious sedation is added. A sterile approach is also required for the second stage.

For the orbital area, the second-stage procedure is similar to the technique described for the oral cavity. The incision is created inferior to the eyebrow and the flap reflected supraperiosteally. The cover screws are located and the periosteum over the implants is removed with a punch blade knife. The overlying soft tissue flap is thinned by removing subcutaneous tissue. This flap is then repositioned and the skin is perforated over the fixtures. The cover screws are removed and the abutments are connected on top of the fixtures. Healing caps are placed and polysporin-impregnated gauze is wrapped around the abutment sleeves in order to compress the soft tissue flap (Fig. 27). Use of free skin grafts has not been necessary for the orbital rim region.

For the nasal area, the second-stage procedure is similar. However, due to the anatomic limitations and close approximation to the oral cavity, extreme care is necessary to avoid a through and through communication from the dermis layer into the oral cavity. A major goal during the second surgical stage is to reduce the thickness of the tissue flap in order to provide a nonmobile tissue bed around the implants and to use as short an abutment sleeve as possible.

Prosthesis Design Considerations

While the details concerning fabrication of facial prostheses are beyond the scope of this chapter, a few basic principles should be mentioned. A resection moulage can be very helpful. Impressions of the defect are usually obtained with elastic impression materials, taking care not to displace the tissues being recorded. The contours of the prostheses are sculpted in wax, both on the cast and on the patient. Surface characteristics, appropriate contour, coloration, and margin placement are equally important factors to be considered. Processing the materials used in facial restoration is complicated and requires special instrumentation. Special large flasks are necessary for processing large prostheses.

The retentive mechanism must be contoured and positioned so as to avoid creating distortions of the facial prosthesis (Fig. 28). The silicone elastomers continue to be the most popular materials used in facial restorations. This material is easy to process, accepts extrinsic coloration, and exhibits acceptable color stability when exposed to the ultraviolet rays of the sun. However, its poor edge strength requires that templates of

acrylic resin be fabricated to house the retentive network. These templates are fashioned to fit within the confines of silicone facial prostheses.

Coloration

Coloration of the prosthesis varies with the materials used and the preference of the clinician. Basic skin tones should be developed into a shade guide for each material. The base shade selected for a patient should be slightly lighter than the lightest skin tones of the patient, because as color is added extrinsically the prosthesis will darken. Color may be applied either intrinsically or extrinsically. Intrinsic coloration is longer lasting and is therefore preferred, but it is more difficult to accomplish than extrinsic coloration.

Maintenance

In implant patients hygiene is achieved by sulcus style toothbrushes, proxy brushes, and other oral hygiene aids. If daily hygiene is not maintained, keratin and debris begin to accumulate on the abutment cylinders, resulting in inflammatory reactions and tissue hypertrophy. Three month follow-up is recommended.

REFERENCES

1. Ordway D. The crisis of cancer—challenge to change. *J Prosthet Dent* 1977;37:184.
2. Curtis T, Beumer J. Restoration of acquired hard palate defects: etiology, disability and rehabilitation. In Beumer J, Curtis T, Firtell D, eds. *Maxillofacial rehabilitation.* St Louis: CV Mosby, 1979;202.
3. Parel S, Branemark P-I, Jansson T. Osseointegration in maxillofacial prosthetics. Part 1: Intraoral applications. *J Prosthet Dent* 1986;55:490.
4. Lang B, Bruce R. Presurgical maxillectomy prosthesis. *J Prosthet Dent* 1967;17:613.
5. Desjardins R. Obturator prosthesis design for acquired maxillary defects. *J Prosthet Dent* 1978;39:424.
6. Curtis T, Beumer J. Speech, palatopharygeal function and restoration of soft palate defects. In: Beumer J, Curtis T, Firtell D, eds. *Maxillofacial rehabilitation.* St Louis: CV Mosby, 1979; 275.
7. Beumer J, Zlotolow I. Restoration of facial defects. In: Beumer J, Curtis T, Firtell D, eds. *Maxillofacial rehabilitation.* St Louis: CV Mosby, 1979;333.
8. Marunick M, Harrison R, Beumer J. Prosthetic rehabilitation of midfacial defects. *J Prosthet Dent* 1985;54:533.
9. Hamada M, Lee R, Beumer J, Moy P. Craniofacial implants in maxillofacial rehabilitation. *J Calif Dent Assoc* 1989;17:25.
10. Jacobsson M, Tjellstrom A, Fine L, Andersson H. A restrospective study of osseointegrated skin penetrating titanium fixtures used to retain facial prostheses. *Int J Oral Maxillofac Implants* 1992;7:523.
11. Nishimura R. Use of osseointegrated implants in restoration of facial defects. Part II. Orbital defects. *J Prosthet Dent (in press).*
12. Tjellstrom A, Lindstrom J, Nylen O, Albrektsson B, Nero H, Sylven C. The bone acnhored auricular episthesis. *Laryngoscope* 1981;XC15:811.

PART V

Related Conditions and Procedures

CHAPTER 31

Transseptal Transsphenoidal Pituitary Surgery

Bruce W. Pearson

Pituitary disorders do not often present to a rhinologist. Rather, the nasal surgeon is drawn into the world of the pituitary specialist by the need for rhinologic access. If we are privileged to be part of the treatment team, it behooves us to know something of the endocrinology.

PITUITARY GLAND AND HYPOTHALAMUS

The word *pituitary,* meaning "pertaining to the secretion of mucus or phlegm" (L. *pituita,* a glutinous mucus), recalls the ancient Vesalian myth that the pituitary gland was the source of our nasal secretions. But it also acknowledged a fact of important anatomy, the accessible position of the pituitary gland, in relation to the subjacent nose. Hypophysis (Gr. *hypo* under + *physis* growth, an outgrowth below the brain) is a safer term.

The popular concept of the pituitary gland as "master gland," somehow functioning autonomously to supervise and coordinate our metabolism, is a contemporary physiologic legend. The pituitary gland is remarkable but not autonomous. Both of its parts, the adenohypophysis and the neurohypophysis, are closely regulated by the hypothalamus (Gr. *hypo* under + *thalamus* compartment, in reference to its position beneath the third ventricle). The hypothalamus, in turn, receives input from virtually the entire central nervous system! Supervision of the anterior pituitary is communicated through a specialized portal vascular system. The posterior pituitary is, in essence, an extension of some specialized hypothalamic neurons whose cell bodies are actually resident in the hypothalamus.

Hypothalamic neurohormones regulate the synthesis and secretion of at least six major peptide hormones produced by the anterior pituitary. These in turn circulate to the thyroid, the adrenals, the gonads, and to several sensitive tissues involved in growth and lactation. The posterior pituitary serves as a storage depot and releasing center for two more peptide hormones, pitressin, or antidiuretic hormone (ADH), and oxytocin. ADH regulates water balance; milk ejection and uterine contractions are influenced by oxytocin. Both peptides are made in cell bodies within the hypothalamus and released from the axons, which have descended to become the neurohypophysis.

As we have noted, the hypothalamus receives neural impulses from virtually all of the central nervous system, which it integrates, to program the synthesis and release of a whole arsenal of hypothalamic neurohormones. These, in turn, regulate the pituitary gland. Virtually all hormones produced in the hypothalamus and the pituitary are secreted in tiny bursts. In addition, adrenocorticotropic hormone (ACTH), growth hormone (GH), and prolactin have a diurnal rhythmicity, and hormones like luteinizing hormone (LH) and follicle-stimulating hormone (FSH), during the menstrual cycle, have longer ultradian rhythms.

The cells of the anterior lobe, which comprise 80% of the pituitary by weight, are particularly interesting to the rhinologist because, like the nose, they originally came from the foregut. An outpouching of primitive ectoderm called Rathke's pouch contacts the underside of the neural tube. This connection persists as the tube develops into the diencephalon. The lower extracranial tissues disappear and the mesoderm taking their place eventually becomes the palate, vomer, and sphenoid.

Hormones secreted by the hypothalamus into the portal vascular system have both releasing and inhibiting effects on the anterior pituitary. They bind to specific receptors on pituitary cell membranes and initiate a sequence of metabolic steps, which either amplify or inhibit the release of intracellular pituitary hormones into the general circulation. Thyrotropin-releasing hormone (TRH) stimulates the pituitary synthesis and secretion of prolactin and thyroid-stimulating hormone (TSH). The rate of GH production depends on the relative strengths of somatotropin (a negative control over GH and TSH) and growth hormone-releasing hormone (GHRH). Corticotropin-releasing hormone (CRH) stimulates the release of ACTH from the pituitary, and gonadotropin-releasing hormone (GRH) stimulates the secretion of LH and FSH.

As you might expect, hypothalamic abnormalities can alter the secretion of hypothalamic neurohormones and thus affect pituitary function. Hypothalamic lesions that lead to hypersecretion of neurohormones may be responsible for some cases of Cushing's syndrome and precocious puberty, and for these, pituitary surgery would, of course, not be therapeutic.

Clinical Presentations of Pituitary Disease

Patients with hypothalamic–pituitary disorders present with the following:

1. Symptoms of a mass lesion, such as a visual field defect.
2. Hypersecretion syndromes, caused by an excess of one or more pituitary hormones, for example, acromegaly, Cushing's disease, or amenorrhea–galactorrhea (Forbes–Albright syndrome).
3. Hyposecretion syndromes involving one or more pituitary hormones, most commonly panhypopituitarism (any of these syndromes may be based on other etiologies, and many presentations are mixtures).
4. Asymptomatic disturbances of the sella.

In the latter case, a mass involving the pituitary is often suggested by the chance finding of an enlarged sella turcica on a skull or sinus radiograph taken for other purposes. An enlarged sella, without any endocrine or visual disorder, may represent a nonpituitary disorder, such as the so-called empty sella syndrome. Pituitary function is usually normal in such a case, and no specific therapy is required. But the actual diagnosis can be difficult, and of course asymptomatic enlargement deserves careful study for a long list of pituitary and nonpituitary possibilities.

Differential Diagnosis

Between 1972 and 1985, Mayo Clinic otolaryngologists assisted their colleagues in neurosurgery in the performance of 1761 transseptal–transsphenoidal procedures on 1689 patients. Of these, 1047 were for functioning pituitary adenomas, and 431 were for nonfunctioning adenomas. There were 66 craniopharyngiomas, 68 empty sellas or cerebrospinal fluid (CSF) rhinorrheas from the sella, and 59 miscellaneous pathologies. Eighteen hypophysectomies were performed for ablative purposes, but this is almost never seen now since the conditions for which it was attempted (diabetic retinopathy and/or metastatic bone pain) are better treated by laser ophthalmologic procedures or, in the case of metastatic bone pain, chemotherapy and specialized analgesia techniques.

Most adenomas presented with endocrine dysfunction (e.g., acromegaly) or mass effects (e.g., visual field defects). The removal of pituitary adenomas was actually more easily accomplished than removal of the normal gland. This was probably because ablative hypophysectomies on normal pituitary glands were performed on brittle diabetics or cancer patients who were much more sick. The sella, of course, was intact in these cases; whereas in many adenomas, it had been thinned and eroded by the tumor, reducing the need for surgical force.

Nonpituitary lesions are important in the differential diagnosis of sellar and parasellar masses. We recognize the following seven categories and try to think of these systematically when we are considering the possible etiology in atypical cases.

I. Cell rest tumors are exemplified by craniopharyngiomas, but chordomas, skull base cholesteatomas, and keratomas are also primitive germ rest possibilities.
II. There are two important primary neural tumors that can erode the sella—gliomas and meningiomas. Gliomas sometimes originate within the optic chiasm. Meningiomas that invade the sella often arise from the sphenoid ridge.
III. Certain malignant tumors can metastasize to the sellar region, such as breast, lung, kidney, and colon.
IV. Vascular lesions, such as an internal carotid aneurysm, rarely occur within the sella.
V. Sphenoid mucoceles and mucopyoceles are the most likely sinus disorders to involve the sella.
VI. Granulomas like sarcoidosis, and even Wegener's granuloma, are not entirely unknown.
VII. A final category of miscellaneous CSF-related entities (such as the empty sella) completes the list of nonpituitary possibilities.

Historical Background

Illustrations from the early German literature show that in the 19th century, the behavior of untreated pituitary tumors was well understood from autopsies. Downward descent into the sphenoid and erosion into the clivus (the solid triangle of basal spheno-occipital skull bone between the sphenoid and the foramen magnum) were clearly depicted. Stretching of the optic chiasm over a superior growth phase and enlargement to disturb the third cranial nerve were well illustrated; preservation of the diaphragm sella, that is, the membranous barrier between the sella and the cranial cavity, was clearly recognized, even in the presence of very extensive tumors.

Extracranial operations made their initial appearances in the first decade of this century. Eiselsberg's (1) approach to the pituitary, through the nose, required a facial incision that ran transversely across the root of the nose, then down the nasofacial groove and finally back across the base of the nose, so the entire external nasal pyramid could be turned aside like a lid, hinged on the soft tissues of the remaining side (Fig. 1). Another approach was offered in which the entire external nose was freed, superiorly and on both sides, to be turned downward based on the upper lip.

The object of these rather drastic rhinotomies was to allow the contents of both nasal cavities, the turbinates, and the septum—in fact everything between the eyes—to be exenterated! Open access to the anterior cranial fossa, the optic nerves, and the hypophysis was required, of course, because conditions of magnification and illumination were limited, tumors were large, often blinding, and sophisticated preoperative imaging and planning procedures had yet to make their appearance. Unfortunately, experience soon showed that crusting and infection were overwhelming whenever the midfacial anatomy was deemed expendable, an intolerable and sometimes fatal complication in the absence of antibiotics.

As early as 1909, Hirsch (2), in Vienna, reported that a submucosal, transseptal approach to the anterior wall of the sphenoid could be achieved through the septal mucosal incision, described by Killian (3), and chisels directed posteriorly through this approach could open both the sphenoid and the sella. Kanavel (4) (Fig. 2) had diagramed the necessary septal framework dissection that same year; so separation and deflection of the septal cartilage from the ethmoid plate and vomer, resection of the bone in the way of the sella (i.e., the lower half of the ethmoid plate and the upper half of the vomer), and, finally, removal of the rostrum of the sphenoid are nothing new. In Baltimore the next year, 1910, Halstead (5) approached the septum by raising the lip through the sublabial incision, and had he stayed submucosal instead of resecting the septum entirely, it might not have fallen to Cushing (Fig. 3), employing the sublabial approach of Halstead (5) and the submucosal dissection of Hirsch (2), to pioneer the initial experience with the sublabial transseptal–transsphenoidal approach we currently use today. Interestingly, the illustrations of hypophysectomy in Cushing's publications show that the anesthesia was administered with

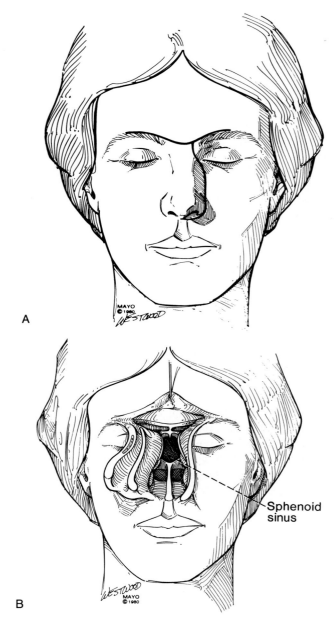

FIG. 1. Eiselberg's extracranial incision providing access to the pituitary gland via the sphenoidal sinus, done around 1910. **A:** Incision outlined. **B:** Sphenoidal sinus exposed. (From ref. 8, with permission.)

a suspended tonsillectomy gag; the septal space was exposed with a bivalved gynecologic speculum, and the whole field was illuminated with the aid of an otolaryngologic headlight.

Unfortunately for this technology, Cushing (6) and Dandy (7) and others soon built a much more attractive infrastructure for transcranial surgery, and although Hirsch kept the faith, an open exposure through the cranial fossae, bypassing the contamination and the vascularity of the nose, became fashionable. Neurosurgical interest in the rhinologic approaches waned,

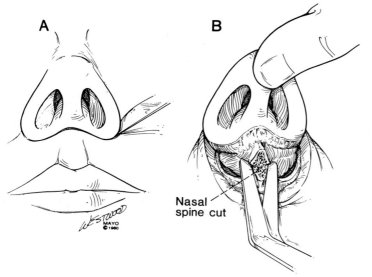

FIG. 2. Kanavel's subnasal incision for transseptal sphenoidal hypophysectomy (about 1909). (From ref. 8, with permission.)

and it is almost a miracle that Cushing's pupil, Dott, Dott's pupil, Guiot, and Guiot's pupil, Hardy, carried the transseptal operation from Baltimore to Edinburgh to Paris to Montreal, where it reemerged in the 1960s (8).

It is interesting to look back at descriptions of neurosurgical approaches to the sellar region. Early on, of course, it was feared by many surgeons that nasal procedures provided exposure that was too limited and contamination that was too dangerous. Consequently, a large frontoparietal bone flap was turned, pedicled on the temporalis muscle; the temporal lobe was elevated; and the sella, hiding beyond the cavernous sinus, the

carotid siphon, and a few major cranial nerves, was approached through the middle cranial fossa. There were also transfrontal approaches, such as the one described by Bronson Ray. The medial anterior portion of the frontal bone flap generally entered the frontal sinus, so mucosal contamination was not truly avoided. At least one olfactory tract had to be transected, and the tissues fixing the optic chiasm over the jugum sellae had to be released to come down on the pituitary. In normal anatomic situations, the prechiasmal space is about 8 mm long, and the length of the tuberculum sellae is 5 mm. With a prefixed chiasm, the space is only about 3 mm long! (Sometimes the chiasm

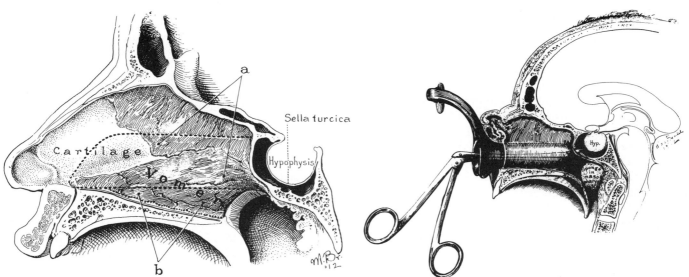

FIG. 3. Cushing's approach to the pituitary through a sublabial submucosal transseptal dissection (about 1912). A: Amount of bone and cartilage removed. B: Speculum in place. (From ref. 8, with permission.)

is much further posterior; in 10% of patients, it lies over the tuberculum sellae.)

The current Mayo Clinic transsphenoidal operation arose primarily through the collaboration of two strong personalities, Dr. Ed Laws and Dr. Eugene Kern, merging the Hopkins tradition of neurosurgery (Dr. Laws) and the Cottle school of rhinology (Dr. Kern). The expertise fostered by Dr. Edward Rynearson and the many pituitary patients treated by Dr. Ray Randle and Dr. Charles Abboud and their colleagues in the Mayo Clinic Endocrine Department fueled demand; and supported, of course, by numerous colleagues, residents, and assistants, these two surgeons launched an experience that now reaches beyond 2000 patients. Most of the information and surgical techniques described in this chapter are based on observations derived as this series evolved. From the viewpoint of one privileged to participate with this team many times, it is recorded here with the wistful reflection that we may never have the opportunity to amass such a concentrated experience again.

Preoperative Consultations

Preoperative consultations are obtained with ophthalmology, radiology, rhinology, neurosurgery, and endocrinology. The ophthalmologist documents visual acuity and maps the visual fields. A radiologist obtains coronal computed tomography (CT) scans and, more importantly, magnetic resonance imaging (MRI) scans, which are of tremendous assistance in localizing the tumor. Full investigation requires arteriography only infrequently—certainly not as a routine study.

The pituitary gland is probably best seen preoperatively on the lateral magnetic resonance imaging (MRI) scan of the head. The gland itself is nestled in the sella turcica (for its resemblance to a Turkish saddle) in the posterosuperior quadrant of the sphenoid sinus (Fig. 4). The upper portion of the pons lies behind the body of the gland and the optic chiasm is generally visible in front of the stalk. Above the pituitary lies the hypothalamus; the downward, funnel-shaped element is called the infundibulum. The division of the pituitary into the adenohypophysis (anterior two-thirds) and neurohypophysis (posterior third) is also usually apparent (Fig. 5).

The rhinologist is concerned with the presence and degree of nasal deformities, nasal infection, and incidental nasal conditions like polyps or chronic ethmoiditis. Regional inflammatory conditions such as active dental abscesses or facial skin infections must be excluded, and intranasal conditions like septal perforations, nasal adhesions, or previous septal surgery need to be recognized and discussed with the patient. The preoperative rhinologic interview gives the surgeon

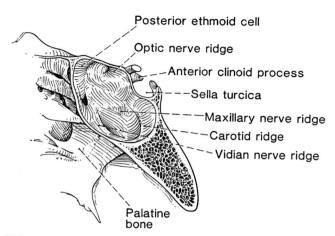

FIG. 4. Anatomy of lateral wall of sphenoid sinus and relations of the sella turcica. (From ref. 9, with permission.

and patient a chance to clarify expectations related to nasal packing and its removal. Standard preoperative photographs are usually obtained. Sometimes this is also an opportunity to address correction or improvement of an external nasal deformity coincident with the surgery at hand.

The preoperative neurosurgical consultation provides an opportunity to determine the status of cranial nerves, the presence or absence of elevated intracranial pressures, and the serious neurologic risks that are being undertaken. Patients need to understand the potential for injury of a cranial nerve, the hypothalamus, or associated vascular structures and to balance this against the morbidity of the disease for which they are considering surgery.

Finally, the endocrinology and laboratory assessments are completed. The complexities of this are well beyond the scope of this chapter, but we will briefly highlight a few of the hyperfunctional endocrine syndromes to at least provide the flavor. Later, we will return to these and mention how each of them impacts on rhinologic aspects of the surgery.

AMENORRHEA–GALACTORRHEA

The most common secretory tumor of the pituitary is one that produces an excess quantity of prolactin. Normally, prolactin plays an important role in the development of the breasts during pregnancy and in promoting lactation after the baby is born. Serum prolactin levels normally range below 20 ng/ml by radioimmunoassay.

The majority of prolactinomas seem to occur in women, and many are so-called microadenomas, that is, tumors less than 10 mm in diameter. The association of amenorrhea, galactorrhea, and a microadenoma of

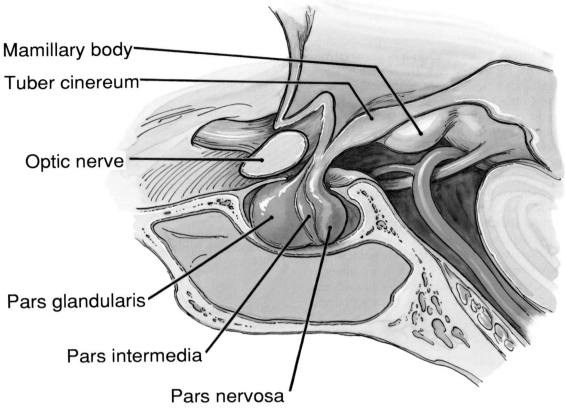

Mamillary body

Tuber cinereum

Optic nerve

Pars glandularis

Pars intermedia

Pars nervosa

FIG. 5. Anatomy of pituitary gland.

the pituitary is called the Forbes–Albright syndrome. Affected women also frequently complain of symptoms of estrogen deficiency, including hot flashes and dyspareunia (even though estrogen production may be normal).

Controversy exists about the optimum treatment of pituitary tumors associated with hyperprolactinemia. Patients with prolactin levels below 100 and normal CT scans have the option to be treated with bromocriptine and kept under surveillance. Even though endocrine symptoms will be controlled, patients treated with bromocriptine must be monitored regularly for the development of mass effects. Small tumors continue to grow and macroadenomas eventually may supervene. For those who are also hypoestrogenic and at risk of developing osteoporosis, surgical treatment is preferred. Surgery is clearly recommended in patients desiring pregnancy and those with embarrassing galactorrhea. To achieve cure with preservation of normal pituitary function, microsurgical removal with conservation of the remaining normal gland is probably the best treatment for patients with a microadenoma.

ACROMEGALY

Syndromes of excessive growth hormone secretion are nearly always due to a functioning pituitary adenoma. Hypersecretion in childhood is uncommon, but prior to closure of the epiphyses, it leads to exaggerated skeletal growth causing so-called pituitary gigantism. Excess growth hormone production occurs more often between the third and fifth decades, resulting in coarse facial features and soft tissue swelling of the "acral" or peripheral parts (i.e., the hands and feet). The size and function of sebaceous and sweat glands increase. Overgrowth of the mandible causes prognathism (Fig. 6). The tongue, which is enlarged and furrowed, constitutes a hazardous obstacle at intubation. Proliferation of the laryngeal cartilages deepens the voice. The effects on costal growth alter the shape of the chest. Articular cartilage proliferation leads to degenerative arthritis. Peripheral neuropathies are common. Many patients have impaired glucose tolerance, and clinically significant diabetes occurs in 10%. Since growth hormone itself is a weakly lactogenic hormone, inappropriate lactation is sometimes seen. Nearly all acromegalic women develop menstrual abnormalities with amenorrhea, and one-third of men develop sexual dysfunction.

Plasma growth hormone levels, measured by radioimmunoassay are typically elevated above 5 ng/ml in acromegaly. Skull roentgenograms show characteristic bony changes, cortical thickening, and frontal sinus enlargement. These features of the disease increase the

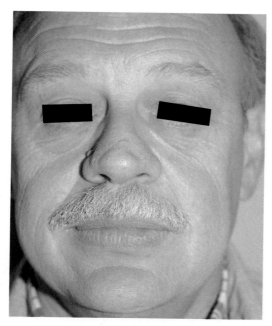

FIG. 6. Acromegaly.

difficulty of transfrontal craniotomy, which was once used more commonly than the rhinologic routes to gain surgical access to the tumor.

Transsphenoidal resection of the functioning adenoma is the preferred treatment today, but radiation therapy may also play a helpful role. Sometimes growth hormone levels are not lowered to normal despite both surgery and radiotherapy, and patients may require medical suppression with bromocriptine mesylate, up to 15 mg/day orally, in divided doses, to help control elevated levels.

CUSHING'S SYNDROME

The term Cushing's syndrome refers to the clinical state resulting from cortisol excess, regardless of the source of the cortisol. Hyperfunction of the adrenal cortex may depend on excess stimulation by ACTH, or cortisol may be produced autonomously by adrenocortical tumors. When excess ACTH is the cause, the source may be the pituitary, an ectopic nonpituitary tumor, or exogenous administration of ACTH. Hyperfunction of the adrenal cortex resulting from pituitary ACTH excess is referred to as Cushing's *disease*. Cushing's disease is generally due to a basophilic adenoma or chromophobe adenoma of the pituitary. When evidence of ACTH overproduction is found in the absence of an obvious sellar lesion, microadenomas are still the usual cause.

The altered general health of Cushing's disease patients adversely impacts on their surgical risk. Patients typically suffer unstable hypertension and osteoporosis, and psychiatric disturbances are not at all uncommon. Temporal balding, hypertrichosis, and other signs of virilism in the female may contribute a bit to this problem; they result from an increasing production of androgens. The skin and mucous membranes are thin and friable in Cushing's disease. Excessive ecchymosis of the cheek and upper lip is often produced by transseptal surgery, and wound healing is mildly retarded.

Patients with Cushing's syndrome usually exhibit elevated levels of morning cortisol, and they lack the normal diurnal decline. Medical therapy includes replacement of potassium, a high protein intake, and sometimes chemical blockade of steroid secretion with aminoglutethimide. Transsphenoidal exploration of the pituitary and excision of the tumor if found are probably best performed in experienced centers. If no tumor is found, the decision between hypophysectomy and irradiation may be problematic. Bilateral adrenalectomy is generally reserved for patients who fail to respond to these measures. Adrenalectomy requires steroid replacement for the remainder of the patient's life, and it also carries a serious risk of developing Nelson–Salassa syndrome. In this disorder, the pituitary gland continues to expand, which produces visual defects, pressure on the hypothalamus, and other local complications. But the most striking phenomenon of Nelson–Salassa syndrome is severe hyperpigmentation of the skin. β-Melanophore stimulating hormone secretion is increased, and darkening of the skin is the clinical consequence.

MULTIPLE ENDOCRINE NEOPLASIA

A group of genetically distinct familial diseases is now recognized in which benign adenomatous hyperplasia and malignant tumor formation involving several endocrine glands occur in characteristic patterns. These are known as the multiple endocrine neoplasia (MEN) syndromes. MEN-1 includes hyperparathyroidism and pancreatic islet cell tumors (often with severe peptic ulceration, i.e., Zollinger–Ellison syndrome). In 65% of cases, a pituitary tumor also occurs, usually a chromophobe adenoma, and often with prolactin and growth hormone hypersecretion. As in Cushing's disease, safe perioperative management surrounding the pituitary surgery of MEN-1 patients requires a well-coordinated team and an extensive medical infrastructure.

TECHNIQUE OF TRANSSPHENOIDAL HYPOPHYSECTOMY

Transsphenoidal hypophysectomy has three components: exposure of the sellar floor by the nasal surgeon,

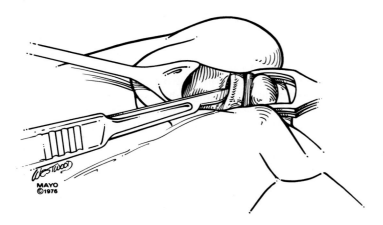

MAYO ©1976

FIG. 7. Surgeon (who is right-handed) holds Cottle columellar clamp in left hand and assistant holds alar protector. After columella clamp has been applied to identify caudal end of septum, right hemitransfixion incision is made about 1 to 2 mm behind caudal end of nasal septum with No. 15 blade. (From ref. 10, with permission.)

removal of the pituitary pathology plus repair of the sellar defect by the neurosurgeon, and closure and repair of the nasal and sublabial wounds by the nasal surgeon again.

Transseptal Exposure

The opening nasal procedure is performed using a headlight and standard methods of general anesthesia and nasal decongestion. The free caudal end of the septal cartilage is sharply exposed in the right nostril through a *right* septal mucosal incision, the so-called hemitransfixion incision of the Cottle septoplasty (Fig. 7). The free mobile edge of the cartilage is hooked to the right, a columella clamp is used to draw the columellar soft tissues to the left (Fig. 8), and the tension necessary to support the opening of a submucosal plane ("anterior tunnel") between the septal cartilage

and the *left* mucoperichondrial flap is generated. Careful sharp dissection with a Cottle knife through the tough subperichondrial planes over the first 1½ to 2 cm of the septal cartilage rewards the operator with wide access into the much more favorable plane behind it (Fig. 9), in which the mucoperichondrium strips up very easily, requiring only a tapered Cottle suction, and the short, then medium, nasal specula for exposure.

At this point, there is no need to extend this dissection all the way posterosuperiorly past the ethmoid plate. It is better to gain more anterior exposure first. Inferiorly, the anterior tunnel is limited, at the junction of the septal cartilage with the septal crest of the premaxilla, by the tough perichondrium that follows the septal cartilage around its inferior edge, passing beneath the cartilage and fused to the periosteum covering the bone. This layer of connective tissue, which will be referred to later as the "transverse aponeurosis" of

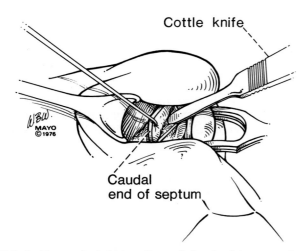

Cottle knife

Caudal end of septum

FIG. 8. Through right hemitransfixion incision, quadrangular septal cartilage is retracted to right with hook, and Cottle knife is used to begin left anterior tunnel by sharp dissection beneath mucoperichondrium of septal cartilage. (From ref. 10, with permission.)

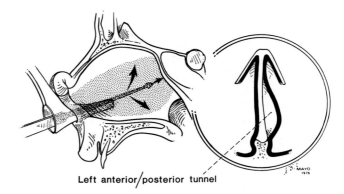

Left anterior/posterior tunnel

FIG. 9. As dissection continues, left anterior tunnel becomes left anterior/posterior tunnel with elevation of mucoperiosteum of perpendicular plate of ethmoid and vomer in posterior portion of nose. With nasal speculum placed through incision into left anterior tunnel, Cottle suction is used to continue mucoperichondrial and mucoperiosteal elevation back to face of sphenoid. (From ref. 10, with permission.)

the septum, is the sheet that connects the right and left septal mucosa across the septo-premaxillary suture line. The left anterior tunnel is considered complete just as soon as the left side of the septal cartilage is bared, and before the very tough transverse aponeurosis is incised.

The next technique of the nasal dissection, generally attributed to Cottle, is known as the maxilla–premaxilla approach. This step, initiated behind the top of the filtrum of the upper lip, but through the septal incision, can make the difference between a safe, dry nasal operation and a septal injury with bleeding. Turn the points of a small, blunt Knapp scissor downward, hug the bony premaxilla, and spread open a plane in the connective tissues directly anterior to the nasal spine (Fig. 10). The "prespine" fascia is exposed by this maneuver, a tough layer of shaggy periosteum coating the entire face of the premaxilla. Incise it sharply on either side of the anterior nasal spine, and then contact the bone of the premaxilla directly with the tip of a Mackenty elevator. Use this to strip the periosteum off the upper anterior surface of the premaxilla to visualize the inferior margin of the piriform aperture. This is the sharp bony rim between the premaxilla and the nasal cavity floor, on either side of the spine. There is no need to remove bone here, as some surgeons advocate, or to destroy the anterior nasal spine.

One advantage (besides familiarity to most rhinologists) with approaching the septal dissection through the nose this way, instead of up under the lip, is that neither the pyriform margin or the anterior nasal spine is in the way. A "full-curve" Cottle elevator can be curled over the pyriform margins, under direct vision now, to strip up the mucoperichondrium of the right and left nasal cavity floors. These are the so-called bilateral inferior tunnels (Fig. 11). Thus three separate anterior nasal submucoperiosteal tunnels have been created—two on the floor and one on the left side of the septal cartilage—and all that is needed is to connect them up by working in the following manner.

Elevate the periosteum fused to the flaring septal crest of the premaxilla by extending the inferior tunnels medially and upward until you reach the out-turned "wings" of the crest. These "support" the lowest margin of the septal cartilage but remain separated from it by the dense aponeurosis of investing periosteum. The anterior terminations of the septal sphenopalatine arteries pass from the septal mucoperiosteum behind the premaxilla wings into the incisive foramina on either side, and these will be stretched or divided.

Successful transseptal exposure now rests on the skill of the rhinologist in connecting the left inferior and left anterior tunnels, then connecting this in turn to the right inferior tunnel (Fig. 12). Rather tortuous bony irregularities and asymmetry are usual in the septal crest of the premaxilla. This is where the opportunity to initiate a tear in the septal mucoperichondrium is greatest. The sharp, spade-shaped end of a Cottle dissector and a No. 15 blade are now the right tools, plus a nasal speculum, to maintain the necessary tension. Cut the transverse aponeurosis sharply on the upper surface of the septal crest of the premaxilla, before its action as a fixation point results in a tear of the mucosa.

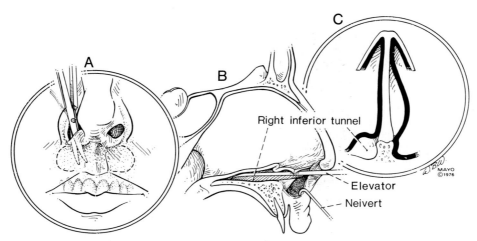

FIG. 10. A: Lip is undermined by elevating tip of nose with left hand and placing Knapp scissors into hemitransfixion incision between oral mucosa and orbicularis muscle anterior to nasal spine. Nasal spine and floor of nose are exposed (within limits of *dotted lines*) so that right inferior tunnel can be created. **B:** Narrow Neivert retractor is inserted into hemitransfixion incision and used to retract soft tissues to expose anterior nasal spine, pyriform aperture, and floor of nose on right. **C:** Curved Cottle elevator is used to elevate mucosa along floor of nose and to develop inferior tunnel. (From ref. 10, with permission.)

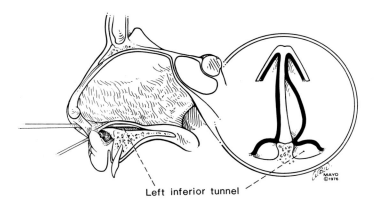

FIG. 11. Development of left inferior tunnel. Crest of pyriform aperture is identified, and curved Cottle elevator is used to elevate mucosa along floor of nose on left. Three tunnels have now been developed—left anteroposterior, right inferior, and left inferior. Note that left-sided tunnels are not connected, for tissue is firmly adherent to region of osseous and cartilaginous joint between quadrangular septal cartilage and crest of premaxilla. (From ref. 10, with permission.)

Eventually, the left anterior and inferior tunnels are connected, and the cartilage is dislocated to the right, adding the right inferior tunnel to the common exposure of the newly bared septal crest of the premaxilla.

From this point onward, use the tapered Cottle suction tube as the dissector. The right and left septal mucosal coverings are no longer fastened to each other by a transverse aponeurosis, as only the septal cartilage–septal crest suture line had one. The posterior edge of the septal cartilage can be dislocated off the vertical plate of the ethmoid under direct vision (Fig. 13), and bilateral submucosal tunnels ("posterior tunnels") can be extended back, straddling the ethmoid

plate with the speculum, all the while resecting bone as you go (Fig. 14). Dislocate the septal cartilage from the vomer and the premaxilla so that the posterior submucosal tunnels reveal the remaining ethmoid plate and the vomer. The slightly thickened ridge of bone representing the fusion line between the vomer and the ethmoid plate is the line of sight to the sphenoid rostrum. The septal cartilage, which is flexible and remains attached to its right nasal mucoperichondrium, is displaced to the right by the progressively longer specula, which are inserted astride the remaining bony ethmoid plate and vomer (Fig. 15).

The bony septum, which lies exposed, should be removed progressively with biting instruments, keeping at least one large bony "batten" to use later in supporting the sellar soft tissue graft (Fig. 16). When the posterior tunnels flare laterally, you are reaching the rostrum

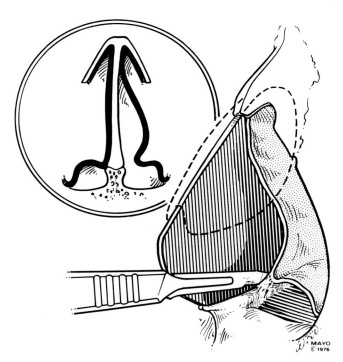

FIG. 12. Illustration of the development and joining of left anterior and left inferior tunnels by sharp dissection of fibrous tissue that binds mucosa in this area to crest of premaxilla. Care is taken not to perforate mucosa. (From ref. 10, with permission.)

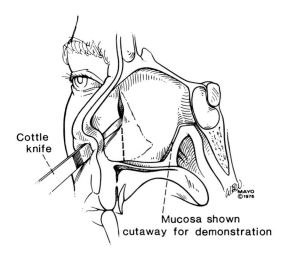

FIG. 13. Either with Cottle knife or Cottle suction tip in left anterior tunnel, posterior edge of quadrangular septal cartilage caudal to perpendicular plate of ethmoid is either incised or subluxed. Care is taken not to perforate mucosa. This allows access to right side of septum so that right posterior tunnel can be elevated before posterior portion of septum is removed. (From ref. 10, with permission.)

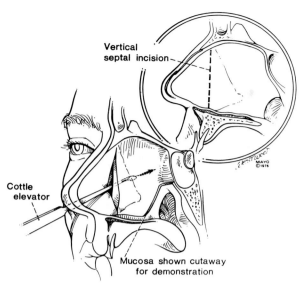

FIG. 14. Development of right posterior tunnel. With Cottle elevator placed through junction of cartilage and ethmoid plate, elevation begins on right side to create right posterior tunnel beneath mucoperiosteum. (From ref. 10, with permission.)

of the sphenoid. If the thin blades of the longest nasal speculum are inserted to the rostral level and cranked laterally, they will lightly crush the supreme turbinates outward, which allows visualization of the medial inferior margin of the sphenoid ostia. When these landmarks are identified, the *transnasal* (transnostril) portion of the dissection is complete.

Elevate the lip next, and make a transverse incision

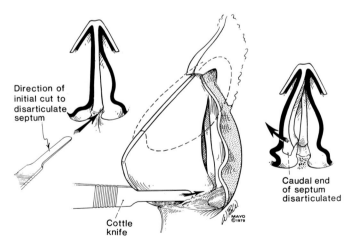

FIG. 15. By sharp dissection, caudal end of septum is disarticulated from attachment to anterior nasal spine and crest of premaxilla and vomer. This allows caudal end of septum, with mucosa attached on right side anteriorly, to be swung into right nasal chamber. Mucosa has been elevated away from both sides of posterior septum. Latter can now be removed back to face of sphenoid. (From ref. 10, with permission.)

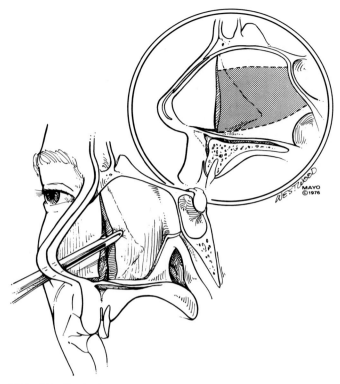

FIG. 16. Posterior septum, bony perpendicular plate of ethmoid, and vomer are removed back to face of sphenoid *(shaded area)* with Lillie–Koeffler bone forceps. (From ref. 10, with permission.)

in the gingivolabial mucosa just below the reflection of the labial mucosa and directly above the attached gingiva superior to the four anterior incisor teeth (Fig. 17). The scalpel blade quickly comes down on bone, bone that has already been uncovered by the anterior premaxilla dissection. Generous sublabial access is thus created into the nasal dissection (the "septal space"), and if the prespine fascia has been incised, the lip can be distended with ease. Now you can insert

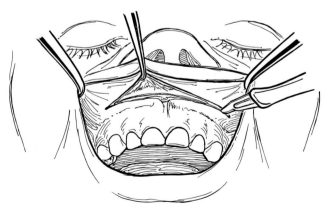

FIG. 17. Sublabial incision made from lateral incisor to lateral incisor.

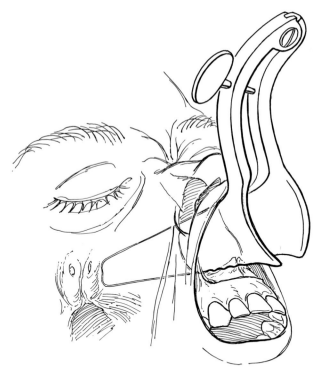

FIG. 18. Pituitary retractor in place anchored on the pyriform crest.

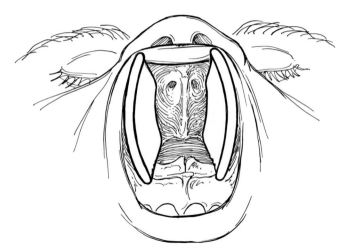

FIG. 19. Exposure of sphenoid rostrum and sphenoid ostia.

the self-retaining bivalved septal–pituitary speculum under the lip and into the septal space (Fig. 18). This bypasses the limitation that would otherwise be imposed by the small size and indistensible character of the external nostril. It avoids having to enlarge the nostril with any external cut, such as the transcolumellar or alar–facial groove incisions others have advocated.

As the speculum is inserted, the considerable advantages of having no mucosal perforation are apparent. The field is dry. As the blades of the speculum advance, they remain submucosal, with no tendency to pass out through a perforation into the nasal cavity. When the speculum tips are opened posteriorly, they create tension on the mucosal flaps. This prevents the flaps from bulging into the field between the bony face of the sphenoid and tips of the speculum blades. Clean, dry exposure of the sphenoid rostrum begets visualization of the sphenoid ostia (Fig. 19). Now use strong rongeurs like the Ferris–Smith and the Hajek to resect the rostrum and enter the sphenoid sinus. Small osteotomes or the drill can be used as well (Fig. 20). Initially, just remove the bone between the two ostia and strip out the sphenoid mucosa with cup forceps to stop it from fouling the suction. Laterally, use the Hajek to enlarge the opening as far as the nasal cavity will allow the speculum blades to go. Inferiorly, remove sufficient bone to visualize the sphenoid recess, the part of the sinus cavity that extends back below the sella tur-

cica. Save the highest resection until last. Stop when your recognize the angle between the ceiling of the sphenoid sinus and the anterior wall of the sella itself (Fig. 21). These landmarks are usually not visible unless the mucosa is removed. Sometimes, the tumor itself will be evident. If not, remember the sellar floor itself can be parchment thin because of the slow erosion from within.

It used to be claimed that anatomic deficiencies in sphenoid pneumatization would sometimes get in the way of a transseptal–transsphenoidal operation. However, even when pneumatization is poor, the sella can still be approached in the manner described. After the sphenoid rostrum is removed, the cancellous bone filling the interval between the sphenoid face and the sella can be removed with a mastoid curet. By manufactur-

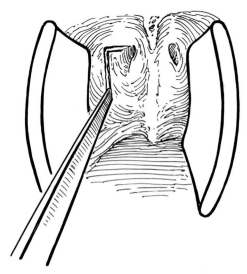

FIG. 20. Osteotome used to enter sphenoid sinus.

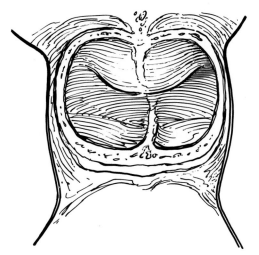

FIG. 21. Sella exposed.

ing a small pseudosphenoid sinus at surgery this way, pituitary access is possible. Orientation is facilitated by the fact that the transseptal approach identifies the midline, the nasal cavity projects the plane of the sphenoid roof, and the rostrum designates the level of the floor of the sella. The image intensifier ("C arm") is also brought into play.

REVIEW OF SURGICAL ANATOMY OF THE SEPTUM IN RELATION TO TRANSSEPTAL DISSECTIONS

Septal perforations are probably avoidable if the surgical anatomy of the septum is clear. The bony palate anterior to the incisive foramen came from the collision of the premaxillary elements of the palatine processes of the maxillae. The separate identity of the premaxilla is obliterated in adult life, but when the premaxillary processes meet in the midline, they deflect up to produce the lower anterior portion of the bony septum, the septal crest of the premaxilla. This is the anvil on which the transverse aponeurosis is divided, releasing the septal mucosa so it can be elevated without being torn. Anatomically, the premaxilla is also the bone of the pyriform margin and anterior alveolus, the bone from which the four incisor teeth have arisen. The septal component is unique because it is normally irregular and asymmetric and its mucoperiosteum is so densely adherent. Behind the incisive foramen, there are septal processes from the maxillae and palatine bones, but they contribute to a much smoother, thinner component to the septum.

The fibrous layer of the septal mucosa is continuous from one side to the other over the premaxillary portion of the septum (the transverse aponeurosis, Cottle's "decussating fibers"), whereas at all other suture lines (e.g., between the *maxillary* palatal elements of the septum and the vomer) and at the joints between the vomer on the ethmoid plate with the septal cartilage, no fibrous aponeurosis binds the right and left mucoperiosteal coverings together. The incisive foramen itself is originally a large midline passageway in the bony nasal floor just back of the septal crest of the premaxilla. The vomer articulates with the septal crest of the premaxilla, and a little flat tab projects downward from the vomer to divide the incisive foramen (on its nasal side) into two channels, through which the main arteries of the septum anastomose with the main arteries of the palate.

The septal arteries enter the nasal cavity through the sphenopalatine foramina, behind the posterior end of the middle turbinates. They cross the upper margin of the choana, turn downward and forward within the septal mucosa, parallel the anterior upper edge of the vomer, and leave the mucosa only when they reach the incisive foramen. Thus the septal mucosa is additionally bound to the junction of the nasal floor and the septum, just behind the septal crest of the premaxilla. Excessive bleeding from the septal arteries or the bone in the region of the incisive foramen may require cautery. An insulated Frazier suction tip works well.

The septal cartilage itself descends to articulate with or subluxate on the irregularities of the septal crest of the premaxilla. The normal anatomic, deformed developmental and post-traumatic vagaries of this cartilage and this articulation are countless. Sometimes the septal cartilage is midline and flat and fits nicely into the grooved upper surface of the crest. But very commonly, it curls off the one side or the other to create a minor or major subluxation or dislocation. These variations add interest to the submucosal dissection, but it is primarily the adhesions from one side to the other by the transverse aponeurosis that are important in terms of their tendency to invite a perforation.

Further anteriorly, in fact anterior to the plane of the premaxilla but arising from it, a sharp bipartite bony protuberance projects. This is the anterior nasal spine. Triangular in cross section, flat, not grooved, on its upper surface and sharply crested in the midline inferiorly, its downward and laterally facing concave surfaces are smoothly continuous with the anterior bony surface of the premaxilla. The right and left ridges continue out to become the sharp pyriform margins of the bony nasal aperture. The anterior nasal spine and the septal crest of the premaxilla both make contributions to the septum, but they are separate in function and concept. The septal crest, for example, is expendable; the nasal spine is not.

Trouble in transseptal surgery is initiated early by impatient technique during the exposure of the septal premaxillary crest. If the techniques of the crest are clear, the safety and satisfaction of transseptal exposure for hypophysectomy are greatly improved. The decision to operate on the nasal septum first, not elevating the lip until later, is based on the following facts. The premaxilla is better exposed first through the nose, so the hardest part of the dissection is simplified. The Cottle nasal instrument set is adapted to the septal hemitransfixion approach; why shouldn't patients with pituitary adenomas benefit from the extensive experience of septum reconstruction accumulated by rhinologic surgeons? The nasal spine can be preserved without compromising access since it does not fall into the line of vision during the transnasal dissection. The nasal approach starts immediately with orientation to the caudal border of the septal cartilage, a familiar sight in septoplasty operations. Finally, working through the nose maintains excellent proprioceptive feedback for the surgeon; there is no pressure from an elevated lip on the shafts of the instruments of dissection.

Introduction of the Pituitary Speculum

A number of transseptal pituitary specula are available. We use the Hubbard speculum for its powerful opening mechanism (it can compress the turbinates) and the slightly outcurved blades at the tip. The metal is strong, so the blades themselves can be thin, which reduces the room taken up by blade thickness. The speculum is introduced through the sublabial incision in the closed position, then parted slightly to straddle the anterior nasal spine. The direction of introduction is backward, not up, parallel to the direction of the upper edge of the vomer. Advance the speculum back through the septal space under direct vision, using a suction and headlight, and search out the sphenoid rostrum. If a small portion of the posterior end of the ethmoid plate was left in place, positive identification of the midline will prove easier. When the speculum tips contact the face of the sphenoid, they are gradually opened while the pressure of advancement is maintained. In this way, as the speculum tips diverge, they slide back into the sphenoethmoidal recess, still under cover of the septal mucosa.

If a large mucosal perforation is present, it can be helpful to prepare two stiff "insulating" plates of thin polyethylene and place them in the septal space to guide the speculum without enlarging the perforation. A little "step" is cut on the lower edge of the plates to hook them onto the pyriform aperture. Otherwise, as the speculum is advanced between them, it is hard to prevent them from being displaced backward. Once advanced, the speculum can be opened without punching into the nasal cavity because now the plates carry the mucosa aside.

The lower aspect of the face of the sphenoid is extremely heavy bone, composed of the sphenoid floor, the medially arching sphenoid processes of the palatine bones, and the thick flared posterior wings of the vomer. Slightly higher, the face is thin and the bone around the sphenoid ostia is actually fragile. By removing the bone between the two ostia, including the midline rostrum, with rongeurs connecting the ostia in fact, access to the sphenoid cavity is achieved without risking entry into the anterior cranial fossa. By entering the weak face instead of the heavy floor, transnasal drills, chisels, and mallets are all unnecessary. Clear orientation to the rostrum and the sphenoid ostia is essential for safety, superiorly, of course, but also because it directs the entry to the midline. Incidentally, if the mucosa of the sphenoethmoid recess bulges into the field just beyond the speculum tips, try advancing the tips of the sphenoid speculum just inside the sphenoid *sinus*, then open them in the normal fashion.

The lateral walls of the sphenoid remain out of view (even after the entry into the sinus is suitably enlarged). The sphenoid sinus contains several vital ridges in its lateral wall, raised by the optic nerve and the carotid artery, and in some cases the vidian nerve. They *can* be viewed with a 70-degree telescope, but the transseptal approach forces the operator to hew to the midline, and the contours raised by these important anatomic neighbors of the sphenoid are not particularly evident in the usual surgical case.

Sellar Dissection

With the speculum in place and a dry field, the operating microscope, the image intensifier, and the neurosurgeon all enter the field. Some tumors are already exposed in the sphenoid, having eroded through the posterior wall. Others, such as microadenomas, offer no evidence of their presence. The sella is opened by cracking its bone with a chisel and flaking away the necessary portions of the anterior wall and floor (Fig. 22). A needle aspiration is performed to alert the surgeon to the presence of an empty sella. The dura is cauterized, then opened with a scalpel (Fig. 23). The dural opening must be bold enough to penetrate right through to the gland. Otherwise, danger exists that a plane of dissection will be established within the dura, and as this is followed superiorly, inferiorly, and laterally, it can only lead to venous bleeding from the dural sinuses, particularly the intercavernous sinuses that connect the right and left cavernous sinuses within the sellar dura. Once the dura is open, a special set of pituitary curets and spoons, as well as an insulated suction cautery are available to manage tumor removal (Fig. 24). For this, neurosurgical skills are obviously mandatory. Decisions have to be made about the proximity of the carotid artery, the risks to the third cranial nerve, the completeness with which tumor is extruding

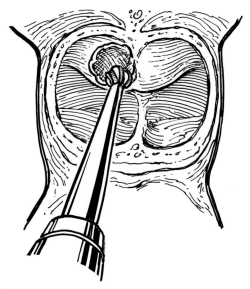

FIG. 22. Bone of sella being removed with drill.

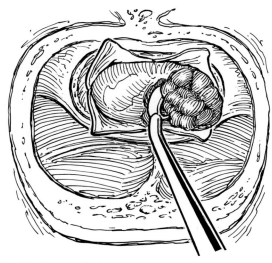

FIG. 24. Tumor being removed with pituitary curet.

into the sella from its suprasellar extensions, the potential for hypothalamic injury, and, in the case of microadenomas, when to quit searching.

It is interesting to recognize that the internal carotid arteries lie beside the sella and that, unlike the sphenoid sinus, the sella itself has no lateral bony walls. There are cases recorded in which these arteries were so large and tortuous and bulged so far medially that the right and left internal carotid siphons were only 4 mm apart. The medial edges of the tentorium, as they swing around the brain stem, come forward to attach to the anterior clinoid processes. The third cranial nerves, which emanate from the base of the brain, course for-

ward lateral to the necks of the posterior clinoid processes and run under the free edge of the tentorium in their medial intracavernous course forward to the superior orbital fissures. Thus an oculomotor nerve is "caught" in the triangular field between the free edge of the tentorium and the posterior clinoid process. Here, it is the most vulnerable of the cranial nerves whenever dissection extends out laterally in the pursuit of lateral extrasellar tumor. In view of these anatomic considerations and the familiarity and expertise of neurosurgeons in the middle fossa approaches to the root of the sphenoid wing, sometimes lateral tumor extension may be better managed by a middle fossa procedure.

At the conclusion of the intrasellar ablation, the pituitary defect is refilled with a small fat–muscle autograft, taken from the right abdominal wall. A small batten of bone derived from the septum is placed transversely in the sellar opening, and this supports the autograft in place.

Septal Reconstruction and Closure

After the neurosurgical portion of the procedure is concluded, search the wound carefully for two items—a perforation and cottonoid patties. The patties are no problem; they just have to be remembered and removed. The perforations are no problem if the mucosa has only been lacerated and not avulsed. With the method of dissection described, the mucosa of the septum in the floor is completely mobile. Therefore the edges of the septal perforation can be approximated with little tension and sutured together with catgut. I prefer 4-0 chromic on a G2 needle. The needle is small and at least a full half circle. The Castrovjejo needle

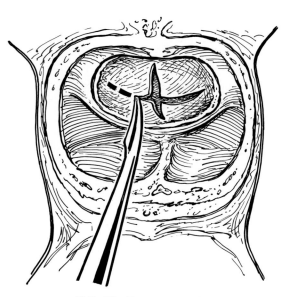

FIG. 23. Dura opened.

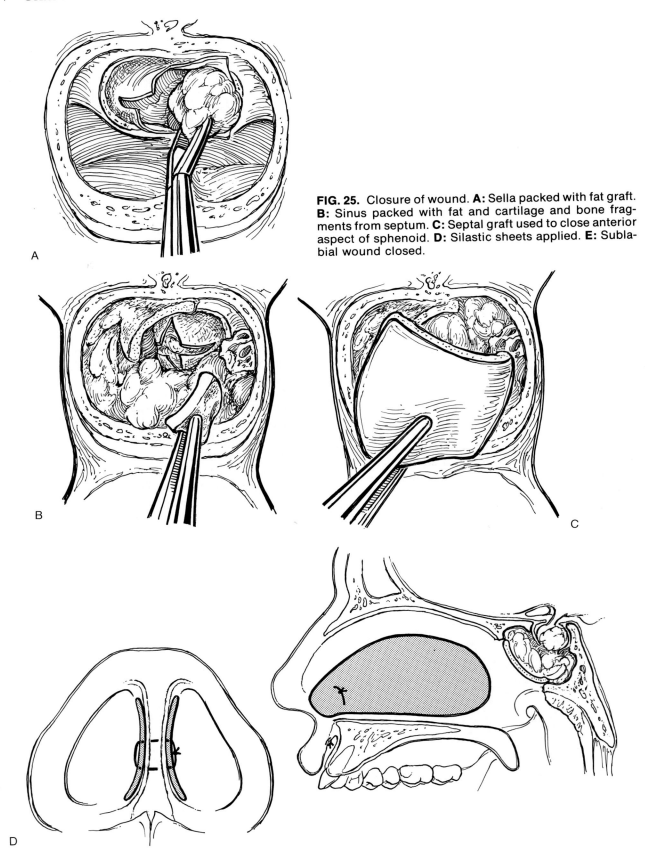

FIG. 25. Closure of wound. **A:** Sella packed with fat graft. **B:** Sinus packed with fat and cartilage and bone fragments from septum. **C:** Septal graft used to close anterior aspect of sphenoid. **D:** Silastic sheets applied. **E:** Sublabial wound closed.

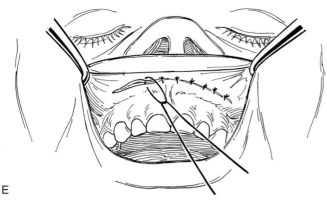

E

FIG. 25. *Continued.*

holder is used to drive the needle through the edges of the perforation while visualization is maintained with a nasal speculum. Retrieve the needle with an otologic alligator forceps, tie the knot outside the nostril, and then set it down with the aid of the alligator forceps. This is a two-handed maneuver, so the nasal speculum should be kept open by its set-screw, and it is supported in place by the assistant. In this manner, the edges of the septal perforations can be reapproximated and usually no more than three sutures are ever required. This procedure takes a little extra time, but it is well worth the result. In the case of large bilateral perforations, place a temporary polyethylene sheet in the septal space as you sew, to help you avoid catching the mucoperichondrium of the opposite side.

Now fix the septal cartilage in the midline. It is not uncommon, especially when the mucoperichondrium has only been elevated from the left side, to find the cartilage wants to dislocate into the left nostril. Pass a single 4-0 vicryl suture through some of the midline fibrous tissue on the undersurface of the nasal spine. Then pass it through the cartilage, around the undersurface of the *cartilage,* and back through again. This provides satisfactory fixation, and the suture does not cut out through the inferior margin of the cartilage.

Snug these sutures up using the excellent direct visualization afforded by the sublabial incision. Then close the sublabial incision with 3-0 chromic catgut sutures, which are expected to dissolve on their own.

Turn your attention back to the septal space, which can be reimplanted with a few thin spicules of bone saved from the earlier approach. The object of this is to maintain a little guide to the plane of separation between the mucoperichondrium flaps, in case reexploration ever becomes necessary. Of course, only a small portion of the posterior half of the septal space need be reimplanted, since the septal cartilage remains in place. Introduce small pieces of crushed cartilage or bone with a thin bayonette forceps and place them like postage stamps on the deep surface of the septal mu-

cosa, where they tend to adhere immediately. Close the transfixion incision with interrupted 4-0 chromic sutures, and place precut polyethylene sheet splints in each nasal cavity to clasp the mucosa to the midline. Use a single nylon mattress suture to transfix the splints to the anterior septum, being careful that the edge of the splint does not actually abrade the hemi-transfixion incision (Fig. 25).

Like many rhinologists, we used to complete the procedure by packing the nose with Cortisporin ointment-soaked half-inch gauze. However, patients would spread horror stories from one case to the next regarding the impressive length of this packing when it was removed, and the marked nasal discomfort this incurred. At present, our patients seem to be much more satisfied with the use of polyamide gel (Vigilon) nasal packs. Fold each pack lengthwise to make an 8 × 1½ cm pad and augment it with a black silk retrieval suture. Remove the external plastic "skin" so that the polyamide gel itself will be the only substance contacting nasal mucosa. Each pack is soaked in Cortisporin suspension before insertion, and each one can remain in place in these patients for 4 days. The primary purpose of the pack is to center the splints, but they also assist in hemostasis.

An external tape and mustache dressing is finally applied with several objectives in mind. The first is to limit the stretch in the upper lip skin and soft tissues so that swelling in the nasolabial area is minimized. The second is to occlude the nostrils completely, so that drainage flows back into the nasopharynx and throat instead of constantly dripping in front. Cut a soft mustache dressing from an ophthalmologic eye pad, apply it after the tape dressing is affixed, and this completes the surgery.

HOW CERTAIN SYNDROMES INFLUENCE TRANSSEPTAL SURGERY

Because the indications for transseptal–transsphenoidal hypophysectomy include several endocrine syndromes, otolaryngologists need to have some working knowledge of the ways in which these syndromes influence the surgery.

Acromegaly

In acromegaly, the nostrils are sometimes large enough that the whole operation can be done through one nostril and a sublabial incision is unnecessary. The septum itself is frequently overgrown with extensive folding and wrinkling above the premaxillary wings. Stand by to assist the anesthesiologist since these patients are typically quite difficult to intubate. The jaw is large but the tongue is even larger. Anticipate a difficult intubation in acromegalics and allow for it in your timing and in the selection of the anesthesia personnel. The nasal cavity in acromegaly can be quite long. The speculum must be at least 11 cm to be inserted transnasally; otherwise, it may not reach all the way back to the sphenoid rostrum.

The nasal spine is routinely removed in some surgical techniques, but, in general, we usually can avoid it. We have removed it, on occasion, in acromegalics, where it can be huge. In these cases, leave it attached to the septal cartilage. Free it with a formal bony saw cut through the spine and nasal bones to which it is attached, and fix it back in place at the end of the procedure using maxillofacial wiring techniques. In general, the nasal spine does not compromise visualization of the sella with the microscope because both the optical axis of each eyepiece and the coaxial illumination tend to straddle the nasal spine, and place it well out of focus in the lower parts of the field.

Prolactinomas

Prolactinomas raise different problems. The patients are often undergoing surgery so that they can regain normal menstrual function and ultimately become pregnant. Cosmesis is quite important and they appreciate an operation that produces no facial scars and no external nasal deformity. If the slight widening of the nasal base that can occur from an extensive premaxillary approach could pose problems, it may be helpful during closure to place a figure-of-eight stitch out into the lateral premaxillary soft tissues and, working in the space in front of the nasal spine, draw these tissues together. Microadenomas (defined as pituitary adenomas under 10 mm) are more common in patients with amenorrhea–galactorrhea, so make doubly sure you achieve excellent exposure and a dry field. This helps the neurosurgeon to be conservative in his/her management. Conservative means the microadenoma can be identified and removed by itself, while the rest of the pituitary gland remains, avoiding the problems of diabetes insipidus and long-term dependence on replacement steroid hormones.

It has been argued that prolactinomas can be followed and their endocrine effects treated with the dopamine agonist bromocriptine. This inhibits prolactin and the growth of the adenoma; in larger doses, it also inhibits the production of growth hormones. However, it has side effects, commonly including nausea and hypotension. The risk, of course, is reduced tumor vigilance, since the tumor itself may be slowed but is not eliminated. Pregnancy accelerates some adenomas.

Cushing's Disease

Cushing's disease presents more serious problems for the nasal surgeon. Cushinoid patients are typically ill. Their facial skin may be characterized by acne rosacea. Most tissues, including their blood vessels, are extremely friable and this, coupled with hypertension, can make the control of bleeding and the avoidance of septal perforations more challenging. The tissue and capillary fragility is often quite noticeable during the dissection. Bony resections (such as the rostrum) are sometimes enhanced by the fact that the bone is often more fragile.

Craniopharyngioma

Craniopharyngiomas are very persistent adherent multicystic tumors that usually begin in a suprasellar location. They tend to affect young, preadolescent patients, causing both mass and endocrine effects. The purpose of transseptal operations on craniopharyngiomas is to obtain material for biopsy, achieve intrasellar removal when appropriate, and, in some cases, simply accomplish some element of decompression and sometimes even intentional fistulization of a few of the larger cysts.

Sphenoid Mucoceles

Sphenoid mucoceles can be approached and drained by the same transseptal procedure outlined here, and, interestingly, mucopyoceles in the sphenoid sinus can produce endocrine deficits, cranial neuropathies, and orbital effects that mimic pituitary tumors in many respects. Through the transseptal approach, resect the entire sphenoid face and the posterior septum. When the bony resection is complete, then resect the soft tissues of the sphenoid face and the posterior septum, working through the nasal cavities. Sphenoid mucoceles often coexist with ethmoid mucoceles and transnasal ethmoidectomy can be undertaken at the same operation.

Empty Sella Syndrome

The empty sella syndrome is an interesting condition in which the patient suffers sellar ballooning (without erosion) and progressive hypopituitarism due to an apparent arachnoid cyst of cerebrospinal fluid accumulating within the sella. This can follow previous surgery or irradiation or simply arise on its own. It is prone to lead to "spontaneous" cerebrospinal fluid leak and is rarely coexistent with an adenoma. Surgery is restricted to the treatment of complications. The associated optic prolapse may produce an opportunity for inadvertent injury to the optic nerves during exploration for a presumed adenoma.

RELATIONSHIP BETWEEN MUCOSAL PERFORATIONS AND ADVERSE RHINOLOGIC SEQUELAE

Otolaryngologists make a big issue of avoiding septal mucosal perforations intraoperatively. Why is this? We have already noted some reasons.

Tears rob mucosal flaps of tension, and tension is important for exposure. Mucosal perforations bleed copiously at their edges and obscure the conduct of the operation. They complicate insertion of the pituitary speculum, as mentioned above, by providing an opening through which the blades pass into the nasal cavity. Perforations of the nasal septal mucoperiosteum are sometimes enlarged by the pituitary speculum. Sometimes new ones are actually created when vigorous opening of the speculum crushes friable septal mucoperiosteum against a strong inferior turbinate. Thus, even if the septal dissection was perfectly done, check the flaps for crush injury perforations as soon as you reenter the case to close.

After the pituitary speculum is removed, perforations increase the time taken in closure. Bleeding persists, and they may require intranasal suturing. Postoperative symptoms are prolonged because healing mucosal lacerations crust and promote secondary turbinate congestion. Of course, a permanent septal perforation is risked; the edges of bilateral septal mucosal perforations prefer to join each other rather than converge across the open space.

A permanent septal perforation causes whistling if it is small, chronic nasal obstruction with bleeding and crusting if it is large, and if it is truly enormous, retraction and an external nasal deformity. Finally, the presence of a chronic septal perforation makes revision pituitary surgery much more difficult, and in cases where only partial removal or decompression could be accomplished, this is a distinct liability.

Complications Including Cerebrospinal Fluid Leak

We reviewed the complications in our first 582 transsphenoidal operations. Fatalities occurred in 1.2%, but with time and exclusion of the first year, this is under 1%. Deaths were caused by hypothalamic injury, vascular injury, and meningitis. Nonfatal complications occurred in approximately 7% of patients. These included permanent diabetes insipidus, cerebrospinal fluid leaks, septal perforation, and other miscellaneous problems.

In most instances following transseptal transsphenoidal hypophysectomy, postoperative care by the otolaryngologist is focused on the nose, while neurosurgery monitors for progressive neurologic dysfunction, and endocrinology manages the metabolism. Otolaryngology's obligation is to determine when to remove the nasal dressing and splints and accomplish this in an expeditious fashion. Be alert to the possibility of a postoperative cerebrospinal fluid leak also. We have come to feel that the best management of this uncommon complication is immediate reexploration and grafting. Return the patient to the operating room and reopen the sublabial incision (only). The septal flaps are not yet adherent, and reimplanted bone and cartilage are still available in the septal space. The sella is simply regrafted by the neurosurgeon with autogenous muscle and refixed in place with a transverse batten. The morbidity of reoperation done this way is low, and the chance of controlling the leak is high. This seems to be preferable to prolonged hospitalization, hoping the leak will somehow seal spontaneously. It often does not seal, and reexploration once the nasal septal flaps are adherent is not nearly as easily performed. Prolonged hospitalization combined with repeated spinal taps, especially taps that drop intracranial pressure enough to reverse the pressure gradient across the leak, risks meningitis and/or tension pneumocephalus, two subjects covered elsewhere in this book.

CONCLUSIONS

Current experience with transsphenoidal procedures gradually leads one to recognize that some concepts regarding the pituitary are better described as myths. The first is that pituitary adenomas are extremely rare; so rare, we have little obligation to know their management. This is clearly not the case for surgeons working in a tertiary care center with endocrine and neurosurgical services. The second is the fear that the nasal approach will provide poor exposure and cause meningitis. This has not been our experience; the nasal route provides visualization of the entire sella, unimpeded by the optic nerves or the carotid artery. Pre-, intra-, and postoperative use of systemic antibiotics curtails most pathogens, the nasal packing is impregnated with antibiotics, and natural lysozymes are prominent in the nasal mucosa. Next, suprasellar extension is not a clear contraindication to transseptal surgery. Many patients in our series had suprasellar tumor extensions, and the natural tendency at surgery was for these rather soft tumors to decompress inferiorly and gradually be delivered into the field. Finally, contrary to what one might predict, hypophysectomy does not necessarily cause permanent diabetes insipidus. In most of these patients, antidiuretic hormone continues to be released.

In careful hands, the transnasal sublabial transseptal transsphenoidal approach to the pituitary is safe and effective in providing excellent exposure and a minimum of operative risk. It leaves no facial scars and no nasal defects and preserves the option of revision. Nowhere in surgery is the team approach more rewarding; working in concert with neurosurgery and endocrinology, nasal surgeons have something legitimate to offer pituitary patients and much to learn in return.

REFERENCES

1. Von Eiselsberg AF. My experience about operation about the hypophysis. *Trans Am Surg Assoc* 1910;28:55.
2. Hirsch O. Demonstration eines nach einer neuenMethode operiten Hypophysentumors. *Veh Dtsch Ges Chir* 1910;39:51.
3. Killian G. Die submucöse Fenesterresktion der Nasenscheidewand. *Arch Laryngol Rhinol* 1904;16:362.
4. Kanavel AB. The removal of tumors of the pituitary body by an infranasal route. *JAMA* 1909;53:1704.
5. Halstead AE. Remarks on the operative treatment of tumors of the hypophysis: with the report of two cases operated on by an oronasal method. *Trans Am Surg Assoc* 1910;28:73.
6. Cushing H. Partial hypophysectomy for acromegaly: with remarks on the function of the hypophysis. *Ann Surg* 1909;50:1002.
7. Dandy WE. A new hypophysis operation: devised by Dr. G. J. Heuer. *Bull Johns Hopkins Hosp* 1913;29:154.
8. McDonald TJ, Laws ER. Historical aspects of the management of pituitary disorders with emphasis on transsphenoidal surgery. In: Laws ER, Randall RV, Kern EB, Aboud CF, eds. *Management of pituitary adenomas and related lesions with emphasis on transsphenoidal microsurgery*. New York: Appleton-Century-Crofts, 1982;1–14.
9. Pearson BW, Laws ER. Anatomical aspects of the transsphenoidal approach to the pituitary. In: Laws ER, Randall RV, Kern EB, Aboud CF, eds. *Management of pituitary adenomas and related lesions with emphasis on transsphenoidal microsurgery*. New York: Appleton-Century-Crofts, 1982.
10. Kern EB, Laws ER. The rationale and technique of selective transsphenoidal microsurgery for the removal of pituitary tumor. In: Laws ER, Randall RV, Kern EB, Aboud CF, eds. *Management of pituitary adenomas and related lesions with emphasis on transsphenoidal microsurgery*. New York: Appleton-Century-Crofts, 1982.

CHAPTER 32

Facial Pain

Jack L. Gluckman and James E. Freije

No book dedicated to disorders of the paranasal sinuses is complete without discussion of the differential diagnosis of facial pain. This is because most facial pain is at some stage attributed to sinus dysfunction not only by the patient but frequently by the primary care physician. This diagnosis invariably sets up a cycle of nonproductive therapy geared to "sinus treatment," consisting of various decongestants and antibiotics with resultant patient and physician frustration and, of course, delay in establishing the true diagnosis. This chapter attempts to outline the major causes of facial pain (Table 1) and presents a practical approach to diagnosis and management of patients with this symptom complex.

PATIENT EVALUATION

Although we have come to rely on sophisticated radiographic and laboratory testing to assist in the diagnosis of complex conditions of the head and neck, the patient with facial pain is best evaluated by a comprehensive and detailed history-taking and physical examination. In no other disorder does the age old axiom, "The patient will tell you the diagnosis," more obviously apply. The patient with facial pain requires at least a half-hour to one-hour consultation for adequate evaluation.

The history should elicit a very detailed description of the pain in terms of its character, location, onset, duration, and frequency, as well as aggravating and relieving factors. Any precipitating events or associated symptoms should be noted. A careful past history is essential to determine the patient's general emotional status, past history of analgesic use and abuse, or any other factors in the past history that may aid one in determining how seriously the pain interferes with the patient's quality of life.

Physical examination consists not only of a complete head and neck examination, including adequate visualization of the whole upper aerodigestive tract, but a comprehensive and careful assessment of the cranial nerves. At least a rudimentary general examination is also recommended. A psychologic profile should be obtained if indicated, particularly in the chronic pain patient and those patients where secondary gain is suspected.

At this stage, the diagnosis should be obvious or at least a general sense of the pathologic process should be apparent. Further testing, for example, computed tomography (CT) scan, magnetic resonance imaging (MRI), or Panorex, should be ordered only as indicated. The concept of obtaining a blanket scan of the head and neck without attempting to exclude specific pathology or, worse still, without performing an adequate physical examination is to be condemned! More

TABLE 1. *Classification of causes of facial pain*

Sinus pain
Odontogenic pain
Orbital pain
Neural pain
  Primary neuralgias
    Trigeminal neuralgia
    Glossopharyngeal neuralgia
    Sluder's neuralgia
  Secondary neuralgias
    Compression and infiltration
    Multiple sclerosis
    Postherpetic neuralgia
Vascular pain
  Migraine
  Cluster headache
  Carotidynia
  Temporal arteritis
Muscle and joint pain
  Muscle contraction headaches
  Temporomandibular joint dysfunction
Atypical facial pain

sophisticated testing (e.g., angiography) should be obtained when appropriate. Occasionally, local anesthetic nerve blocks may be useful in localizing causes of facial pain and aiding in the diagnosis.

A psychogenic etiology or functional overlay is always a consideration, particularly in dealing with chronic pain patients. On the other hand, chronic pain that is very real to the patient may induce significant psychologic dysfunction, which may mask the underlying diagnosis and be misinterpreted as hysteria or malingering for secondary gain. It may be very difficult, if not sometimes impossible, to unravel this complex web. Thus the diagnosis and management of chronic facial pain pose a dilemma to even the most experienced clinician. A final if obvious point that further complicates the management of facial pain is the fact that pain is a purely subjective symptom with difficulty in establishing objective criteria to determine the severity of the symptom and the effectiveness of treatment.

PARANASAL SINUS PAIN

Diseases of the paranasal sinuses have been dealt with elsewhere in this text and the clinical features for each process will not be discussed in detail in this section. Suffice it to state that facial pain due to acute infection of the sinuses usually does not pose a diagnostic problem as clinical evidence of the infection is usually obvious and, together with the radiographic changes, leads to the correct diagnosis being established. Usually multiple sinuses are involved by the infection. On the other hand, pain due to chronic sinus disease is more difficult to diagnose as the clinical and radiographic findings are more difficult to interpret.

Pain from acute maxillary sinusitis is usually predominantly felt in the cheek over the sinus but may radiate into the teeth or the eye. It is intense, throbbing, and exacerbated by sudden movement and bending forward. The sinus is tender to palpation and pus can be identified in the middle meatus on nasal examination.

Acute ethmoiditis typically causes pain in the frontoethmoidal, periorbital, or retro-orbital areas and is likewise characterized by a throbbing intense pain. Examination of the nose reveals purulence in the meatus and varying degrees of mucosal thickening. Periorbital edema may develop and the patient is tender over the ethmoid sinuses. Routine sinus radiographs may be difficult to interpret with changes in the ethmoid best detected on CT scan.

Acute frontal sinusitis results in a severe throbbing or aching pain in the frontal area, which radiates superiorly to the vertex or occiput. The pain is exacerbated by percussion of the sinus, sudden head movement,

and bending over. The sinuses will be tender to palpation and pus will be identified in the middle meatus.

Acute sphenoid sinusitis usually develops in conjunction with infection of the other paranasal sinuses but may occur as an isolated entity. It is characterized by severe retro-orbital pain but may present as frontal, temporal, or occipital pain (1). This is usually throbbing in nature and is worse in the early morning. Changes in vision, particularly diplopia, should make one suspicious for sphenoid pathology. Radiographs of the sinuses may confirm the diagnosis, but frequently a CT scan is necessary.

The real dilemma confronting the clinician is ruling out sinus disease as a cause of chronic facial pain. Unfortunately, many patients with chronic facial pain are labeled as suffering from "sinus" and this diagnosis is reinforced if there should be any radiographic change at all in the sinuses. It is true that "vacuum headaches" may result from impaired aeration of the sinus with either completely normal radiographs and scans or minimal mucosal changes. The pain classically is a dull ache over the sinuses, which is worse in the morning and late at night and is fairly constant. Diagnostic aids include placing the patients on topical nasal decongestants to determine whether the symptoms improve or even marsupializing the affected sinus into the nose to improve aeration (e.g., sphenoidotomy, frontal sinusotomy, nasoantral window). The key, however, to establishing whether sinus disease is the cause of facial pain is a careful history and physical examination and not to overinterpret the minimal radiographic findings that may be encountered.

While inflammatory disease of the sinus is the most common sinus cause of facial pain, obviously other pathology involving the paranasal sinuses can cause pain, for example, tumor, both benign and malignant, or cysts.

ODONTOGENIC PAIN (ODONTALGIA)

Dental pathology is a common cause of facial pain with the pain usually caused by inflammation of the dental pulp or peridontal tissue. This pain often is confined to the tooth but may radiate into the upper or lower jaws and is exacerbated by pressure or thermal stimulation. Usually, the affected tooth can easily be identified either clinically or radiographically.

Pain, however, may occur in normal teeth and be induced by very cold food or even rarely by cold air encountered after leaving a warm building (2). The hypothesis for this phenomenon is that the crowns on these teeth are small and the enamel is thin, rendering the tooth more vulnerable to temperature changes. Extremely sensitive dentine or cementum can cause pain while brushing apparently normal teeth.

Another condition that may present as severe pain in a normal appearing tooth is *atypical odontalgia*, which is a subgroup of atypical facial neuralgia localized to the teeth. This disorder is characterized by throbbing, aching pain in clinically and radiographically normal teeth. The pain lasts from days to years, radiates to the face or neck, does not have a trigger point, and occurs most commonly in middle-aged women (3). This condition is accompanied by depression in nearly two-thirds of cases and migraine in one-third (4). The main concern in dealing with these patients is inadvertently subjecting them unnecessarily to extensive dental procedures that are invariably ineffective. Appropriate therapy consists of recognition of the condition, avoidance of dental procedures, and psychiatric evaluation and therapy, including antidepressants (5). The "cracked tooth syndrome" is a not infrequent cause of dental pain radiating to the face. Clinically, these patients present with pain induced by pressure or thermal stimulus. The crack may be obvious or subtle. Repair of the tooth prevents further cracking and exposure of the pulp (6).

Finally, one should always be aware that dental pathology may precipitate trigeminal or atypical facial neuralgia (7,8). Even an empty socket at the site of previous tooth extraction may cause atypical facial pain. The cavities are detected on dental radiographs and treatment consists of thorough curettage of the bony cavities with complete resolution of pain in the majority of cases (7).

ORBITAL PAIN

Pain of orbital origin is usually in the distribution of the ophthalmic division of the trigeminal nerve and, if severe, may cause spasm of the ipsilateral frontal and occipital musculature. There are three main subgroups of pain of ocular and periocular origin (9):

1. Eye strain (refractive errors and muscle imbalance).
2. Intraocular inflammation and hypertension.
3. Diseases of the external eye and adnexa.

Pain from refractive errors and extraocular muscle imbalance are probably rare and overdiagnosed. The headache or facial pain that results increases with use of the eyes and occurs after prolonged use. It is characterized by periorbital aching radiating to the frontal and temporal areas and rarely the occiput and may be associated with blurred vision. The refractory disorders are usually uncorrected hyperopia and astigmatism, which depend on ciliary muscle contracture for accommodation, particularly while reading. Refraction will reveal the problem and treatment is by corrective lenses. Muscle imbalance (e.g., due to convergence in-

sufficiency) also may cause pain and headache, particularly after reading. This type of discomfort is relieved by covering one eye. Treatment consists of prisms or exercises designed to strengthen the ability of the eye muscles to converge.

As has already been stated, the clinician should take great care not to overdiagnose these abnormalities as a cause of facial pain. In fact, refraction and muscle balance disorders may cause symptoms in one individual and not in the next. Likewise, one should not overreact to commonly occurring occasional, fleeting uniocular stabbing pains (ophthalmalgia) (10), which are of no significance.

Intraocular inflammation and increased intraocular pressure cover a broad range of disorders that are a definite cause of ocular pain. Acute uveitis (inflammation of the iris, ciliary body, and/or choroid) results in severe throbbing periorbital pain and may radiate inferiorly and be misdiagnosed as dental or sinus disease. Photophobia is characteristic, together with blurring of vision and tearing. The eye is injected, the globe tender to palpation, and the pupil constricted because of spasm of the iris sphincter. While anterior uveitis may be due to contusion or some collagen disorders, in 90% of cases no etiology is obvious (9). The condition is often self-limiting and is treated with atropine and steroid drops. If this condition is suspected, ophthalmology consultation is imperative.

Optic neuritis may be secondary to intraocular inflammation, sinusitis, meningitis, or sarcoidosis. In a significant percentage of cases, it may be the first sign of multiple sclerosis (11). Clinically, there is severe periorbital pain, which may be predominantly retro-orbital, aggravated by extreme movement of the eye and tenderness of the globe is noted. Vision deteriorates a few days later and may progress to total visual loss or recover over weeks to months.

Rapid elevation of intraocular pressure with associated ocular damage (e.g., glaucoma, primary or secondary) may cause pain. This is characteristically periorbital and may be accompanied by nausea and vomiting. There may be associated conjunctival and lid congestion and tearing. Vision may deteriorate.

The diseases of the external eye and adnexae (e.g., conjunctivitis, episcleritis, corneal abrasion, dacryocystitis, and styes and chalazia) are all relatively easily diagnosed with a history of pain aggravated by lid movement together with the obvious clinical findings of the disease process.

More rarely, it should be remembered that orbital tumors or pseudotumors may cause facial pain and should strongly be suspected in cases of unilateral proptosis. Diagnosis is confirmed by CT scan. Thyroid-induced exophthalmos does not usually cause significant eye pain but may cause discomfort on eye movement (12).

It should be remembered that occasionally orbital pain may not be due to ocular or periocular pathologies per se but is referred from a distant source. Therefore, if pathology is not evident on ophthalmologic evaluation, the underlying etiology should be sought elsewhere.

FACIAL NEURALGIAS

Trigeminal Neuralgia

Of the cranial neuralgias, trigeminal neuralgia or tic douloureux is the most common. It usually occurs in patients over 50 years of age in a 2:1 female to male predominance.

The syndrome consists of spasms of unilateral, recurrent, excruciating pain lasting seconds to minutes confined to the distribution of the trigeminal nerve usually the second or third divisions. The pain often is initiated by stimulation of trigger points especially around the infraorbital and mental foramina. Stimuli include speaking, chewing, shaving, or simply lightly touching the face. The patient characteristically does anything possible to avoid these precipitating events. Between episodes, the patient is pain free. The attacks are episodic, occurring many times a week then disappearing for weeks to months. Primary trigeminal neuralgia is *not* associated with any objective neurologic deficit.

The pathophysiology of primary trigeminal neuralgia is complex and poorly defined. It is thought that there is an excitatory state built up by temporal summation of afferent impulses, together with reduced inhibitory mechanisms (13). Secondary trigeminal neuralgia due to involvement of the nerve by other pathologies needs to be excluded before making the diagnosis of tic douloureux. Clinically, a sensory deficit in the distribution of the nerve, persistent dull aching pain following the paroxysm, or pain beyond the distribution of the trigeminal nerve should make one suspicious. Causes of secondary neuralgia include compression by intracranial tumors, for example acoustic neuromas, trigeminal neuromas, meningiomas, and congenital cholesteatoma; invasion by malignant tumors of the nasopharynx; brain stem vascular anomaly; syringomyelia; and multiple sclerosis. Multiple sclerosis should be thought of in atypical trigeminal neuralgia in young patients.

While the classic case of trigeminal neuralgia requires no more than an adequate history and normal physical examination to establish diagnosis, a CT scan of the head and neck and/or MRI and even possibly angiography should be performed to rule out causes of secondary neuralgia if this possibility is even remotely considered.

The initial treatment of primary trigeminal neuralgia

is carbamazepine (Tegretol). This has proved to be extremely effective by reducing the temporal summation of afferent impulses that precipitate the attacks (13). It is so effective that some authorities advocate the use of the drug as a diagnostic test, and if the neuralgia does not response in 24 to 48 hr, the diagnosis is in doubt. The drug can be used continuously or intermittently to precipitate a remission; while in remission the drug can be stopped. The usual dosage is 100 to 200 mg twice or three times daily, but the dosage should be titrated against the patient's symptoms. Unfortunately, in some patients, it loses its effectiveness with time while in others, the symptoms return after cessation of the drug. In some patients, the sedative effect and occasionally nausea and vomiting, vertigo, and even ataxia preclude the use of the drug. Renal and hepatic toxicity have rarely been reported. Regular blood counts should be performed to detect the development of another serious complication—agranulocytosis—although this is extremely rare. If symptoms persist on carbamazepine, phenytoin should be added and if there is no response to both drugs, chlorphensin can be added (13).

If the condition proves refractory to medical therapy (25% of cases) some form of ablative therapy should be considered. Division of the posterior root in the middle fossa has been proposed but results in significant loss of touch perception; therefore sectioning of the posterior root in the posterior fossa was advocated. A number of less complicated and less hazardous procedures, however, have been developed in recent years. Injection of neurotoxic agents into the gasserian ganglion has proved effective and simple to perform. Alcohol, phenol, and even boiling water have been used. Unfortunately, a high incidence of complications related to loss of sensation (e.g., keratitis and anesthesia dolorosa) have been noted using this technique (14). Stereotaxic coagulation of the gasserian ganglion is extremely safe and reliable and seems to spare the loss of proprioception encountered with the other techniques (15,16). The hypothesis that vascular compression of the nerve root at the pons is a major etiologic factor and therefore can be relieved by vascular decompression remains controversial (17). Unfortunately, it remains difficult to predict which patients will benefit from this approach prior to craniotomy (13).

Glossopharyngeal Neuralgia

Weisenberg (18), in 1910, was the first to recognize that pain could arise from irritation of the glossopharyngeal nerve; however, Harris (19), in 1921, first described the syndrome of glossopharyngeal neuralgia. Some authors have used the term vagoglossopharyngeal neuralgia, implying that the pain can radiate in the distribution of the vagus as well, but the more accurate term remains glossopharyngeal neuralgia.

Primary glossopharyngeal neuralgia occurs characteristically in patients over 40 years of age with an equal male to female incidence. Unilateral stabbing pharyngeal pain is the dominant complaint; however, it may be referred to the ear and lower jaw and therefore present as facial pain with the character of the pain being highly diagnostic. Its onset is sudden and unexpected and is violent and intense with the attacks lasting 20 to 30 sec. A sensation of burning may persist for several minutes after the acute attack. The first attack can be isolated and followed by a period of remission lasting for years; however, eventually a pattern of recurring attacks begins with variable frequency. The recurrent episodes may last for several days or weeks with the remission periods becoming less frequent and increasingly shorter. Associated symptoms include salivary disturbances with a dry mouth and vasomotor phenomena, including syncope and even cardiac arrest (20). These attacks are characteristically precipitated by stimulation of a trigger zone (usually in the oropharynx) by swallowing, yawning, coughing, opening the mouth, or extending the tongue.

Essential to the diagnosis of glossopharyngeal neuralgia is the characteristic history, together with isolation of the trigger zone. Stimulation of this area will initiate the symptoms and injection or application of a local anesthetic should provide temporary relief.

In the differential diagnosis, it is important to exclude secondary causes of glossopharyngeal nerve irritation (e.g., intracranial and head and neck tumors). The distinguishing feature of these secondary causes is the almost continuous pain without the characteristic "on and off pattern" seen with primary glossopharyngeal neuralgia. Therefore a careful head and neck examination is mandatory and head CT scan should be performed if there is a high index of suspicion. An elongated styloid process also may cause secondary glossopharyngeal neuralgia.

Therapy is initially with carbamazepine, and phenytoin can be added if complete control is not achieved. Anticholinergics may be helpful for the vasomotor symptoms.

Ultimately, if the condition proves refractory to conservative treatment, surgery may become necessary. Glossopharyngeal neurectomy may be performed via an extracranial transcervical approach or by an intracranial approach. These procedures usually result in permanent cure.

Sluder's Neuralgia

Sluder's neuralgia almost defies classification because of confusion as to its etiology. This symptom

TABLE 2. *Various names for Sluder's neuralgia*

Sluder's neuralgia
Sphenopalatine neuralgia
Sluder's lower-half headache
Ciliary neuralgia
Vidian neuralgia
Pretrosal neuralgia
Histamine cephalgia
Autonomic faciocephalgia
Periodic migrainous neuralgia
Nasal vascular headaches
Charlin's syndrome
Erythromyalgia of the head
Atypical vascular cephalgia
Lower-half headaches
Vail's neuralgia of the vidian nerve
Syndrome of Mondrum Benisty

complex has been described and redescribed through the years and labeled with various names (Table 2).

Evaluation of the clinical features of these various described syndromes confirms the similarity with only the names and theories regarding the pathogenesis being different. As Sluder first described (21) and subsequently elaborated on (22–24), the features of this syndrome, and in the absence of any more appropriate name, it seems reasonable for this syndrome to be named "Sluder's neuralgia."

Sluder postulated that the condition was due to an irritation of the sphenopalatine ganglion based on its close relationship with the sphenoid, ethmoid, and maxillary sinuses. This theory was supported by the observation that the symptoms were relieved by local anesthesia applied to the ganglion (25). Even if correct, the exact triggering mechanism for these headaches remains obscure.

Another possibility is that the pain is due to a nasal reflex secondary to the middle turbinate impinging on the nasal septum due to mucosal congestion. In support of this concept is the work of McAuliffe and Goodell (26), who demonstrated that stimuli applied to the various areas of the nasal cavity caused referred pain to different parts of the head. This in fact results in all the classical features of Sluder's neuralgia, including the lacrimation and injection of the eye. It was also observed that the pain of nasal origin may outlast the period of stimulation; and adequate anesthesia and decongestion of the nose abolish these headaches.

While a combination of these hypotheses probably plays a role in the development of this syndrome, the exact etiology remains as obscure today as it did to Sluder 70 years ago

Irrespective of its etiology, this syndrome is easily recognizable and is characterized by two major features:

1. *Pain.* This is always unilateral and is usually in the distribution of the ophthalmic and maxillary

divisions of the trigeminal nerve, particularly in the periorbital area. It may radiate occasionally to the ear and rarely to the neck and shoulder (25). The pain is usually stabbing but occasionally aching in nature and usually lasts from ½ to 2 hr and rarely a whole day.

2. *Associated vasomotor changes.* Ipsilateral nasal obstruction, rhinorrhea, and lacrimation almost always accompany the pain. Increased salivation and even changes in taste have been reported but are extremely rare (25).

Characteristically, the attacks occur at random with no obvious precipitating factor or trigger mechanism. The time interval between bouts also is variable with attacks occurring every day in some patients and only a few times a month in others. Clinical examination during an acute episode confirms the vasomotor changes, but no other abnormalities are present. Comprehensive neurologic evaluation is noncontributory. A frequent finding is a deviated nasal septum often impinging on the middle turbinate on the ipsilateral side (25–29).

Most patients have consulted a multitude of physicians in a vain attempt to obtain cure. Simple analgesics and antimigrainous and antineuralgic drugs usually have been attempted to alleviate their symptoms. A significant percentage of patients will seek psychiatric evaluation to help them cope with their problem.

Once the diagnosis of Sluder's neuralgia is suspected, careful nasal examination is imperative to determine the relationship between the septum and the middle turbinate. If these structures are noted to be in close approximation, surgery is considered only if the following criteria are met:

1. Classical clinical history of Sluder's neuralgia.
2. Anatomic evidence of the septum impinging on the middle turbinate.
3. Positive vasoconstrictor test; that is, during an acute episode the insertion of cocaine or any other local anesthetic/vasoconstrictor combination between the middle turbinate and septum results in dramatic relief of the pain. This technique may be used to relieve symptoms during the acute episode. An alternate technique to relieve the pain is to inject local anesthetic up the palatine canal.

Another diagnostic test is to stimulate the middle turbinate during remission and attempt to provoke the pain (29).

In refractory cases, if the above criteria have been met, septoplasty and/or middle turbinectomy can be performed with excellent results (25,28). Why surgery should be successful in some cases only is obscure.

SECONDARY NEURALGIAS

Facial pain can result from direct invasion or compression of cranial nerves intracranially, at the skull base or in their peripheral distribution. The trigeminal nerve and glossopharyngeal nerves are particularly vulnerable with subtle clinical differences in symptomatology and objective findings on examination making the clinician suspicious for an underlying etiology.

Perineural invasion by high-grade malignancies including adenocystic carcinoma and squamous cell carcinoma may affect these nerves in their peripheral course, particularly at the skull base (30). Certainly, facial pain is a well-established symptom of nasopharyngeal carcinoma (31), but almost any skull base cancer can cause pain by direct invasion (32).

Intracranial tumors, an elongated styloid process, and multiple sclerosis are all causes of secondary neuralgias.

It is therefore imperative that if there should be any suspicion of an underlying tumor, a CT scan or MRI of the head and neck should be performed.

Postherpetic Neuralgia

Postherpetic neuralgia is an occasional sequela of herpes zoster infection occurring more frequently in older patients (33,34). Herpes zoster primarily affects the posterior spinal root and cranial nerve ganglia. It occurs in adults who have had chickenpox and lies dormant until it is reactivated, particularly in an immunocompromised patient or if there is an underlying malignancy. In 15% of cases the ophthalmic division of the trigeminal nerve is affected. Postherpetic neuralgia may persist for months or years after the infection although rarely, in young patients, it may last only a few weeks (35). The pain is unilateral and follows the distribution of the cranial or cervical nerve involved. It is constant, never varying, and sometimes is described as giving a feeling of heat. Light pressure may aggravate the pain. The mechanism for the pain in postherpetic neuralgia has never been explained fully, with numerous hypotheses being presented.

The diagnosis of postherpetic neuralgia is usually not difficult except when the vesicular eruptions have gone unnoticed. Once the lesions have resolved, examination reveals areas of hyperesthesia and paresthesia and occasional scarring and/or pigmentation of the skin in the distribution of the affected nerve. There also may be an associated weakness of the muscles of mastication on the ipsilateral side. In most instances, postherpetic neuralgia resolves spontaneously over several weeks to months. The elderly and immunocompromised patients are exceptions and may have a more prolonged course. If it fails to settle within 6 months, spontaneous resolution is most unlikely.

Antiviral agents have no role in the treatment of postherpetic neuralgia (36). Analgesics are necessary but should be used judiciously as long-term usage is most likely. If possible, narcotics or any other addictive drugs should be avoided but, if required to control pain, the patient should be monitored carefully. Antidepressants and tranquilizers are most useful in conjunction with analgesics and aid the patient in coping with the pain. Anticonvulsants (e.g., phenytoin and carbamazepine) may occasionally help in eliminating the sharp neuralgic type pain.

The infiltration of steroids subcutaneously in the area of maximal pain has been used successfully and certainly is a simple procedure with no known complications and is well worth attempting if drug therapy fails (37,38).

The role of stellate ganglion block is still unclear. Some authors claim excellent results while others demonstrate no effect (39). The best results are obtained in patients with postherpetic neuralgia of less than 2 months duration.

Psychosocial counseling is essential, as many of these patients become suicidal. If all else fails, a transcutaneous electrical nerve stimulation (TENS) unit, hypnosis, acupuncture, or even ice therapies can be tried and they all have their proponents. Finally, various destructive surgical procedures can be used but they all have unpredictable responses and of course the sequela of loss of sensation.

VASCULAR PAIN

Migraine

It is certainly beyond the scope of a chapter on facial pain to discuss migraine in any detail. Exactly what syndromes fall into the category of migraine is unclear but the definition from The Ad Hoc Committee of the National Institute of Neurologic Disease and Stroke is as good as any (40). This refers to migraine as recurrent attacks of headache, commonly unilateral in onset, and usually associated with nausea and vomiting, some of which may be preceded by neurologic and mood disturbances. It usually commences in adolescence but may develop at any age. There is frequently a strong family history.

The first phase of vasoconstriction results in the aura or prodromal symptoms while the second phase of vasodilatation results in the headache.

There are several clinical variants of migraine with the pain usually in the form of a headache but occasionally it may present as facial pain. The classic form, which occurs in approximately 10% of patients, is preceded by a well-defined abrupt onset prodrome, which usually consists of seeing bright halos, zigzags, or spots in front of the eyes. These symptoms last for 10 to 30 min and are followed by the typical pulsatile headache, which often is accompanied by nausea and vomiting, fatigue, and photophobia. The headache may last from one to several hours.

The more common form of migraine is characterized by an absence of a well-defined prodrome, but rather vague irritability or gastrointestinal symptoms, which may last hours or even days before the onset of the headache. The headache is throbbing and may even be bilateral and may last hours or days.

A number of less common but more complicated migraine syndromes exist with the symptoms dictated by the site of maximum vascular disturbance. Headaches associated with extraocular muscle paralysis involving the third cranial nerve occur in *ophthalmoplegic migraine*, with the paralysis only becoming obvious after the headache subsides. In *hemiplegic migraine complex*, a transient hemiplegia or hemiparesis of the contralateral face and arm accompanies the throbbing headache. *Basilar artery migraine* consists of bilateral visual field defects followed by a severe headache. This phenomenon often affects young girls and may be associated with menses. Finally, various other disorders (e.g., gastrointestinal disturbances, cyclic edema, bouts of fever and tachycardia) with or without headaches are felt to be migrainous in nature and are included under the category of *migraine equivalents*.

A comprehensive history together with a negative physical exam usually establishes the correct diagnosis and further testing is not usually necessary. However, in a small but significant percentage of patients there may be underlying or associated intracranial pathology (41,42) and more elaborate evaluation by CT scan, MRI, or even carotid angiogram may be indicated. These should be considered, particularly if these are persistent focal neurologic deficits; pain that awakens patients from sleep; and failure of conventional medical therapy.

Many of the patients who present with migraine have their quality of life severely compromised not only by the headache but also by a fear of the headaches developing and therefore need to be treated with empathy and understanding. First, they should be reassured that the headaches can be treated and frequently prevented. The first step consists of attempting to identify any obvious precipitating factor (e.g., diet, allergies). These should be avoided or treated if possible. Symptomatic treatment consists of analgesics to be taken during the acute episode or ergot alkaloids to be taken during the prodromal phase to prevent vasodilatation. If the frequency of the headaches necessitates excessive use of ergot alkaloids, prophylactic medication should be instituted to avoid the development of ergotism, which is characterized by vasoconstriction of the vessels with a Raynaud's disease-like phenomenon. Prophylactic drugs include a combination of low-dose ergotamine with caffeine and phenobarbitol, beta-blockers, calcium channel blockers, tranquilizers, and antidepressants if indicated.

Cluster Headaches

Cluster headaches, like migraines, are classified as vascular headaches but have features that allow them to be distinguished from migraine. Synonyms include periodic migrainous neuralgia and Horton's histaminic cephalgia. Cluster headaches are far less common than migraines, typically affect middle-aged men, and have no specific familial predilection (43,44). Cluster headaches occur more frequently in smokers and drinkers (45) and are associated with an increased incidence of peptic ulcer disease (46). Although vasodilatation generally is accepted to play a role in the mechanism of cluster headaches, the exact pathophysiology of the disorder remains unknown.

The pain is unilateral and characteristically occurs in the temporal and frontal areas and around the eye but can involve any part of the face. It has a boring, stabbing, nonthrobbing character and is associated with ipsilateral lacrimation and rhinorrhea. A partial Horner's syndrome (i.e., ptosis and miosis) may be present. The pain may wake the patient from sleep and last from 20 to 90 min. Classically, there is no precipitating event other than alcohol intake if the patient is in the middle of a "cluster."

The headaches typically occur in "clusters" of 6 to 12 weeks with one to three episodes per day followed by a period of remission that may last for up to 1 year. A chronic form of cluster headaches also may occur with the remission period being absent.

Treatment of cluster headaches is similar to that of migraine with analgesics and ergot alkaloids or the inhalation of 100% oxygen if feasible (47). For chronic cluster headaches, lithium and prednisone have varying degrees of success, but long-term use should be avoided due to the side effects of these medications (48).

Carotidynia

While predominantly a cause of neck and throat pain, the discomfort caused by carotidynia may radiate along the distribution of the branches of the external carotid artery and cause facial pain. This condition was first described by Fay in 1927 (49,50) but only gained acceptance after being redescribed by Hilger in 1949 (51).

It is characterized by episodic neck and throat pain radiating into the face, jaw, and scalp. It lasts under 2 weeks and is self-limiting in 90% of cases (52,53). It may develop at any age, with females being more commonly affected.

The etiology and hence the pathophysiology is not well understood. Theories include an atypical form of migraine (53), an abnormal vasomotor control of the carotid system (51), and a carotid arteritis (54). It is most likely, however, due to overdistension and relaxation of the carotid artery similar to the phenomenon seen in vascular headaches. This is supported by the fact that there is a well-known association between carotodynia and other migrainous disorders (52,53,55). An upper respiratory tract infection has been noted as a preceding incident in 20% of cases (52). Finally, an elongated styloid process may cause carotidynia by pressure on the carotid system (56).

Clinically, these patients complain of a unilateral sore throat and neck pain radiating up the side of the face. It is usually aching or throbbing in nature and aggravated by swallowing, straining, or head motion. While it usually spontaneously resolves, rarely it may become chronic or recurrent. A diagnostic sign is that the patient constantly palpates the neck in the region of the carotid bulb (51). Examination usually is negative with the exception of a swollen tender carotid bulb. Palpation may reproduce or precipitate the pain. Occasionally, the carotid bulb swelling may be so marked that it may be misdiagnosed as a mass or aneurysm.

Diagnosis is made on history and the palpation of the tender carotid bulb. There are no constitutional symptoms or signs with a normal sedimentation rate.

Treatment consists of aspirin or nonsteroidal anti-inflammatory agents and rarely a short course of steroids. Antimigraine therapy (e.g., ergotamine) also may be effective. In refractory cases, an elongated styloid process should be sought, either by palpation in the tonsil fossa or radiographically, and, if thought to be the cause of the pain, surgically removed.

Temporal Arteritis

Temporal arteritis (giant cell arteritis) occurs primarily in the elderly and consists of temporal headaches, together with episodes of ischemia involving various structures in the head and neck. The syndrome is closely related to polymyalgia rheumatica, a musculoskeletal disorder characterized by myalgias of the neck, shoulders, back, and lower extremities. Biopsy-proven temporal arteritis occurs in over 50% of patients diagnosed with polymyalgia rheumatica (57).

Symptoms of temporal arteritis include a throbbing headache in one or both temporal areas, aggravated by local pressure, jaw claudication, dysphagia, lingual

Raynaud's phenomenon, and even lingual infarction, facial palsy, and hearing loss (58). The most feared complication of temporal arteritis is bilateral blindness, which can occur in a significant number of untreated patients. Physical exam reveals tender, nodular temporal arteries, which may become pulseless. There is an elevated sedimentation rate. Biopsy of the temporal artery reveals lymphocytic infiltration early in the disease but later this progresses to necrotic areas surrounded by plasma cells, lymphocytes, multinucleated giant cells, and even amyloid deposits (58). If a negative biopsy is obtained and suspicion is high, the contralateral artery should be biopsied.

Treatment consists of a prolonged course of steroids, which for practical purposes eliminates the risk of blindness. Because of the seriousness of the complications, patients strongly suspected of having temporal arteritis should be given a therapeutic trial of steroids even if temporal artery biopsies are normal.

MUSCLE AND JOINT PAIN

Muscle Contraction Headaches

Muscle contraction or "tension" headaches are probably the most common type of headache encountered and probably occur in varying degrees in most of the general population. The pain typically occurs in the occipital, frontal, or temporal areas, has a squeezing band-like character, and usually is associated with anxiety or stress. The headaches can last from hours to days and are frequently relieved by over-the-counter analgesics.

As the name implies, the mechanism of the headaches is related to chronic contraction of the scalp muscles. Since other disorders in the head and neck (e.g., temporomandibular joint dysfunction) can result in chronic scalp and neck muscle contraction, the diagnosis of tension headache should be made only after other underlying causes have been excluded (59).

Temporomandibular Joint Dysfunction

Disorders of the temporomandibular joint are a common cause of headache and facial pain. While pain may be attributed to abnormalities of the joint itself, in the majority of cases it is due to the secondary myofascial pain dysfunction syndrome that results. The syndrome is characterized by a unilateral, constant, dull pain in the periauricular area, which may radiate to the temporal region or neck. The pain is exacerbated by chewing and may be associated with limitation of jaw motion, deviation of the mandible on opening the mouth, and hypertrophy of the ipsilateral masseter muscle.

There may be a clicking of the joint with crepitus and tenderness to palpation.

Temporomandibular joint disorders can be subdivided into two main groups: extracapsular and intracapsular disorders.

The *extracapsular disorder* is referred to as the temporomandibular joint dysfunction syndrome or myofascial pain dysfunction syndrome. In this condition, pain and dysfunction are caused by fatigue and eventual spasm in the muscles of mastication, resulting from bruxism or clenching (60). Psychological factors are thought to play a significant role in both teeth clenching and grinding, and therefore the myofascial pain dysfunction syndrome can be due to underlying functional disorders. In other cases, malocclusion may be a contributing factor. The diagnosis is confirmed by normal clinical and radiographic evaluation of the joint. Treatment consists of counseling, nonsteroidal anti-inflammatory drugs, soft diet, physiotherapy, splint therapy, and occlusal equilibrium. Transcutaneous electrical nerve stimulation (TENS), myoneural injection therapy, and behavioral modification may be helpful. In a small number of patients, organic joint changes may occur from prolonged joint abuse, requiring surgical intervention (61).

Intracapsular disorders of the temporomandibular joint include traumatically induced internal derangement of the joint, as well as various types of arthritis. Temporomandibular internal derangement is defined as an abnormal relationship of the articular disc to the mandibular condyle fossa and articular eminence (62). Secondary muscle spasm and pain can occur as with the myofascial pain dysfunction syndrome. The diagnosis of internal derangement is confirmed by positive joint findings on physical exam, CT scan, or MRI and/or joint arthroscopy. Conservative measures such as nonsteroidal anti-inflammatory medications, soft diet, and splint therapy can be used initially. If these are unsuccessful, surgical intervention may be necessary.

Temporomandibular joint arthritis and subsequent ankylosis can occur from infectious, traumatic, degenerative, or rheumatoid causes. The temporomandibular joint is affected in over 50% of patients with rheumatoid arthritis (63). The hallmark of these disorders is joint crepitus with limitation of movement, muscle spasm, and pain. The diagnosis is confirmed radiographically and treatment may be conservative or surgical reconstruction of the joint.

ATYPICAL FACIAL PAIN

Although several of the less common facial pain syndromes are categorized as "atypical" facial pain merely because they do not exactly fit the description of the classic facial pain syndromes, the diagnosis of atypical facial pain should be reserved for a select group of patients whose facial pain has a functional etiology. Atypical facial pain was first described by Frazier and Russell (64) in 1924 when these patients were differentiated from those with trigeminal neuralgia. While some of the patients in this series were probably suffering from cluster headaches, the majority fit the criteria of atypical facial pain that is accepted today.

The diagnosis of atypical facial pain can be made only after all possible organic etiologies of the pain have been ruled out. In most instances, this is accomplished by a thorough head and neck exam, as well as ophthalmologic, neurologic, and dental evaluations as indicated. A screening CT scan or MRI of the head and neck will have been obtained in most patients to rule out occult malignancy. Other criteria used to make the diagnosis of atypical facial pain include (a) pain lasting longer than 6 months, (b) a nonanatomic distribution, and (c) symptoms incompatible with any known syndrome (65).

There is a marked female to male predominance of 10:1 with a mean age of onset of 40 years (66). The syndrome is characterized by continuous, deep, nonlocalized pain that may have an aching, sharp, or burning quality. The pain becomes bilateral in approximately one-quarter of patients and is preceded by a minor operative procedure (e.g., dental extraction) or minor facial trauma in approximately half of the cases (66).

Various psychiatric disorders have been identified in patients with atypical facial pain, including depression, anxiety disorders, conversion reactions, personality disorders, and psychoses (66–69). Although it is generally accepted that atypical facial pain has a psychogenic origin, the exact psychologic or psychophysiologic mechanism of the disorder is unknown. In keeping with its psychogenic etiology, tricyclic antidepressants have been shown to be effective in the treatment of these patients (70,71). Routine analgesics are usually ineffective but narcotics or any other addictive drugs should be avoided. Once an organic etiology has been ruled out, psychiatric evaluation is essential.

SUMMARY

As can be seen by this review, a wide variety of disorders can present with facial pain. While these conditions are quite diversified and fall under the jurisdiction of several medical specialities, adhering to a few general principles will facilitate proper management of these patients.

1. A comprehensive history and physical exam are mandatory in evaluating these patients. Allow time for this evaluation.

2. Appropriate neurological, psychiatric, dental, ophthalmologic, and otolaryngologic referrals should be obtained as indicated.
3. Radiographic evaluation including CT scan or MRI should be used if any suspicion exists that an underlying pathology for the pain is present.
4. Every attempt should be made to treat the underlying etiology and avoid the blanket use of analgesics.
5. Surgical ablation of the affected nerves should be performed only when medical therapy has been exhausted.

REFERENCES

1. Wyllie JW, Kern EB, Djalilian M. Isolated sphenoid sinus lesions. *Laryngoscope* 1973;83:1252–1265.
2. Brooke RI. Atypical odontalgia. *Oral Surg* 1980;49:196–199.
3. Reik L Jr. Atypical odontalgia: a localized form of atypical facial pain. *Headache* 1984;24:222–224.
4. Rees RT, Harris M. Atypical odontalgia. *Br J Oral Surg* 1978–79;16:212–218.
5. Remick RA, Blasberg B, Barton JS, et al. Ineffective dental and surgical treatment associated with atypical facial pain. *Oral Surg* 1983;55:355–358.
6. Cameron CE. Cracked tooth syndrome. *J Am Dent Assoc* 1964;68:405–411.
7. Roberts AM, Person P. Etiology and treatment of idiopathic trigeminal and atypical facial neuralgias. *Oral Surg* 1979;48:298–308.
8. Roberts AM, Person P. Further observation on dental parameters of trigeminal and atypical facial neuralgias. *Oral Surg* 1984;58:121–129.
9. Behrens, Myles M. Headaches associated with disorders of the eye. *Med Clin North Am* 1978;62:507–521.
10. Lansche RK. Ophthalmodynia periodica. *Headache* 1964;4:247–249.
11. Percy AK, Nobrega FT, Kurland LT. Optic neuritis and multiple sclerosis: an epidemiologic study. *Arch Ophthalmol* 1972;87:135.
12. Carlow TJ. Headache and the eye. In: Dalessio DJ, ed. *Wolff's headache and other head pain,* 5th ed. New York: Oxford University Press, 1987;305–320.
13. Dalessio DJ. The major neuralgias, post infectious neuritis, and atypical facial pain. In Dalessio DJ, ed. *Wolff's headache and other head pain,* 5th ed. New York: Oxford University Press, 1987;266–289.
14. Miller H. Pain in the face. *Br Med J* 1968;2:577–580.
15. Carron H. Control of pain in the head and neck. *Otolaryngol Clin North Am* 1981;14(3):631–652.
16. Tew JM, Keller JT, Williams DS. Application of stereotactic principles to the treatment of trigeminal neuralgia. *Appl Neurophysiol* 1978;41:146–156.
17. Jannetta PS. Treatment of trigeminal neuralgia by suboccipital and transtentorial cranial operations. *Clin Neurosurg* 1976;24:538–549.
18. Weisenbug TH. Cerebello-pontine tumor diagnosed for 6 years as tic douloureux. The symptoms of irritation of the ninth and twelfth cranial nerves. *JAMA* 1910;55:1600–1604.
19. Harris W. Persistent pain in lesions of the peripheral and central nervous system. *Brain* 1921;44:557–571.
20. Riley HA, Berman WJ, Wortis H, et al. Glossopharyngeal neuralgia initiating or associated with cardiac arrest. *Trans Am Neurol Assoc* 1942;68:28–29.
21. Sluder G. Role of the sphenopalatine (Meckel's) ganglion in nasal headache. *NY Med J* 1908;989–990.
22. Sluder G. The anatomic and clinical relations of the sphenopala-

tine (Meckel's) ganglion to the nose and its accessory sinuses. *NY Med J* 1909;293–298.

23. Sluder G. Further clinical observations on the sphenopalatine ganglion (motor sensory and gustatory). *NY Med J* 1910; 850–851.

24. Sluder G. Etiology, diagnosis, prognosis, and treatment of sphenopalatine ganglion neuralgia. *JAMA* 1913;1201–1205.

25. Aubry M, Pialoux P. Sluder's syndrome. In: Vinken PJ, Bruvn GW, eds. *Handbook of clinical neurology.* Amsterdam: North-Holland Publishing, 1968; chap 30.

26. McAuliffe GW, Goodell H. Experimental studies on headache: pain from the nasal and paranasal structures. *Res Publ Assoc* 1945;23:185.

27. Eagle WW. Sphenopalatine ganglion neuralgia. *Arch Otolaryngol* 1942;35:66.

28. Danforth HB. Nasal vascular headache. *Laryngoscope* 1964;74: 151–161.

29. Slalom AA. Otorhinological headaches. In: Vinken PJ, Bruvn GW, eds. *Handbook of clinical neurology.* Amsterdam: North-Holland Publishing, 1968; chap 19.

30. Carter RL, Pittam NR, Tanner NSB. Pain and dysphagia with squamous cell carcinomas of the head and neck: the role of perineural spread. *J R Soc Med* 1982;75:598–606.

31. Thomas JE, Waltz AG. Neurological manifestations of nasopharyngeal malignant tumors. *JAMA* 1965;192:103–106.

32. Greenburg HS, Deck MDF, Vikram B, et al. Metastasis to the base of the skull: clinical findings in 43 patients. *Neurology* 1981; 31:530–537.

33. Hines JD, Nankervis G. Herpes zoster infection. *Hosp Med* 1977;8:72–84.

34. Frengly JD. Herpes zoster. A challenge in management. *Prim Care* 1981;8:715–731.

35. Mayme GE, Brown M, Arnold P, et al. Pain of herpes zoster and post herpetic neuralgia. In: Raj P, ed. *Practical management of pain.* Chicago: Year Book, 1986;345–364.

36. McKendric MS, McGill JI, White JE, et al. Oral acyclovir in acute herpes zoster. *Br Med J* 1986;293:1529–1532.

37. Erstein E. Triamcinolone-procaine in the treatment of zoster and post-zoster neuralgia. *Calif Med* 1971;115:6–10.

38. Tio R, Moya F, Vorasaron S. Treatments of post-herpetic neuralgia. *Anaesthesiol Sinica* 1978;16:151–153.

39. Colding A. The effect of regional sympathetic blocks in the treatment of herpes zoster. *Acta Anaesthesiol Scand* 1969;13: 133–141.

40. Friedman AP. Classification of headache. *JAMA* 1972;222: 1400–1402.

41. Friedman AP. Migraine. *Med Clin North Am* 1978;62(3): 481–494.

42. Joseph R, Cook GE, Steiner TJ, et al. Intracranial space-occupying lesions in patients attending a migraine clinic. *Practitioner* 1985;229:477–481.

43. Caviness VS, O'Brien P. Headache. *N Engl J Med* 1980;302: 446–449.

44. Kudrow L. Cluster headache: diagnosis and management. *Headache* 1979;19:142–150.

45. Kudrow L. Physical and personality characteristics in cluster headache. *Headache* 1974;13:197–201.

46. Kudrow L. Prevalence of migraine, peptic ulcer, coronary heart disease, and hypertension in cluster headache. *Headache* 1976; 16:66–69.

47. Fogan L. Treatment of cluster headache: a double-blind comparison of oxygen versus air inhalation. *Arch Neurol* 1985;42: 362–363.

48. Ekbom K. Lithium for cluster headache: review of the literature and preliminary results of long term treatment. *Headache* 1981; 21:132–140.

49. Fay T. Atypical neuralgia. *Arch Neurol Psychiatry* 1927;18: 309–315.

50. Fay T. Atypical neuralgia: a syndrome of vascular pain. *Ann Otol* 1932;41:1030–1062.

51. Hilger JA. Carotid pain. *Laryngoscope* 1949;59:829–838.

52. Roseman DW. Carotidynia. *Arch Otolaryngol* 1967;85:103–106.

53. Loushin L. Carotidynia. *Headache* 1977;17:192–195.

54. Pearse HE, Hinshaw JR. Bilateral arteritis simulating carotid body tumors. *Surg Gynecol Obstet* 1956;103:263–266.

55. Raskin NH, Prusiner S. Carotidynia. *Neurology* 1977;27:43–46.

56. Gluckman JL, Wolf BA. When a sore throat is not just a sore throat. *J Respir Dis* 1986;7(9):7–10.

57. Ettlinger RE, Hunder GG, Ward LE: Polymyalgia rheumatica and giant cell arteritis. *Annu Rev Med* 1978;29:15–22.

58. Sofferman RA. Cranial arteritis in otolaryngology. *Ann Otol Rhinol Laryngol* 1980;89:215–219.

59. Robinson CA. Cervical spondylosis and muscle contraction headaches. In: Dalassio DJ, ed. *Wolff's headache and other head pain,* 4th ed. New York: Oxford University Press, 1980; 362–380.

60. Laskin DM. Etiology of the pain dysfunction syndrome. *J Am Dent Assoc* 1969;79:147–153.

61. Guralnick W, Kaban LB, Merrill RG. Temporomandibular-joint afflictions. *N Engl J Med* 1978;299:123–129.

62. Dolwick MF, Riggs RR. Diagnosis and treatment of internal derangements of the temporomandibular joint. *Dent Clin North Am* 1983;27(3):561–572.

63. Blozis GG. Evaluation of patients with maxillofacial pain. *Dent Clin North Am* 1973;17(3):379–390.

64. Frazier CH, Russell EC. Neuralgia of the face: an analysis of 754 cases with relation to pain and other sensory phenomena before and after operation. *Arch Neurol Psychiatry* 1924;11: 557–563.

65. Mock D, Frydman W, Bordon AS. Atypical facial pain: a retrospective study. *Oral Surg Oral Med Oral Pathol* 1985;59: 422–474.

66. Solomon S, Lipton RB. Atypical facial pain: a review. *Semin Neurol* 1988;8(4):332–338.

67. Remick RA, Blasberg B, Campos PE, et al. Psychiatric disorders associated with atypical facial pain. *Can J Psychiatry* 1983;28: 178–181.

68. Gayford JJ. Atypical facial pain. *Practitioner* 1969;202:657–660.

69. Lascelles RG. Atypical facial pain and depression. *Br J Psychiatry* 1966;112:651–659.

70. Feinmann C, Harris M, and Conley R. Psychogenic facial pain: presentation and treatment. *Br Med J* 1984;228:436–438.

71. Sharav Y, Singer E, Schmidt E, et al. The analgesic effect of amitriptyline on chronic facial pain. *Pain* 1987;31:199–209.

CHAPTER 33

Orbital Decompression for Dysthyroid Optic Neuropathy

Dwight R. Kulwin and Robert C. Kersten

Thyroid-associated eye disease (thyroid ophthalmopathy) is a poorly understood immunologic phenomenon of the orbital structures that is frequently associated with thyroid endocrinopathy. It consists of proptosis (orbitopathy), eyelid retraction, and extraocular muscle dysfunction. This association is not well linked, as many patients with hyperthyroidism do not exhibit any eye findings and some patients with clinical thyroid ophthalmopathy do not have a measurable thyroid abnormality, or are hypothyroid.

The orbital immune reaction primarily affects the orbital musculature, particularly the extraocular muscles and the eyelid retractors. Thyroid ophthalmopathy may also result in enlargement of these muscles, with some associated edema of the orbital fat as well, thus increasing total orbital volume.

HISTOPATHLOGY

The histopathological changes in thyroid ophthalmopathy demonstrate a predominantly mononuclear inflammatory reaction consisting of lymphocytes, plasma cells, and occasional mast cells, consistent with an immune reaction. The inflammation is usually restricted to the extraocular muscle bellies, sparing the insertions. A mononuclear inflammatory response with edema may also be noted in orbital fat and the lacrimal gland.

It is theorized that extraocular muscles are involved in an organ-specific immune-mediated reaction. The muscle fibers are pathologically separated by mucopolysaccharides and collagen, causing increased volume of the extraocular muscles and leading to fibrosis, scarring, and interfascicular fatty infiltration. Extensive fibrosis can result in the failure of orbital decompression surgery, as such abnormal orbital tissues may not readily prolapse into a space that is opened.

The cause of thyroid-associated eye disease remains speculative, yet the growing body of knowledge points to an autoimmune etiology. A high incidence of autoimmune disorders such as myasthenia gravis, pernicious anemia, vitiligo, Sjögren's syndrome, and Addison's disease, occurring in conjunction with Graves' disease, lends support to an autoimmune etiology.

A leading hypothesis holds that Graves' thyrotoxicosis and thyroid ophthalmopathy may frequently be associated diseases resulting from different autoimmune reactions directed against the thyrotropin receptor of the thyroid cell on the one hand, and against orbital tissue on the other. There is evidence that aberrations in both humoral and cell-mediated immunity exist as noted by the fact that plasma cells are a major component of inflammatory infiltrates in extraocular muscles, and that, in some patients, thyroid ophthalmopathy has been noted to improve with plasmapheresis.

EVALUATION OF THE ORBITAL DECOMPRESSION PATIENT

Patients considered for orbital decompression need a thorough ophthalmic examination to aid in the diagnosis of thyroid disease, to evaluate the state of the eye and orbit, and to rule out other conditions that can masquerade as thyroid ophthalmopathy, such as orbital pseudotumor, neoplasms, cellulitis, carotid cavernous fistula, and axial myopia (a big eye). The ophthalmologist plays a key role in staging the disease and determining the effect of orbitopathy on ocular structures so as to advise when medical or surgical intervention such as orbital decompression is indicated.

The Werner classification, adapted and modified in 1977 by the American Thyroid Association (ATA) with further changes in 1981, is an attempt at classification of orbital changes in dysthyroid orbitopathy. Although useful in categorizing findings, it does little to meaningfully stage the disease or determine treatment.

External examination should note any eyelid or conjunctival edema, lagophthalmos, retraction of the upper or lower eyelids, injection over the extraocular muscle insertions, and proptosis.

Proptosis may be unilateral or bilateral and is usually measured with a Hertel exophthalmometer fixed at the lateral orbital rim. A difference of 2 mm or more between the two eyes is considered abnormal. Greater than 17 mm on exophthalmometry readings may represent proptosis, but there is great variability in development of the orbital rims between males and females, as well as between the races. Thus the upper limits of normal extend up to almost 25 mm for black males.

Grossly, proptosis can be assessed by viewing the cornea from either above the brow, or below, by looking up toward the patient's eyes with the neck extended. In evaluating proptosis, resistance to retropulsion should be assessed with gentle digital ballottement.

The single most common ocular motility abnormality encountered is an inability to elevate the eye, causing vertical diplopia. This is due to fibrotic shortening of the inferior rectus muscle. When medial rectus fibrosis occurs, a sixth nerve palsy can be mimicked, as the patient is unable to abduct the eye.

On computed tomography (CT) scanning, the belly of the extraocular muscle is enlarged, with the tendinous insertion on the globe being spared. The pattern of extraocular muscle involvement in order of frequency is inferior rectus, medial rectus, superior rectus, and rarely lateral rectus. It is unknown why some muscles are involved more than others.

At the slit lamp, signs of corneal exposure such as superficial punctate keratopathy can best be noted with placement of fluorescein dye in the eye. Also, assessment of intraocular pressure is important as it is well recognized that the inelasticity and fibrosis of the extraocular muscles and tightness of the orbit may produce pressure elevations.

From 3% to 8.6% of patients with thyroid ophthalmopathy develop optic neuropathy. Therefore the examination must include a thorough evaluation of optic nerve function. Visual acuity, light brightness comparison, color vision testing, assessment of pupillary reaction and relative afferent pupillary defect, ophthalmoscopy, and visual field testing are mandatory.

It is theorized that the optic neuropathy most commonly results from dysthyroid orbitopathy with compression of the optic nerve at the orbital apex by the enlarged extraocular muscles converging at the an-nulus of Zinn. Support for this theory is generated by numerous CT studies showing extraocular muscle enlargement at the orbital apex, and extraocular muscle volume studies showing a quantitative increase within orbits of patients with dysthyroid optic neuropathy. Patients with mild to moderate proptosis may be at a greater risk for optic neuropathy than more proptotic patients as they have not autodecompressed their orbits by expanding orbital volume through the development of proptosis.

A thorough medical evaluation is essential to establish the diagnosis of a dysthyroid state, so that appropriate therapy can be instituted. It should be kept in mind that patients may be euthyroid, hyperthyroid, or even hypothyroid at the time of presentation. Endocrine evaluation should include serum triiodothyronine (T_3), tetraiodothyronine (T_4), and thyroid-stimulating hormone (TSH) radioimmunoassays as well as T_3 resin uptake, which is of value in computing free T_4 index (FT_4I).

A CT scan of the orbit and sinuses should be obtained both to evaluate the orbit and to assure that no sinus abnormality or acute sinus disease is present.

INDICATIONS FOR SURGICAL ORBITAL DECOMPRESSION

Orbital decompression may be used to treat the sequelae of thyroid orbitopathy. Corticosteroids, radiation therapy, and chemotherapy are current modalities available to medically decompress the orbital contents. The traditional indication for surgical orbital decompression is compressive optic neuropathy unresponsive to medical therapy. In addition, corneal decompensation from exposure due to severe proptosis and disfigurement from exophthalmos are also indications for surgical decompression.

Although we have discussed the indications for orbital decompression surgery with regard to its most common use in thyroid ophthalmopathy, one should not be left with the impression that the procedure lacks application in other clinical settings. Efficacy of decompression has been well documented in the following clinical settings: (a) intraorbital hemorrhage related to trauma, blepharoplasty, retrobulbar anesthesia, and sinus surgery; (b) traumatic optic neuropathy with bone fragments impinging on the optic nerve; (c) in medial wall fractures with entrapment, medial wall decompression may be performed to extricate the entrapped tissue; (d) craniofacial dysostosis (Crouzon's and Apert's syndromes) with exorbitism may be treated with orbital decompression combined with infraorbital augmentation or midfacial advancement; (e) palliative treatment for selected cases of compressive optic neuropathy due to meningioma compressing the posterior orbit; and (f) granulomatous disease with involvement of the sinuses and contiguous orbit with exophthalmos and optic nerve dysfunction (primarily sarcoidosis).

Orbital decompression is performed to counter the effects of increased orbital volume caused by enlargement of the orbital structures from thyroid ophthalmopathy. Expansion of the bony orbit can be used for those people in whom the contents of the orbit remain permanently enlarged, or in whom severe functional problems develop during the acute stage of the disease.

In our practice, 70% to 80% of patients undergo orbital decompression as part of a sequence of procedures to provide them with a more normal appearance, while 20% to 30% of patients undergo orbital decompression to treat a functional abnormality such as optic nerve compression, exposure keratitis, or severe strabismus.

SURGICAL ORBITAL DECOMPRESSION

An orbital decompression should enlarge the bony orbit in such a way as to allow maximal displacement of the eye posteriorly, while minimizing displacement along the other spatial axes. Additionally, since compression of the optic nerve by hypertrophied extraocular muscles is most severe in the posterior aspect of the orbit, where the orbital walls come together, it is crucial to remove bone to the very back of the orbit in order to remove any pressure on the optic nerve.

Various approaches for decompressing the orbit in thyroid ophthalmopathy have been described. These include transcranial, transantral, frontoethmoidal, and periorbital approaches.

Of the four walls of the orbit, two of them, the medial and inferior, are surrounded by large well-aerated sinuses, affording a major avenue for substantially enlarging the orbit. Superiorly, the orbital roof is directly adjacent to the frontal lobe. Therefore potential space for herniation of orbital tissues is minimal. Similarly, the lateral orbital wall is adjacent to the temporalis muscle so that there is less potential space for orbital decompression. Hence the most substantial effect from orbital decompression can be achieved by removing the medial and inferior orbital walls.

In the transantral approach, decompression of the orbit is obtained by removing the floor and medial orbital wall. Access to these orbital areas is through a Caldwell–Luc approach, with removal of most of the anterior maxillary face up to the level of the infraorbital nerve (Fig. 1). This provides excellent exposure of the posterior two-thirds of the orbit and the medial orbital wall. However, because of the soft tissues overlying the anterior maxillary face and the presence of the infraorbital rim, exposure to the anterior portion of the orbital floor and to the bone surrounding the nasolacrimal duct is poor.

Another problem with the transantral approach is that it can sometimes be very difficult to visualize the infraorbital neurovascular bundle as it transverses the orbital floor. Additionally, as bone is removed in the transantral approach, if any rents develop in, or if there is a preexisting dehiscence of, the periorbita, orbital fat can herniate into the sinus and impede visualization (Fig. 2).

The periorbital approach to the orbital floor and medial orbital wall, whether transcutaneous or transconjunctival, affords an excellent view of the anterior two-thirds of the orbital floor and the area around the nasolacrimal duct (Fig. 3). However, visualization of the most posterior centimeter of the orbital floor is very

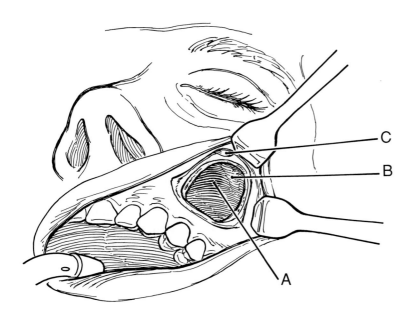

FIG. 1. Transantral approach to orbital decompression: roof of maxillary sinus (orbital floor) (*A*); infraorbital nerve pathway (*B*); and infraorbital nerve (*C*).

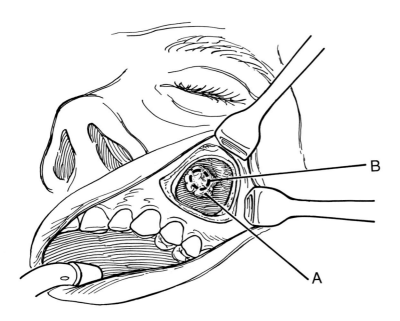

FIG. 2. Transantral approach. Fat (*A*) is herniating through the bony opening (*B*) in the orbital floor.

difficult. Likewise, visualization of the medial orbital wall is suboptimal. As with the transantral approach, at times it can be very difficult to identify the infraorbital neurovascular bundle.

In our experience with over 250 eyes, we have found that a combined approach to orbital decompression, utilizing both the periorbital and transantral approaches, is the safest and most effective way to decompress the orbit. When used in combination, these approaches complement each other, compensating for areas of poor visualization, minimizing the difficulty in

delineating the neurovascular bundle, and helping to avoid tearing the periorbita (Figs. 4 and 5). Through the periorbital incision, one can actively elevate the orbital contents, thus preventing orbital fat from herniating down into the sinus as the bone along the orbital floor is removed. Through transillumination of the orbital floor from above and below, one can accurately visualize the entire course of the infraorbital neurovascular bundle.

In our hands, this combined approach is as fast as either one of the separate approaches. In addition, we have yet to encounter any serious complication of orbital decompression, such as injury to the eye, optic nerve, lacrimal system, and infraorbital neurovascular bundle, or a cerebrospinal fluid leak, or the need for reoperation because of inadequate bone removal or periorbital excision. These complications are reported with a frequency of 2% to 20% when the orbit is decompressed through either approach alone.

As the combined approach to orbital decompression takes no more time than either single approach, provides superior visualization and better access to the orbital bones, and results in a complication rate lower than that reported for either single technique, it is, in our opinion, the safest and most effective way to perform a surgical orbital decompression.

SURGICAL TECHNIQUE

After the ophthalmologist has determined that orbital decompression is indicated, the patient is seen by an otolaryngologic surgeon. The patient is then scheduled for surgery.

Surgery is performed with the patient under general endotracheal anesthesia, with the tube fixated to the

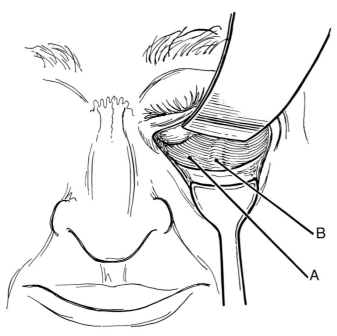

FIG. 3. Transcutaneous approach to orbital decompression: orbital floor (*A*) and infraorbital nerve pathway (*B*).

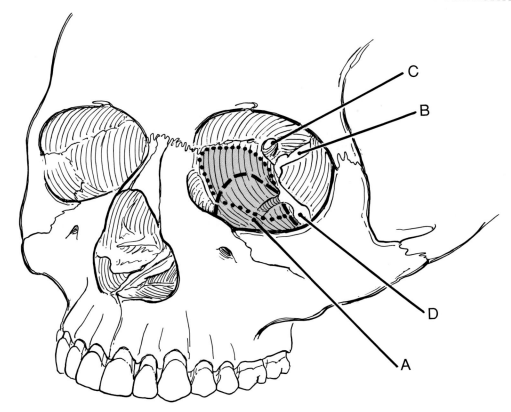

FIG. 4. Superimposing the areas of good visualization through the periorbital (---) and transantral (···) approaches shows that by combining both techniques all of the orbital floor and medial orbital wall are well visualized: infraorbital nerve (A); superior orbital fissure (B); optic canal (C); and inferior orbital fissures (D).

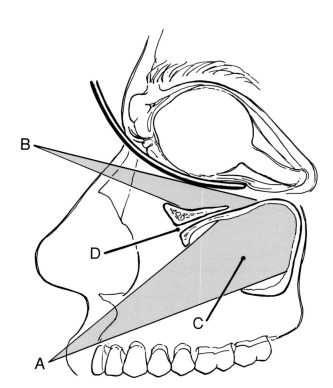

FIG. 5. Sagittal view of the orbit and maxillary sinus during a combined approach orbital decompression showing the areas best visualized by the transantral (A) and periorbital (B) approach: maxillary sinus (C) and infraorbital nerve (D).

contralateral side of the mouth. The ipsilateral nostril is packed with a nasal decongestant, and the lower ipsilateral eyelid and buccal sulcus are each infiltrated with 1% lidocaine with epinephrine.

Although a transconjunctival approach can be used, we prefer an infraciliary incision in the lower eyelid, extending just beyond the lateral canthus. After the initial incision has been made, a 6-0 silk temporary tarsorrhaphy is placed between the upper and lower eyelids at the lateral limbus. If needed, a temporary tarsorrhaphy is placed through the contralateral eyelids to prevent exposure of the eye during surgery, as lagophthalmos is frequently seen in thyroid ophthalmopathy. A skin muscle flap is then developed and dissected from the underlying orbital septum down to the inferior orbital rim. In patients with thyroid ophthalmopathy, the orbital septum may have numerous festoons and may be scarred to the orbicularis. However, the septum can usually be kept intact.

The periosteum is incised at the infraorbital rim. The periorbita is then elevated from the orbital floor going back about 2 cm, where, variably, a single arterial vessel comes up from the infraorbital neurovascular bundle into the orbit. This vessel is placed on a gentle stretch, cauterized and then cut. Elevation of the periorbita is then carried back to the level of the inferior orbital fissure laterally and the orbital apex medially.

After the orbital contents have been elevated, the otolaryngologist performs an ipsilateral Caldwell–Luc approach to the maxillary sinus, elevating the soft tissues of the cheek from the anterior maxillary face up to the level of the infraorbital neurovascular foramen. The bone of the anterior maxillary face is removed to this level. It is crucial to create a large bony opening to allow adequate visualization.

At this point, the nasal packing is removed and a nasoantral window is created. As one of the major purposes in performing an orbital decompression is to allow orbital fat to herniate into the maxillary sinus, obstruction of the nasoantral ostium frequently occurs.

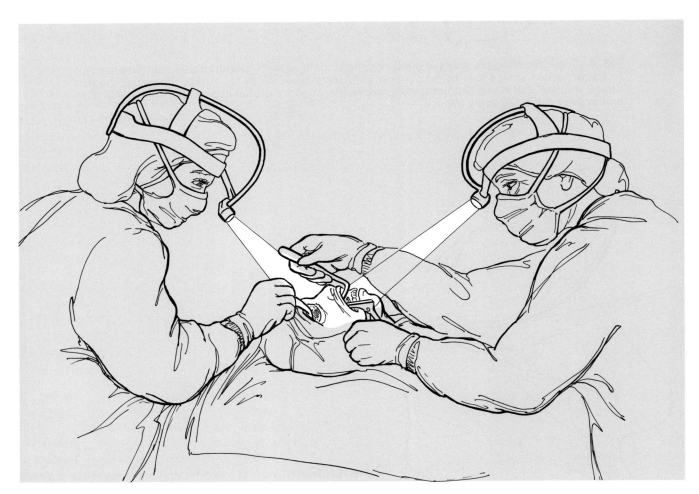

FIG. 6. Operating positions for combined approach decompression. Surgeons are using transillumination to identify the course of the infraorbital nerve.

The nasoantral window ensures aeration and drainage of the maxillary sinus.

The maxillary sinus mucosa is decongested with topical application of ½% Neo-Synephrine and then the mucosa from the top half of the maxillary sinus is stripped and removed.

At this point, the two surgeons begin to operate concurrently.

The ophthalmic surgeon elevates the orbital contents from the orbital floor with a malleable retractor. His/her assistant then pulls the skin muscle flap inferomedially with a Ragnell retractor. The otolaryngologist arranges for his/her assistant to retract the cheek.

The ophthalmic surgeon, wearing a fiberoptic headlight, looks down onto the bony orbital floor while the otolaryngologic surgeon, also wearing a headlight, looks up from below. Through transillumination, the course of the infraorbital neurovascular bundle can be confidently identified (Fig. 6). The ophthalmic surgeon then uses a 4-mm osteotome and hammer, at the direction of the otolaryngologic surgeon, to create an opening in the orbital floor medial to the infraorbital neurovascular bundle, pushing a large flap of bone down into the maxillary sinus. The two surgeons remove the bone of the orbital floor medial to the infraorbital neurovascular bundle.

The ophthalmic surgeon removes the anterior portion of the orbital floor, proceeding forward to the infraorbital rim (Fig. 7). The bone lateral to the nasolacrimal duct is also removed. The ophthalmic surgeon then retracts the orbital contents to improve surgical exposure, while the otolaryngologic surgeon removes the orbital floor back to the posterior wall of the maxillary sinus (Fig. 8). With a vantage point superiorly, the ophthalmic surgeon may be able to provide guidance as to how far posterior bone removal should be performed. As the posterior portion of the orbital floor curves around to the posterior wall of the maxillary sinus, there is a firm bony buttress; this is the posterior limit of the floor removal.

At this point, the otolaryngologic surgeon performs a transantral ethmoidectomy, removing the medial wall of the orbit to just above the medial rectus muscle. Several millimeters of intact bone are left beneath the anterior and posterior ethmoidal vessels.

We typically leave the orbital floor lateral to the infraorbital neurovascular bundle intact, as the amount of floor that can be removed lateral to the infraorbital neurovascular bundle (and anterior to the infraorbital fissure) is small and does not provide significant additional decompression. In addition, we feel that this portion of the floor provides important support for the globe, minimizing hypo-ophthalmus.

When an especially large decompression is needed,

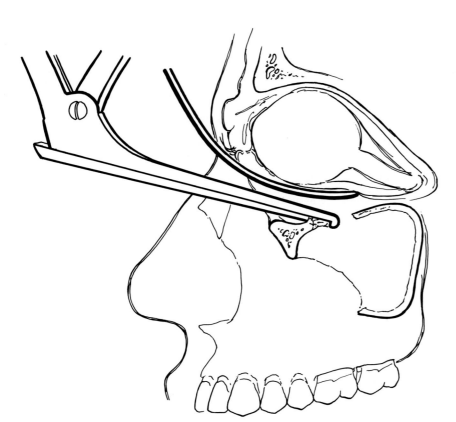

FIG. 7. Removal of the anterior orbital floor through a periorbital incision.

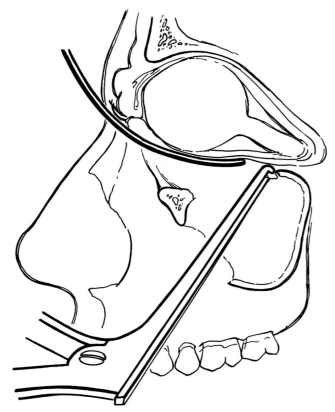

FIG. 8. Removal of the posterior orbital floor. A malleable retractor is positioned through the eyelid incision to elevate the orbital contents, preventing herniating orbital tissues from obstructing visualization and impeding bone removal.

one can work from both above and below to remove all the bone surrounding the infraorbital neurovascular bundle. On those rare instances of extreme proptosis, the lateral portion of the orbital floor and even the lateral orbit rim and wall are removed.

After this joint bone removal has been completed, the ophthalmic surgeon then approaches from below, and looking up through the anterior maxillary bony opening, incises periorbita. The incision is made with a large curved Church scissors along the medial edge of the infraorbital neurovascular bundle, from the infraorbital rim posteriorly to the back wall of the maxillary sinus. A parallel incision is made medially, and a large block of periorbita is excised, allowing herniation of the orbital fat. The medial periorbita is stripped so that it hangs loosely from its medial attachment, thus allowing it to bulge into the ethmoid sinus. Gentle pressure is placed on the globe to identify any residual periorbital bands, which are then cut.

As long as periorbita hangs limply and does not provide any interference to orbital fat herniation into the maxillary or ethmoid sinuses, it does not need to be removed.

After stripping the inferior periorbita, one will frequently see that the posterior one-third of the orbit contains residual tissue that appears to be periorbita. However, careful inspection will usually demonstrate this structure to have anteroposterior striations and a reddish tinge, indicating that it is a hypertrophied inferior rectus muscle.

A substantial change in the position of the eye compared with the preoperative position should be obvious at this time. The Caldwell–Luc and lower eyelid incisions are then closed in an appropriate fashion. The contralateral tarsorrhaphy is removed, while the ipsilateral tarsorrhaphy is left in place for 3 days to keep the lower eyelid stretched superiorly to prevent the development of cicatricial eyelid retraction.

At the end of the procedure, iced dressings are applied and continued for 48 hr postoperatively.

One gram of a first-generation cephalosporin is given to the patient intravenously at the beginning of surgery and the patient is continued on a dosage of 500 mg four times a day by mouth for 5 days thereafter.

If the patient is to undergo a contralateral orbital decompression, this procedure is usually performed on the second postoperative day, both to allow the patient to recover and also to ensure that no complication has occurred to the initially operated orbit.

The patient typically goes home the day after surgery. Unless indicated, steroids are not usually given during the procedure or postoperatively.

SELECTED REFERENCES

1. Calcaterra TC, Thompson JW. Antra-ethmoidal decompression of the orbit in Graves' disease: ten years' experience. *Laryngoscope* 1980;90:1941.
2. Colvard DM, Waller RR, Neault RW, et al. Nasolacrimal duct obstruction following transantral–ethmoidal orbital decompression. *Ophthalmic Surg* 1979;10:25.
3. Gorman C, Waller R, Dyer J. *The eye and orbit in thyroid disease.* New York: Raven Press, 1984.
4. Koornneef L, Mourits M. Orbital decompression. *Orbit* 1988;7:225.
5. Leone CR, Bajandas FJ. Inferior orbital decompression for dysthyroid optic neuropathy. *Ophthalmology* 1981;88:525.
6. Leone CR, Piest KL, Newman FJ. Medial and lateral wall decompression for thyroid ophthalmopathy. *AJO* 1989;108:160.
7. McCord CD. Current trend in orbital decompression. *Ophthalmology* 1985;92:21.
8. McCord CD. Orbital decompression for Graves' disease. *Ophthalmology* 1981;88:533–541.
9. Merritt JH, Schaeffer SD, Close LG. Orbital decompression for optic neuropathy secondary to thyroid eye disease. *Laryngoscope* 1988;98:712.
10. Moran RE, Letterman GS, et al. The surgical correction of exophthalmos. *Plast Reconstr Surg* 1972;49:595.
11. Mourits M, Koornneef L, et al. Orbital decompression for Graves' ophthalmopathy by inferomedial plus lateral, and by coronal approach. *Ophthalmology* 1990;97:636.
12. Ogura JH, Lucente FE. Surgical results of orbital decompression for malignant exophthalmos. *Laryngoscope* 1974;84:637–644.

13. Riddick FA. Immunologic aspects of thyroid disease. *Ophthalmology* 1981;88:471.

14. Sergott RC, Felberg NT, Savino PJ, et al. The clinical immunology of Graves' ophthalmopathy. *Ophthalmology* 1981;88:484.

15. Shorr N, Seiff S. The four stages of surgical rehabilitation of the patient with dysthyroid ophthalmopathy. *Ophthalmology* 1986;93:476.

16. Small RG, Meiring NL. A combined orbital and antral approach to surgical decompression of the orbit. *Ophthalmology* 1981;88:542–547.

17. Von Haache NP, Wilson JA, Dale BA, et al. The Patterson operation for decompression of the orbit. *Clin Otolaryngol* 1986;11:365.

18. Wilson WB, Manke WF. Orbital decompression in Graves' disease. The predictability of reduction of proptosis. *Arch Ophthalmol* 1991;109:343.

CHAPTER 34

Cerebrospinal Fluid Rhinorrhea

Bruce W. Pearson

In the second century A.D., Galen, like Hippocrates 600 years before him, believed the mucus found in the respiratory tract originally arose in the brain. Respiratory secretions were thought to be strained through the ethmoid bones, and into the passageways of the nasal cavity (1). Perhaps an enlarged pituitary, dipping down into a sphenoid sinus, suggested this. Maybe the olfactory foramina that were evident in the cribriform plate fostered this idea. Lacking preservation, microscopy, and biochemical knowledge, postmortem neural tissues and mucus may have shared many physical features!

Today, of course, the separate origins of nasal fluid and "brain fluid" are considered obvious. Some may find it surprising that there are still situations faced by clinicians where the source of a clear rhinorrhea is not so apparent. The distinction between serous nasal secretions and fluids that leak down into the nose from the "water" supporting the brain, through a pathologic opening in the skull base dura and bone, can perplex the most intrepid physician. Moreover, the challenge to localize and repair the site of communication after the diagnosis is made can prove even more formidable. Failure to acknowledge a cerebrospinal fluid (CSF) leak, until a bout of meningitis demands it, risks brain damage, cranial neuropathy, and death. Preventing these outcomes and meeting this challenge is the goal of this chapter, in which the diagnosis and treatment of cerebrospinal fluid rhinorrhea will be described.

BACKGROUND

Traumatic CSF rhinorrhea has been recognized since the 17th century. Bidloo the Elder, a Dutch surgeon, described a case in which intracranial fluid "flowed from the nose like a clear fountain" (2). "High-pressure" CSF rhinorrhea, due to hydrocephalus, was reported by Miller in 1826 (3). In 1884, the phenomenon of air within the cranial cavity, from an ethmoid defect, was reported at autopsy by Chiari (4). St. Clair Thompson (5) described the first important clinical series, 20 patients with "spontaneous" CSF rhinorrhea, at the turn of the century and, in doing so, established appropriate respect for the dangerous significance of this deceptively innocuous symptom.

In this century, several important issues pertinent to CSF leakage have been elucidated by various investigators. The incidence of meningitis in patients with *untreated* CSF rhinorrhea was shown to be 50% by Calvert and Cairns (6) in the preantibiotic era. After antibiotics became available, however, meningitis was not eliminated; the mortality rate was still found to be 20% by Levins et al. (7) in 1972. During the 1920s, Dandy (8) described the first successful intracranial repair, and this was the principal method of approach until Dohlman's (9) report of an extracranial technique in 1948. Trauma was recognized as the commonest cause of CSF rhinorrhea once patients began to survive head injuries in significant numbers, but in 1968, the special diagnostic significance of "spontaneous" CSF rhinorrhea was redefined by Ommaya et al. (10). Numerous authors have described specific tests for both identification and preoperative localization of a source of CSF rhinorrhea. By the 1970s the technical aspects and long-term failure rates [27% initial failure and 10% overall in the Ray–Bergland (11) 1967 series] of repair by intracranial operative techniques had been clarified. Transethmoid and transfrontal repairs gained in credibility with reports by Calcaterra (12) and others, aided by the development of ingenious new nasal flaps (13,14), the adaptation of old ones (15), and magnificent advances in computed tomography (CT) scans of the sinuses (16). More recently, with improved comprehension of when an extracranial approach is appropriate and when an intracranial operation is more advisable, excellent levels of safety and success in controlling leaks and preventing meningitis are attainable.

PHYSIOLOGY OF CEREBROSPINAL FLUID

Cerebrospinal fluid is a clear, watery liquid produced by the choroid and lateral ventricular plexi, at the rate of approximately 20 ml/hr in adults. This amounts to nearly 500 ml/day, or roughly four times the normal volume of the CSF compartment, which is 90 to 150 ml. The normal pressure of CSF, 100 to 200 mmHg, supports the brain and spinal cord with a uniform force. Lower "opening" pressures (of around 20) are not uncommon when lumbar punctures are performed on patients with CSF leakage. The glucose content in CSF runs around two-thirds of that in blood; it is rarely below 50 mg/dl (providing meningitis is absent). The level of 50 mg/dl is higher than the glucose levels found in mucus, lacrimal secretions, or serous fluid. Therefore quantitative glucose determinations were once used to prove a clear fluid from the nose was CSF. Subsequently, numerous observers have shown that contemporary glucose oxidase based tests, like Clinistix or Testape, are invalid when used for this purpose. The combination of their high sensitivity and the genuine presence of some glucose in nasal or lacrimal secretions yields false-positive rates up to 40% (17). When patients insist they have CSF rhinorrhea, but the sole positive finding is their own unsupported contention, I have sometimes given them a test strip to take home and report. Their repeated experience of a negative result will sometimes convince them their obsession is false. However, it must be confessed that even this use is not entirely reliable; false-negative results are possible with real CSF, when, for example, both an intermittent leak and cholinergic rhinorrhea are present.

Cerebrospinal fluid functions to cushion the brain from mechanical trauma; the brain weighs 1500 g in air but only about 50 g in CSF. Having no lymphatics to absorb and drain away noxious metabolites, the brain also depends on CSF to act as a metabolic "sink," helping dilute unwanted substances so effective neuronal activity is preserved.

Devoid of platelets, leukocytes, or fibrin precursors, CSF is singularly lacking in either the humoral or cellular elements of self-repair. No wonder even pinpoint defects can be so agonizingly recurrent and persistent! What tissue repair mechanisms do exist are certainly a poor substitute for the regeneration of healthy dura. These processes, which are often visualized at the time of a surgical repair, include (a) arachnoid/glial scar formation, (b) atrophic brain "plugs," (c) incomplete osteogenesis, and (d) nasal mucosal hyperplasia and granulation.

CLINICAL APPROACH TO CEREBROSPINAL FLUID LEAKAGE

The discovery of a suspected CSF leak should always draw prompt and critical attention on the part of the otolaryngologist. I find it helpful to build my own responses around the answers to five key questions:

1. Is the fluid the patient reports actually cerebrospinal fluid?
2. If yes, what would be the etiology of the hole or holes in the dura?
3. What is the site? Specifically, can we exclude (a) the ear, (b) the upper two-thirds of the frontal sinus, or (c) the midline of the sella. If one of these is the source, the transethmoidal approach will clearly not be appropriate. A nonethmoid extracranial approach might be possible, however. Mastoid/transtemporal surgery is effective for the ear, a frontal–osteoplastic flap for the frontal sinus, and transseptal transsphenoidal repairs for the sella.
4. Is it out in the lateral recesses of a well-pneumatized sphenoid sinus, are there large multiple defects, or is this a high-pressure leak? If so, call the neurosurgeon. An intracranial (middle fossa) repair will be required for the sphenoid wing, a bicoronal intradural repair may be needed for extensive bilateral anterior cranial fossa dural repairs, and the control of concomitant intracranial pressure elevation is mandatory for success in cases where high-pressure leakage is the problem.
5. If the leak *is* apparently ethmoid or cribriform, on which *side* is it most likely to be found? This is all you can hope for in many cases. Fortunately it is all you need to know, because the ethmoid roof, the lower part of the frontal sinus, the cribriform plate, and much of the sphenoid sinus can all be visualized simultaneously through the exposure afforded by a transethmoidal exploration. In fact, in a normal well-pneumatized sinus, an effective exploration can be performed without sacrificing flaps, or any of the patient's other options for repair.

IS THE FLUID IN QUESTION REALLY CEREBROSPINAL FLUID?

Several clinical features of CSF influence the typical history. CSF is, of course, water clear, but more importantly, it lacks the viscosity of mucus. This makes it hard for the patient to control. It drips from the nose without warning. The nasal cavity is unnaturally wet (usually only on one side), despite the tendency to sniffle or blow. Positions may aggravate the leak, as may straining or the Valsalva maneuver. Antihistamines do nothing, of course, and nasal obstruction is usually lacking. The same injury that caused the leak may also be the cause of anosmia, which is found in 78% of traumatic cases (18). The major defect may be on the side opposite the dripping or bilateral rhinorrhea may occur. The same injury that causes a frontal sinus fracture, for example, can break the intersinus septum. An injury that breaches the cribriform not infrequently extends across the midline. In spontaneous CSF rhinorrhea, particularly, more than one site may be leaking. One can never assume that a leak has stopped just because the history of trauma is remote. Complications of CSF fistula, such as recurrent meningitis, or an air–fluid level (demonstrating pneumocephalus) on a plain skull radiograph denote a persisting leak until proved otherwise.

CHEMICAL TESTS

Probably the most specific method of identification of CSF is to collect some fluid and test for the presence of beta II transferrin (19). Transferrins are detected by gel electrophoresis, immunofixation, and silver staining. Beta I transferrin can be identified in normal tissue and secretions, but when two bands (beta I and beta II transferrin) are identified, an unknown fluid can be reported as positive for CSF. The advantage of this test is not only its specificity, but the fact that it can be performed on an extremely small volume of fluid. The disadvantage is its lack of wide availability outside large reference laboratories, but perhaps this is currently undergoing change.

If 0.5 cc or so of bloodless fluid can be collected in a glass tube (ask the patient to lean forward and strain), fluid chloride content is the most available practical chemical test and quite a useful one. While chlorides in serum range from 98 to 112 mEq/liter, the chloride content of CSF is higher, above 120 (up to 130 mEq/ liter). Thus an elevated chloride value in an unknown sample of drippage from the nose is highly presumptive evidence of CSF.

WHY IS A CEREBROSPINAL FLUID LEAK PRESENT?

Cerebrospinal fluid rhinorrhea is a process, not an etiologic diagnosis. The diagnosis of the *cause* of the leak requires a careful history and physical examination, including examination of the nasal cavity and ear. Once the diagnosis of CSF rhinorrhea is recognized, there is no point limiting one's investigative focus to the discovery of the site of a bony hole! Holes in the cribriform are normal (the olfactory foramina); bone can be thinned to the point of radiolucency in numerous other locations (e.g., where the anterior ethmoid arteries branch off into the anterior meningeal arteries at the front of the cribriform plate) and suture junctions

between the frontal, ethmoid, and sphenoid bones can all look like fracture lines on a CT scan. The "holes" of concern are really the ones in the dura (and arachnoid). The question that must therefore be answered is: What tore, punctured, thinned, or eroded the dura? Trauma is usually the likeliest reason for a defect, blunt head trauma, in which plain film evidence of a gross fracture is often lacking. The heavy exterior buttresses of the bony skull, the orbital margins, the glabella, and the frontal processes of the maxillae stand up to a blow, but they transmit the energy more deeply into the skull, where it encounters and disrupts the thin delicate laminae of the ethmoid roof and the cribriform plate. The attached dura is generally torn as well, and a leak or meningitis or both may ensue, at any time after continuity between the normally sterile subarachnoid space and the intermittently contaminated nasal or sinus cavities is established.

The pathology of immediate traumatic CSF leakage, in the acute stage of trauma, is different from that of delayed CSF rhinorrhea, a late or persistent complication of trauma. Acute cases may heal and resolve; delayed cases are destined to persist and recur. CSF rhinorrhea following rhinologic, otologic, or skull base surgery is a special category of trauma. Here again, diverse etiologic factors, including the concomitant disease, are pertinent to the prognosis and management. Sometimes there is no history of trauma or surgery at all, just the development of so-called spontaneous CSF rhinorrhea. This suggests several etiologic possibilities (20):

1. An intracranial or a skull base lesion is present that has breached the dura. This process must be discovered and investigated before further steps are taken.
2. Intracranial CSF pressure is increased, locally or diffusely. This process also must be understood before a successful repair can be planned.
3. Proof of an accidental injury, sometimes an ancient one, will be discovered in the course of the management, even though the episode of trauma has long been forgotten or denied.

REGION OR SITE OF LEAKAGE: THE FLUORESCEIN TEST

The history and physical findings remain the most reliable factors in establishing whether or not a leak is present, and of course they often suggest the site. Anterior rhinoscopy is improved by cocainization, trimming the vibrissae, and palpating with a cotton wool applicator. Intranasal examination with a 2.7-mm 30-degree and 70-degree rigid nasal telescope is highly recommended, and examination of the ears with an otologic microscope and tympanometry should never be overlooked.

To confirm the leak and assist with its localization, the most useful study in our practice is probably the fluorescein dye test (21). All dyes carry a risk of reaction, but the risk is small and acceptable if certain precautions are taken. A proper neurologic examination is first completed, then a spinal tap is created through the L3–L4 or L4–L5 lumbar interspace. Next, 0.5 cc of sterile 5% fluorescein dye is instilled, *after it has been diluted* in 10 cc of CSF. This mixture is *slowly* injected in the subarachnoid space of the spinal canal, over 5 min. Depending on the rate of the leak, a wait of 20 min to 3 hr is required for the dye to rise through the spinal subarachnoid space to be present in the cranial cavity. Seven tiny labeled cottonoid pledgets are placed in the decongested and topically anesthetized nasal cavity to absorb the dye. A rigid 0-degree 2.7-mm nasal telescope and its tiny cup forceps attachment can be useful instruments in this task. Before placement, each retrieval string is tagged with a special label to indicate the side and location of each pledget. The sites of placement are as follows: the right and left cribriform (nasal roof), the right and left middle meatus (posterior half), and the true right and left sphenoethmoidal recesses (above and behind the posterior end of each middle turbinate). A seventh pledget can be placed in an inferior meatus to serve as a "control" for lacrimal secretions. Insertions should be scrupulously atraumatic, to avoid blood contamination. One hour later, remove the cottonoids and examine them under an ultraviolet light. Examine the eardrums also, under the bright light of an operating microscope, to detect fluorescein fluorescence in middle ear cavity. If the source is middle ear or mastoid, traveling to the nasal cavity through the eustachian tube, the dye may otherwise be missed.

Fluorescein dye is gentle enough to be instilled in the eye and is commercially available as an intravenous agent for fundoscopic examination. Nevertheless, dilution and slow instillation are mandatory for a safe fluorescein dye test. A two-way stopcock should be connected to the spinal needle, to allow the infusion of a diluent (saline) as well as prompt withdrawal of dye, in case a reaction is recognized. Sensitivity reactions affect the lower spinal cord; patients who have experienced such a reaction developed acute burning pain in the lower trunk and lower extremities, followed by tonic and clonic seizures of the muscles in the legs (22). The use of fluorescein to stain CSF represents an "unapproved" use of a Food and Drug Administration (FDA) approved medication. Used wisely, with support from the literature, and on an ethical and logical basis, we feel it certainly can be justified in these life-threatening situations. Our own experience, adhering rigorously to the dilution and timing described, has been that no reactions have occurred in an estimated experience of over 60 fluorescein injections. From the published reports of reactions others have studied, no permanent disabilities have occurred.

RADIOLOGIC LOCALIZATION OF THE SOURCE OF CEREBROSPINAL FLUID RHINORRHEA

The maxillary antrum does not contact the skull base, of course, but it sometimes acts as a dependent repository for fluid dumped into the middle meatus from a frontal or ethmoid source. There, a plain film showing an opaque antrum, especially with a air–fluid level on the Waters view, can be helpful. On a brow-up lateral plain film of the skull, a fluid level in the sphenoid sinus may be recognizable when the sphenoid is the site of a leak (Fig. 1). In upright films, the fluid has less chance to collect. Plain skull radiographs do not image a leak by themselves but they may show intracranial air. This constitutes proof of a fistula and, more importantly, a clinical emergency. Air in the head may act as an expanding intracranial mass (tension pneumocephalus), with all the danger that progression implies, including permanent neurologic deficit or even death. Plain sinus radiographs do not show much detail of the ethmoids (Caldwell view and lateral view), and, of course, the cribriform and the frontal sinuses are very poorly evaluated by this modality.

Presently, metrizamide computed tomographic cisternography (MCTC) is the radiologic study most likely to localize the site of CSF leakage. Consequently, it has displaced most other radiologic tests (16). The contrast agent, metrizamide, is an nonionic triiodinated water-soluble compound that is instilled into the subarachnoid space via lumbar puncture. This is generally followed by careful tipping and positioning of the patient so as to guide the contrast medium into the head, often with fluoroscopic control. Coronal high-resolution CT scans are then taken through the sinuses, attempting to catch some dye in the leak. Under ideal conditions, metrizamide within the cranial cavity can actually be followed right through a dural and bony defect, thus pinpointing the exact site of a leakage and outlining the pathway of the fistula. In other cases, it will simply be seen within the nasal cavity, or within a particular sinus, confirming the presence of a leak and suggesting its probable location. Unfortunately, in 20% to 40% of cases, even with provocative measures like intrathecal saline infusion, coughing, and decubitus positioning, metrizamide fails to show the site of leak (23). As in many tests in medicine, absence of proof does not constitute proof of absence, and further study is necessary. If the fluorescein test *and* MCTC

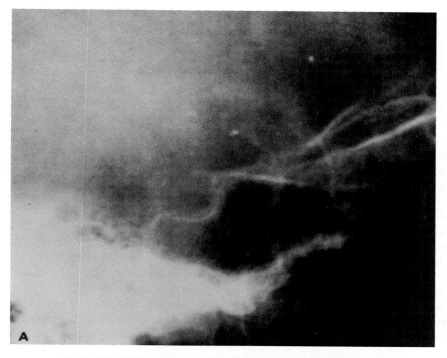

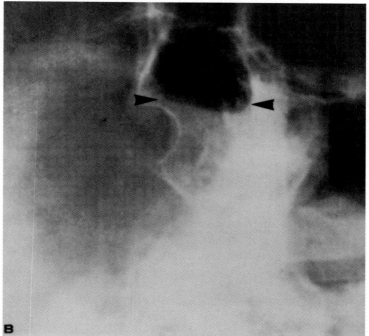

FIG. 1. A: Lateral plane film of sphenoid sinus demonstrating a CSF leak with a corresponding fluid level. **B:** Brow-up view demonstrating a shift in the fluid level (*arrows*).

are both negative, but clinical indications are strong (e.g., recurrent meningitis, intracranial air, fluid with a chloride level over 120 mEq), we are sometimes dependent on surgical exploration itself to localize the leak.

EXTRACRANIAL EXPOSURE OF THE SITE OF CEREBROSPINAL FLUID RHINORRHEA

Anyone who has witnessed the extensive adhesions that can form inside the nose after intranasal trauma, such as repeated polypectomy, ethmoidectomy, or even just prolonged intranasal packing, can appreciate the ease with which tissue from one wall of the nasal cavity can be tranposed to another. The pattern of blood flow through turbinate mucosa and nasal septal mucosa is so rich that almost any random flap will survive. Furthermore, the highly irregular surfaces of the nasal interior ensure that an excess of mucosa is available, and the base of a flap can be planned near enough the fistula site that the reach is always sufficient.

Three main intranasal mucoperiosteal flaps and one frontal pericranial flap are available for extracranial repairs. These are, in order of use in our practice, the middle turbinate flap, the anterior lateral (atrial) nasal flap, the upper septal flap, and the frontal pericranial flap. The middle turbinate flap is based posteriorly, on a lateral posterior nasal branch of the sphenopalatine artery, and is very useful for resurfacing both the denuded cribriform and much of the ethmoid roof (13). It can be completely detached anteriorly and superiorly and can even be turned back into the sphenoid sinus if necessary. The loss of a middle turbinate would, of course, constitute a serious physiological deficit and possibly increase the danger of secretional crusting and infection. But the mucosa of the mobilized middle turbinate flap is completely preserved, not lost. No scar actually crosses the posterior pathway of its pattern of mucociliary flow, because the posterior attachments are retained. In practice, the functional deficit is minimal. The postoperative appearance is rather arresting, however. A visible ridge of cavernous erectile tissue persists at the site of the repair—an aberrant miniturbinate, in effect, displaced to the roof of the common nasoethmoidal cavity.

The anterior intranasal (Boyden) flap, which was originally described to reconstruct the nasofrontal duct (15), can be useful in sealing CSF leaks situated anterior to the anterior ethmoid artery. The anterior ethmoid artery is picked up passing from the orbit into the ethmoid complex, where it angles forward and medially across the roof of the ethmoidectomy cavity. Here, its passage marks the junction between the most anterior ethmoid cell and the true frontal sinus. Sometimes, if the bony cover under which it runs is greatly thinned, it serves as a signpost to the possible site of a leak. Middle turbinate flaps based posteriorly cannot be drawn far enough forward to provide satisfactory cover this far anteriorly, whereas the Boyden flap, pedicled anterior to the turbinates, easily reaches this region without tension.

The third source of mucosa within the nose is the upper septum. A very serviceable septal mucoperiosteal flap can be raised from the ethmoid plate, based on the face and rostrum of the sphenoid sinus (14). The typical dissection used to develop a septal flap from the underlying cartilage and bone is borrowed from submucosal resection surgery. Once created, the septal flap is transposed or rotated up to its destination, leaving the donor site open to granulate.

In many ways, "extracranial repair of a CSF leak" is just a fancy name for a well-planned and slightly extended external ethmoidectomy, combined with one of these flaps, and sometimes supplemented with telescopic and/or microscopic visualization. The entire ethmoid roof, the cribriform plate, much of the sphenoid, and the lower one-third of the frontal sinus can all be visualized simultaneously through an external ethmoidectomy approach. All you need to know is which side to try: this is usually obvious from the history and the findings. However, if the slightest doubt exists about which side to try, one can go to the operating room with permission for bilateral ethmoidectomies. In this way, if a leak was certain, but the initial side explored proved negative, or the injury was found to extend to the other side, repetition of the preparation, anesthesia, and healing period could be avoided, and the maximum chance of success could be ensured with an extracranial approach.

TECHNIQUE OF TRANSETHMOID REPAIR, INCLUDING ENDOSCOPIC ASSISTANCE

The actual conduct of an extracranial transethmoidal repair is as follows. After induction of anesthesia, surgery begins with the placement of a lumbar catheter in the subarachnoid space. All pertinent scans and radiographs are posted in the operating room. Fluorescein dye is administered with the same care (instill it slowly and dilute it carefully) as was mentioned in the previous discussion. The nose is decongested thoroughly, then carefully inspected with a 4- or 2.7-mm intranasal telescope. Sometimes it is possible to visualize the leak directly. For example, a pulsating arachnoid plug may be visible in the roof of a previously operated ethmoid cavity or in the region of the fractured cribriform plate.

If the leak can be visualized endoscopically, it may also be amenable to transnasal repair *without* an external ethmoidectomy (24). A septoplasty is used both to donate a flap and to improve access. The bone around the site is denuded with fine elevators and forceps and an autogenous graft of muscle and connective tissue from the platysma and cervical fascia can then be obtained. Under direct endoscopic visualization, the tissue plug is tamped into the site of leakage transnasally. A septal flap, developed as an extension of the septoplasty, is then used to complete the repair (Fig. 2). Submucosal "tunnels" are simply extended upward to the top of the septum and the posteriorly based flap is cut with nasal scissors and rotated up over the autograft. Pressed Gelfoam and a carefully positioned, Cortisporin-suspension-soaked polyamide gel (Vig-

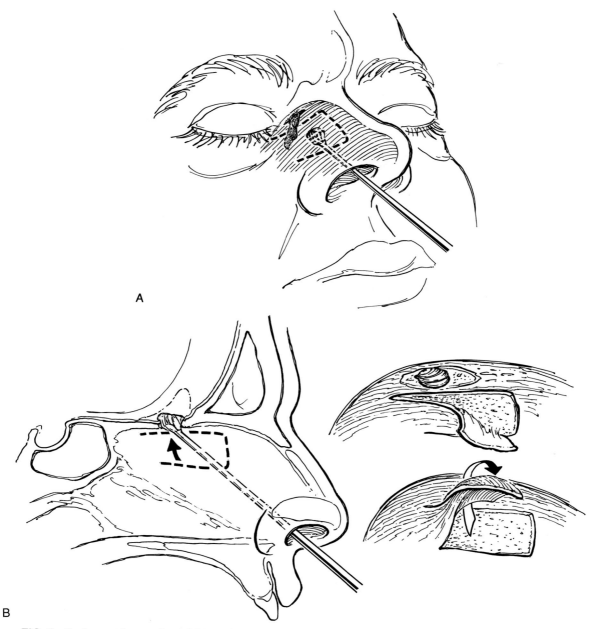

FIG. 2. Endoscopic repair of CSF leak. **A:** A muscle plug is used to plug the hole in the cribriform area. The septal flap is outlined. **B:** The septal flap is turned into place.

ilon) (25) intranasal dressing are used to support the flap in place for 4 or 5 days. The lumbar drain can be continued also, to reduce pressure on the repair, but only while the nasal packing is present. During this same period, the patient should be placed on strict bed rest; at the time of discharge, stool softeners are prescribed and the patient is requested to refrain entirely from blowing the nose and, if a sneeze is imminent, to remember to do it through an open mouth.

In most of our cases, suitable conditions for an endo-

scopic repair are not found to be present. Therefore we usually carry on with a formal classical transethmoidal repair. An external ethmoidectomy is initiated in an orderly and delicate manner through a stepped medial canthal incision (Fig. 3A). The frontal process of the maxilla, which forms the very solid bony barrier immediately anterior to the ethmoid sinus, is removed. The medial canthal ligament-bearing periosteum over the frontal process must be incised and elevated, and the medial orbital periosteum can then be separated from

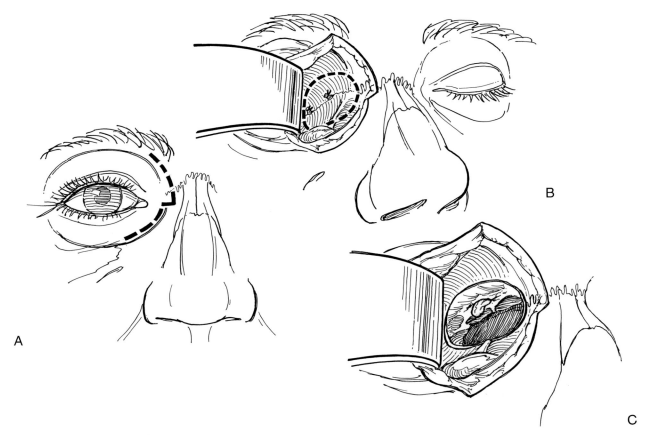

FIG. 3. External ethmoidectomy approach. **A:** Stair-stepped incision. **B:** Lamina papyracea exposed, lacrimal sac retracted. **C:** Careful removal of the ethmoid cells is done through this external ethmoidectomy approach, preserving the mucoperiostium anterior to the posterior lacrimal crest, especially if a Sewell–Boyden flap is to be used.

the lamina papyracea. The lacrimal bone is resected, and the anterior ethmoid artery is interrupted with a bipolar cautery and divided. Judicious exenteration of the ethmoid septa can now proceed, working carefully back to the sphenoid, with loupes or microscopic magnification (Fig. 3B). Avoid avulsing any mobile fracture fragments and, of course, do not create a leak in the act of trying to find one. Acknowledge any fracture lines, and be aware that a low-hanging post-traumatic arachnoid encephalocele can quickly present itself in an ethmoid cell.

If a unilateral ethmoid CSF leak is present, it is generally discovered in the roof or, more commonly, in the thin vertical supracribriform lamina of the most medial part of the roof, during the course of this dissection. There are at least five signs:

1. Pulsations, transmitted from the cranial cavity.
2. A thin steam of clear fluid spurting out into the blood, which is slowly welling up in the field of dissection.

3. An arachnoid diverticulum, truly a mini-encephalocele.
4. A dark black hole, small, but stark in contrast to the white denuded bone.
5. A definite wisp of fluorescein-stained CSF, which looks like bright yellow-green automotive antifreeze. Fluorescein-stained CSF is generally bright enough to be seen without ultraviolet illumination, especially under the intense light of an operating microscope or a rigid nasal endoscope. To enhance identification of an intermittent leak, the anesthesiologist can raise CSF pressure. The stopcock on the lumbar catheter extension set affords access to inject 20 or 30 cc of saline, 10 cc at a time.

If the leak is not discovered with these maneuvers, it is appropriate to extend the dissection beyond the ethmoid. The next field of interest is the nasal cavity and inspection of the cribriform plate. With an intranasal instrument, feel the level of the cribriform, which is lower than the normal roof of the ethmoid, and puncture laterally (and carefully) from the nose into the ethmoid. The lateral nasal wall structures can then be progressively detached from the cribriform level, and from the anterior nasal vault in front of the cribriform, to be displaced downward and into the nose. This preserves all the tissue useful for repair, while it extends the exposure to include the cribriform plate and the upper septum. The middle turbinate remains pedicled on its posterior neurovascular supply, the lateral nasal wall mucosa anterior to the middle turbinate is preserved and better visualized, and an excellent view of the mucosa of the upper septum is obtained simultaneously. At this point the cribriform and upper septum are still covered with mucosa. In dissecting this off, one will inevitably transect one or two of the many tiny arachnoid sheaths that accompany the olfactory nerve fibers through their foramina. This is not very consequential, as long as it is recognized and the cribriform bone itself is preserved. Arachnoid sheath leaks are pinpoint openings, which seal themselves rather spontaneously. Sometimes, they actually serve to indicate the presence and appearance of the fluorescein. As long as they are not mistaken for the pathological leak, no problem seems to arise.

If both the ethmoid and the cribriform inspections are negative, the sphenoid sinus cavity should be better visualized, by removing the bony sphenoid rostrum and the posterior portion of the septum (submucosally). This "cross-court" approach through the ethmoids gives a better view of the lateral aspect of the contralateral sphenoid than the ipsilateral one. It should also be appreciated that, depending on the extent of pneumatization, lateral sphenoid leaks are very challenging to find (Fig. 4). If the operating microscope has been the only visual aid up to this point, don't forget that the 2.7-mm 30-degree and 70-degree nasal telescopes are also particularly useful. They allow laterally directed and "around-the-corner" views not possible with the operating microscope alone. A tangential leak in the ethmoid roof or the cribriform may even be detected at this point, because of the new viewpoint or the extra lighting intensity introduced by the additional fiberoptic illumination.

When a leak is identified (hopefully not one *created* by the operator), the microscope or the telescope is carefully repositioned and visualization is optimized. Usually, in longstanding traumatic leaks, the dural hole is single and small. If a miniature graft of autogenous muscle and/or fibrofatty tissue is pushed upward into the site with a blunt otologic instrument, the leak can usually be plugged (Fig. 5). The 45-degree Lillie attic hook, a blunt mastoid probe, or a Derlaki mobilizer are all useful instruments for this purpose. The primary role of the free graft is to stop the flow of CSF intraoperatively, to sustain a CSF-free wound while the next

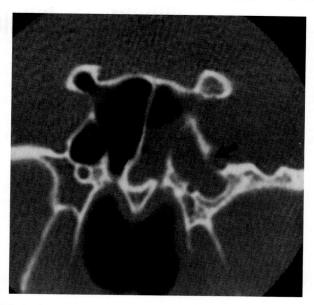

FIG. 4. CT scan in coronal plane, demonstrating a sphenoid sinus fluid level as well as a lateral wall CSF leak (*arrow*). Leak was plugged using the 30-degree angled telescope.

layer, the living intranasal flap, is carefully secured in place. The secondary role is to continue this seal during the few weeks it takes to heal to the surrounding bone. Cribriform leak sites need to be denuded of surrounding mucosa, of course, to bare the viable bone to which

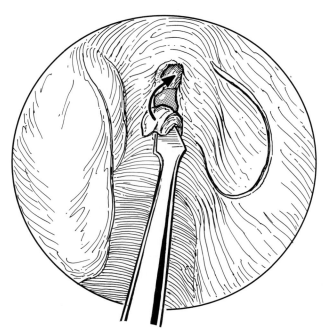

FIG. 5. Using the operating microscope, the area of CSF leak in the fovea ethmoidalis is identified. The leak is plugged with autogenous muscle manipulated by an otologic dissection instrument (see text).

TABLE 1. *Cerebrospinal fluid rhinorrhea: the concept of a four layered repair*

Layer	Rationale	Transnasal, transeptal or transethmoid extracranial repair	Transfrontal extradural extracranial repair	Transfrontal intradural intracranial repair
I	*Hydraulic plug:* to stop the flow, so the surgeon can work and the repair can heal	Free soft tissue autografts (fibrin glue?)	Dural homograft or direct suturing of the dural defect	CSF is automatically evacuated by the intradural approach
II	*Structural support:* to support the dura and avoid a delayed encephalocele	Existing bony support is usually adequate	Septal bone, thin calvarial graft, or an acrylic cranioplasty	Calvarial bone grafts or acrylic cranioplasty
III	*Living layer:* to supply fibroblasts, capillaries and fibrin, a scaffold for the dural repair, and a living layer that will actively seal to the bone	Middle turbinate flap, septal mucosal flap, or nasal atrium flap	Pericranial flap, tissue from the underside of the coronal anterior scalp flap	Free fascia lata, free pericranium, a pericranial flap from the undersurface of the anterior scalp flap, or direct suture of the dural defect
IV	*Dressing:* to support layers I, II, and III and reduce the risk of pneumocephalus, hemorrhage, or flap displacement	Cortisporin-suspension-soaked Vigilon intranasal dressing	Cortisporin suspension soaked Vigilon intranasal dressing	Free soft tissue autograft stuffed into the "funnel" defect in the dura, below layer III

the mucosal flap can seal. Since the free "plug" may die or shrink, and lead to recurrence of the leak, the living layer is important (Table 1).

If a middle turbinate flap is to be used, stabilize it with two forceps and dissect out the inner bony architectural support. Then evert the mucosa and move it up against the denuded site of the intended repair (Fig. 6). Alternatively, the newly exposed mucosa of the upper septum can be elevated, as in a submucous resection (SMR), and tailored to produce a flap (see Fig. 2). Its margins are the denuded bony cribriform plate, the anterior nasal vault, and a horizontal incision back toward the sphenoid rostrum. In reach and extent, it is rather similar to the middle turbinate flap. If the leak lies too far anterior for a middle turbinate flap or a septal flap, use the Boyden flap of anterior nasal mucosa. This comprises a rectangle of nasal mucoperiosteum, which is elevated from the lateral nasal wall, that is, from the agger nasi and the atrium of the nose. Based anterior to the middle turbinate, as previously mentioned, it can easily be turned and then rotated up into an anterior frontoethmoidal defect (Fig. 7; see also chapter by Donald, Surgical Management of Frontal Sinus Infections, Figs. 28, 29, and 30).

These methods of repair are satisfactory for small defects in which most of the bony anatomy is retained, but sometimes the bony defect is large enough to merit structural repair. A third or supporting rigid layer is required if, in the operator's judgment, long-term development of a delayed meningocele is possible. A suitable batten of septal bone from the ethmoid plate or

vomer should be used to reconstitute the roof of the ethmoid or the nasal cavity (Fig. 8). The middle turbinate flap can be tailored to retain some of its intrinsic bone too (26), of course, but if this is done, care must be taken to avoid the potential disruptive effects of an overlooked concha bullosa. If the mucosa within the "bullosa" is inadvertently preserved, it will interfere with subsequent adhesion of the flap and compromise the longevity of the repair. These details can be anticipated by studying the preoperative CT scan, to define the problem mucosa ahead of time and plan to remove it during surgery.

Once the bony support layer is assured, the living intranasal flap is carefully positioned and a final temporary seal, the nasal packing, is inserted. We believe nasal flaps are best supported and maintained in position with Cortisporin-suspension-soaked polyamide gel (Vigilon) packings (25). With this material, which is slippery, swells, and holds an antibiotic, the subsequent removal proves both atraumatic and comfortable. Repair the periosteal/medial canthal ligament layer with 2-0 or 3-0 absorbable suture to preserve a level palpebral axis. The facial cutaneous wound can be closed with 6-0 plain or mild chromic catgut so no suture removal is later required near the eye. The packing should probably remain in place for 4 or 5 days postoperatively, and once again, if the patient is given a stool softener and cautioned not to strain or blow his or her nose, the pressure on the repair after packing removal will be reduced.

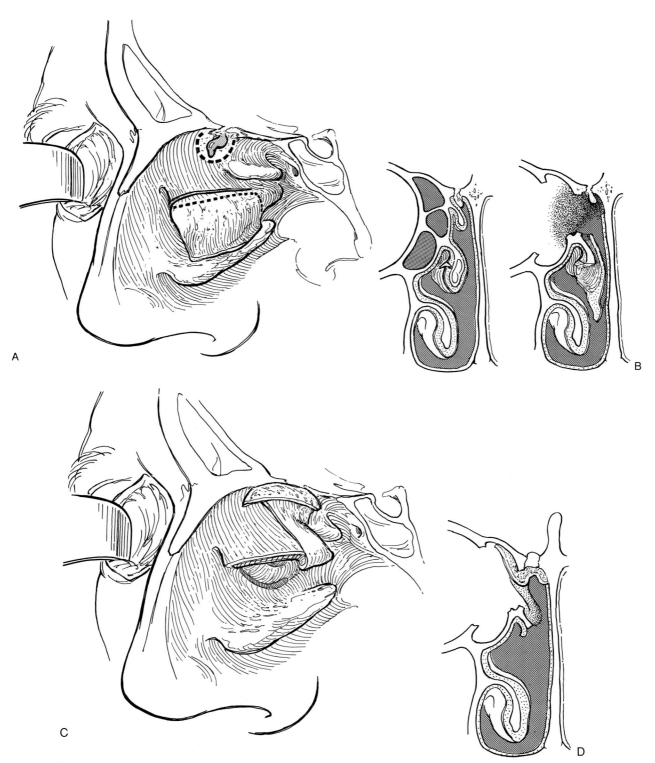

FIG. 6. Middle turbinate flap used for repair. **A:** Area of proposed ethmoidectomy for CSF leak is outlined and the laterally based middle turbinate flap is also outlined. **B:** Coronal view showing flap elevation. **C:** Flap being turned into defect. **D:** Coronal cut showing flap in place.

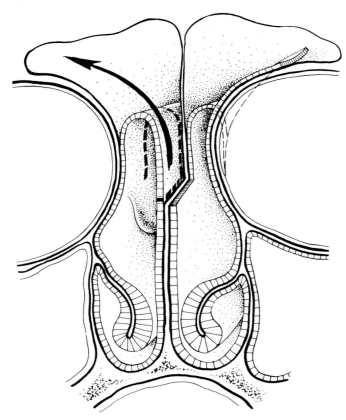

FIG. 7. Sewell–Boyden flap (see also chapter by Donald, Surgical Management of Frontal Sinus Infections; and Figs 28, 29, and 30).

INTRACRANIAL REPAIR

In extensive traumatic craniofacial injuries, with accompanying intracranial pathology, direct closure of a CSF fistula will fail unless the increased intracranial pressure is simultaneously rectified. In nontraumatic leaks, predisposing intracranial lesions, such as tumors, are not uncommon, and concomitant recognition and management of the associated increase in intracranial pressure are mandatory.

Intracranial repair has been criticized because the division of the olfactory tracts results in anosmia. However, unilateral division is of minimal significance, and after trauma, 78% of patients present with anosmia anyway. The transcranial intradural approach may be performed with a bicoronal incision for optimal cosmesis, and a bony glabellar trephine may be employed in contrast to a more extensive frontal craniotomy. Hyperventilation and osmotic diuresis are used to diminish the morbidity of frontal lobe elevation. One rationale for the intracranial approach is the extensive exposure it affords for intradural inspection and the broad access it provides for direct suture repair of the dura, which may be very valuable in multiple nontraumatic defects or extensive injuries that cross the floor of the anterior cranial fossa.

Middle fossa craniotomy is often the only way to visualize and repair a lateral sphenoid leak. The same is true of medial temporal bone defects when hearing preservation makes translabyrinthine approaches contraindicated.

CEREBROSPINAL FLUID RHINORRHEA FROM AN OTOLOGIC SOURCE

Autopsy studies in normal individuals indicate an incidence of osseous defects in the temporal bone of 0.6% (27). A congenital dehiscence of the dura must be much less common. CSF from a middle or posterior fossa defect into the temporal bone air cell system can pool in the mastoid and middle ear and flow down the eustachian tube to produce a unilateral rhinorrhea, which is almost indistinguishable from that of a primary sphenoethmoidal or a cribriform leak. Patients typically complain of a moist nostril, and dripping tends to occur only in certain positions. As in the nose, traumatic etiologies are commonest, but mastoid and middle ear surgery, attic cholesteatomas, and intracranial or otologic tumors can also penetrate the middle or posterior fossa dura and cause leakage. Meningitis is more likely to be the signal event if middle ear pathology is the cause, but all cases of CSF rhinorrhea merit careful examination of the ears. Otologic symptoms may not be volunteered if CSF rhinorrhea occurs, and the ears are always suspect in cases of unknown origin.

Sometimes CSF flow is delayed in the middle ear, and it accumulates to give the typical appearance of serous otitis media, even to the replication of a Type B tympanogram. However, the negative pressure usually associated with a genuine case of inflammatory serous otitis media is absent in cases of CSF in the middle ear. If CSF in the middle ear were misdiagnosed and treated as serous otitis media, that is, a tympanostomy tube was placed, the history will reveal that the ear continued to drain until the tube was removed.

While the detailed surgical treatment of CSF rhinorrhea of temporal bone origin is beyond the scope of this chapter and the mission of this book, the general principles of suspicion, diagnosis, localization, and repair are comparable to those for leaks originating in the nasal and sinus cavities. Fluorescein dye tests and MCTC are the principal diagnostic devices used to identify and demonstrate the leak. Of course, oval or round window leakage of perilymph can produce a clear fluid in the middle ear, but only in the rare instance of a patent cochlear aqueduct is the volume of perilymph sufficient to mimic CSF from a nasal source (28). Transtemporal otosurgical explorations are particularly indicated in patients who are already deaf (e.g., from the original temporal bone fracture or the otologic or neurological pathology or surgery). Mas-

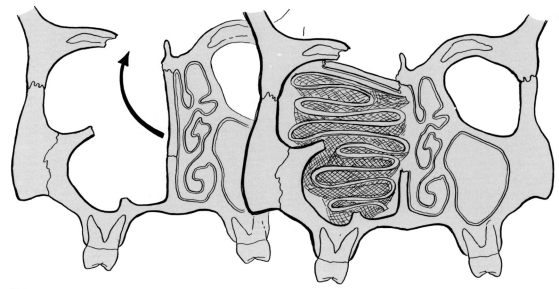

FIG. 8. Septal flap complete with septal cartilage and bone for large CSF leaks. (From ref. 36, with permission.)

toid approaches to the tegmen and the posterior plate may also be attempted in patients where hearing preservation is desirable, but transcranial neurosurgical middle fossa or posterior fossa procedures may be more prudent and reliable, especially when accompanying encephaloceles complicate the presentation.

TENSION PNEUMOCEPHALUS

When air accumulates and expands in the intracranial cavity, especially the ventricles, the brain is forced downward. The medial part of the temporal lobe herniates through the tentorial opening, compressing the upper midbrain (a "pressure cone") and the patient gradually becomes obtunded. A breach in the dura, which is complicated by tension pneumocephalus, is thus a true neurologic emergency. Pneumocephalus automatically implies tension. The air must be pumped in continuously just to be sustained (Fig. 9). Unreplenished air in the cranial cavity (e.g., after neurosurgical procedures) is relatively rapidly absorbed. In persistent or progressive pneumocephalus, air is introduced into the cranial cavity at a faster rate than reabsorption can accommodate.

Tension pneumocephalus can occur even in the patient who does not cough, sneeze, or blow the nose. Theories explaining the pathophysiology of pneumocephalus remain hypothetical. It seems likely a ball-valve mechanism is operating at the site of the CSF leak or air enters, and CSF leaves, but the air rises into the cranial cavity and cannot escape, much like air entering an inverted bottle of fluid. Perhaps arteries inside the head create a pulsating intracranial pressure

gradient, which then plays a role. Several authors have noted that when air enters the cranial cavity in quantities sufficient to elevate intracranial pressure, an exit site for CSF, separate from the fistula itself, is often present (29). This might be the lumbar puncture wound, a lumbar catheter placed to help a fistula close, or a lumboperitoneal shunt. If a rhinologic fistula admits air into the cranial cavity, which eventually enters

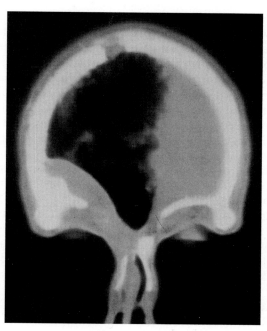

FIG. 9. Large tension pneumocephalus in a patient, following anterior fossa skull base surgery, who developed a ball-valve effect in a dehiscent anterior fossa floor.

the ventricles, it appears particularly difficult to reabsorb. There seems to be a virtual intracranial and/or intraventricular airlock. The ventricles are progressively enlarged and the brain is progressively compressed as more and more CSF is displaced. The air, of course, entered the head at room temperature, but as it rapidly warms, it expands, accelerating the course of events. Patients at risk for tension pneumocephalus should carefully be followed by sequential skull films or CT scans, and if air is present with a spinal catheter in place, the catheter should probably be removed. The rate of drainage of CSF could also simply be restricted, as described under another section of this chapter, when CSF leakage from a planned intraoperative dural defect is the problem.

ACUTE TRAUMA: THE MANAGEMENT OF CSF LEAKAGE DETECTED IMMEDIATELY AFTER INJURIES TO THE HEAD

Acute traumatic CSF rhinorrhea has a reasonable chance of stopping on its own. It is generally not warranted, nor is it very feasible, to attempt an acute-phase formal transethmoidal or extracranial repair. Mucosa in the nose and sinuses cannot be removed from the unstable bony fragments with any degree of control. The site of the leak is very difficult to identify and, moreover, is easily misinterpreted. What intranasal soft tissues would normally be used for repair will be found to be hemorrhagic or inflamed, unreliable, and unsuited for surgery. Reduction of the associated facial fractures is appropriate immediate treatment; 85% of acute traumatic leaks will stop within 1 week with fracture reduction alone (30).

Two or three weeks after the acute phase, one is sometimes confronted with the decision to undertake an extracranial repair, or not, in a patient who continues to leak after head trauma but remains in a comatose state. Despite the coma, it is probably best to agree to undertake the repair. The patient may ultimately recover very satisfactory cerebral function, or it may be diminished, but all the while, meningitis and pneumocephalus will remain constant dangers. A comatose patient is subject to nasal instrumentation, assisted ventilation, and long-term care in an institutional or hospital environment so the obligation to avoid these complications is particularly relevant. If an extracranial repair is not undertaken, this may prejudice the recovery—or seem to do so in the minds of relatives and loved ones, especially if they are disappointed with a suboptimal neurologic recovery.

INADVERTENT IATROGENIC LEAKS PRODUCED DURING NASAL OR SINUS SURGERY

Deliberate surgical dissection along the cribriform plate is rarely performed. If tumor surgery was the indication, an anterior craniofacial approach is more likely to have been performed. Nevertheless, sometimes it does occur, at maxilloethmoidectomy, for example. Separation of the olfactory mucosa from its cribriform bed shears the arachnoid sleeves that tend to accompany the olfactory nerve fibers as they pass down through their numerous foramina. Sometimes a tiny leak is observed, but if this is the only injury, atraumatic nasal packing will soon establish adequate control.

If the cribriform plate itself is perforated, fate and packing cannot be trusted and the principles of layered closure should be instituted. The first thing to overcome is any sense of denial or inertia. A leak sustained during endoscopic sinus surgery, for example, may tempt one to minimize the injury, but this is not appropriate. How can the patient be protected from pneumocephalus, meningitis, a delayed leak, or encephalocele if corrective action is ignored? Access will be limited and it may be difficult to employ the microscope, but surgeons who operate on the nose and sinuses generally have both the skills and the tools to undertake a satisfactory transnasal repair. Start by taking a culture, then institute an antibiotic IV. A small soft tissue autograft can be pressed up into the defect with otologic instruments like the 45-degree Lillie attic hook, a blunt mastoid probe, or a Derlaki mobilizer, and the effectiveness of the seal can be observed with a 30-degree nasal telescope. It is generally possible to transpose some regional septal mucosa over a cribriform defect and maintain it in position with a small pad of compressed Gelfoam. This in turn can be supported with Vigilon, as described in a previous section.

A slightly different hazard exists in frontal sinus surgery. If the true interfrontal sinus septum is off center, and pneumatization extends up into the crista galli, the intracranial sulcus between the crista and the anterior frontoethmoid roof on the other side may present into the frontal sinus as a partial vertical posterior bony ridge (31). This can look like a second, albeit rudimentary, intrasinus septum. Removal during frontal sinus surgery is sure to result in a dural dehiscence, again requiring primary repair. If the frontal sinus surgery is being done through the coronal approach, with an osteoplastic flap, generous exposure is available for the repair. On the other hand, frontal sinus mucosa is unsuitable for a flap, and nasal flaps can be difficult to elevate into this area, especially if the nasofrontal duct is to remain patent. It may be better to resect more bone, and suture the dura directly, or to plug the hole with a small graft and obliterate the sinus with abdominal fat. If obliteration is undertaken, it is crucially important to remove every last vestige of frontal sinus mucosa to avoid a delayed frontal mucocele. A pericranial flap can be helpful to seal off the nasofrontal ducts and prevent remucosalization from below.

Sometimes the problem at surgery is to determine if in fact a CSF leak has been produced. This might be important, for example, after the removal of a congenital nasal mass. Limited access and expected blood staining may make the visual confirmation of fluorescein rather difficult. In this case, one can inject 200 to 500 μCi of indium-111 diethylenetriamine pentaacetic acid (DTPA) by lumbar puncture (32). Pledgets can be left in the nasal cavity for about 1 min, and a control can be soaked in the patient's blood elsewhere in the wound. The pledgets are sent to the Nuclear Medicine staff, who soon report counts six to seven times greater than the blood count in cases they deem to be positive. A negative test may save much unnecessary concern and a positive one gives the surgeon and the patient an excellent opportunity for primary intraoperative repair.

DELAYED POSTOPERATIVE CEREBROSPINAL FLUID LEAKS AFTER TRANSSPHENOIDAL HYPOPHYSECTOMY

The arachnoid descends as a pouch below the diaphragma sellae in up to 40% of normal individuals. A CSF leak is therefore sometimes produced by transsphenoidal hypophysectomy. Large tumor size and previous radiotherapy probably contribute to the risk. The surgeon working in the sella has usually tried to repair the leak with an intrasellar free graft, often maintained in place by a batten of septal bone, turned transversely, just inside the sella opening. After the intranasal packing is removed, however, it is recognized that a CSF leak is persistent. It is tempting to wait, hoping the leak will stop, or to attempt to control the flow with serial lumbar punctures. However, it is usually better to return to the operating room and effect a new transeptal repair. Early on, this is simply a matter of proceeding back through the septal approach via the original nasal incision, without even reopening the sublabial incision, regrafting the sella, restoring the batten, and repeating the intranasal dressing. The septal flaps are easily separated at 1 week, whereas if you wait, the septal flaps will become readherent. Not only is the risk period increased and the hospitalization prolonged by the wait-and-see approach, but a much more difficult nasal septal dissection is likely.

CEREBROSPINAL FLUID LEAKAGE FROM PLANNED INTRAOPERATIVE DURAL DEFECTS

Anterior craniofacial and infratemporal skull base procedures create deliberate intraoperative CSF leaks by the very nature of the surgical resections. To be successful, surgical planning must anticipate this fact and incorporate every possible strategy for successful healing. This may include planning the skin incision to lie at a distance from the site of the dural defect and preserving pericranium for intraoperative use as a flap. Sometimes a pericranial flap should be replanned to include the galea and frontalis layer with the pericranium (33). This is a less natural scalp dissection than the usual separation plane through the loose areolar layer, between the galea and the cranial periosteum. The galea is attached to the dense subdermal connective tissue layer of the scalp and a galea–frontalis myofascial flap dissection must take into account the strength and rich vascularity of this tissue as well as preservation of the blood supply of the overlying skin.

Dead space is an important factor in many craniofacial cases; dural repairs need support. With proper planning, the temporalis muscle can be mobilized on its deep temporal blood supply, detached from both the skull and the coronoid process, and rotated into a region such as the infratemporal fossa to give support to a middle fossa repair, with separation from the sphenoid sinus. The frontal sinus can be cranialized to reduce the area of frontal dura at risk for a leak, and the separation between dura and the nasal cavity can be increased by the interposition of a pericranial flap roofing the former nasofrontal ducts and underlying an anterior cranial fossa dural defect. Dural repairs can be planned with precision, using homograft dura and/or temporalis fascia. Fibrin glue may be useful to temporarily seal dural needle holes and help fill minor interstices (34). Drains are best avoided in the presence of major dural wounds; the chance of leading CSF to the outside—or worse, allowing fistulization with pneumocephalus—is too great. Probably the single most contributory factor in the production of postoperative CSF leakage and skull base resections is suboptimal wound closure at the conclusion of the operative procedure. In this regard, exhaustion of the surgeon probably plays a significant and underrecognized role. Thought should be given to appropriate scheduling, to minimize the impact of this factor.

SPINAL DRAINAGE

After extensive cranial base operations in which a CSF fistula has been produced, the risk of returning to the operating room for repairs may be too high, and the chance of success may seem low. Since the wound is still healing, this may be the time to try a special strategy—"flow-regulated" continuous spinal drainage. Flow-regulated continuous spinal drainage can sometimes help seal a difficult (and recent) CSF leak without reoperation. CSF is normally produced at around 18 cc/hr in an adult. By incorporating an Imed 350 gravity infusion system into the spinal catheter drainage line, and setting the flow regulator to no more than 15 cc/hr, continuous spinal drainage can be maintained, without the usual dangers (35). An unregulated lumbar catheter would siphon CSF off at a faster rate, creating the negative gradient between atmospheric air and intracranial cavity pressure mentioned earlier, with a heightened risk of pneumocephalus and meningitis.

SPONTANEOUS CEREBROSPINAL FLUID RHINORRHEA

In 1985, my colleagues and I had an opportunity to review 28 patients with "spontaneous" CSF rhinorrhea (20). This was a challenging group because of the difficulty in diagnosis and the problems of localization. Three major diagnostic categories emerged: (a) congenital anomalies of the skull base; (b) delayed post-traumatic CSF leaks, in which the history of trauma was remote and thus sometimes obscure; and (c) intracranial tumors with dural invasion, plus or minus elevated intracranial pressure.

Depending on the suspected cause and location of a spontaneous leak, these fistulas were variously approached with extracranial or intracranial procedures. Only 22 patients treated achieved control of the leakage, 17 after one operation and 5 after multiple procedures. Of the patients who were known to continue leaking despite surgical treatment, three died of intracranial tumors and two others died from intracranial complications of their persistent fistulas. Overall, intracranial repair techniques were successful in less than 60% of cases, whereas 16 of 20 extracranial transethmoidal operations were successful in controlling the leak. Transseptal repair of a sphenoid leak was the least successful approach (3 out of 10), but leakage after transseptal operations is often successfully handled via the transethmoidal operation. Failed extracranial operations were rarely salvaged by an intracranial repair, whereas the opposite was not at all rare.

CONCLUSIONS

Once the presence and correct side of an intranasal or sinus CSF leak have been established, and a primary intracranial etiology has been excluded or managed, extracranial methods of dural repair seem to offer excellent success rates and lower morbidity and mortality rates than intracranial operations have achieved. There are exceptions, of course, especially in the lateral sphenoid recesses, in the temporal bone leak with preserved hearing, and in cases with intracranial pathology. The transethmoidal procedure is reliable in its ability to expose most nonotologic leaks, other than high frontal and lateral sphenoid, and is effective in obtaining their closure. Extracranial repairs have established themselves as the initial procedures of choice in small and medium, delayed post-traumatic, and many so-called spontaneous CSF rhinorrhea cases, but thoughtful preparatory investigation and meticulous execution of the surgery are necessary to ensure their long-term success.

REFERENCES

1. Taylor J. A case of cerebrospinal fluid rhinorrhea following multiple fractures of the skull which involved the left frontal sinus and the left orbit. *Trans Ophthalmol Soc UK* 1934;54:312–315.
2. Morgagni G. *De Sedibus et Causio Morborum: Liber I*, No XV, Art 21. Padua, 1762.
3. Miller C. Case of hydrocephalus chronicus, with some unusual symptoms and appearances on dissection. *Trans Med Chir Soc Edinb* 1826;2:243–248.
4. Chiari H. Ueber einer Fall, von Luflonsammlong in Der Ventrikeln des Menschlichen Gehoins. *Z Heirk* 1884;5:383–384.
5. Thomson St C. *The cerebrospinal fluid; its spontaneous escape from the nose.* London: Cassel & Co, 1899.
6. Calvert CA, Cairns H. Discussion on injuries of the frontal and ethmoidal sinuses. *Proc R Soc Med* 1942;35:805–810.
7. Levins S, Nelson KE, Spies HW, et al. Pneumococcal meningitis. *Am J Med Sci* 1972;264:319–322.
8. Dandy WD. Pneumocephalus (intracranial pneumocele or aerocele). *Arch Surg* 1926;12:949–982.
9. Dohlman G. Spontaneous cerebrospinal rhinorrhea. *Acta Otolaryngol Suppl* 1948;67.
10. Ommaya AK, Dichiro G, Baldwin M, et al. Nontraumatic cerebrospinal rhinorrhea. *J Neurol Neurosurg Psychiatry* 1968;31:214–255.
11. Ray BS, Bergland RM. Cerebrospinal fluid fistula: clinical aspects, techniques of localization and methods of closure. *J Neurosurg* 1967;30:399–405.
12. Calcaterra TC. Extracranial surgical repair of cerebrospinal rhinorrhea. *Ann Otol Rhinol Laryngol* 1980;89:108–116.
13. Vrabec DP, Hallberg OE. Cerebrosinal rhinorrhea. *Arch Otolaryngol* 1964;80:218–229.
14. Montgomery WW. Cerebrospinal rhinorrhea. *Otol Clin North Am* 1973;6:757–771.
15. Boyden GL. Surgical treatment of chronic frontal sinusitis. *Ann Otol* 1952;61:558–563.
16. Naidich T, Moran C. Precise anatomic localization of atraumatic sphenoethmoidal cerebrospinal fluid rhinorrhea by metrizamide CT cisternography. *J Neurosurg* 1980;53:222–228.
17. Hull HF, Morrow G. Glucorrhea revisited. *JAMA* 1975;234:1052–1053.
18. Ommaya AK, et al. Cerebrospinal fluid fistula. In: Wilkins, Rengachary SS, eds. *Neurosurgery*, vol 2. New York: McGraw Hill 1985.
19. Yokoyama K, Hasegawa M, Shiba KS, et al. Diagnosis of CSF rhinorrhea: detection of tau-transferrin in nasal discharge. *Otolaryngol Head Neck Surg* 1988;98:328–332.
20. Hubbard JL, McDonald TJ, Pearson BW, et al. Spontaneous cerebrospinal fluid rhinorrhea: evolving concepts in diagnosis and surgical management based on the Mayo Clinic experience from 1970 through 1981. *Neurosurgery* 1985;16:314–321.
21. Charles DA, Snell D. Cerebrospinal fluid rhinorrhea. *Laryngoscope* 1979;89:822–826.
22. Moseley JI, Carton CA, Stern WE. Spectrum of complications in the use of intrathecal fluorescein. *J Neurosurg* 1978;48:765–767.
23. Manelfe C, Cellerier P, Sobel D, et al. Cerebrospinal fluid rhinorrhea: evaluation with metrizamide cisternography. *Am J Neuro Radiol* 1982;3:25–30.
24. Papay FA, Maggiano H, Dominquez S, et al. Rigid endoscopic repair of paranasal sinus cerebrospinal fluid fistulas. *Laryngoscope* 1989;99:1195–1201.
25. Salassa JR, Pearson BW. Polyethylene oxide gel. *Arch Otolaryngol Head Neck Surg* 1991;117:1365–1367.

26. Yessehow RS, McCabe BF. The osteo-mucoperiosteal flap in repair of cerebrospinal fluid rhinorrhea: a 20 year experience. *Otolaryngol Head Neck Surg* 1989;101:555–561.

27. Adams GL, McCoid G, Weisbeski D. Cerebrospinal fluid presenting as serous otitis media. *Minn Med* 1982;July:410–415.

28. Binhammer RT. CSF anatomy with emphasis on relations to the nasal cavity and labyrinthine fluids. *Ear Nose Throat J* 1992;71:292–299.

29. Davis DH, Laws ER, McDonald TJ, et al. Intraventricular tension pneumocephalus as a complication of paranasal sinus surgery: case report. *Neurosurgery* 1981;8:574–576.

30. Lewin W. Cerebrospinal fuid rhinorrhea in closed head injuries. *Br J Surg* 1954;42:1–6.

31. Denecke HJ. *Die Otorhinolaryngologischen Operationen. Die Allgemein-Chirurgischen Einegriffe am Hals,* II Aufl. Berlin: Springer, 1953.

32. Grundfast KM, Mihail R, Majd M. Intraoperative detection of cerebrospinal fluid leak in surgical removal of congenital nasal masses. *Laryngoscope* 1986;96:211–214.

33. Jackson IT, Adham MN, Marsh WR, et al. Use of the galeal frontalis myofascial flap in craniofacial surgery. *Plast Reconstr Surg* 1986;77:905–910.

34. Nishihira S, McCaffrey TV. The use of fibrin glue for the repair of experimental CSF rhinorrhea. *Laryngoscope* 1988;93:625–627.

35. Swanson SE, Chandler WF, Kocan MJ, et al. Flow-regulated continuous spinal drainage in the management of cerebrospinal fluid fistulas. *Laryngoscope* 1985;95:104–106.

36. Donald PJ. *Head & neck cancer: management of the difficult case.* Philadelphia: Saunders, 1984;176.

CHAPTER 35

Fibro-osseous Diseases

Paul J. Donald

The fibro-osseous diseases of the facial bones, and thus indirectly the sinuses, are uncommon disorders that are generally completely unrelated but have similarities in how they affect the sinuses. They are grouped together only because of some commonality in histology and pathophysiology in terms of sinus involvement and because there is a modicum of similarity in the methods of treatment. Batsakis describes these lesions as a group of lesions afflicting the skeleton where the normal bony architecture is replaced by collagen, fibroblasts, and varying amounts of calcified tissue (1).

FIBROUS DYSPLASIA

Fibrous dysplasia is an uncommon disorder characterized by lesions of the skeleton in which specific sites experience a disorganized growth of fibrous and osteoid tissue in the medullary bone. It is a rare disease with an incidence of around 1 in 17,000 admissions to hospital (2). It has two forms, monostotic, in which solitary lesions are seen, and polyostotic, in which multiple sites are identified. Albright's syndrome is a triad of symptoms characterized by polyostotic fibrous dysplasia, cutaneous pigmentation, and sexual precocity. These lesions have an autonomous growth pattern, producing tumorous masses in bone causing facial abnormality and sinus dysfunction.

The term fibrous dysplasia was initially coined by Lichtenstein (3) in 1938, and 6 years later Lichtenstein and Jaffe (4) gave a concise clinical description of the entity. The etiology is entirely unknown except in the case of Albright's syndrome. With this last exception, there is no familial or hereditary basis for this disease. The original theory of Lichtenstein that postulates the genesis of the process as a hamartoma that develops in primitive mesenchyme is still adhered to. The notion of the lesion arising as the result of past trauma and

representing an aberration of the healing process (5) is given little credence today (6).

The monostotic form accounts for 75% to 80% of the cases. Series of cases tend to be dominated by reports from large centers, which often are referred the worse cases, and so the series would tend to have an inflated number of the polyostotic variety. The actual incidence of the monostotic form is probably higher than the 80% reported. Reed (7) reported 9 of 25 cases who had the polyostotic form, but Schlumberger found only 2 of 69 cases with this form, probably more representative of the general frequency. Table 1 illustrates an analysis of sites of involvement in these two series. Only 14 of 84 sites involved sites juxtaposed to the sinuses. The area above the first molar is the commonest site in the maxilla (Fig. 1) (6). The frontal bone is the commonest in the calvarium with the ethmoid–sphenoid much less commonly involved (Figs. 2 to 4).

The polyostotic disease tends to be confined to multiple sites in one bone or on one side of the body. In the most severe cases, bilateral involvement is seen and in the worst case every bone in the skeleton can be afflicted. Approximately 40% to 50% of cases with

TABLE 1. *Sites of involvement of fibrous dysplasia (5,7)*

Site	Number of cases
Maxilla	11
Zygoma	2
Frontal bone	1
Mandible	3
Skull	5
Femur	11
Tibia	10
Humerus	3
Pelvic bones	1
Metatarsal	0
Hand bones	0
Vertebrae	1

581

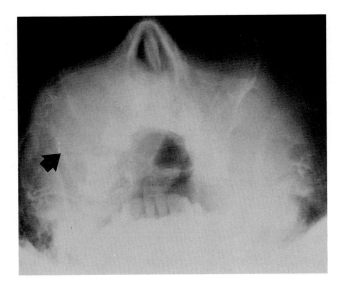

FIG. 1. Maxilla and zygoma above the first molar tooth involved with fibrous dysplasia *(arrow)*. Radiograph demonstrates the usual ground glass appearance, covered in a thin cortical plate.

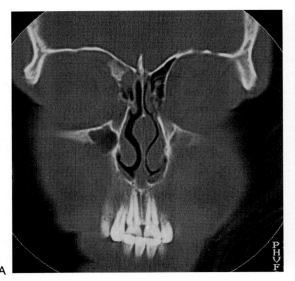

A

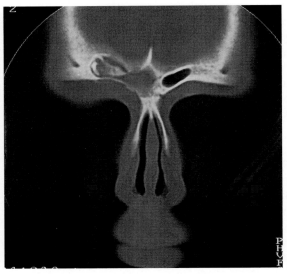

B

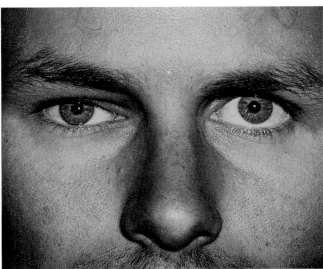

C

FIG. 2. Fibrous dysplasia of frontal bone invading the frontal sinus. **A:** Tumor in orbital plate. **B:** Lesion invading frontal sinus. Note opacification of sinus. **C:** Mass in frontal bone depressing right eyelid.

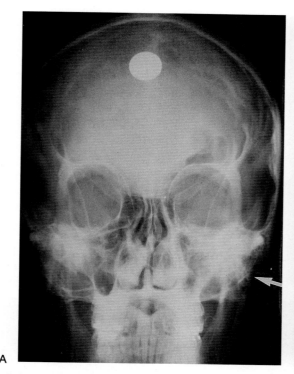 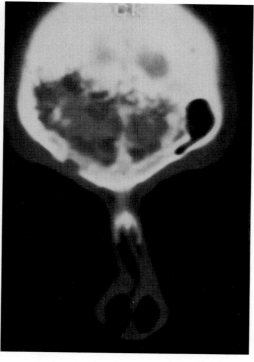

FIG. 3. Fibrous dysplasia of frontal bone invading frontal sinus. **A:** Caldwell view showing ground glass appearance (see *arrow*). **B:** Coronal computed axial tomography (CAT) scan showing frontal sinus invasion.

polyostotic disease have facial or cranial bone involvement in addition to other skeletal sites (6).

Albright's syndrome, sometimes called Albright–McCune–Sternberg syndrome, is composed of a triad of polyostotic fibrous dysplasia, cutaneous pigmentation, and precocious puberty. It is nonhereditary but has been seen in monozygotic twins. The cutaneous lesions have a dark brown to tan coloration, are usually more than 1 cm in diameter, consist of fewer than six in number, and have jagged, irregular edges. The sexual precocity is seen most often in females and uncommonly in males. Affected individuals are often tall in early life, but at adulthood are generally short in stature because of premature closure of the epiphyses. Occasionally, the disease is accompanied by other abnormalities such as hyperthyroidism, hyperparathyroidism, diabetes mellitus, Cushing's syndrome, acromegaly, coarctation of the aorta, hypertension, rudimentary kidneys, and mental retardation (6).

The lesions of facial bones usually appear in the first and second decade of life. However, in one patient in Harris' series (8) the first manifestation of disease was not until she was 68 years of age. Most patients are under 30 years of age at presentation. Those with polyostotic disease usually present in childhood. Most facial lesions are monostotic in type.

Clinically, the lesions frequently present as an asymptomatic mass. Pain, however, is common and

with extremity of disease the patient may suffer a pathological fracture as the initial manifestation of disease. In the frontal bone, the lesion may encroach on the nasal frontal duct, plug off the sinus, and cause mucocele formation (Fig. 3). Involvement of the ethmoid and maxillary sinuses may impede drainage from these sinuses. Facial deformity without other symptomatology is the commonest manifestation. Nasal obstruction, recurrent sinusitis, dental malocclusion, gum and palatal swelling, and proptosis are other symptoms of disease. In the mandible and maxilla, bulging of the gingival mucosa is seen, but the soft tissue itself is normal. Lesions generally stop growing in adulthood (9). There may be the appearance of intramuscular myxomas in the muscle adjacent to the affected bone. This phenomenon is more common in monostotic than the polyostotic variety. These lesions tend to occur 20 to 30 years after the diagnosis of fibrous dysplasia is made (10).

The usual radiographic manifestation is a lesion of ground glass appearance covered by a thin shell of cortical bone (Fig. 1). There are no perforations of the cortex. The ground glass appearance is reflective of a homogeneous mixture of fibrous and osseous elements. If the fibrous component is predominant, then the lesions appear radiolucent like a cyst with either a unilocular or polylocular appearance (11). Lesions have been variously described as pagetoid, chalky,

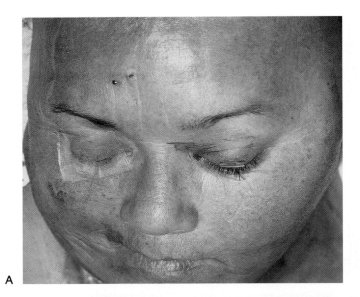

A

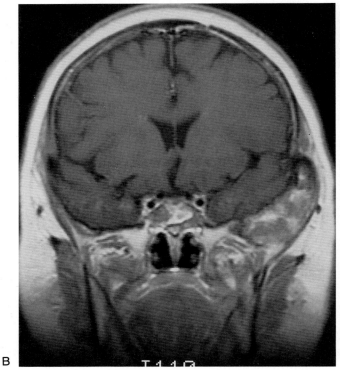

B

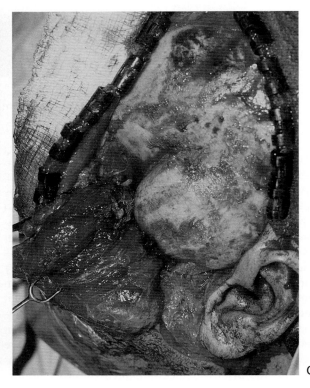

C

FIG. 4. **A:** Patient with fibrous dysplasia of the sphenoid bone. **B:** Radiograph showing typical ground glass appearance of lesion. **C:** Lesion exposed at time of surgery.

sclerotic, whorled plaque, and cyst-like (10,12). A common scenario is for early lesions to have a cyst-like quality, but as more osteoid is added to the lesion as it matures with time it takes on more of a ground glass or peau d'orange type of appearance (13) due to the finely speckled calcification.

The gross appearance of the lesion is a pink to gray-white color and firm but soft enough to cut with a knife. It is rubbery in consistency and may contain small clear fluid-filled cysts. A gritty sensation as the knife cuts through the lesion may be experienced and is due to

the variable amount of osseous material within. In the maxilla, the lesion may be too hard to cut because of the amount of osteoid. Those particular masses are often sclerotic on radiographs. There may be a grossly laminar appearance to the lesion resembling the rings of a tree stump. The histological picture of fibrous dysplasia is characterized by a whorling, haphazard array of fibrous tissue interspersed with bony spicules. The oxytalan fiber is characteristic of the lesions of fibrous dysplasia. As distinct from collagen, reticulin, or elastic fibers, this fiber resists acid hydrolyses. Under nor-

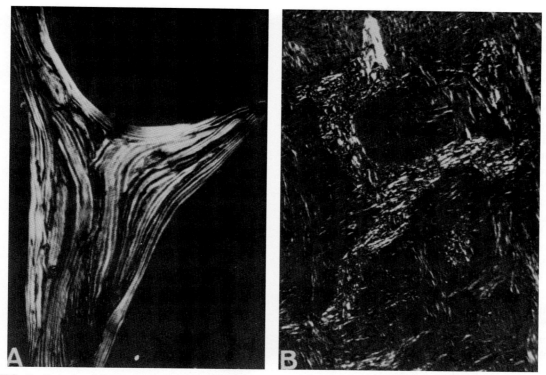

FIG. 5. Polarized light examination of collagen fibers of lamellar bone **(A)** compared to that of fibrous dysplasia **(B)**. Note the regularity and parallel disposition of fibers in (A) compared to the random, haphazard arrangement in (B). (From ref. 7, with permission.)

mal circumstances, oxytalan fiber usually is found in the periodontal membrane. It is found to be closely related to the elastic fibers (14). Unlike the regularity of collagen disposition within normal lamellar bone, that of fibrous dysplasia is random and haphazard (Fig. 5). The bony spicules have a characteristic shape described as "Chinese character," "C&S," or "jigsaw puzzle" in configuration. The bone is much more cellular than normal cancellous bone spicules, is thinner in width, and has highly irregular margins (Fig. 6). There is an absence of osteoblasts around the rim of these woven bone segments. There are no inflammatory cells and no osteoclasts seen in the lesion.

Treatment is directed at eliminating sinus dysfunction by removing disease that obstructs sinus drainage, restoring normal ocular function, and correcting or at least improving visible facial deformity. Cranial foramina that may be encroached upon by the disease, producing cranial nerve dysfunction, must be decompressed. Complete resection of the lesion is the most desired treatment. However, because this is basically a benign process, total exenteration that will result in a decrease in function, disturbance, or major deformity must be avoided. Since oftentimes the patient does not seek medical attention until the lesion achieves considerable size, total resection without incurring significant deformity and morbidity is impossible. In these cases,

the relief of sinus obstruction and a contouring of the bone are done to achieve symmetry. Surgery prior to adolescence is inadvisable because the stripping of the periosteum and excision or curettage of the lesion may stimulate it to grow (15). In this age group, treatment

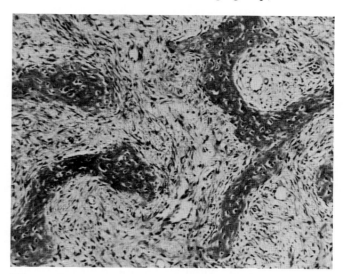

FIG. 6. Spicules of bone from a lesion with fibrous dysplasia showing the characteristic irregular "Chinese character" type of configuration. Note the cellularity of the bone and the irregular margins (H&E, ×100). (From ref. 7, with permission.)

should be limited to a small incisional biopsy unless severe functional impediments occur. In the postadolescent period, the small lesion should be excised completely. Incomplete removals tend to recur, albeit slowly. Fibrous dysplasia patients require close periodic follow-up for a protracted time. Recurrent lesions will require intermittent recontouring and there is the risk, although very small, of malignant degeneration. Dahlin (9) describes three cases of malignant degeneration in nonirradiated cases in his large series from the Mayo Clinic. However, he has had seven malignancies that arose in fibrous dysplasia that had been irradiated. Any rapid or sudden growth in a site of fibrous dysplasia must be viewed with much suspicion.

CHERUBISM

Cherubism is a genetically determined condition of the jaws where there is a relatively symmetrical deposition of fibrous tissue within the bone. The condition is an autosomal dominant condition with 100% penetrance in males and 60% to 70% in females (1). There are varying degrees of expressivity.

This disorder was first described by Jones et al. (16) in 1950. It is characterized by a symmetrical swelling at the angle of the jaws and, in about two-thirds of the cases, in the maxillae. It usually appears in the second or third year of life and grows rapidly for the next 2 years or so, then slows down for about 5 years, arrests, then regresses following puberty (1). The lesion may disappear completely during adulthood, but it is not uncommon for the person to be left with some residuum.

Histologically, the lesion has a large fibrous tissue component that may be densely packed or loose. The more loosely arranged pattern with more in the way of blood vessels seem to be associated with a more rapid growth rate (7). There are aggregates of giant cells with some possessing up to 50 nuclei. There are occasional areas of hemorrhage with hemosiderin deposits. Some osteoid may be present, but it is important to emphasize that there is no relationship to fibrous dysplasia.

The clinical appearance is pathognomonic. The mandibular angles, and oftentimes the cheeks, are swollen, giving the child a visage resembling the plump-cheeked angelic cherubs characteristic of the art of the Renaissance period (Fig. 7). The maxillary swellings produce a tightness of the cheek skin with retraction of the lower lid and enlargement of the maxillary sinus roof and infraorbital rims. The aforementioned factors elevate the globe and withdraw the lower eyelid, creating a scleral show below the corneal limbus. This produces the "looking toward heaven" appearance described originally by Jones et al. (16). The palate is often V-shaped and thickened. The alveolar bone may be in-

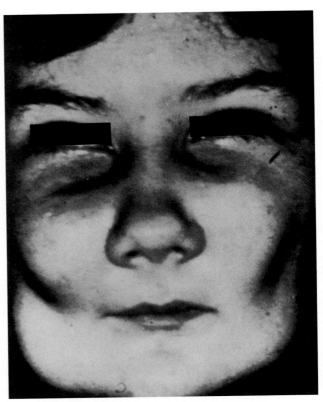

FIG. 7. Child with the characteristic facial appearance of cherubism with symmetrical cheek and jaw swellings. Note the "looking toward heaven" appearance. (From ref. 30, with permission.)

vaded and the process may even engulf the teeth. The maxillary sinus may become completely filled with the lesion and bulge the floor of the orbit upward.

The radiographic appearance initially is of multilocular cysts. The cortex becomes thin but does not perforate. As the cysts mature while the child grows to adolescence, the cysts take on a ground glass appearance as the lucent areas fill with more dense fibrous tissue and osteoid. The risk during the cystic stage for the active child involved in contact sports is pathological fracture. A very early sign on lateral plane films is the "hard palate" sign, which is produced by the thickening of palatal bone, producing a line that is not seen in the normal child because of its usual thinness.

Treatment is delayed, with few exceptions, until adulthood because of the natural history of the disorder. Surgery in childhood is fraught with problems such as intensive hemorrhage brought about by the extensive vascularity of the early lesion. Additionally, fracture of the bone may occur and stimulation of the mass to undergo accelerated growth has been reported (17). Radiation therapy is clearly contraindicated. Induction of malignancy later in life and osteoradionecrosis as well as perturbations in growth may occur. If treatment is necessary, curettage and replacement of the defect by calvarial or hip graft bone may be done.

OSSIFYING FIBROMA

This somewhat confusing lesion is probably best understood as a spectrum of disease. The origin is in the primitive mesenchymal cells in the periodontal connective tissue of the jaws. They can occur in either the maxilla or the mandible, being most common in the latter. Hamner et al. (18) described the lesions as cementoid, osteoid, cemento-osteoid, and fibroid in type. This study provides some order and clarity to the comprehension of these lesions as perhaps a spectrum of disease rather than a single entity. This group of abnormalities includes ossifying fibroma, cementifying fibroma, benign cementoblastoma, and periapical fibrous dysplasia.

In contrast to fibrous dysplasia, which is seen princi-

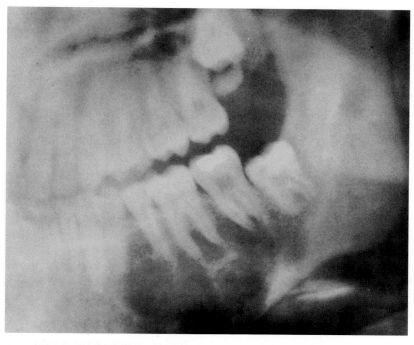

A

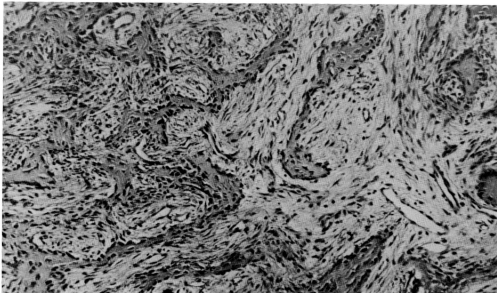

B

FIG. 8. A: Radiograph of ossifying fibroma of mandible. (From ref. 20, with permission.) **B:** Histologic appearance of ossifying fibroma. Note the contrast with fibrous dysplasia: peripheral lamellar bone in the bony spicules that are in turn lined by osteoblasts (H&E, × 140). (From ref. 19, with permission.)

pally in the young, these lesions of the ossifying fibroma group have the highest incidence in the third and fourth decades of life. The lesions are usually solitary and slow growing. However, rapid growth can occur especially in younger patients and when the tumor-like growth is located in the maxilla. It can assume an aggressive behavioral pattern, causing local destruction and rapid local recurrence after incomplete resection (1,19). The lesion may invade both the maxillary and ethmoid sinuses and the teeth may be displaced.

Histologically, the lesion is different from fibrous dysplasia. The bony spicules are similar to those in the latter lesion except that, although the central part is of woven bone, the periphery is lamellar bone. Furthermore, the rims of these spicules are lined with osteoblasts (Fig. 8B). In some areas inflammatory cells, hemosiderin deposits, and giant cells are found.

The radiographic appearance of the lesion is variable (Fig. 8A). The early lesions appear as a clearly outlined radiolucency that with maturity becomes less discrete. An area of radiodensity with occasional flecks of calcification may be seen. In a mature ossifying cementoma, there is a clear, well-demarcated radiolucency with a radiodense regular area internally. Invasion of the maxillary sinus with partial or complete opacification and even involvement of the ethmoid sinuses may be seen.

Local resection with assurance that there is a complete removal is done. If only a thin shell of bone is left, bone grafting may be necessary. Complete resection is absolutely essential in the maxilla.

DESMOPLASTIC FIBROMA

Desmoplastic fibroma is a very rare condition that is seen mostly in extremity bones and only occasionally in the head and neck. In the Barnes et al. review (6) of the literature, only two cases were reported in the maxilla and 24 in the mandible. In the AFIP series (19) and Dahlin's (9) collection, none were reported in the maxilla. There have been sporadic reports of lesions affecting the nasal cavity and paranasal sinuses (21,22).

The desmoplastic fibroma is in the class of extra-abdominal desmoid tumors. They are usually slow growing, hard, painless tumors that infiltrate surrounding structures but never metastasize. However, because of their locally invasive quality, they may be thought of as a low-grade type of fibrosarcoma. They are histologically bland and show no hallmarks of malignancy. They are hard, white, solid tumors with only the very occasional cyst. When cut with a knife, they have a white glistening surface and occasionally a gritty feel. The fascicles of fibrous tissue take on a whorled

and trabeculated pattern. They may completely replace the bone they invade.

Under microscopic examination (Fig. 9), the lesions show dense cartilaginous fibrous tissue with numerous fibroblasts. The bone often shows fingers of fibrous tissue extending into it. The fibroblasts are characterized by their high cytoplasmic content. The nuclei are not hyperchromatic. The lesion is differentiated easily from fibrous dysplasia or ossifying fibroma in that it has no osseous component. Electron micrographs (Fig. 10) show a prominent rough endoplasmic reticulum with numerous collagen fibrils in the extracellular spaces. The cellular outline is elongated and tapered. The Golgi apparatus is prominent and the nucleus has a rough outline with prominent nucleoli. Numerous actin bundles often are seen within the cytoplasm (24).

Clinically, as mentioned, they usually present as a slow-growing painless mass. However, the tumors in the head and neck are usually much faster growing than the extra-abdominal desmoids of other sites. In the series of 34 patients reported by Masson and Soule (25), 21 (62%) were aware of their mass for less than 1 year. The lesions may be painful and tender. They may achieve considerable size, with patients presenting with lesions as large as 20 cm in diameter (22).

The radiographic appearance is usually of a unilocular or multilocular cyst, oftentimes with trabeculations. The overlying cortical bone is expanded and thinned or penetrated with tumor advancing into adjacent soft tissue. Tooth roots adjacent to the tumor often are eroded.

Treatment is by radical excision because of the infiltrative nature of the lesion. A cuff of uninvolved tissue must be taken for a tumor-free margin around the mass because of the particular aggressiveness of the head and neck lesions compared to other bodily sites. Local recurrences are reported in 20% to 77% of cases. One of the six patients with nasal and sinus tumor in the series of Fu and Perzin (21) died of local recurrence. Cytotoxic drugs and irradiation therapy are not recommended.

Periosteal desmoids show little difference from desmoplastic fibroma except for their origin in subperiosteum. The tumor erodes into the cortical bone and expands into overlying soft tissue.

CHONDROMYXOID FIBROMA

Chondromyxoid fibroma is a rare benign tumor of putative cartilaginous origin. The tumor usually is seen in the tibia (33%) and only 0.6% are found in the facial skeleton (26). In Dahlin's series (27) of 30 such lesions, he found none in the head and neck. Table 2 lists the anatomic distribution of 16 cases of head and neck

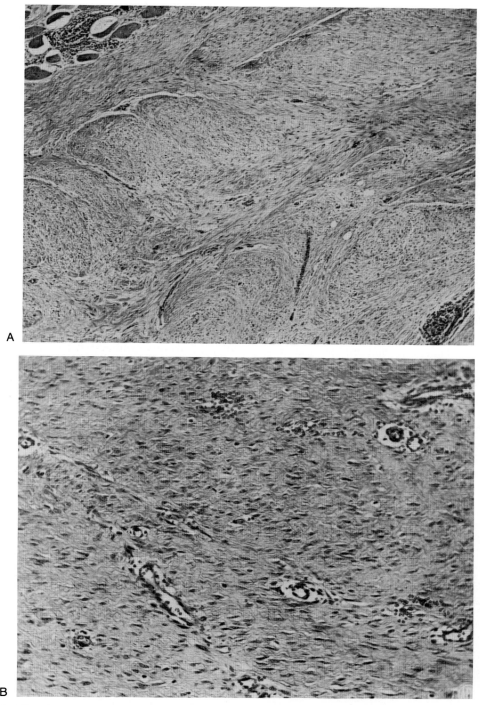

FIG. 9. Histologic appearance of desmoid fibroma. **A:** Whorling pattern of collagen bundles (×35). **B:** Characteristic fibroblastic cells with abundant cytoplasm and uniform spindle-shaped nuclei (×145). (From ref. 24, with permission.)

chondromyxofibroma and it is remarkable that only three could possibly involve the sinuses.

It presents as a slow-growing, tender, and painful mass that usually begins before the age of 30. Patients complain of progressive swelling of the bony part, loos-

ening of the teeth, trismus, sometimes headache, and even vertigo.

Radiographically, the mass presents as a punched-out lesion in the bone with a bulging, thinned, and sometimes eroded overlying cortex. There may be tra-

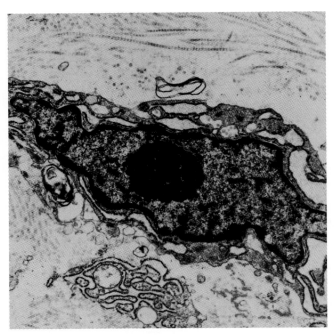

FIG. 10. Electron microscopic appearance of fibroblast from an extra-abdominal desmoid, demonstrating prominent rough endoplasmic reticulum and collagen fibrils in the extracellular spaces (×11,400). (From ref. 23, with permission.)

TABLE 2. Anatomic distribution of 16 cases of chondromyxoid fibroma of the head and neck

Site	Number of cases
Mandible	5
Frontal bone	2
Skull (not otherwise specified)	2
Parietal bone	1
Occipital bone	1
Mastoid	1
Petrous pyramid	1
Base of skull—foramen magnum area	1
Pterygopalatine space	1
Cervical spine	1

From ref. 6, with permission.

The gross specimen is firm, gray or gray-white in appearance, and closely resembles fibrocartilage, but it does not have the mucinous slimy consistency of the myxoid component or the blue-gray color of cartilage. Hemorrhage and cyst formation are quite common. There is a lobulated appearance brought about by bundles of fibrous connective tissue. The tumor appears to be restricted by the presence of the periosteum. A thin cortex of bone often is seen around the lesion and occasionally this bone is seen to be eroded.

Histologically, it is essential to differentiate between this lesion and chondrosarcoma. The characteristic histological picture is that of lobules of myxoid material surrounded by bands of collagenous material and fibroblasts. The myxoid cells are stellate in appearance, often multipolar, and more dense in the periphery of

beculations within and an often stippled appearance secondary to small calcific deposits within the substance of the tumor. The overlying cortical bone tends to be scalloped and sclerotic but may be eroded through (Fig. 11).

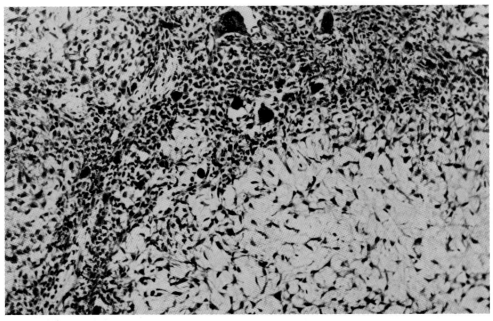

FIG. 11. Microscopic appearance of chondromyxoid fibroma. Note the lobular pattern with increased cellularity at the extremity of a lobule. (From ref. 19, with permission.)

the lobule than centrally. As the lesion matures, the myxoid material becomes more replaced by fibrous tissue. Chondrocytes can be identified in all specimens but vary greatly in their amount and never exceed 75% of the tumor volume. Treatment is by resection with a narrow margin of healthy tissue. Recurrences are related most commonly to incomplete excision, which usually have been done by curettage.

FIBROMA

The notion of a facial bone "fibroma" is discussed and argued extensively throughout the literature and the condition probably represents a spectrum of disease rather than a specific isolated entity. Batsakis (1) describes the entity of "central fibroma" as a lesion in an intraosseous location in the jaws that is nonossifying in type. He includes three basic variants: nonossifying fibroma, desmoplastic fibroma, and odontogenic fibroma. In his notion of fibroma, Dahlin includes myxoma, cortical desmoid, fibromatosis, and xanthoma. The latter is a variant that contains a considerable amount of lipoid material. Fibromatosis as he describes it is not self-limiting like the usual fibroma, is often multiple, and increases in size as the child matures. Curiously, in Dahlin's series of 72 cases of fibroma, none affected the facial or cranial skeleton, speaking to the rarity of this lesion in the head and neck (29).

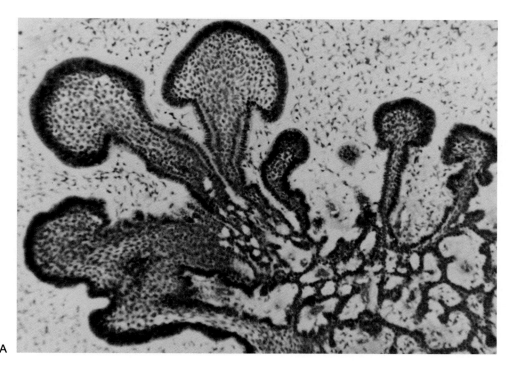

A

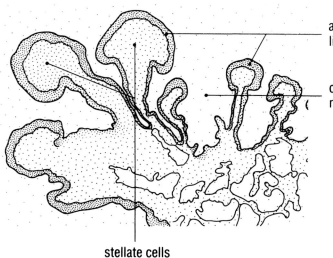

B

ameloblast-like cells

cellular mesoderm

stellate cells

FIG. 12. Histological appearance of ameloblastic fibroma with frond-like projections of ameloblastic tall palisaded cells. Note stellate reticulum-like tissue in the central areas and a background of mesenchymal cells (H&E). **A:** Histological photomicrograph. **B:** Explanatory diagram. (From ref. 13, with permission.)

In the AFIP description (30), the fibroma is assigned to a cell of origin usually from the odontogenic cell series. They describe fibromas as ameloblastic, mesenchymal, odontogenic, and cementifying. Clearly, the pure "central fibroma" of the maxilla and sinuses is a distinctly rare lesion.

The odontogenic fibroma, while still extremely uncommon, is thought to arise from either the epithelial element or connective tissue cells associated with the dental anlage. The ameloblastic fibroma is comprised of primitive dental epithelium arranged in papilliferous fronds, solid balls, or flat sheets. The central areas beneath these tall palisaded areas look like primitive stellate reticulum. The stroma in which it lies is full of stellate mesenchymal cells in a loose collagenous matrix (Fig. 12). The lesion presents as a slow-growing, painless mass most commonly in the mandible but occasionally in the maxilla. It may or may not be encapsulated and is seen as a unilocular or multilocular radiolucency on radiography. It may be associated with an unerupted tooth. Male and female incidence is the same and it is found usually in patients under the age of 20.

A seemingly related lesion that is more of a hamartoma (31) than a true neoplasm is the ameloblastic fibro-odontoma. In addition to the ameloblastic elements, enamel, dentin, cementum, and the components of the pulp space may be found (30). They are found almost always associated with an unerupted, often impacted, molar tooth. The tumor is commonest in the under-20 age group, with the average age of 8.1 years (31). It is most usual in the mandibular molar area but may be found also in the maxilla, protruding into the maxillary sinus (Fig. 13).

Both lesions can be treated by enucleation with some additional curettage of the ameloblastic fibroma because of its slightly more invasive character. The hamartomatous ameloblastic fibro-odontoma, with its more benign course, is treated by simple enucleation and moreover even the underlying tooth can be successfully preserved (32).

The odontogenic fibroma is a benign tumor, found mainly in the mandible, that has a dense background of fibrous tissue with some strands of inactive odontogenic epithelium (Fig. 14). Occasional small foci of cementum-like material are seen. These lesions probably are related to the odontogenic myxoma and indeed have ultrastructural similarity (30). They have separate designations because of light microscopic differences. The lesions can vary from small to quite large and deforming, with those in the maxilla extending into the antrum. Radiographs show a unilocular or multilocular "soap bubble" pattern of lucency adjacent to an unerupted tooth. Treatment is by conservative local excision.

The cementifying fibroma is usually a small innocuous asymptomatic lesion seen in persons over the age of 40 and seen as an incidental finding on a dental radio-

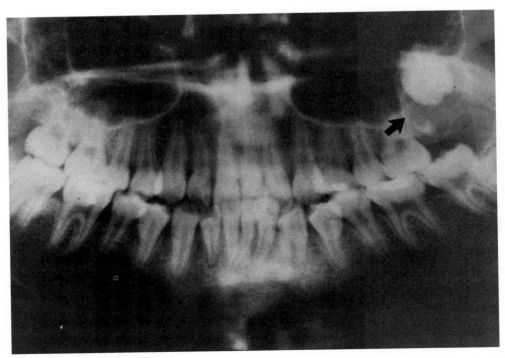

FIG. 13. Panorex radiograph showing cyst-like lesion in the left upper distal maxilla *(arrow)*. A radiodensity is seen within the more apical portion of the lesion. The lesion histologically was an ameloblastic fibro-odontoma. (From ref. 32, with permission.)

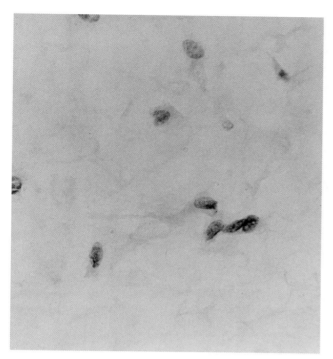

FIG. 14. Histologic pattern of odontogenic fibroma. (From ref. 13, with permission.)

graph. They are seen as radiolucencies or radio-opacities at the apices of the teeth. It is considered by Hamner et al. (18) to be the commonest fibro-osseous lesion in the jaws. This tumor can occur even in the frontal bone. It is thought to arise from the cells of the periodontal ligament. In the beginning, the lesion is made up mainly of fibrous tissue but as the tumor matures, islands of cementum appear (Fig. 15). Although usually small and asymptomatic, some lesions may become large, deforming, and painful. Treatment is by simple conservative excision.

FIBROMYXOMA

Unlike the more benign odontogenic fibromas, the fibromyxoma is clinically more aggressive. This is especially true of this lesion when found in the paranasal sinuses (1). They generally are seen in teenagers and young adults. This is called by some authorities an odontogenic myxoma because of its putative origin in the mesenchyme of the dental papilla (30). It is a loose gelatinous tumor more commonly found in the mandible than the maxilla. The tumor is grayish to yellow in color, often bosselated on the periphery, and may even be very firm in consistency if there is a predominant fibrous component.

Histologically (Fig. 16), the tumor is comprised of a background of collagenous fibrous tissue varying in amount from tumor to tumor, but uniform within each

individual lesion (30). The cellular component is a loose arrangement of variable stellate cells with round well-formed nuclei and rare mitotic figures. Although odontogenic epithelial nests are seen occasionally, no differentiation of these cells is seen.

On radiographic examination, the tumors are radiolucent with fine, lacy trabeculations across the lesion, giving the appearance of tennis racquet strings (Fig. 17). The lucency may be outlined sharply or indistinctly, the latter pattern suggestive of malignancy. It may be unilocular or multilocular in configuration. They often are associated with an unerupted tooth.

Treatment needs to be a little more aggressive than for most benign odontogenic tumors. There is a tendency to recur after simple curettage. Because of the amorphous gelatinous nature of the tumor, complete excision is very difficult. A narrow margin of healthy bone must be excised with the lesion in order to prevent local recurrence.

FIBROSARCOMA

Fibrosarcoma is distinctly rare in the head and neck and accounts for only 5% of fibrosarcomas from all sites (33,34). Fibromatosis may be considered to be a well-differentiated fibrosarcoma because of its aggressive behavior, ability to invade local tissues, and frequency of recurrence after conservative local resection (21). Fibrosarcoma of the head and neck is not uncommonly found in the nose and paranasal sinuses. In the Mark et al. series (35) of 29 head and neck fibrosarcomas, 33% were found in these sites. In the Fu and Perzin series (21), there were six cases that took origin in the paranasal sinus area. Dahlin (9) had 158 fibrosarcomas in his collection, but only 27 involved the head and neck, with only three of these involving the sinuses and those all involved the maxillary sinuses.

According to Batsakis (1), many early descriptions of fibrosarcoma were of tumors whose cellular differentiation was problematic and were thus dubbed with this diagnosis. In more enlightened times, by using increasingly sophisticated diagnostic tools and stains, a more accurate diagnosis can be made. The degree of cellular differentiation dominant throughout the tumor is an important determinant of prognosis. Figure 18 is a clinical example of a young woman with a well-differentiated fibrosarcoma of the ethmoid sinus who has survived tumor-free for 5 years following an aggressive but ocular-sparing procedure. Figure 19 illustrates a patient with an aggressive poorly differentiated fibrosarcoma who rapidly succumbed to her disease.

Conley (36) described the natural history of 124 cases of fibrosarcoma of the head and neck. Well-differentiated tumors comprised 87% of the total and the prognosis was excellent with an 83% cure rate. There were

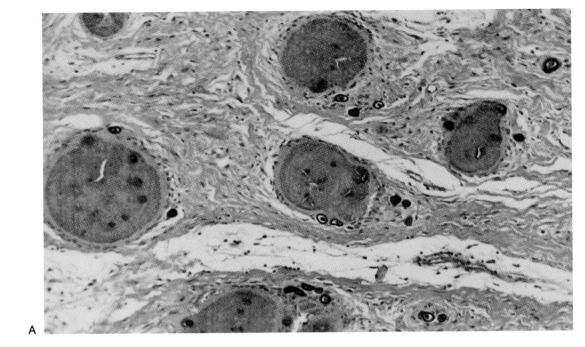

A

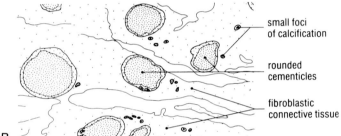

small foci
of calcification

rounded
cementicles

fibroblastic
connective tissue

B

FIG. 15. Histologic appearance of cementifying fibroma. Note the presence of cementicles in a background of dense fibrous connective tissue (H&E). **A:** Photomicrograph. **B:** Explanatory diagram. (From ref. 13, with permission.)

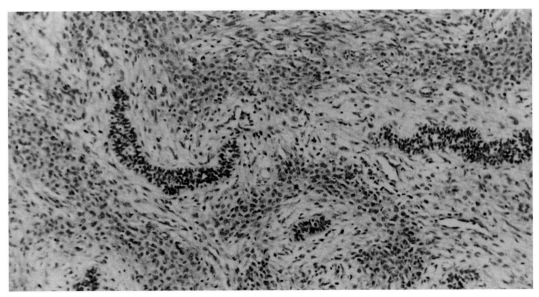

FIG. 16. High-power photomicrograph of myxoma. Note the stellate mesenchymal cells in a loose collagenous background. (From ref. 13, with permission.)

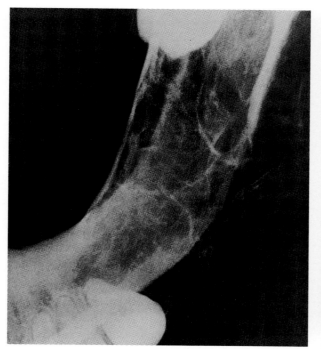

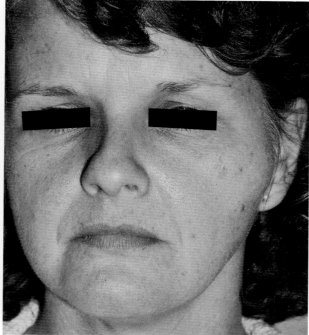

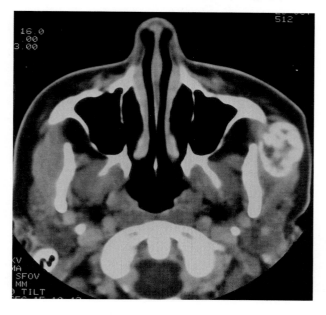

FIG. 17. A: Radiograph of fibromyxoma of mandible showing multiloculated appearance as well as the "tennis racquet string" trabeculations within the lesion. (From ref. 13, with permission.) B: Patient with fibromyxoma of zygoma. C: CAT scan of fibromyxoma of zygoma.

only two cases of metastasis in this group. On the other hand, only 25% of the 16 patients with a poorly differentiated lesion survived. They tended to die from local recurrence and distant metastases. There were a few cases of recurrent well-differentiated fibrosarcoma that became poorly differentiated on recurrence. One patient in my experience escalated into a poorly differentiated tumor after radiation therapy for a residual well-differentiated tumor (Fig. 20).

In the Mark et al. series (35), 17 patients were low grade and 11 patients were high grade, possibly reflecting the referral pattern of a large tertiary care univer-

sity hospital. The 5-year actuarial relapse-free survival was 58%. Of the nine cases of fibrosarcoma of the sinuses, five were free of disease with a minimum of 2-year follow-up. There were two patients dead of local disease, one of local and distant metastases, and another alive with distant disease. All the patients with high-grade disease were dead and all the patients with low-grade tumors were alive, one surviving with distant metastatic disease.

Well-differentiated lesions are usually hard, white, and fibrous, invading the bony walls of the sinus and even the overlying soft tissue. The poorly differen-

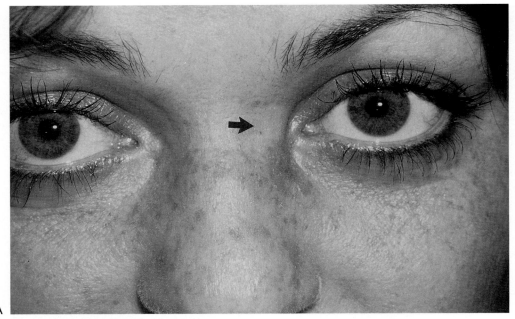

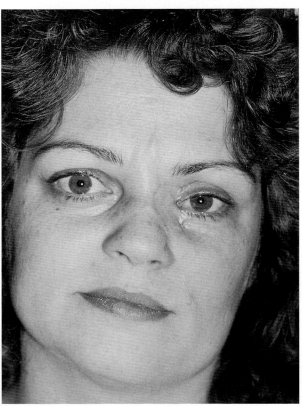

FIG. 18. Young woman with a well-differentiated fibrosarcoma of the left ethmoid sinus. **A:** Tumor in left inner canthal region *(arrow).* **B:** Patient is tumor-free 5 years postoperatively following resection of inner canthal skin, conservative resection of the orbit, and reconstruction with midline forehead flap.

tiated variety varies from firm to soft and myxoid. Bone erosion and soft tissue invasion are common. The histological features of the well-differentiated lesion often present the classical dilemma of distinction between fibrosarcoma and so-called fibromatosis—spindle-shaped cells with little variation in size and shape, few to no mitotic figures, and regular bands of tightly woven collagenous tissue. The mark of malignancy is the extension of tumor into adjacent tissues. The more poorly differentiated tumors are more cellular, and the cells are pleomorphic with more mitotic figures. The stroma is less obvious and more disorganized, occasionally osteoid, and new bone induced at the edge of the tumor's progression through existing bone is seen.

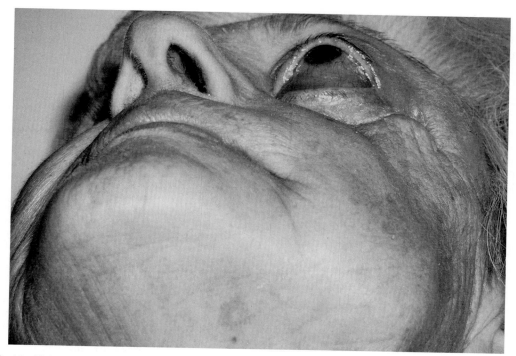

FIG. 19. Elderly female with a highly aggressive fibrosarcoma recurrent after total maxillectomy. Note proptosis produced by orbital invasion of tumor.

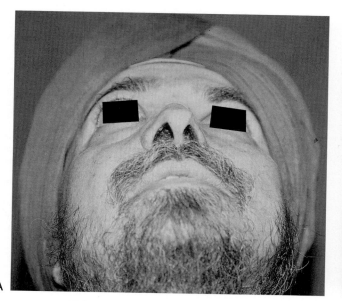

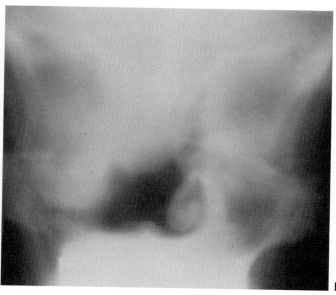

A

B

FIG. 20. A: Middle-aged man with a highly aggressive, poorly differentiated fibrosarcoma of the sphenoid, ethmoid, and maxillary sinus beginning in the nasopharynx. The tumor invaded the orbit, causing proptosis and extensive invasion of the anterior and middle cranial fossa. **B:** Tomograph of poorly differentiated fibrosarcoma, showing extensive sinus erosion and extension into the intracranial cavity.

Radiographs show a homogeneously radio-opaque mass without calcification, invading adjacent sinus bone and sometimes overlying soft tissue (Fig. 20B).

Treatment is with resection whose extent varies with the degree of differentiation and the degree of tumor extension. Generally, well-differentiated lesions can be excised with a narrow margin. More extensive and poorly differentiated tumors need radical resection with wider margins of healthy tissue surrounding the lesion. The place of radiation is unclear, but in Conley's (36) and my experience, the tumors are not radio-sensitive and they are responsible in some instances for malignant transformation.

REFERENCES

1. Batsakis JG. Non-odontogenic tumors of the jaws. In: *Tumors of the head and neck: clinical and pathological considerations,* 2nd ed. Baltimore: Williams & Wilkins, 1984;381–419.
2. Houston WO Jr. Fibrous dysplasia of maxilla and mandible. Clinicopathology study and comparison of facial bone lesions with lesions affecting general skeleton. *J Oral Surg* 1965;23:17–39.
3. Lichtenstein L. Polyostatic fibrous dysplasia. *Arch Surg* 1938;36:874–898.
4. Lichtenstein L, Jaffe HL. Fibrous dysplasia of bone. A condition affecting one, several, or many bones, the graver cases of which may present abnormal pigmentation of the skin, premature sexual development, hyperthyroidism or still other extraskeletal abnormalities. *Arch Pathol* 1942;33:777–816.
5. Schlumberger HG. Fibrous dysplasia of single bones (monostotic fibrous dysplasia). *Milit Surg* 1946;99:504–527.
6. Barnes L, Peel RL, Berbin RS, Goodman MA, Appel BN. Diseases of the bones and joints. In: Barnes L, ed. *Surgical pathology of the head and neck,* vol. II, New York: Marcel Dekker, 1985;884–1044.
7. Reed RJ. Fibrous dysplasia of bone. A review of 25 cases. *Arch Pathol* 1963;75:480–495.
8. Harris WH, Dudley HRJ, Barry RJ. The natural history of fibrous dysplasia. An orthopedic pathological and radiographic study. *J Bone Joint Surg* 1962;44A:207–233.
9. Dahlin D. *Bone tumors: general aspects and data on 6,221 cases,* 3rd ed. Springfield, IL: Charles C Thomas, 1981;362–367.
10. Enzinger FM, Weiss SW. *Soft tissue tumors.* St. Louis: CV Mosby, 1983;762–763.
11. Fries JW. The roentgen features of fibrous dysplasia of the skull and facial bones. *Am J Roentgenol Radium Ther Nuclear Med* 1957;77:71–88.
12. Obisesan AA, Lagundoye SB, Daramola JO, et al. The radiologic features of fibrous dysplasia of the craniofacial bones. *Oral Surg* 1977;44:949–959.
13. Cawson RA, Wveson JW. *Oral pathology & diagnosis.* Philadelphia: Saunders 1987;8.3–8.5

14. Bhasker SN, ed. *Orban's oral histology & embryology,* 9th ed. St Louis: CV Mosby, 1980;226–227.
15. Dierks E, Caudill LJ, O'Leary JD. Surgical recontouring of a panfacial fibro-osseous deformity. *J Oral Surg* 1979;37:682.
16. Jones WA, Gerrie J, Pritchard J. Cherubism: a familial fibrous dysplasia of the jaws. *J Bone Joint Surg* 1950;32B:325.
17. Scott RF, Ellis E. Surgical treatment of non-odontogenic tumors. In: Thawley SE, Panje WR, Batsakis JG, Lindberg RD, eds. *Comprehensive management of head & neck tumors,* vol. 2. Philadelphia: Saunders, 1987;1559–1577.
18. Hamner JE, Scofield HH, Cornyn J. Benign fibro-osseous jaw lesions of periodontal membrane origin. An analysis of 249 cases. *Cancer* 1968;22:861.
19. Spjut H, Dorman HD, Fechner RE, Ackerman LV. Tumors of bone and cartilage, In: *Atlas of tumor pathology,* fascicle 5. Washington D.C.: AFIP, 1971;260–262.
20. Regezi JA, Sciubba JJ. *Oral pathology—clinical pathological correlations.* Philadelphia: Saunders, 1989;370.
21. Fu Y-S, Perzin KH. Nonepithelial tumors of the nasal cavity, paranasal sinuses and nasopharynx. A clinico-pathological study. VI. Fibrous tissue tumors (fibroma, fibromatosis, fibrosarcoma). *Cancer* 1974;37:2912.
22. Kyriakos M. Pathology of selected soft tissue tumors of the head and neck. In: Thawley SE, Panje WR, Batsakis JG, Lindberg RD, eds. *Comprehensive management of head & neck tumors,* vol 2. Philadelphia: Saunders, 1987;1241–1297.
23. Toxy JB, Battifora H. The electron microscope in the study and diagnosis of soft tissue tumors. In: Trump BE, Jones RT, eds. *Diagnostic electron microscopy.* New York: Wiley, 1980.
24. Enzinger FM, Weiss SW, eds. *Soft tissue tumors.* St. Louis: CV Mosby, 1983;56–5.
25. Masson JK, Soule EH. Desmoid tumors of the head and neck. *Am J Surg* 1966;112:615.
26. Huvos AG. *Bone tumors, diagnosis, treatment, & prognosis.* Philadelphia: Saunders, 1979;190–198.
27. Dahlin D. *Bone tumors: general aspects and data on 6,221 cases,* 3rd ed. Springfield, IL: Charles C Thomas, 1981;57–70.
28. Mirra JM, Gold RH, Marcove RC. *Bone tumors, diagnosis & treatment.* Philadelphia: Lippincott, 1979;190–198.
29. Dahlin D. *Bone tumors: general aspects and data on 6,221 cases,* 3rd ed. Springfield, IL: Charles C Thomas, 1981;122–136.
30. Hoffman S, Jacoway JR, Krolls SO. Intraosseous and periosteal tumors of the jaws. In: *Atlas of tumor pathology* 2nd ed., fascicle 24. Washington D.C.: AFIP, 1987.
31. Slootweg PJ. An analysis of the inter-relationship of the mixed odontogenic tumors—ameloblastic fibroma, ameloblastic fibro-odontoma and the odontomas. *Oral Surg* 1981;51:266.
32. Okura M, Nakahara H, Matsuya T. Treatment of ameloblastic fibro-odontoma without removal of the associated impacted permanent tooth: report of cases. *J Oral Maxillofac Surg* 1992;50:1094–1097.
33. Figueiroda MTA, Marques LA, Camphos-Filho N. Soft tissue sarcomas of the head and neck in adults and children: experience at a single institution and a review of the literature. *Int J Cancer* 1988;41(2):198–200.
34. Freeman AM, Reiman HM, Woods JF. Soft tissue sarcomas of the head and neck. *Am J Surg* 1989;158:367–372.
35. Mark FR, Sercary A, Tran L, et al. Fibrosarcoma of the head and neck: the UCLA experience. *Arch Otol* 1991;117:396–401.
36. Conley J. *Concepts in head & neck surgery.* Stuttgart: G Thieme Verlag, 1970;201–202.

CHAPTER 36

Oroantral Fistula

Jack L. Gluckman

An oroantral fistula is by definition an abnormal communication between the oral cavity and the maxillary sinus. It can be classified as *acute* or *chronic* with the vast majority falling into the acute group secondary to dental extraction. The acute variety tends almost invariably to heal spontaneously within a few weeks and only rarely progresses to chronicity. Once a fistula has become chronic, however, an underlying cause should be suspected, for example, persistent infection, neoplasm, or epithelialization of the tract. Oroantral fistulas are more common in men than women perhaps because dental extraction is more common and more difficult in men (1).

ETIOLOGY

Extraction of teeth closely related to the floor of the maxillary sinus is by far the most common cause of an oroantral fistula (Table 1). This particularly follows extraction of the first and second molars and rarely the third molar and second premolar (1–3). These almost always spontaneously heal in 2 to 3 weeks and require no treatment other than packing of the socket with Gelfoam or oversewing the socket, if feasible. Factors that predispose to the development of a chronic fistula include the presence of a retained dental root within the maxillary sinus with local infection; the development of secondary maxillary sinusitis; focal osteomyelitis of the bone surrounding the tooth; and epithelialization of the fistula tract. Finally, the larger the bony defect, the greater the likelihood of failure to heal. Fistulas larger than 5 mm in diameter are unlikely to heal spontaneously (4). A large defect may result from a particularly traumatic extraction, where a significant portion of the floor of the antrum is fractured. In addition, any systemic disease that may impair healing (e.g., diabetes, malnutrition) may predispose to chronicity. Other iatrogenically induced oroantral fistulas in-

clude failure of the gingivobuccal sulcus incision to heal following a Caldwell–Luc procedure. This may be because of inadequate suturing or wound infection. Some surgeons feel that it is unnecessary to suture the incision at all, and while this would seem likely to predispose to the development of an oroantral fistula, proponents of this technique vigorously deny that this is a factor. Obviously, resection of the palate for malignancy will result in a significant oroantral fistula. While various flaps have been described to close these defects, the most simple and effective technique is to use a prosthesis. Oronasal fistulas are a common complication of cleft palate repair (5). Finally, facial trauma may result in the development of an oroantral fistula secondary to a palatal fracture.

Dental infection, which usually is the indication for the dental extraction, may result in a chronic fistula after extraction. This may be due to a focal area of osteomyelitis. Maxillary sinusitis per se will not result in an oroantral fistula, but if it complicates an acute fistula, it may predispose to chronicity and will need to be treated as an integral part of the management of the fistula. Osteomyelitis of the maxillary sinus, which rarely is seen today, may result in the development of a chronic oroantral fistula. Chronic granulomatous disease of the maxillary sinus may present with an oroantral fistula (e.g., fungus infections, midline granuloma).

Cysts and neoplasms, both benign and malignant, may cause a fistula by bony erosion. In fact, one of the first signs of a maxillary sinus carcinoma may be the development of loose teeth and an oroantral fistula.

PATHOLOGY

An oroantral fistula may present anywhere on the alveolar ridge or hard palate, depending on the underlying etiology. The usual site follows extraction of the

TABLE 1. *Etiology of oroantral fistula*

Trauma
    Iatrogenic: Dental extraction, Caldwell–Luc, palatal re-
        section, cleft palate repair, radiation
    Accidental: Maxillofacial injuries
Infection
    Nonspecific: Dental abscess, osteomyelitis
    Specific: Granulomas
Cysts
Neoplasms
    Benign
    Malignant

first and second molars, because the apices of these teeth are separated from the antral cavity by only a thin layer of bone varying in thickness from 0.1 to 0.7 cm in that region (6). A traumatic extraction may result in a fracture of this floor with a significant defect resulting. Factors that predispose to chronicity of the fistula include focal osteomyelitis, maxillary sinusitis, retained roots in the antral cavity itself, and epithelialization of the tract.

The most common complication of a fistula is maxillary sinusitis, which occurs to a varying extent within 48 hr (7) and is probably present to some degree in all patients with chronic fistulas (1).

CLINICAL FEATURES

The diagnosis of an oroantral fistula is usually not difficult. The patient may complain of a strange taste in the mouth and may actually feel the discharge. On eating, fluid or air may pass into the sinus and/or the nose, and if the defect is large, food may be forced into the sinuses. Many patients may present with recurrent unilateral maxillary sinusitis and this may become the dominant problem. If a retained root is present within the sinus, the odor may be particularly foul.

Examination will reveal a fistula, which, depending on the size, may easily be identified or may only be apparent on probing if small. The presence of granulations in the tooth socket or related to the Caldwell–Luc incision may help identify a subtle, small fistula. Likewise, if the patient blows his/her nose or performs a Valsalva maneuver, this may force secretion or air through the fistula and help with identification.

PATIENT EVALUATION

If the patient is referred during the acute phase, that is, within the first few days of the dental extraction, the fistula tract needs to be inspected to ensure the absence of any malignancy or untoward disease process. A sinus radiograph also should be taken to exclude the presence of any retained roots and the patient should be followed carefully to ensure satisfactory progress.

If the fistula is still present at 2 to 3 weeks or the patient is seen *ab initio* at this time, the fistula should be identified, probed to determine the extent of the bony defect, and a sinus radiograph taken to evaluate the status of the sinus cavity mucosa and exclude any underlying disease process. A biopsy of the tract is desirable, if in any way suspicious.

Radiographically, focal polypoid reaction around the fistula is commonly present; however, a diffuse mucosal thickening or even an air–fluid level may be apparent, indicating diffuse antral infection. If the history is the classic form for fistula development following dental extraction, and the radiographs are nonsuspicious, a computed tomography (CT) scan is not indicated. If, however, the fistula becomes chronic and the plain radiographs show significant sinus disease or suggest underlying pathology, then a CT scan should be ordered. This should be helpful in delineating the extent of the sinus infection, the size of the bony defect, and, of course, whether there is an underlying cyst or neoplasm.

MANAGEMENT

Acute

The vast majority of oroantral fistulas present following dental extraction and will heal spontaneously. After the patient has been evaluated in the routine manner and a sinus radiograph has been taken, the socket should be packed with Gelfoam and/or oversewn. The patient is placed on antibiotics and advised to keep the mouth clean using a cleansing mouthwash. A follow-up visit is scheduled for 2 weeks and in the vast majority of cases, the fistula will heal with no sequelae.

If retained roots are noted in the antrum on a routine radiograph, these should be removed. These may be extracted successfully through the socket. If not, a simple nasoantral window may suffice to extract this foreign body or a Caldwell–Luc procedure may become indicated. If this foreign body is left *in situ*, it will almost certainly lead to infection and a chronic fistula. If the retained root is small, it is conceivable that it can be removed by an endoscopic technique.

Chronic

If when seen at 2 to 3 weeks the fistula remains patent, or if seen for the first time at this stage, the fistula is deemed chronic and the approach is more aggressive.

The fistula is carefully inspected and probed to determine the extent of the bone defect. The fistula should be debrided to remove any epithelialization of the tract, and a specimen is sent for histology to exclude any unsuspected granuloma or malignancy. A sinus radiograph should be obtained and a CT scan, as indicated. If, as expected, there is evidence of focal mucosal reaction around the fistula, or if there is diffuse maxillary sinusitis, a course of antibiotics should be commenced. If there is obvious sinusitis, an antral lavage should be performed through the fistula or, if too small, through the inferior meatus of the nose. This should be performed two to three times per week until the return is clear. Occasionally, the patient may be taught to perform the lavage personally through the fistula on a daily basis. In addition, the tract should be freshened using silver nitrate. If the fistula is small, a certain percentage will heal using these conservative measures.

If the maxillary sinusitis fails to resolve and/or the fistula persists, surgical intervention is indicated.

SURGICAL MANAGEMENT OF OROANTRAL FISTULAS

The surgical closure of an oroantral fistula, while apparently quite simple, may be extremely challenging with the choice of procedure depending on the size and site of the defect, the presence of surrounding teeth, the health of the surrounding tissues available for repair, and whether there is associated maxillary sinusitis. In general, if the fistula is closed during the acute phase, the success rate is 90% to 95% probably because of the high incidence of spontaneous closure, whereas once the fistula is chronic, the success rate drops to 60% to 70% depending on the technique (6,8).

Management of Maxillary Sinusitis

If overt maxillary sinusitis is present at the time of closure of the fistula, this needs to be eliminated as an integral part of the repair. This is accomplished by performing a Caldwell–Luc procedure through a gingivobuccal incision, removing the unhealthy mucosal lining and/or bone, and creating a nasoantral window for permanent drainage. In addition, the fistulous tract may be debrided through the sinus and any foreign body can be removed.

Because the gingivobuccal incision may compromise the creation of a buccal flap, it has been argued that if there is no overt sinus disease either clinically or radiographically, a Caldwell–Luc procedure is not necessary and a simple nasoantral window will suffice. Some authors feel that it is very rare that surgical therapy for the sinus is indicated (6). In general, however, it is probably better to explore the sinus than chance failure due to chronic sinusitis.

Techniques for Repair of Fistula

Techniques for surgical repair can be divided into local flaps, tongue flaps, distant flaps, and grafts. In general, the small fistulas can be closed using a single flap with a simple single-layered closure. Moderate sized defects, on the other hand, require a combination of local flaps with a double-layered closure if feasible (9).

LOCAL FLAPS

Buccal Flaps

The most common technique for closure of a *small* oroantral fistula is the buccal mucoperiosteal flap. These flaps are not very useful for larger defects because they are thin and have a somewhat precarious blood supply. These may take the form of a simple advancement flap, rotational flap, and a transversal or sliding flap.

The simple advancement flap was first described by Rehrmann (10) (Fig. 1). It is broad based and mobility can be improved by making an incision in the periosteum at the base of the flap. This technique is not only technically simple but is very successful in closing small fistulas (11). One disadvantage is that the gingivobuccal sulcus is compromised by this procedure, rendering placement of dentures difficult in the edentulous patient (12). Others have not noted this as a problem and feel that the sulcus reforms in 4 to 8 weeks (11). Some authors recommend the placement of dentures in the immediate postoperative period (13), although it would appear prudent to delay denture placement for at least 6 to 8 weeks to avoid compromising the flap (14). In addition, this flap may be compromised by the gingivobuccal incision of a Caldwell–Luc operation.

A variation of this simple advancement flap has been described, which is essentially a sliding mucoperiosteal flap with the periosteum once again being incised at the base to improve mobility (15,16) (Fig. 2). The disadvantages of this flap include the presence of a denuded raw donor site area and significant gingival undermining, which may predispose to periodontal disease (13).

A further variation described in the edentulous patient is the transversal flap, which is in essence a bipedicled advancement flap (17) (Fig. 3). This, unfortunately, does not allow much mobility and has not proved very useful in our experience.

Postoperatively, all patients are placed on antibiotics for 7 days and kept on a soft diet. The patient is instructed not to forcibly blow the nose until the flap has healed.

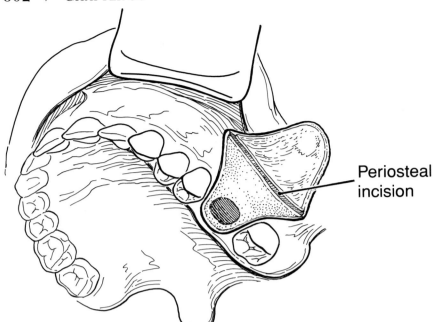

FIG. 1. A simple broad-based buccal advancement flap. Note the release incision in the periosteum to improve mobility.

Palatal Flaps

The various palatal flaps can be divided into advancement, rotational, and island flaps. The mucoperiosteum of the palate is abundant and vascular and therefore is an ideal tissue for closure of oroantral fistulas. It is, however, less elastic and thicker than buccal mucosa and thus less mobile in creating an adequate flap. It is the flap of choice for closure of *small to moderate* sized oroantral fistulas in many surgeons' hands.

A simple advancement flap of the palate really is quite unsatisfactory because little mobility can be obtained; thus it has no real place except perhaps in the closure of extremely small fistulas (Fig. 4).

A posterior-based rotational flap, on the other hand, is an excellent flap, obtaining its blood supply from the ipsilateral palatine artery (Fig. 5). It does, however, require significant mobilization of the mucoperiosteum of the palate to obtain adequate tissue. The flap is designed to include the fistulous tract so that the closure is performed as a simple transposition flap (Fig. 6). The donor site is allowed to heal in by secondary intention, which usually takes 4 to 8 weeks depending on the size

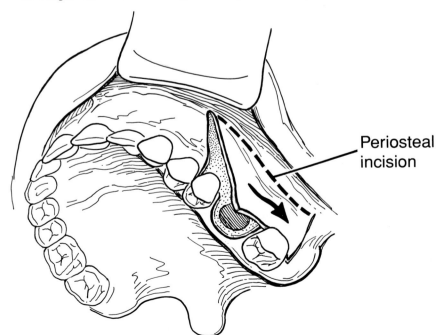

FIG. 2. A sliding mucoperiosteal buccal flap. This leaves a denuded donor site. Note the periosteal release incision.

of the defect. Its disadvantages include a tendency of the thick unwieldy pedicle to kink and the weight of the pedicle to pull away from the repair because of gravity. To overcome the tendency to kink, it has been suggested that the "dogear" be excised from the pedicle (18), but this is probably more likely to result in a compromised blood supply and further problems. To negate the tendency of the flap to pull away, it has been recommended that a bridge of tissue be left between the fistula and the donor site under which the flap can be placed to secure it in position (19) (Fig. 7). This too has proved impractical in our hands because of the thickness of the flap and the tenuous nature of the mucoperiosteal bridge.

In order to overcome many of the problems relating to lack of mobility and thickness of the palatal flaps, the use of an island-pedicled flap base on the greater palatine vessels has been described and evaluated

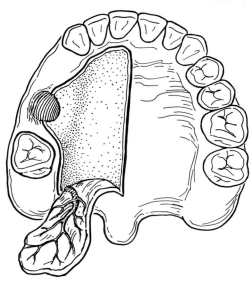

FIG. 5. Design of the palatal flap based on the palatine artery.

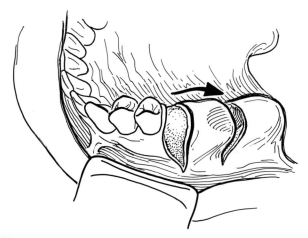

FIG. 3. Transversal flap. This is a bipedicled advancement flap (*arrow*).

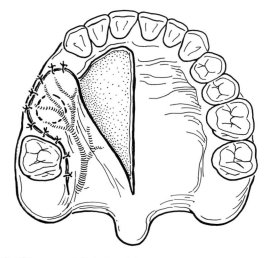

FIG. 6. Closure of fistula with a simple transposition flap.

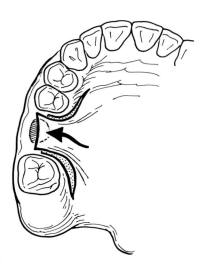

FIG. 4. Simple palatal advancement flap (*arrow*). This is very unsatisfactory as little mobility can be obtained.

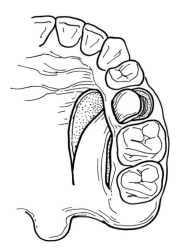

FIG. 7. Palatal flap secured by bringing flap under retained strip of mucoperiosteum.

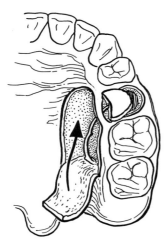

FIG. 8. Island-pedicled palatal flap (*arrow*). Note that the proximal mucosal flap is sutured back over the donor site defect.

(20–22). This technique is performed by developing a posterior-based rotational flap, taking great care not to compromise the greater palatine vessels. These are isolated carefully and the area of mucoperiosteal flap to be used is isolated and sutured into position (Fig. 8). The proximal pedicle mucosal flap is separated from the underlying vessels and placed back over the donor site defect. While technically a little more intricate, this is an excellent technique with significant advantages over the simple rotational flap. Care must be

taken not to stretch the vessels, and therefore it should not be used for anterior defects.

Postoperatively, the patient is placed on antibiotics for 7 days and instructed not to blow the nose and to maintain a soft diet until the wound has healed.

Combination Local Flaps

In the moderate to large defects, it is probably better to try and obtain a double-layer closure by developing a circumferential flap around the fistula and inverting this over the fistula, closing this with absorbable suture and then using either a buccal or palatal flap as a second layer (9) (Fig. 9). The advantage of this is that it gives epithelial coverage on both sides of the reconstruction, which lessens the chances of infection of the flap and diminishes flap contraction. In delineating this circumferential flap, it is important to define the bony defect, which is always larger than the soft tissue defect.

Tongue Flaps

In dealing with even larger defects, there may not be adequate local tissue to obtain satisfactory closure. In this situation, one of a variety of tongue flaps may be used. These flaps are well vascularized and reliable and supply enough tissue to close almost any sized defect. The major disadvantage is the mobility of the

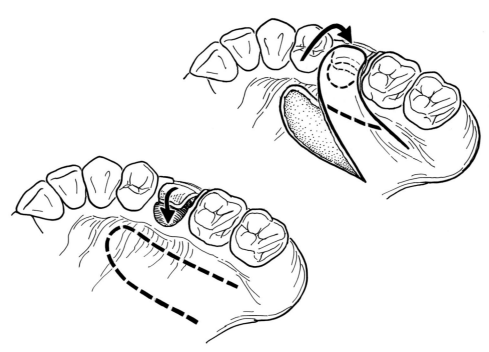

FIG. 9. First-layer closure performed by inverting the flap created from local tissues (*arrows*). The second layer usually is formed by a palatal flap.

tongue, which may require stabilization in some manner to prevent the flap from pulling away. This may take the form of placing the patient in intermaxillary fixation (23) or suturing the tongue to the maxillary premolars (24,25). In general, it is better to use a posterior-based flap because this flap originates from the less mobile posterior third of the tongue. Once the flap has taken, the pedicle is divided under local anesthetic.

Distant Flaps

Various distant flaps have been used for closure of larger defects of the palate, particularly after radical ablative surgery (26,27). These include various pedicled flaps and even free flaps. These may vary from nasolabial flaps to chest flaps and forehead flaps. While these procedures can be accomplished successfully, in general, closure using a prosthesis is far more successful and simple.

GRAFT PROCEDURES

Bone

Rarely, in a large defect where it is felt that solid support is needed to ensure success, a bone graft harvested from the anterior face of the maxillary antrum may be used with a local or tongue flap employed for soft tissue coverage. A technique for pedicling the bone of the anterolateral wall of the maxillary antrum or periosteum and rotating it into the defect has been described (28). Iliac crest may be a useful donor site for a free bone graft.

Synthetic Materials

The use of these materials requires minimal mobilization of regional tissues and has been described as being relatively easily performed with good results. Gold foil (29), gold plate (30), tantalum (31), and polymethylmethacrylate (32) have been used but are no longer in vogue.

Lyophilized collagen (33) has enjoyed recent popularity and has the advantage over other materials in that it becomes incorporated into the tissues and thus does not have to be removed. Lyophilized human fibrin seal has been used with excellent results (34). This simple nonsurgical technique consists of the application of this material to the defect after it is mixed with a solution of thrombin, calcium chloride, and aprotinin. The mixture is injected into the socket just above the floor of the maxillary antrum. It appears particularly useful in sealing acute fistulas after extraction.

In conclusion, while most acute fistulas close spontaneously, closure of chronic fistulas requires careful planning and meticulous technique with attention given to the frequently associated maxillary sinusitis.

REFERENCES

1. Amaratunga NA. Oroantral fistulae—a study of clinical, radiological and treatment aspects. *Br J Oral Maxillofac Surg* 1986; 24:433–437.
2. Killey HC, Kay LW. *The maxillary sinus and its dental implications*. Bristol: John Wright, 1975;40–70.
3. Ehrl PA. Oroantral communication: epicritical study of 175 patients with special concern for secondary operative closure. *Int J Oral Surg* 1980;9:351.
4. Skolnick EM, O'Neil JV, Baim HM. Closure of oroantral fistula. *Laryngoscope* 1979;89:844–845.
5. Campbell Reid DA. Fistula in the hard palate following cleft palate surgery. *Br J Plast Surg* 1962;15:377–381.
6. Yih WY, Merrill R, Howerton D. Secondary closure of oroantral and oronasal fistulas. *J Oral Maxillofac Surg* 1988;46:357–364.
7. Valderhaug J. Reaction of mucous membrane of the maxillary sinus and the nasal cavity to experimental periapical inflammation in monkeys. *Int J Oral Surg* 1973;2:107.
8. Haanaes HR, Pedersen KW. Treatment of oroantral communication. *Int J Oral Surg* 1974;3:124.
9. Quayle AA. A double flap technique for the closure of oronasal and oroantral fistulae. *Br J Oral Surg* 1981;19:132.
10. Rehrmann A. Eine methade zur Schliessung von Kieferhohlen perforationen. *Deutsch Zahnarztl* 1936;39:1136–1139.
11. Killey H, Kay L. An analysis of 250 cases of oroantral fistulas treated by buccal flap operation. *J Oral Surg* 1967;24:726–739.
12. Wowern NV. Treatment of oroantral fistula. *Arch Otolaryngol* 1972;96:99–104.
13. Awang MN. Closure of oroantral fistula. *Int J Oral Maxillofac Surg* 1988;17:110–115.
14. Del Junco R, Rappaport I, Allison G. Persistent oral antral fistulas. *Arch Otolaryngol Head Neck Surg* 1988;114:1315–1316.
15. Moczair L. Nuovo methodo operatiopela chisura derre fistole del sena mascellase di origina dentale. *Stomatologiia (Mosk)* 1930;28:1087–1088.
16. Wowern NV. Closure of oroantral fistula with buccal flap. Rehrmann versus Moczair. *Int J Oral Surg* 1982;11:156–165.
17. Schuchardt K. Methodik des Verschlusses von Defekten im alveolarforsate zahnlose oberkiefer. *Deutsch Zahn Mund Kieferheilk* 1953;17:366–369.
18. Kruger GO. *Textbook of oral and maxillofacial surgery*, 6th ed. St Louis: CV Mosby, 1984;291–293.
19. Choukas NC. Modified palatal flap technique for closure of oroantral fistulas. *J Oral Surg* 1974;32:112–113.
20. Hendersen D. Palatal island flap closure of oroantral fistula. *Br J Laryngol Otol* 1974;75:744–746.
21. Gullane PJ, Arena S. Palatal island flap for reconstruction of oral defects. *Arch Otolaryngol* 1977;103:598–599.
22. James RB. Surgical closure of large oroantral fistula using a palatal island flap. *J Oral Surg* 1980;38:591–595.
23. Steinhauser EW. Experience with the dorsal tongue flap for closure of defects of the hard palate. *J Oral Maxillofac Surg* 1982; 40:787–789.
24. Guerrero-Santos J, Artimirano JT. The use of lingual flaps in repair of fistulas of the hard palate. *Plast Reconstr Surg* 1966; 38:123–128.
25. Kruchinskyi GV. New method of palatal defect repair. *Acta Chir Plast* 1972;14:23–27.
26. Bakamjian V. A new technique for primary reconstruction of the palate after radical maxillectomy for cancer. *Plast Reconstr Surg* 1963;31:103–108.
27. Skolnick EM, Yee K, Keyes G. Flap reconstruction in major surgery of the head and neck. *Laryngoscope* 1976;86:1584–1587.

28. Brusati R. The use of an autogenous osteoperiosteal flap to close oroantral fistulas. *J Oral Maxillofac Surg* 1982;40:250–251.

29. Mainous EG, Hammer DD. Surgical closure of oroantral fistula using gold foil technique. *J Oral Surg* 1974;32:528–530.

30. Steiner M. Oroantral closure with gold plate. *J Oral Surg* 1952;18:513–515.

31. Budge CT. Closure of oroantral opening by the use of tantalum plate. *J Oral Surg* 1952;10:32–33.

32. Al-Sibahi A, Ameen S. The use of soft polymethlymethacrylate in the closure of oroantral fistula. *J Oral Maxillofac Surg* 1982;40:165–166.

33. Mitchell R, Lamb J. Immediate closure of oroantral fistula with collagen implant. A preliminary report. *Br Dent J* 1983;154:171–173.

34. Ztajcic Z, Todorovic LJ, Petrovic V. Tissuecol in closure of oroantral communication. A pilot study. *Int J Oral Surg* 1985;14:444–446.

CHAPTER 37

Congenital Lesions

Dale H. Rice and Paul J. Donald

A congenital disorder is one that has its inception prior to birth. It may be either inherited or acquired and may either be manifest at birth or become apparent later. Acquired disorders may arise through sporadic gene mutations or by direct injury to the fetus. The risk in the general population for congenital defects of the paranasal sinuses is unknown, but major defects appear to be uncommon. The embryology of this region has been covered in a previous chapter. It is well to remember that development of the paranasal sinuses cannot begin until the intranasal structures are well established. In the third to fourth month of fetal development, mucous membranes begin to infiltrate the cartilaginous structures of the lateral nasal wall by a process of primary pneumatization. As growth continues, secondary pneumatization occurs, with infiltration of the bony structures of the lateral nasal wall. The maxillary sinus initially pneumatizes the ectethmoid cartilage at about 10 weeks with secondary pneumatization beginning around the fifth month. The ethmoid sinuses begin with primary pneumatization of the ectethmoid also at about 4 months of gestation. Secondary pneumatization occurs largely after birth. Primary pneumatization seems not to occur in either the frontal or sphenoid sinuses.

CONGENITAL DISORDERS

Absence of the paranasal sinuses is extremely rare, with only one reported case (1). There has also been one reported case of unilaterally absent paranasal sinuses (2). There has been a single family reported with the constellation of microcornea, glaucoma, and absence of the frontal sinuses. The type of transmission is unknown since there was no male-to-male transmission. The frontal sinuses are, however, quite variable in size and agenesis in isolation is not unusual. A small or absent frontal sinus may be seen in patients with otherwise normal sinuses. Unilateral maxillary sinus aplasia or hypoplasia is unusual, but not rare, and is usually seen in otherwise normal patients (Fig. 1).

Hereditary hyperostosis frontalis has been reported (3). It is an unusual disorder characterized by marked thickening of the posterior wall of the frontal sinus. It has been claimed by some to occur in 12% of females (4). The patient is usually asymptomatic and it most often presents as an incidental, if not startling, finding on a radiograph. It occurs with a female predominance of 9:1, suggesting sex-linked or cross-linked transmission, while some will show other modes of transmission. It is noted most commonly in middle-aged females but has been reported in adolescents. A variety of endocrine, neuropsychiatric, and gonadal disturbances have been related to this disorder. It is important to differentiate this entity from the generalized hyperostosis of the frontal bone seen in such congenital conditions as Crouzon's disease, craniometaphyseal dysplasia, and Steinert's myotonic dystrophy. It is not uncommon in these latter syndromes to have no frontal sinus at all.

Monostotic fibrous dysplasia (Jaffe–Lichtenstein syndrome) has been reported in a number of bones, but the most common are in the craniofacial region. The maxilla and mandible are most frequently involved (Figs. 2 and 3). This diagnosis can only be absolutely established with a biopsy and the lesion is treated only to maintain an acceptable cosmetic appearance. Monostotic fibrous dysplasia may not be strictly congenital but appears early in life and is probably hamartomatous (5). There are three types by activity. The most active form has a richly cellular connective tissue matrix with frequent mitoses. The bone itself is abnormal, occurring in a myriad of sizes and shapes, and predominates in the preadolescent. The quiescent form is seen in the adolescent or near-adolescent. The connective tissue matrix is more mature, with few mitoses and a

607

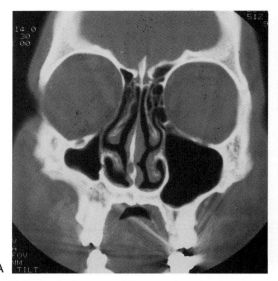
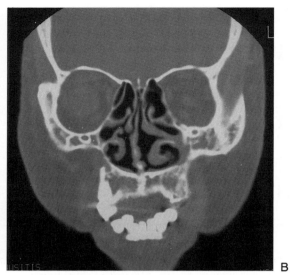

FIG. 1. **A:** Coronal CT scan showing hypoplasia of the right maxillary sinus. **B:** Coronal CT scan showing bilateral aplasia of the maxillary sinuses.

more conspicuous bony component. The third or inactive stage is least common. There is degeneration of the connective tissue matrix and bone islands may be absent. Fibrous dysplasia may be distinguished from the other fibro-osseous lesions by the absence of lamellar bone formation. The computed tomography (CT) scan appearance is diagnostic. Treatment is indicated only to maintain a satisfactory cosmetic appearance or a functionally acceptable child. (A more complete discussion of this entity is found in the chapter by Donald, Fibro-osseous Diseases.)

NASAL DERMOIDS

The nasal dermoid sinus or cyst is lined by epithelium, which includes adnexal structures (hair, hair follicles, eccrine glands, sebaceous glands). They account for approximately 10% of all the dermoid cysts in the head and neck (6). Dermoids can occur anywhere in the periorbital or nasal area (Fig. 4). In a retrospective series of 84 such lesions (7), 54 (64%) occurred in the frontotemporal region, usually around the brow, 21 (25%) were in the orbital region, and 9 (11%) were in the nasal area. This lesion must be distinguished from the epidermoid cyst. The dermoid cyst is of mixed ec-

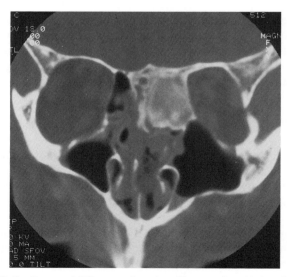

FIG. 2. Axial CT scan showing dense fibrous dysplasia of the right maxilla.

FIG. 3. Coronal CT scan showing fibrous dysplasia of the left ethmoid.

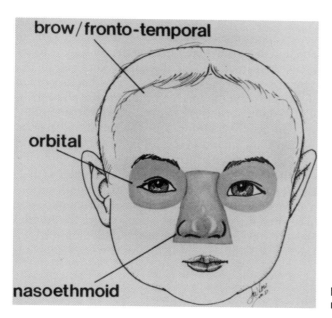

FIG. 4. Areas of potential involvement with periorbital and nasal dermoids. (From ref. 7, with permission.)

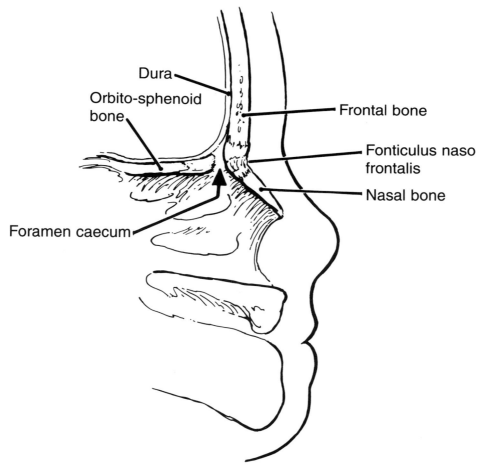

FIG. 5. The fonticulus nasofrontalis, the site of emergence of glabellar–nasal dermoids, is between the cartilaginous precursor of the frontal and nasal bones.

todermal and mesodermal elements in contrast to the epidermoid cyst, which is derived from only ectoderm. The latter is lined by a simple squamous epithelium without skin appendages.

The embryonic origin of nasal dermoids begins in the second and third months of fetal development. At this stage, the nasal and frontal bones begin their ossification process. The membranous viscerocranium of the nasal bone inferiorly is connected to the membranous neurocranium of the frontal bone above by a firm membrane called the fonticulus nasofrontalis (Fig. 5). The horizontally disposed cartilaginous neurocranium behind this region possesses a gap called the foramen caecum (6). During embryologic development, a prolongation of dura extends through the foramen caecum,

traverses the prenasal space below the neurocranium and behind the nasal bone, through the fonticulus nasofrontalis, and tracks under the nasal skin (Fig. 6). As the embryo matures, the dura retracts back through the fonticulus and the foramen caecum and all remaining dural elements and the sinus tract resorb and obliterate. The fonticulus closes as the nasal and frontal bones close together and the foramen caecum shrinks down to a small aperture through which eventually passes the dorsal nasal vein. The latter develops superiorly as the superior sagittal sinus. If the dura retraction draws in epidermal and dermal elements along with it, then a nasal dermoid persists with a potential connection through the nose to the dura (Fig. 6B).

The nasal dermoid generally presents as a subcuta-

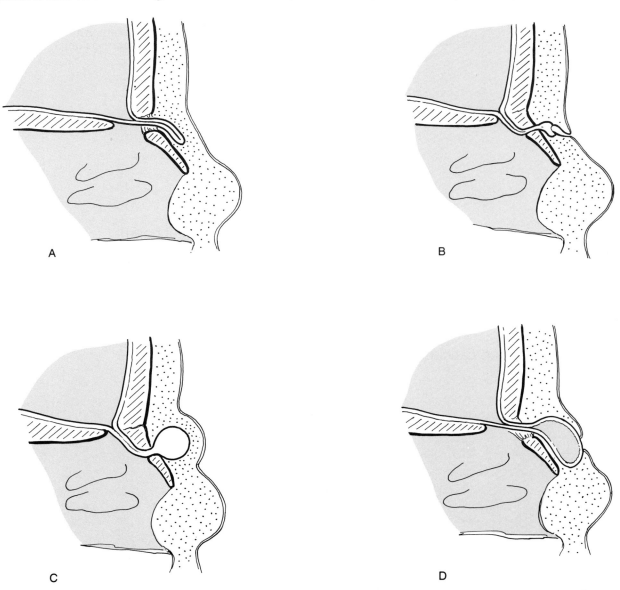

FIG. 6. Connection of nasal dermoid from the skin to the dura through the foramen caecum of the cartilaginous neurocranium. **A:** Emergence of the dural elements through the fonticulus nasofrontalis. **B:** Connection to the skin. **C:** Nasal glioma. **D:** Nasal meningocele.

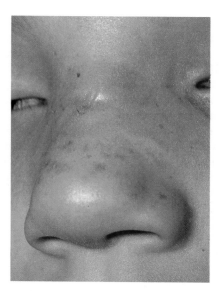

FIG. 7. Dermoid cyst located on nasal dorsum with hairs protruding.

neous mass or as a sinus tract, with or without an external opening. Nasal dermoids can occur anywhere from the anterior cranial fossa to the base of the columella, and if large may cause a widened nasal dorsum. In most series, the cysts commonly occur in the medial canthal region or in the supratip area. Typically, an external opening will be in the supratip region, with one or two hairs protruding (Fig. 7). These lesions may extend in to the cartilaginous and bony areas of the paranasal region, usually passing through a suture line, and may also extend intracranially. The cystic component may be expandable. In Bartlett's series (7), four of nine lesions had intracranial extension. Those presenting in the glabella were simple and did not extend beyond the nasal–frontal suture line. Those farther down the nose often had a punctum and were more complex in their

extension. Most of the stalks that went intranasally were purely fibrous tissue and did not contain dural or neural elements. Prior to excision, the lesion must be accurately evaluated by direct coronal CT to determine if there is an intracranial connection. Occasionally, un-ossified areas in the floor of the anterior cranial fossa (cribriform plate, fovea ethmoidalis) may make the CT scan difficult to interpret. If the CT scan is indeterminate, magnetic resonance imaging (MRI) with the added advantage of a sagittal projection, will usually delineate both components if they exist.

If an intracranial connection is present, a combined neurosurgical and transfacial approach is indicated. The neurosurgical component should be performed first. This usually involves a bifrontal craniotomy and extradural exploration of the floor of the anterior cranial fossa. If the dura is involved, it may be excised and repaired at this time. The head and neck surgeon completes the excision. Lesions confined to the nasal cavity may be managed without neurosurgical intervention. For those in the lower two-thirds of the nose, a single midline vertical incision including the fistula, or exposing the cyst, is probably the approach of choice. For cysts over the nasion, a horizontal incision probably gives the best cosmetic result (Fig. 8). For cysts off the midline or with considerable overlying skin involvement, the creative use of local flaps must be employed for the best possible results, bearing in mind the lines of minimum tension.

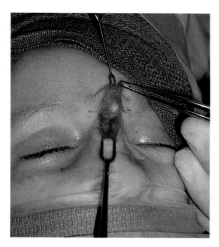

FIG. 8. Horizontal incision in glabellar region with exposure of dermoid cyst and connection to the nasal–frontal suture line.

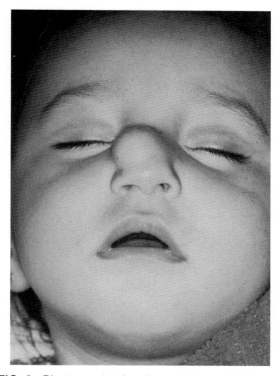

FIG. 9. Photograph of patient with nasal glioma.

NASAL GLIOMAS

The nasal glioma is a rare nasal tumor (8) of which 60% to 65% are located extranasally while the remainder are intranasal. They, as well as encephaloceles, have the same embryological origin as dermoids. Gliomas generally lack an intracranial connection although 15% to 20% have a fibrous connection to the dura. Histologically, they are comprised of heterotopic neural tissue that is predominantly glial and are not true neoplasms. When they connect intracranially, they do so through a stalk of fibrous tissue with some interspersed glial elements. Because of the patent foramen caecum, manipulation of the mass may cause rupture of the dural connection and a subsequent cerebrospinal fluid (CSF) leak. Extranasal gliomas are generally located at the side of the bridge of the nose, are firm, lobular, and noncompressible (Fig. 9). They will not pulsate or transilluminate. Often the nasal dorsum is broadened and the eyes are more widely separated than normal. The male to female ratio is approximately 3:2. The intranasal glioma is usually situated high in the nasal fossa, may be mistaken for a polyp, and may cause nasal obstruction. A glioma may be difficult to

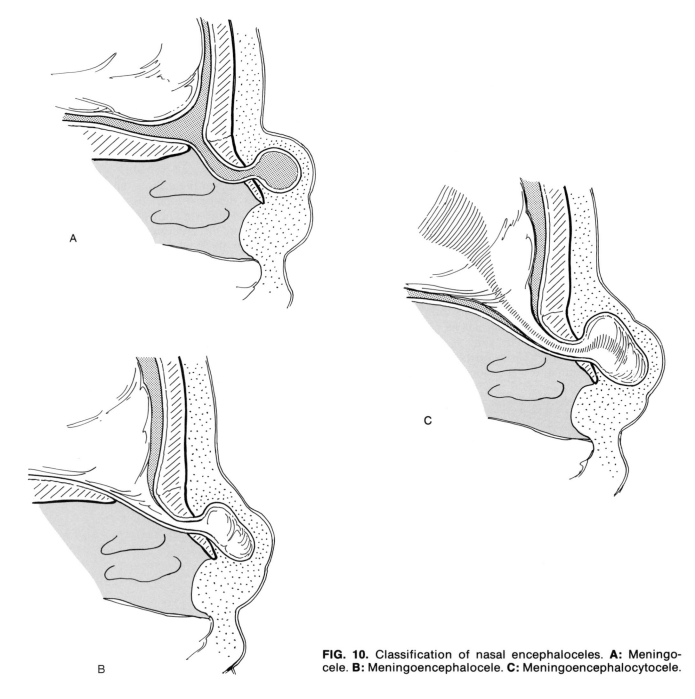

FIG. 10. Classification of nasal encephaloceles. **A:** Meningocele. **B:** Meningoencephalocele. **C:** Meningoencephalocytocele.

differentiate from an encephalocele. There may be an associated bony defect in the anterior cranial fossa floor. Gliomas are best treated by excision. Early excision of the extranasal type may serve to prevent subsequent deformity of the nasal bones. Recurrence is rare. The intranasal variety should be biopsied to confirm the diagnosis. But first, a CT examination should be performed to detect any bony defect in the base of the anterior cranial fossa. In addition, direct intracranial communication must be excluded before excision is attempted. If an intracranial communication exists, a combined approach should be performed. Intranasal lesions may be removed directly intranasally, if possible through a lateral rhinotomy, or approached through a facial degloving incision.

NASAL ENCEPHALOCODES

The nasal encephalocele has an origin similar to the nasal dermoid (Fig. 10). These are rare lesions, occurring once in 20,000 to 40,000 live births (9). Hughes et al. (10) have classified encephaloceles (although they are usually lumped together) as (a) meningoceles—containing only meninges, (b) meningoencephaloceles—containing brain and meninges, and (c) meningoencephalocytoceles—containing a part of the ventricular system, brain, and meninges. All encephaloceles contain CSF. They are commonest in the lumbosacral region with a frequency five times greater than the cranial type. The anterior variety of cranial encephaloceles make up only 25% of the total.

Anterior or sincipital encephaloceles are commonest in Russia and Southeast Asia (9). The lesion is associated in 30% to 40% of cases with other congenital craniofacial anomalies (11) such as Crouzon's disease, Apert's syndrome, and various types of facial clefts (Fig. 11). Hypertelorism is extremely common.

Encephaloceles of the anterior cranial fossa are of two types according to their point of exit from the cra-

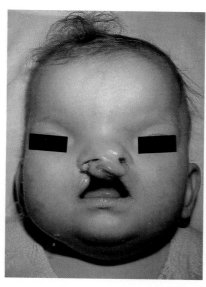

FIG. 11. Congenital ethmoidal meningoencephalocele with marked hyertelorism and associated cleft lip and palate.

nial floor (11). The most anterior group exit the foramen caecum and are called frontoethmoidal and those that exit at a point from the anterior cribriform plate to the posterior clinoids and from the superior orbital fissure are called basal encephaloceles. The anterior frontoethmoidal type are further classified into nasofrontal, nasoethmoidal, and naso-orbital. Tables 1 and 2 summarize the point of exit in the sutural elements of the facial skeleton, external site of appearance, and percentage of frequency (10) of both frontoethmoidal and basal encephaloceles. The former present primarily extranasally and the latter intranasally. The sincipital encephaloceles rarely present intranasally when they are confined to the embryonic prenasal space.

Encephaloceles then, like gliomas, may present externally, intranasally, or as a combination of both. In fact, encephaloceles may be difficult to distinguish

TABLE 1. *Frontoethmoidal encephaloceles*

Type	Point of bony sutural exit	External site of presentation	Frequency
Nasofrontal	Nasal and frontal	Nasion	39%
Nasoethmoidal	Nasal and upper lateral cartilages	Low nasal dorsum	41%
Nasal orbital	Frontal and lacrimal	Medial orbit	20%

TABLE 2. *Basal encephaloceles*

Type	Point of bony sutural exit	Site of presentation	Frequency
Transethmoidal	Cribriform plate	Intranasal	70%
Sphenoethmoidal	Sphenoid and ethmoid	Intranasal and nasopharynx	20%
Transsphenoidal	Craniopharyngeal canal	Nasopharynx and sphenoid	5%
Spheno-orbital	Superior orbital fissure	Infratemporal fossa	5%

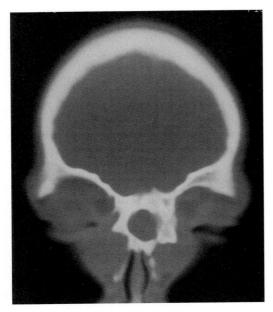

FIG. 12. Meningoencephalocele expanding nasal bones on CT scan.

from gliomas. Both are congenital and occur in similar locations (Fig. 12). Unlike the glioma, however, the encephalocele contains an ependyma-lined space and is filled with CSF that communicates directly with the ventricles of the brain (Fig. 13). On CT scan, an encephalocele will always demonstrate a defect through the floor of the anterior cranial fossa in the region of the anterior neuropore (Fig. 14). Furthermore, the mass will often, but not always, increase in size and tension with straining or crying.

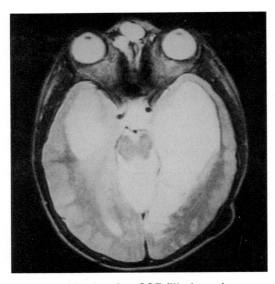

FIG. 13. Axial MRI showing CSF-filled meningoencephalocele.

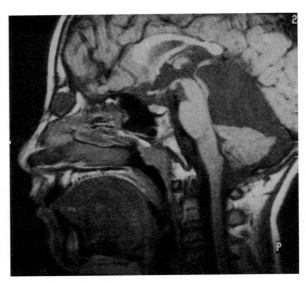

FIG. 14. Sagittal MRI showing herniation of meningoencephalocele through floor of anterior cranial fossa.

Frontoethmoid encephaloceles typically appear in the region of the glabella, are soft and compressible, bluish in color, and transilluminate. Basal encephaloceles appear similarly, but intranasally, and may be mistaken for a nasal polyp. They are soft and compressible and usually present by age 5. Either type should be investigated with a CT scan and MRI to adequately plan the excision. All encephaloceles require a combined intracranial and transfacial approach. The treatment of choice involves complete excision with closure of the dural defect. The excision may be staged if necessary with the intracranial part always done first.

LACRIMAL DUCT OBSTRUCTION

Congenital nasolacrimal duct system obstruction may occur at any place along the length of the system, from the canaliculi to the intranasal opening. Depending on the site of obstruction, these infants may present with dacryocystitis, epiphora, or an intranasal mass, causing nasal obstruction and respiratory distress. A variety of terms have been used to describe a cystic lesion if it occurs, but the preferred current terminology is congenital nasolacrimal duct drainage system (NLDS) cyst. The treatment of epiphora or dacryocystitis is conservative, with massage and antibiotics if indicated. If the infant presents with life-threatening nasal obstruction from an intranasal mass, the initial therapy should include marsupialization of the cyst to relieve the obstruction and to allow the resumption of obligate nasal breathing. This will generally suffice as the definitive treatment as well. Healing is uneventful, but nasal irrigation and cleaning may be required for a time.

TERATOMA

Approximately 50% of all teratomas that occur in the head and neck involve the nose, paranasal sinuses, and nasopharynx (12). For the nasal types, there is a 6:1 female predominance. True teratomas contain all three germ layers, unlike the nasal dermoid, which contains only ectodermal and mesodermal components. Unlike the situation in other parts of the body, teratomas in the nasopharynx never become malignant. However, in the nose and paranasal sinuses, a tumor comprised in part of teratomatous elements, called a teratocarcinosarcoma, can be seen. This is extremely rare, seen in adults, highly aggressive, and has a poor prognosis (13). Teratomas in the nose are described by Barnes as "vanishingly rare" (14). Head and neck teratomas are extremely rare. In a series of 578 cases involving the head and neck and central nervous system by Gonzales-Crussi (15), only 1.7% occurred in the head. They differ from harmartomas in that the three germ layers represented differentiate into tissue not indigenous to the area. The usual presentation is that of airway obstruction, rhinorrhea, or cough with a nasal or nasopharyngeal mass. Nasopharyngeal teratomas may erode intracranially, or intracranial tumors may erode into the nasopharynx. There may be significant associated deformities. Excision is the treatment of choice. These can be approached through a transpalatal or facial degloving approach in most instances.

Congenital absence of the nose is rare, with only 13 cases in the English literature (16). Usually agenesis of the nose is associated with monstrosity and death. The embryologic nasal placode fails to develop. There is a concave soft tissue obturation anteriorly and choanal atresia posteriorly. There are no paranasal sinuses and a high arched palate. Lack of development of the olfactory area leads to absence of the rhinencephalon. Because of the close relationship of orbital and nasal development, there are often abnormalities of the eyes.

CT scan and MRI in one case reported showed complete absence of the anterior soft tissues of the nose with thin anterior and thick posterior atretic plates. A soft tissue mass filled the single hypoplastic nasal cavity, which did not communicate with the brain. There was no evidence of paranasal sinus development. In a recent report, a child with congenital absence of the nose survived, bearing many of the above listed anomalies (Fig. 15).

PROBOSCIS LATERALIS

Proboscis lateralis was first described in 1884. It is quite rare with approximately 42 reported cases (24). The usual appearance is a soft, movable appendage several centimeters long arising near the medial canthus. The ipsilateral anterior nares are usually atretic while the sinuses are normal. The proboscis drains

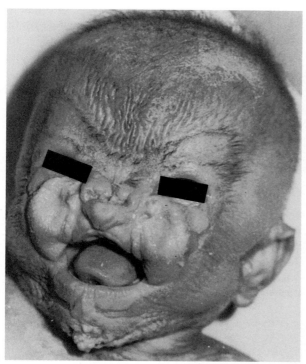
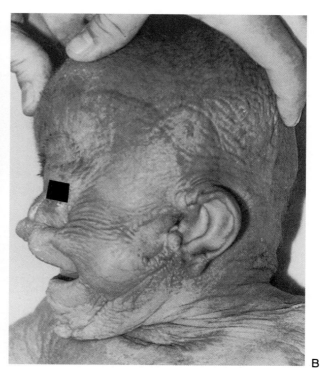

FIG. 15. A: Congenital absence of nose in Beare–Stevenson syndrome. (From ref. 17, with permission.) **B:** A severe case of Beare-Stevenson syndrome and associated congenital deformities.

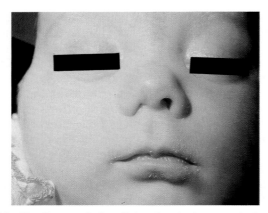

FIG. 16. Congenital unilateral anterior nasal atresia.

tears and can be shown to be connected to the lacrimal sac. Kirkpatrick (25) proposed an operative correction to join the proboscis to a newly formed nasal cavity on the same side.

Cleft nose is also a rare congenital deformity that usually occurs as an isolated event but may be hereditary (26). The cause is unknown and the cleft may occur in several sites. In general, repair should be delayed until about age 4 if possible (27).

NASAL ATRESIA

Congenital anterior nasal atresia occurs with failure of absorption of epithelial plugs, which normally close the anterior nares from the second through the sixth month of fetal life. The atresia is usually unilateral (Fig. 16) and may be either bony or membranous. If bilat-eral, the newborn may have respiratory distress. CT scanning may reveal underdevelopment or occasional absence of the anterior ethmoid and maxillary sinuses. The treatment is to reconstruct the anterior nares in such a way as to achieve an epithelial lined vestibule with cosmetically acceptable nostrils.

CHOANEAL ATRESIA

Congenital posterior choanal atresia may also be unilateral or bilateral. The most common theory to explain this deformity is persistence of the buccopharyngeal membrane. If bilateral, it will present as airway obstruction immediately after birth, as newborns lack mouth breathing reflexes and are obligate nasal breathers. This is aggravated by the fact that in newborns the epiglottis is close to the soft palate and the tongue is close to both the hard and soft palates. These features make oral respiration difficult at best. The obstructing barrier may be membranous or bony with bony obstruction occurring in 90% of cases. The bony obstruction is generally not a flat plate, per se, but a lateral encroachment and thickening of the posterior lateral nasal walls into the choana (Fig. 17). The membrane varies in thickness from 1 to 10 mm and generally lies anterior to the posterior border of the hard palate. It is said to occur in one in every 5000 live births and is twice as common in females as in males. When unilateral, it is usually right-sided. Twenty-five percent of these patients have a single minor or a single major associated anomaly, while 50% have multiple associated abnormalities. Diagnosis can be made by the inability to pass a rubber catheter through the infant's

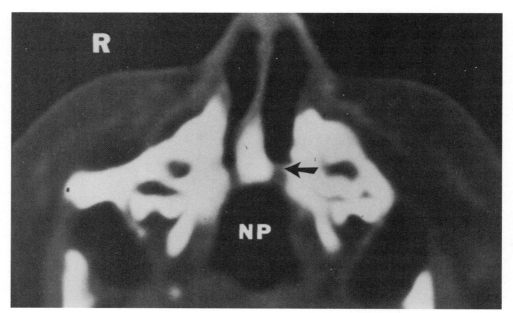

FIG. 17. Axial CAT scan of bilateral choanal atresia showing bony atresia plate (arrow). (From ref. 18, with permission.)

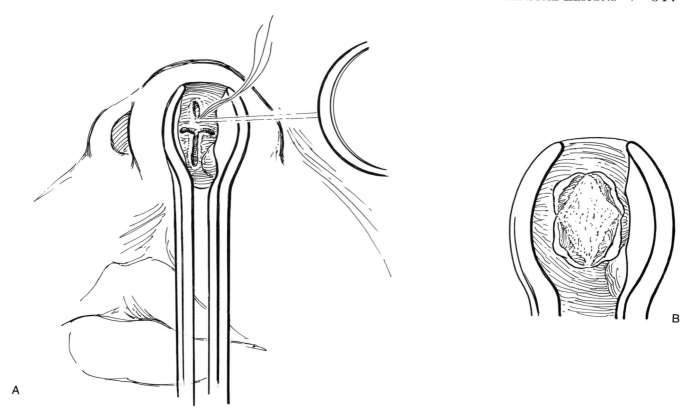

FIG. 18. Laser used to create a cruciate incision on the nasal side of the atresia. **A:** Transnasal view. **B:** Flaps cut.

nose to a distance of more than 3 cm. It can also be confirmed by radiographic studies, injecting contrast material into the infant's nose. Unilateral atresia should be suspected in an infant with persistent unilateral nasal rhinorrhea. Treatment depends on the type of obstruction and the patient. In unilateral obstruction, where the infant is doing well, treatment is best postponed. In bilateral atresia, treatment may be life-saving and should be performed early. With modern instrumentation, it should be possible to operate safely on either unilateral or bilateral atresia through a transnasal or transpalatal approach.

Congenital atresia must often be treated early in order so save the newborn's life. Because infants are obligate nose breathers, the insertion of an oral airway is essential to allow the infant to sleep and feed. Definitive early intervention usually involves some break through the atresia plate and the placement of a stent. With thin bony or membranous atresia plates, penetration can be achieved transnasally with the laser. This allows the construction of offset flaps from the nasal and nasopharyngeal sides that may be interdigitated across the excised atresia plate area. The procedure is difficult to perform because of the extremely confined space of the infant nasal cavity.

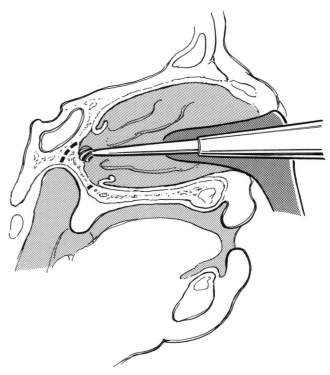

FIG. 19. Pituitary drill used to excise bony atresia plate.

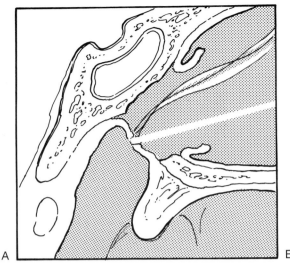

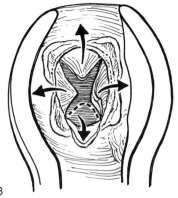

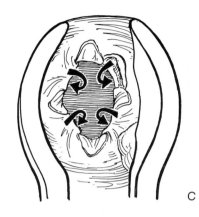

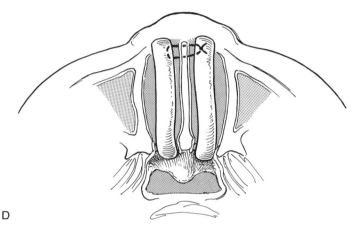

FIG. 20. Cruciate incisions are made with the CO_2 laser in the nasopharyngeal side with the axis at 90 degrees to the flaps of the nasal side. **A:** Side view with laser cutting flaps. **B:** Intranasal view with flaps cut. **C:** Flaps transposed. **D:** Stents placed.

SURGICAL TREATMENT CHOANEAL ATRESIA

Under general anesthesia, the nose is cocainized for maximal mucosal shrinkage. A nasopharyngeal pack of wet gauze is placed to avoid accidental laser injury to the nasopharynx. A self-retaining nasal speculum is placed through the nares and the turbinates are gently but firmly compressed against the lateral nasal wall until the point where the nasal cavity funnels into the area of atresia. The technique similar to that described by Healy et al. (19) and Davis (20) is used. A cruciate incision is made in the nasal mucosa with the CO_2 laser under microscopic control (Fig. 18). The bony atresia plate, if very thin, can be removed with the laser. The low water content of bone leads to considerable heat generation by the laser, hence its limited applicability in osseous excision. A pituitary drill can be used to drill away the plate (Fig. 19). The mucosal flaps are tucked under the retractor blades for retraction to avoid catching them in the drill bit. Once the bone has been removed, the mucoperiosteum facing the nasopharynx is seen.

Cruciate incisions are made in an axis corresponding to the midportion of the flaps on the nasal side (Fig. 20). An attempt is made to interpose these flaps across the atresia site, then fix them in place by a nasal stent of soft Silastic. Unfortunately, some flap destruction occurs with the laser vaporization during flap creation despite the microspot size and low wattage of 4 to 6 watts used (20). The pulsed rather than continuous mode also helps to diminish laser damage. Despite these precautions and the diminutive size of this area in infants, laser damage and often flap injury accidentally engendered by the drill result in small and often damaged flaps. However, any transposition of mucosa across the new areas will be beneficial to healing and a deterrent to cicatrization. Rolled Silastic or a preformed tube helps to maintain patency. The tube is removed at 3 to 6 weeks.

The transnasal approach is often a temporizing measure. Restenosis is not uncommon. Richardson and Osguthorp (21) report a restenosis rate of 36% and Healy et al. (19) 33%. Laser vaporization can be reinstituted for fibrous restenosis but definitive repair by a trans-

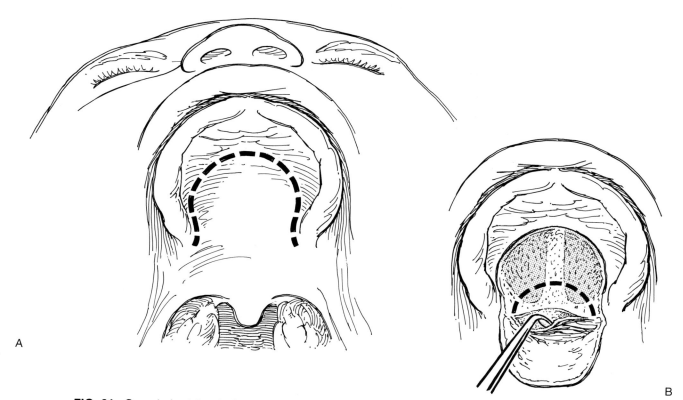

A

B

FIG. 21. Owen's incision in hard palate. **A:** Flap outlined. **B:** Flap retracted and palatal muscles dissected from insertion on posterior surface of palatine bone. Note projected area of bone excision outlined.

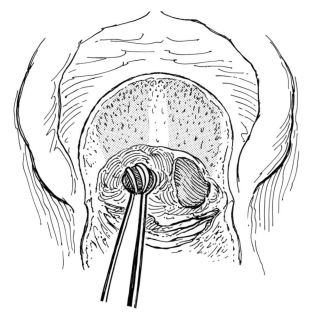

FIG. 22. Hard palate bone is drilled, exposing area of atresia.

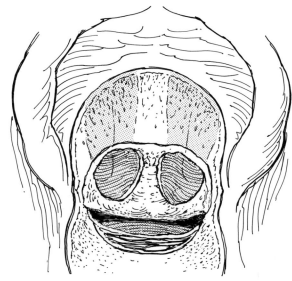

FIG. 23. Area of atresia removed with bur, exposing mucoperiosteum of septum and atresia site.

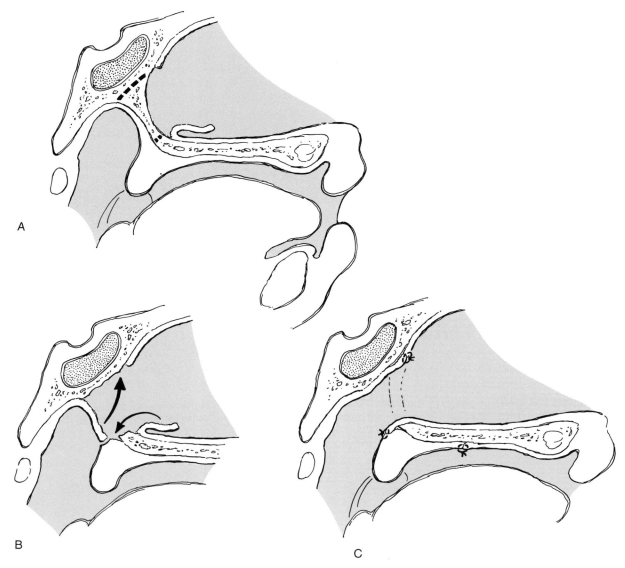

FIG. 24. Paired mucoperiosteal flaps are constructed on the nasal and nasopharyngeal sides. **A:** Flaps on nasal side are retracted and bony resection is outlined. **B:** Lateral view showing the direction in which both sets of flaps will be transposed across the defect. **C:** Flaps in place.

palatal route is delayed until near the end of the first year of life.

The most successful form of surgical treatment is the transpalatal resection. Oral endotracheal intubation is performed and the head dropped into the Rose position. A mouth gag such as the Dingman is placed intra-orally and the palate exposed. The technique used is similar to that described by Montgomery (22).

After local infiltration of the hard palate with 0.50% xylocaine and 1/100,000 epinephrine, an Owen's incision is made (Fig. 21). The palatal mucoperiosteum is dissected posteriorly to the insertion of the soft palate onto the posterior edge of the palatine bone. If additional freedom is needed, one or both of the greater palatine vessels are ligated.

The bone is drilled away down to the mucoperiosteum of the nasal side. During the dissection and drilling, the atresia plate becomes obvious (Fig. 22). It is seen as a widening of the vomer and an encroachment on the expanded vomer by the root of the medial pterygoid plates. The bone of the vomer is drilled away until normal septal architecture is encountered. Lateral bone is drilled away until a choana of optimal size is constructed on each side. During this procedure, the integrity of the mucoperiosteum is carefully protected. The bone should be drilled with a diamond bur, which is much kinder to the mucoperiosteum.

Once the area of atresia and septum have been sufficiently drilled away (Fig. 23), the nasal mucoperiosteum is incised to produce paired flaps based on the nasal floor (Fig. 24). The posterior mucoperiosteal flaps pedicled on the nasopharyngeal roof are then cut and placed across the raw edge of the atresia plate resection site superiorly. These latter flaps will then be laid in a posterior to anterior direction. The flaps on the nasal pedicle will be laid inferiorly in an anterior to posterior direction. Any soft sutures that can be used to tack the flaps *in situ* are placed. The soft Silastic stenting tubes are placed in the defects helping to hold the flaps in place. The tubes are sutured together behind the septum posteriorly and then through the cartilaginous septum anteriorly.

The Owen's incision is sutured shut with absorbable sutures. The stents are removed in about 3 months or more. Patency rates are very high.

Congenital nasal stenosis, as contrasted to choanal atresia, is quite rare and seems to have been only recently recognized. A recent report documented 16 cases (23). All patients had bony nasal obstruction not due to the choanal atresia, but secondary to a bony stenosis in the inferior nasal meatus. Approximately half of these patients will have associated anomalies, usually of the midface. The majority will outgrow the problem in 2 to 3 months with conservative treatment.

CONCLUSION

Congenital lesions affecting only the sinuses are either rare or rarely recognized. More common congenital lesions involve the nasal cavity. For intranasal masses, care should be taken to exclude an intracranial component.

REFERENCES

1. Gebhart RN, Acquarelli MJ. Absence of the paranasal sinuses. In: Bergsma D, ed. *Birth defects atlas and compendium*, 2nd ed. Baltimore: Williams & Wilkins, 1979;854–855.
2. Goh AS, Acquarelli MJ. Unilateral absent paranasal sinuses with hypertrophic middle turbinate. *West J Med* 1966;7:239.
3. Rimoin DL. Hyperostosis frontalis interna. In: Bergsma D, ed. *Birth defects atlas and compendium*, 2nd ed. Baltimore: Williams & Wilkins, 1979;550.
4. English GM. Congenital anomalies of the nose, nasopharynx and paranasal sinuses. In: English GA, ed. *Otolaryngology*, vol. 2. Philadelphia: Lippincott, 1992;11–37.
5. Batsakis JG. *Tumors of the head and neck*. Baltimore: Williams & Wilkins, 1979.
6. Hengerer AS, Newburg JA. Congenital malformations of the nose and paranasal sinuses. In: Bluestone DB, Stool SE, Scheetz MD, eds. *Pediatric otolaryngology*, 2nd ed. Philadelphia: Saunders, 1990;719–722.
7. Bartlett SP, Lin KY, Grossman R, Katowi BJ. The surgical management of orbitofacial dermoids in the pediatric patient. *Plast Reconstr Surg* 1993;91:1208–1215.
8. Gorenstein A, Kern EB, Facer GW, Lawo ER Jr. Nasal gliomas. *Arch Otolaryngol* 1980;106:536.
9. Shugar JMA. Embryology of the nose and paranasal sinuses and resultant deformities. In: Goldman JL, ed. *The principles and practice of rhinology*. New York: Wiley, 1987;113–131.
10. Hughes A, Sharpino A, Hunt W, et al. Management of the congenital midline nasal mass: a review. *Head Neck Surg* 1980;2:222.
11. Charoonsmith T, Suwanwela C. Frontoethmoidal encephalomeningocele with special reference to plastic reconstruction. *Clin Plast Surg* 1974;1(1):27.
12. Batsakis JG, Farber ER. Teratomas of the head and neck. *EENT Digest* 1968;30:67.
13. Batsakis JG. Pathology of lesions of the nose and paranasal sinuses: clinical and pathological considerations. In: Goldman JL, ed. *The principles and practice of rhinology*. New York: Wiley, 1987;27–28.
14. Gnepp DR. Teratoid neoplasms of the head and neck. In: Barnes L, ed. *Surgical pathology of the head and neck*. New York: Marcel Dekker, 1985;1416–1433.
15. Gonzales-Crussi F. Extragonadal teratomas. *Atlas of tumor pathology*, Ser II, Fasc 18, Washington, DC: AFIP, 1982.
16. Cole RR, Myer CM III, Bratcher SO. Congenital absence of the nose: a case report. *Int J Pediatr Otorhinolaryngol* 1989;17:171–177.
17. Andrews JM, Martins DMFS, Ramos RR, Ferrieira LM. A severe case of Beare–Stevenson syndrome and associated congenital deformities. *Br J Plast Surg* 1993;46:443–446.
18. Osguthorpe JD, Richardson MA. Surgical management of choanal atresia. In: Johnson JT, Blitzer A, Ossoff R, Thomas JR, eds. *Instructional courses*, vol 1. Rochester, MN: American Academy of Otolaryngology–Head & Neck Surgery, 1988;39.
19. Healy GB, McGill T, Strong MS, Jako GJ, Vaughan CW. Management of choanal atresia with the carbon dioxide laser. *Ann Otol Rhinol Laryngol* 1978;87:658.
20. Davis KR. *Lasers in otolaryngology–head and neck surgery*. Philadelphia: Saunders, 1990;147–148.
21. Richardson MA, Osguthorpe JD. Surgical management of choanal atresia. *Laryngoscope* 1988;98:915.
22. Montgomery WW. *Surgery of the upper respiratory tract*, vol I, 2nd ed. Philadelphia: Lea & Febiger, 1982;460–465.
23. Knept-Junk KJ, Bos CE, Berkowits RWP. Congenital nasal stenosis in neonates. *J Laryngol Otol* 1988;102:500–502.
24. Mugaddu EG. Proboscis lateralis—a rare congenital anomaly. *S Afr Med J* 1985;68:45.
25. Kirkpatrick TJ. Lateral nasal proboscis. *J Laryngol Otol* 1970;84:83–89.
26. Khoo BC. The bifid nose with a report of three cases in siblings. *Plast Reconstr Surg* 1965;36:626.
27. Mullin WR, Millard DR Jr. Management of congenital bilateral cleft nose. *Plast Reconstr Surg* 1985;75:253–257.

CHAPTER 38

Epistaxis

Jack L. Gluckman and Egbert J. de Vries

Epistaxis is an extremely common occurrence that rarely requires medical intervention. As most nose bleeds are self-limiting, the true incidence is unknown; however, most adults have experienced at least one nose bleed during their life and over half of children have had at least one episode by the age of 10 (1). Only a miniscule percentage, however, experience significant epistaxis requiring the care of an otolaryngologist. On the other hand, from the otolaryngologist's perspective, epistaxis can vary from a routine problem requiring a simple solution, to an extremely frustrating, difficult to manage, potentially life-threatening condition that taxes his/her ingenuity and clinical expertise to the maximum.

Epistaxis can be classified by etiology, anatomic location, or severity. The vast majority, however, are the result of relatively minor trauma due to violent sneezing, nose blowing, or following intranasal digital manipulation and arise from the anterior septum. Epistaxis that warrants medical attention may be because the bleeding persists and proves refractory to pressure or routine remedies or because the episodes are recurrent.

ANATOMY

The branches of the internal and external carotid arteries supply the mucosa of the nose. The rich anastomoses between these two systems and between the right and left sides result in the bleeding occasionally being extremely difficult to control.

The *internal carotid artery* supplies the upper nasal vault via the anterior and posterior ethmoid arteries, which are major branches of the ophthalmic artery. The ophthalmic artery enters the orbit with the optic nerve through the optic foramen. Of its ten branches, two, the posterior and anterior ethmoid arteries, leave the orbit through foramina along the frontoethmoid su-

ture line (Fig. 1). Occasionally, these foramina may lie just above the suture line (2). The foramen of the anterior ethmoid artery is approximately 1.5 cm from the posterior lacrimal crest with the foramen of the posterior ethmoid artery lying a further 1 cm posterior to this (2). The posterior ethmoid foramen is extremely close to the optic foramen (4 to 7 mm) and any surgical manipulation of this vessel should be performed with great caution. An even greater reason to be concerned is that the posterior ethmoid artery itself exits from the periorbita only 1 to 2 mm from the optic nerve. The *posterior ethmoid artery* traverses the ethmoid sinus in the posterior ethmoid canal, enters the anterior cranial fossa giving off a meningeal branch, and then descends between the cribriform plate and the fovea ethmoidalis to enter the nose where it divides into medial and lateral branches supplying the roof of the nose down to the superior turbinate and corresponding portion of the septum. The *anterior ethmoid artery* likewise passes through the ethmoid sinus via the anterior ethmoid canal, intracranially sends off a dural branch and then enters the nose between the cribriform plate and ethmoid cells and supplies the anterior superior portion of the septum and lateral wall via a medial and lateral branch. The terminal branches of the anterior ethmoid artery anastomose with branches of the sphenopalatine artery at the anterior aspect of the septum (Kiesselbach's plexus). Also, a branch emerges between the nasal bones and upper lateral cartilages and supplies the tip of the nose. Absence of the posterior ethmoid and rarely the anterior ethmoid arteries has been described (2).

The *external carotid artery* is the blood supply to the rest of the nose by way of the external maxillary artery (*facial artery*) and the internal maxillary artery. The *superior labial artery* is a branch of the facial artery and primarily supplies the upper lip; however, two of its branches, the septal and the alar branches, supply

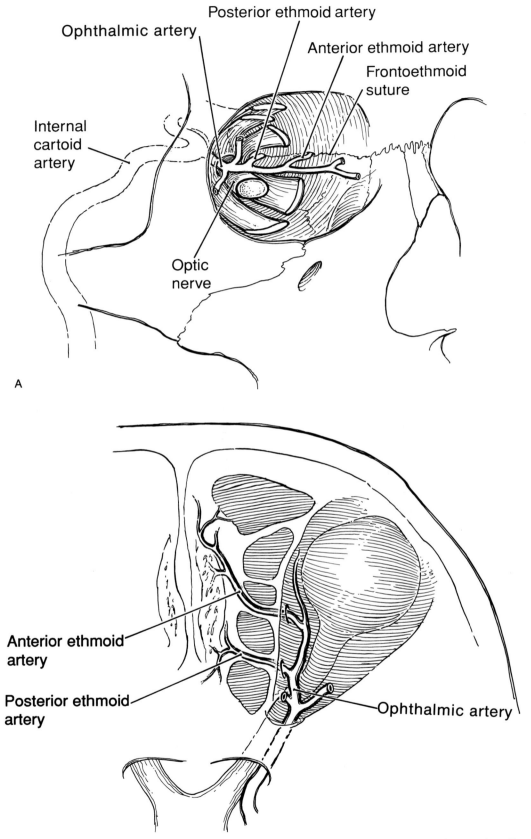

FIG. 1. The intraorbital relationships of the anterior and posterior ethmoid arteries as visualized from an anterolateral view **(A)** and superior view **(B).**

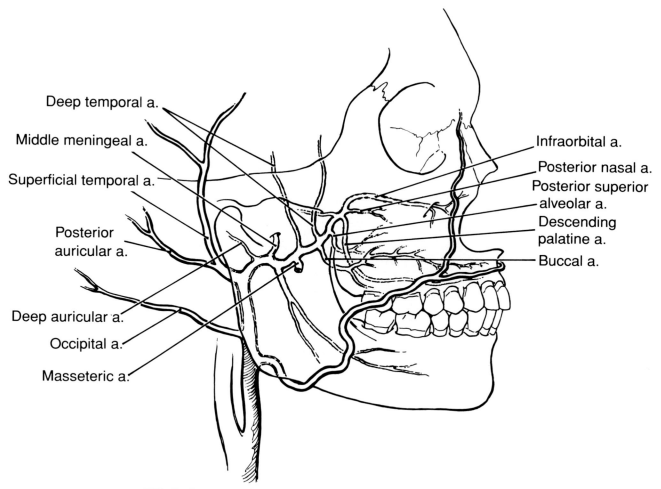

FIG. 2. Anatomy of the internal maxillary artery and its branches.

blood to the mucosa of the anterior septum and the mucosa of the nasal vestibule.

Branches of the *internal maxillary artery* supply the majority of the vasculature to the nasal cavity (Fig. 2). This artery passes through the infratemporal fossa and enters the pterygopalatine fossa via the pterygopalatine fissure. In this fossa, it gives off multiple branches. These branches may exit the fossa anteriorly (infraorbital and greater palatine), laterally (superior alveolar), posteriorly (branch to the foramen rotundum, artery of the pterygoid canal, and the pharyngeal artery), and medially (posterior nasal and sphenopalatine). The two terminal branches of the maxillary artery are the sphenopalatine artery and the posterior nasal artery. They enter the nose through the sphenopalatine canal to supply the posterior septum and the lateral nasal wall. The greater palatine artery descends within the greater palatine canal to the hard palate. It then proceeds anteriorly to the incisive foramen where it enters the nose and contributes branches to Kiesselbach's plexus.

The internal maxillary artery and its branches share the pterygopalatine fossa with the pterygopalatine ganglion and the second division of the trigeminal nerve. These structures are encased in fibroadipose tissue, which fills this space. The variability of the branching and the tortuosity associated with atherosclerosis result in significant variation in the anatomy (3). The maxillary artery and its branches, however, always lie anterior to the nerves.

A free anastomosis of end-arterioles of branches of the anterior ethmoid artery, sphenopalatine artery, and superior labial artery occurs on the anterior septum (Little's area). This is known as Kiesselbach's plexus and is subject to minor trauma because of its location and troublesome bleeding because of the complicated blood supply (Fig. 3).

The *venous drainage* in general follows the course of the arteries. The anterior and posterior ethmoid veins drain to the cavernous sinus; the sphenopalatine veins to the maxillary vein or cavernous sinus via the emis-

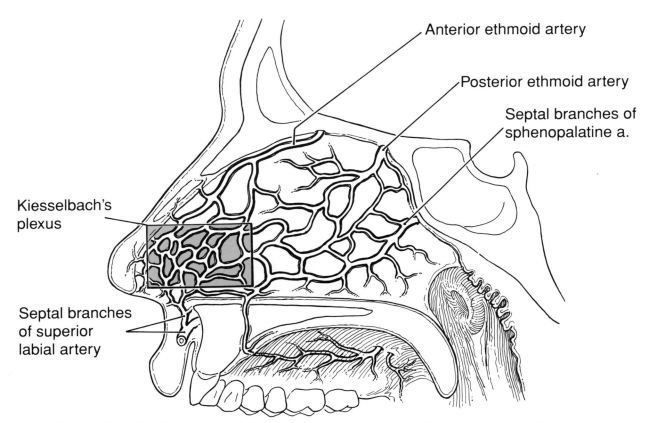

FIG. 3. Kiesselbach's plexus and the main vascular supply contributing to its formation on the anterior aspect of the nasal septum (Little's area).

sary veins; the greater palatine veins to the maxillary veins to the posterior facial veins or cavernous sinus; and the septal veins to the anterior facial vein.

The lining of the nose consists of mucoperichondrium or mucoperiosteum. This is a ciliated pseudostratified columnar epithelium in all but the upper portion of the nose, where olfactory epithelium predominates. The submucous connective tissue is richly vascularized, accounting for the heavy bleeding that may occur with even minor trauma.

ETIOLOGY

Local Causes

Trauma

As has been stated already, most cases of epistaxis (Table 1) are secondary to relatively minor trauma due to sneezing, nose blowing, or digital manipulation and are either self-limiting or easily controlled with simple measures. This epistaxis usually arises from the anterior septum. Vascular engorgement of the nasal mucosa due to allergic or infectious rhinitis makes the

mucosa more vulnerable to this type of injury. The cold dry air of the winter months or the central heating used without humidification may exacerbate these conditions. A septal deviation or spur may predispose a certain area of the mucosa to drying, leading to recurrent epistaxis. Nasal continuous positive airway pressure therapy (CPAP), which is increasingly being used for obstructive sleep apnea, also may cause epistaxis once again by the drying effect of the air (4).

A nasal foreign body may cause an intense local reaction, which may result in epistaxis. Topical nasal spray (e.g., decongestant or steroid) and even instilled eyedrops (e.g., antiglaucoma agents) may irritate the nasal mucosa and cause epistaxis (5). Overaggressive treatment of epistaxis with packing or cautery (particularly electric cautery) or cocaine abuse may cause chronic ulcers, which lead to septal perforation, crusting, and repeated epistaxis.

Epistaxis may be the presenting symptom of nasal fracture. This bleeding usually is due to laceration of the mucosa and is self-limiting and rarely requires treatment. Occasionally, it can be quite severe, necessitating cautery or even ligation of the bleeding vessel. Epistaxis due to mucosal disruption secondary to na-

TABLE 1. *Etiology of epistaxis*

Local
  Traumatic
    Digital manipulation
    Drying effect of air
    Foreign body
    Nasal fractures
    Facial fractures
    Iatrogenic: Packing, cautery, surgery, intubation
    Barotrauma
  Inflammatory
    Acute: Viral, bacterial, allergic rhinitis
    Chronic: Nonspecific—chronic rhinosinusitis,
      rhinitis medicamentosa, cocaine, decongestants
          Specific—granulomas
  Deviated nasal septum
  Neoplastic
    Nasal
    Paranasal sinus
    Nasopharyngeal
Systemic
  Bleeding dyscrasia
  Atherosclerosis
  Hereditary telangiectasia (Osler–Weber–Rendu
    disease)
Idiopathic

sogastric tube insertion or nasotracheal intubation, while usually self-limiting, may occasionally be severe.

On the other hand, epistaxis due to mid-third facial fractures may be severe and is more often due to disruption of the internal maxillary artery or its terminal branches (6,7). A telescoping nasoethmoid fracture can disrupt the anterior ethmoid artery with resultant severe epistaxis. Of course, severe epistaxis following base of skull fracture may be due to a carotid–cavernous fistula. Delayed bleeding after a midface fracture may be secondary to a pseudoaneurysm of the maxillary artery.

An aneurysm of the cavernous portion of the internal carotid artery following blunt or penetrating trauma or even spontaneously developing may rupture into the sphenoid sinus with resultant massive and life-threatening epistaxis (8).

Epistaxis as a complication of a surgical procedure can range from minor to major. Epistaxis may result from surgery to the nasal structures (septoplasty, septorhinoplasty, turbinectomy), paranasal sinuses (endoscopic or conventional), or nasopharynx (adenoidectomy or biopsy). Osteotomies for orthognathic surgery may disrupt the arterial supply, leading to immediate or delayed bleeding (9).

Barotrauma involving the paranasal sinuses may result in hemorrhage within a sinus cavity with resultant epistaxis. This may occur during flying or scuba diving, particularly if there is an associated upper respiratory tract infection.

Inflammation

Nasal congestion due to infection, allergy, or rhinitis medicamentosa may predispose to epistaxis. In addition, any of the chronic granulomas that may affect the nasal cavity (e.g., tuberculosis, sarcoid, Wegener's) may present with epistaxis. Obviously, any suspicious area should always be biopsied. Inflammatory processes or trauma may lead to septal perforation, which may be a major source of epistaxis. These bleed from the exposed margins, which usually crust and have extremely friable granulation tissue.

Deviated Nasal Septum

A deviated septum interferes with the normal flow of air, producing eddying currents that dry the mucosa, resulting in crusting and then epistaxis. While the deviation may be significant and involve a large portion of the septum, small spurs are just as likely to cause problems.

Neoplasm

Epistaxis may be the presenting symptom of a tumor of the nose, paranasal sinuses, or nasopharynx, either benign or malignant. Juvenile angiofibroma may bleed spontaneously and severely, as may the rare solitary angiomas arising from the septum (10). Other tumors, varying from simple papilloma to squamous cell carcinoma, are more likely to cause mild intermittent epistaxis but severe bleeding may occur. The possibility of an underlying malignancy should always be considered and every patient should be evaluated carefully to exclude this possibility.

Systemic Causes

Blood Dyscrasias

Epistaxis may be the presenting symptom or a dominant problem in patients with a bleeding diathesis. While usually there is obvious evidence either on history or examination of a diathesis, occasionally the diagnosis may be more subtle and sought by careful history taking, particularly regarding a family history and examination looking for evidence of bruising and so on. The differential diagnosis of bleeding diathesis is enormous, varying from primary coagulopathies (e.g., hemophilia or von Willebrand's disease), secondary conditions (e.g., leukemia, myeloma, aplastic anemia, hepatic disease) or drug induced conditions, just to name a few. If even remotely suspicious, a hematologic consult should be obtained in order that the appropriate barrage of tests may be performed to establish a diagnosis, preferably prior to any blood transfusion. Occasionally, mild blood dyscrasia may be identified as the etiology of recurrent epistaxis in children (11,12). The treatment of epistaxis due to coagulopathy is fraught with difficulty. The use of cautery is contraindicated and standard packing material may only aggravate the condition by excoriating the mucosa, particularly on removal. Details of management will be discussed under treatment.

Atherosclerosis

With aging, atherosclerosis of the vessels supplying the nose may prevent vascular constriction, leading to uncontrollable hemorrhage. In these patients the epistaxis usually originates in the posterior aspect of the nose (13). Hypertension is often cited as being associated with an increased incidence of epistaxis; however, no significant difference in the prevalence of epistaxis has been found in patients with or without hypertension (13,14). The hypertension noted in older patients with epistaxis is probably related to the age of the patient, the atherosclerosis, and the stress associated with the uncontrolled bleeding.

Hereditary Hemorrhagic Telangiectasia (Osler–Weber–Rendu Disease)

This is an autosomally dominant inherited disease characterized by abnormal subcutaneous and submucosal telangiectasia scattered throughout the body (15,16) (Fig. 4). The telangiectasias are common on the face and on the mucous membranes of the tongue, lips, and nose but can be found almost anywhere on the body. Gastrointestinal, respiratory, and genitourinary systems also may be involved. The most common symptom is recurrent, spontaneous epistaxis that begins at puberty and usually worsens with age, although in a few patients improvement can occur later in life. The vascular anomaly is a small arteriovenous fistula, which on histologic examination demonstrates dilated vessels without elastic or muscular tissue in the vessel wall. Bleeding is caused by a combination of telangiectatic vessels, local trauma, and fragile mucous membranes. Because of the lack of contractile elements in the vessel wall, the bleeding may not stop spontaneously and can be very severe, necessitating multiple transfusions over the years. Treatment is extremely difficult.

Idiopathic

Despite thorough evaluation, in approximately 10% of patients an underlying etiology will not be identified. This may be because of a subtle underlying coagulopathy or a minor trauma that was unrecognized (17).

PATIENT EVALUATION

The evaluation of a patient with epistaxis depends frequently on whether the patient is seen with acute active bleeding, usually in an emergency room, or in the period between bleeds in a nonemergent situation, usually in the office when a more leisurely evaluation can be undertaken.

Most patients seek medical attention between acute

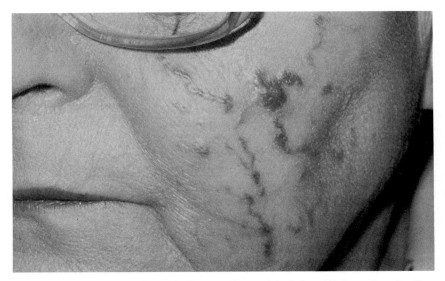

FIG. 4. Cutaneous telangiectasia in a patient with Osler–Weber–Rendu disease.

episodes and are thus seen in a controlled setting usually in the otolaryngologist's office. A careful *history* should be obtained in order to identify any etiologic factor, be it a bleeding diathesis, a history of sinonasal disease, tresis, or sinonasal medication. At the very least, a rudimentary *general physical examination* should be performed, looking for evidence of anemia, stigmata of a bleeding tendency, hypertension, or the presence of telangiectasia elsewhere on the body.

Examination of the nose is facilitated by the use of a topical vasoconstrictor combined with an anesthetic placed on a cotton pledget. A solution of 4% cocaine is ideal for this purpose, but if this is not available, a mixture of lidocaine with epinephrine may be used. This should be left in place for a few minutes and then the interior of the nose carefully inspected. An eschar or prominent vessels on the anterior septum may indicate a common site for bleeding, particularly in children. A septal spur may be identified, which may have an exposed vessel on the prominence or hidden behind it. Of course, every attempt should be made to examine the nose thoroughly in every case to exclude an underlying or coexisting neoplasm or granuloma. Frequently, a marked septal deformity may obscure adequate visualization of the nasal cavities and a fiberoptic examination of the nose and nasopharynx may be required. If no source is identified and paranasal sinus disease is suspected, a radiograph or computed tomography (CT) scan may be performed.

On the other hand, a patient may seek medical attention during an active nose bleed and these patients are seen in the emergency room, where facilities for examining the nose are less than ideal and the active bleed may obviate adequate evaluation. Before patient evaluation can begin, the bleeding needs to be controlled as expeditiously as possible and, if severe, the patient rendered hemodynamically stable by inserting an intravenous line and being carefully monitored. The patient should be sitting or in a semirecumbent position with clothing protected by a waterproof cover. It is better to try and get the patient to spit out and not swallow the blood as this may induce nausea and vomiting. All medical personnel should wear gloves and gowns to protect clothing and eye protection because of the tendency of the patient to cough and splutter. An attempt should be made to suction out the nose or ask the patient to blow their nose prior to identifying the bleeding site. This can then be controlled by packing with gauze or cotton impregnated with a combination of local anesthesia and vasoconstrictor. More definitive packing or cautery would depend on the site of the bleeder. Only now should full patient evaluation be performed including history from patient and family and a general physical examination as well as examination of the nose and pharynx.

Laboratory tests for anemia and coagulopathy should be performed, as indicated, and blood crossmatched for transfusion if necessary. Radiographic studies of the sinuses may be of value, if one is concerned about a paranasal sinus tumor, but usually are not performed on a routine basis. Angiography is reserved for special situations and not routinely performed.

MANAGEMENT

Anterior Epistaxis

It is a fact that most nose bleeds are minor, arising from the anterior aspect of the septum. Therefore, if the physician is required to advise on the emergency care of an epistaxis via the telephone, it is best to advise the patient to pinch the anterior nares to apply pressure to this area and to hold pressure for a few minutes.

Cautery

The most common cause of recurrent anterior epistaxis is bleeding from Kiesselbach's plexus on the anterior aspect of the septum. If the bleeding site is identified, either by noting active bleeding or an eschar or prominent vessels in this area, a cotton pledget or 1-in. ribbon gauze impregnated with a local anesthetic–vasoconstrictor combination is used. Cocaine (4%) is an excellent choice, but alternatively 4% lidocaine with epinephrine 1:100,000, or 4% lidocaine with 0.5% phenylephrine can be used. Once adequate anesthesia has been obtained by keeping the pledget in place for at least 5 min, the bleeding site may be cauterized.

Chemical Cautery

Silver nitrate is the most commonly used chemical cautery. This is best used in the solid state, as using the liquid form on a cotton applicator may result in burns of the anterior nares and upper lip as the liquid runs out of the nose or is sneezed out. The best technique is to cauterize circumferentially around the bleeding site before cauterizing the actual offending bleeding vessel as the act of cautery on the fragile bleeding vessel may precipitate more bleeding, which may be impossible to stop with chemical cautery. Too vigorous or repeated cautery may result in significant ulceration or even septal perforation.

Electric Cautery

If there is an active arterial bleed, silver nitrate will not control the bleeder. In this situation, it is best to inject, submucosally, the area around the bleeding site with local anesthesia, to tamponade the bleeder, and then to cauterize with an electric cautery. Electric cautery should be used with great caution, however, because if too aggressively performed, it may lead to septal perforation. Occasionally, if the bleeding site is further back, the site can be identified with a 30-degree endoscope and treated with electric cautery (18).

After cautery, the patient is advised to apply an antibiotic ointment three times a day for approximately 10 days to keep the eschar soft. In addition, the patient is instructed to keep the mouth open when sneezing and to avoid blowing the nose for the same period. Occasionally, it may be necessary to recauterize the bleeding site.

In children, the most common cause of epistaxis is nasal vestibulitis with crusting and secondary digital manipulation. This can be controlled by daily application of an antibiotic ointment and usually cautery is not indicated. On the other hand, if cautery is indicated, it should be performed under general anesthesia in the younger child.

Anterior Packing

Nasal packing is rarely required to control anterior nasal bleeding; however, if cautery is not feasible because of lack of facilities, if an obvious site cannot be identified, or the bleeding cannot be controlled by conventional means, packing is the treatment of choice. Multiple different materials and different techniques have been described for packing the nose with the procedure of choice dependent on the bleeding site and severity of the bleed. The nasal cavity should be anesthetized adequately prior to placement of the pack using the techniques described above. A $\frac{1}{2}$- to 1-in. ribbon gauze impregnated with antibiotic ointment or vaseline is used most commonly. Oxidized cellulose preparations, absorbable gelatin sponge, and porcine strip packing may be used, particularly if there is an underlying bleeding tendency, or if packing is required for hereditary telangiectasia. The advantage of these materials is that the packing spontaneously dissolves, and therefore the trauma of pack removal is eliminated. Regardless of the type of packing used, the key is to apply adequate pressure to the bleeding site. A poorly placed pack will fail to achieve this goal and, in addition, may fall out sooner than desired. "Blind" packing (i.e., simply stuffing the pack into the nose) should never be attempted as it may be traumatic, ineffective, and occasionally may be pushed into the pharynx. The key is adequate visualization and a layered placement of the pack, filling the nasal cavity (Fig. 5). Occasionally it is possible to place a more localized pack and still obtain adequate pressure on the bleeding site. This is usually feasible in cases of oozing due to a bleeding diathesis, but not when the bleeding is brisk. The packing usually is removed at 5 to 7 days to allow thrombus formation. A simple alternative to anterior packing includes a specially designed balloon that can be inflated to fill the nasal cavity and the nasopharynx (Fig. 6) or a nasal tampon (19).

Complications of nasal packing may be related to placing the pack itself, the presence of the pack in the nasal cavity, and removal of the pack. If inadequate topical anesthesia has been applied, the act of packing may be extremely uncomfortable and may occasionally induce a vasovagal reaction. A nasal–vagal reflex has been described, which may result in profound cardiovascular changes (20). "Blind" packing may aggravate the bleeding by causing mucosal injury, particularly if there is a deviated septum, and occasionally may be pushed into the pharynx. The mucosal damage may ultimately result in synechiae between medial and lateral walls.

The nasal packing, while in place, causes mechanical obstruction of the nasal cavity and may result in epiphora and obstruction of the sinus ostia with secondary sinusitis (21). Therefore, if the pack is to remain in place for more than a few days, prophylactic antibiotics should probably be used. Bilateral nasal packing may result in anoxia, particularly in the elderly patient, and this will be discussed in more detail in the section on posterior epistaxis.

Toxic shock syndrome has been described with intranasal packing, but this is an extremely rare event (22–24). This syndrome is caused by the endotoxin of *Staphylococcus aureus,* which colonizes the packing. It is characterized by a sudden onset of high fever, gastrointestinal upset, myalgia, and, in severe cases, shock. A rash may develop during the acute illness and is later followed by desquamation of the skin, particularly on the palms and soles. Usually the illness commences 12 to 24 hr after insertion of the packs. The use of antibiotic-impregnated gauze may decrease the potential for this complication to occur, but it is better to cover patients with antistaphylococcal antibiotics.

Complications associated with removal of the pack include a vasovagal attack and precipitation of further bleeding because the pack is adherent to the healing underlying mucosa.

Chronic relapsing anterior epistaxis may be an extremely vexing problem, particularly if arising from Little's area. The prolonged use of topical antibiotic ointment to soften and moisturize the area and the use of adequate humidification, as well as an attempt to discourage digital trauma, are the best treatments, par-

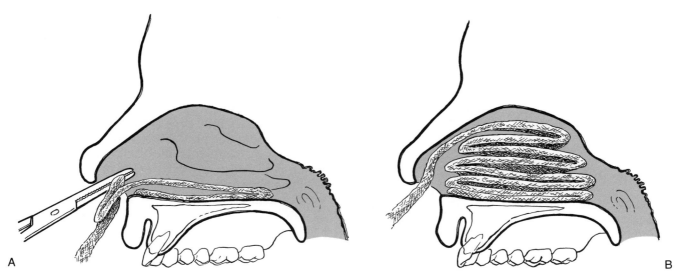

FIG. 5. Layered anterior packing to effectively tamponade the bleeding site.

ticularly in children. If the condition continues in spite of this conservative therapy, a submucosal (not subperichondrial) dissection of the area with the intent to interrupt the blood supply may prove useful.

Posterior Epistaxis

There is no clear-cut definition as to what constitutes "posterior" as opposed to "anterior" epistaxis, but clinically it can best be regarded as bleeding that arises from so far posterior that the bleeding site cannot be identified by anterior inspection or controlled by an anterior pack.

Posterior bleeding is most often arterial in nature, frequently arising from a group of vessels located at the posterior end of the inferior turbinate near the sphenopalatine foramen (Woodruff's nasopharyngeal plexus) (21). The usual clinical picture of posterior epistaxis is of severe bleeding presenting from the front of the nose and the nasopharynx and may even be life-threatening. Occasionally, however, it can be quite occult with the patient swallowing large quantities of blood without being aware of it. These patients usually

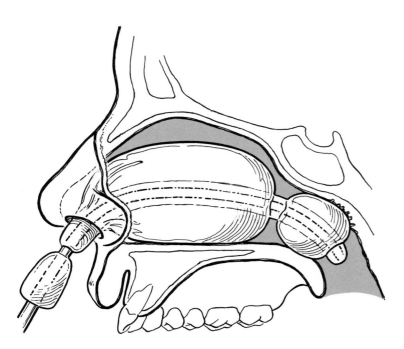

FIG. 6. Customized balloon providing anterior and posterior tamponade.

present to the emergency room and are frequently hemodynamically unstable, requiring resuscitation and careful monitoring. They usually require admission to hospital depending on the severity of the epistaxis, the general condition of the patient, and the therapeutic regimen necessary to attain control. Identification of the bleeding site and the institution of effective treatment can be most frustrating.

Therapeutic Alternatives

Usually these patients require, as an emergency measure, the placement of posterior and anterior packing to obtain control of the acute bleeding. Once this has been accomplished and the patient stabilized hemodynamically, a decision has to be made as to how best to proceed, with this decision depending on the condition of the patient, the facilities available, and the philosophy and experience of the physician in charge of the management of the patient. The alternatives are as follows:

1. It may be decided to leave the packing in place and only remove it at 5 to 7 days and then observe the patient. If the patient should continue to bleed with the packing *in situ* or rebleed after removal of the packs, this patient can be taken to the operating room, the nose and nasopharynx examined, a septoplasty performed if needed to gain access, and any obvious bleeding site cauterized directly. If this is not possible or desirable because a bleeding site is not identified or cautery is not successful, the packs can be replaced and the cycle of events repeated or proceed to vessel ligation. This conventional conservative approach is certainly effective in the vast majority of cases but has the drawbacks of prolonged hospitalization and the discomfort of packing.
2. On the other hand, it may be decided to take the patient to the operating room early, remove the packs, examine the nose and nasopharynx, and perform a septoplasty if needed, not only for access to allow cautery if feasible but to allow the placement of an effective pack if this is not possible.
3. A third alternative is to perform early vessel ligation or, in select cases, embolization to obviate the need for prolonged packing and hospitalization. In favor of early vessel ligation as opposed to the other techniques is a shorter hospital stay, a claimed higher control rate, and the relative comfort of the procedure as compared to prolonged packing. These advantages, of course, need to be weighed against the potential disadvantages of an unnecessary operation and general anesthesia.

Posterior Packing

The first step in the placement of posterior and anterior packs is to suction the nose, then apply a combination vasoconstrictor and topical anesthetic to the nose, and to spray the posterior oropharynx with anesthetic spray to facilitate the placement of the packs. The posterior nasopharyngeal pack is placed initially, then the transnasal anterior pack is buttressed against it. The packing may consist of the traditional gauze pack, which is placed transorally, or an inflatable balloon, which is placed through the nose. The latter method, even though less effective, has become very popular as a first-line treatment because of ease of placement.

Nasopharyngeal Packing

Nasopharyngeal packs are placed to tamponade any bleeder vessel in the nasopharynx or posterior choanae and to act as a buttress against which the anterior pack can be placed. A pack that occludes the posterior choanae unilaterally or bilaterally can be created and customized by folding 2-in. gauze impregnated with an antibiotic ointment and secured using silk suture or umbilical tape (see Fig. 8). It is important that the packing not be too tightly structured in order that it may conform to the dimensions of the nasopharynx and posterior choanae and effectively apply pressure to the bleeding site. The technique to place these packs consists of inserting soft red rubber catheters intranasally, which are retrieved through the oral cavity. A single catheter is used for a unilateral pack and bilateral catheters for bilateral packs. The sutures or umbilical tape on the pack are then attached to the catheter(s) and the pack is then drawn into the nasopharynx by pulling on the catheter(s) (Fig. 7). It may be necessary to manipulate the pack around the soft palate with a finger. The suture or umbilical tape is taped to the side of the cheek to facilitate later removal of the pack. The posterior pack is maintained in position by tying the sutures or tape over a cotton or gauze buttress placed over the columella (Fig. 8). An anterior pack unilateral or bilateral is then placed firmly against the posterior pack. The packing is usually left *in situ* for 5 to 7 days, during which time the patient is kept on broad-spectrum antibiotics. When it is decided to remove the packs, the anterior packs are removed first and if no bleeding is encountered, the posterior pack is removed by pulling on the suture attached to the cheek after dividing the anterior transnasal suture. In general, even though uncomfortable for the patient, these posterior packs can be placed under local anesthesia in most circumstances. Occasionally, however, general anesthesia may be indicated.

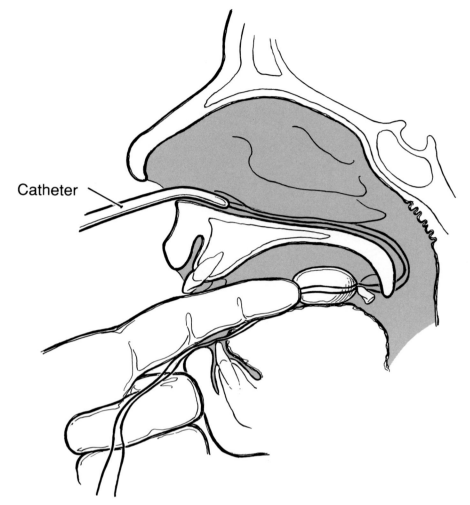

FIG. 7. Placement of nasopharyngeal pack by retracting catheter through nose.

Balloon Techniques

A more convenient, but somewhat less effective, method of placing a nasopharyngeal pack is the use of inflatable balloon packs. While easy to place, they do not exert uniform pressure in the posterior choanae and nasopharynx and therefore are less successful in tamponading an arterial bleed (25). Either a Foley catheter No. 16, together with standard anterior gauze packing, or a specifically designed low-pressure double-balloon tampon may be used. The deflated system is passed into the nasopharynx, where the posterior balloon is inflated using saline. Forward traction is then applied and the anterior balloon then inflated (Fig. 6). If a Foley catheter is used, it is inserted into the nasopharynx transnasally and the balloon is inflated with a volume of saline sufficient to stop the epistaxis, but not enough to cause the patient discomfort (Fig. 9). The catheter is secured anteriorly by using a hemostat or clamp, being careful to interpose padding against the anterior nares to prevent ischemic necrosis. Anterior packing is then placed in the anterior nose buttressed against the balloon, if indicated. At 5 to 7 days, the balloon may be deflated, the anterior packs removed, and, if no bleeding is encountered, the catheter or balloon tampon removed.

In addition to the complications associated with anterior packing, posterior packing has its own set of problems. The pack is uncomfortable to insert and uncomfortable while in place. Eustachian tube dysfunction is a frequent problem with hemotympanum occasionally developing.

The most important and serious complication of posterior packing, however, is hypoxia with secondary myocardial and/or cerebral ischemia and even death (26). The mechanism for this is somewhat controversial and has been attributed to a "nasopulmonary reflex," which lowers the oxygen tension (27), but some studies have failed to document such as reflex (28,29). Most likely, the decreased oxygenation is due to the bulk of the packing per se, aspiration of blood, the use of sedation, and an associated low hematocrit (30). Sup-

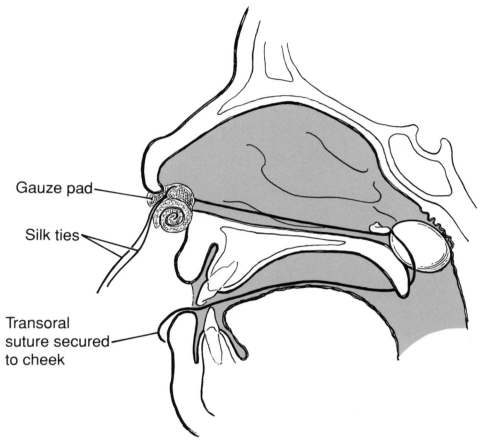

Gauze pad

Silk ties

Transoral
suture secured
to cheek

FIG. 8. Pack secured in position. Note silk suture brought out through mouth and then taped to cheek.

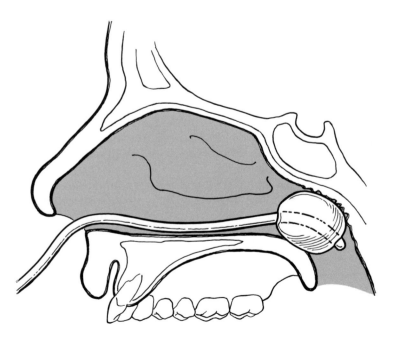

FIG. 9. Foley catheter *in situ.* Anterior packing can now be placed against the balloon.

plemental oxygen is therefore mandatory and medications that depress the respiratory centers should be avoided if possible. Old and frail patients and those with a history of heart or respiratory disease should be monitored in an intensive care unit. If there is a high level of anxiety, a case can be made for a prophylactic tracheostomy.

Arterial Ligation

An alternate first-line method of treatment in severe or recurrent posterior epistaxis, or a backup for epistaxis refractory to conservative treatment, is selective arterial ligation. The decision as to when to perform ligation varies according to the experience and philosophy of the treating physician and the nature of the epistaxis. The decision as to which vessels to ligate is dependent on the site of the bleeding. This may sometimes be difficult to determine and necessitate multiple vessel ligation to obtain control. Angiography to determine the bleeding site is not routinely performed but may be useful in unusual situations, for example, if nasopharyngeal bleeding is encountered, if carotid–cavernous fistula is suspected, or if embolization is to be considered. In general, ligation should be performed as close as possible to the site of bleeding because more proximal occlusion will not control collateral circulation, although this is probably not as important a concept as was once thought.

Internal Maxillary Artery Ligation

This vessel and its branches may be approached via the maxillary antrum or transorally. It is an excellent method of obtaining control if the bleeding can be isolated as arising from one of its branches (31,32).

Transantral Approach

The transantral approach may be performed under local anesthesia, but general anesthesia is preferable. A sublabial incision in the gingivobuccal sulcus is made and the periosteum is elevated to expose the anterior face of the maxilla. The infraorbital nerve is identified and avoided. The anterior face of the antrum is opened widely and an inferiorly based flap in the mucosa of the posterior wall of the antrum is created. The posterior wall of the antrum is removed using chisel, drill, or punch, taking care to leave the periosteum intact. The periosteum is then incised in a cruciate manner using a needle point cautery and reflected to expose the contents of the pterygomaxillary fossa. At this stage, some surgeons use a microscope for the remainder of the procedure, while others use simple loupes. The internal maxillary artery and its branches lie in fibroadipose tissue anterior to the vidian nerve and can be exposed by careful dissection with blunt right-angle hooks, alligator instruments, or hemostats (Fig. 10). Self-locking vascular clips are applied to the internal

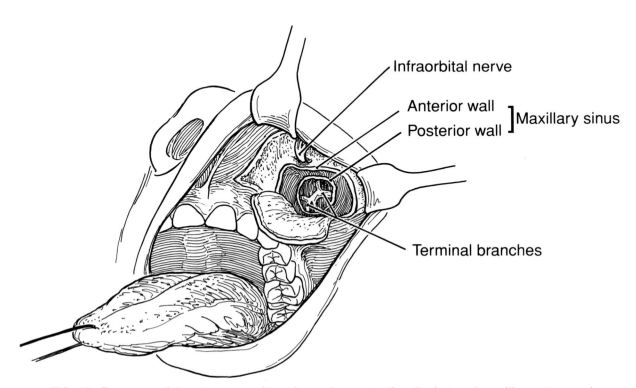

FIG. 10. Exposure of the pterygomaxillary fossa demonstrating the internal maxillary artery and its branches.

maxillary artery and as many of its distal branches as possible. The efficacy of the procedure is now assessed by examining the nose to determine whether the bleeding has stopped. If, as is frequently the case, packing is already in place, this should be removed. A nasoantral window is performed, the inferiorly based posterior wall mucosal flap replaced, and a sheet of Gelfoam placed to secure it. The sublabial incision is then closed using absorbable suture.

Transantral ligation of the internal maxillary artery is successful 90% of the time if performed correctly for the proper indications. Failure may be because of collateral circulation with branches of the ipsilateral internal carotid artery, or facial artery, or with branches of the contralateral maxillary artery or because of incomplete ligation (33). Complications include a temporary loss of sensation to the teeth and cheek, facial swelling, oroantral fistula, and, rarely, injury to the pterygopalatine ganglion.

Transoral Approach

To avoid the potential complications listed above, transoral ligation of the internal maxillary artery has been advocated (34). Under general anesthesia, a gingivobuccal incision is made extending from the upper second or third molar, inferiorly along the anterior aspect of the ascending ramus of the mandible (Fig. 11). The buccal fat pad is removed and can be replaced at the termination of the procedure. The temporalis muscle is identified at its insertion into the medial aspect of the coronoid process of the mandible and is bluntly dissected from the ramus, preserving its inferior attachment. The internal maxillary artery then comes into view and is then divided after placement of vascular clips (Fig. 12). The major advantage of this approach is its simplicity and it is particularly useful if a transantral approach cannot be performed because of sinus trauma, infection, or neoplasm. It is, however, possibly more likely to fail because the artery is ligated more proximally than with transantral ligation. Facial pain and trismus are the most significant complications (34).

Ethmoid Artery Ligation

If the bleeding can be localized to the superolateral aspect of the nose, or if the ethmoid vessels have been

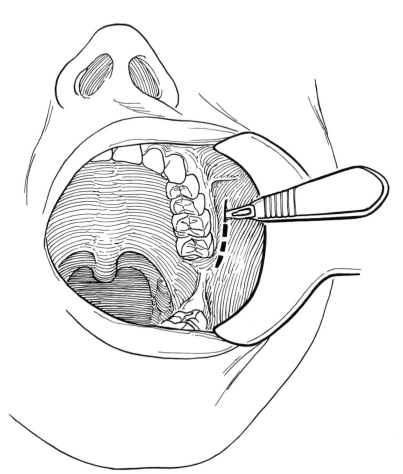

FIG. 11. Incision to expose the internal maxillary artery intraorally.

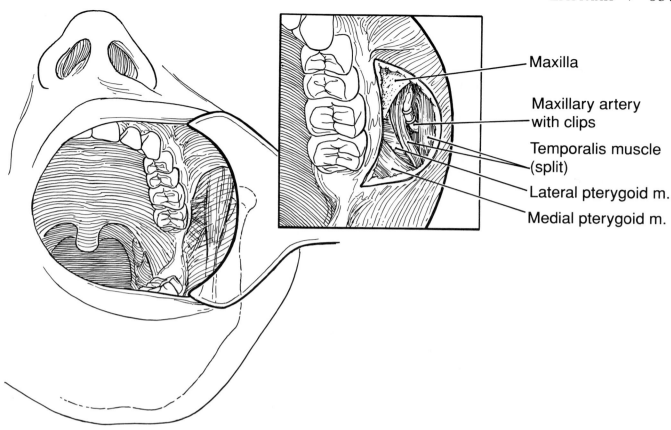

FIG. 12. Identification of the internal maxillary artery via the intraoral approach.

thought to have been severed (e.g., following lateral osteotomies and ethmoidectomy), or if the bleeding site cannot be localized and controlled by internal maxillary artery ligation, the ethmoid vessels need to be addressed. Under local or preferably general anesthesia, an external ethmoidectomy incision is made midway between the medial canthus and the dorsum of the nose. The periosteum is incised and elevated, the lacrimal sac elevated from the lacrimal fossa and the lamina papyracea exposed. The frontoethmoid suture line is identified and the orbital contents are gently retracted. The anterior ethmoid artery, which lies approximately 1.5 cm posterior to the posterior lacrimal crest, is ligated with two self-locking vascular clips and divided. Controversy exists as to whether the posterior artery should be routinely clipped or only if ligation of the anterior artery fails. In general, it is advised to clip this vessel taking special care because of the close proximity of the optic nerve. Under no circumstances should this vessel be cauterized or should undue dissection be performed around this vessel. Complications include optic nerve damage and intraoribtal hemorrhage due to retraction of the ethmoid vessel into the orbit (35).

External Carotid Artery Ligation

While simple to perform, this procedure is possibly more likely to fail because the proximal ligation is unlikely to affect the peripheral collateral circulation; however, excellent results with external carotid ligation alone have been described (36). The artery should be ligated as proximal as possible below the origin of the ascending pharyngeal artery, or this branch should be ligated separately, particularly if the epistaxis is arising from the posterior aspect of the nose or nasopharynx and this vessel is thought to be contributing to the vascular supply.

Embolization

An alternative to ligation of the internal maxillary artery is embolization of this vessel. The advantages of this technique over surgical ligation are that more distal vessels can be obliterated, the pre-embolization angiogram may demonstrate the bleeding site, and finally, if successful, the hospital stay is short. Proponents of this technique suggest early embolization in order to avoid the potential complications of either nasal packing or surgical ligation (37). Others advocate embolization for the treatment of patients who fail posterior packing (38) or for those patients where a surgical procedure is contraindicated (e.g., poor general health or local disease precluding ligation via a transoral or transantral approach). Yet another approach would be to perform embolization early and combine it with ethmoid artery ligation if this failed to control bleeding.

This procedure is performed by an invasive radiologist in the radiology department. Access is obtained by percutaneous catheterization of the femoral artery under local anesthesia. The catheter is then directed to the internal maxillary artery under fluoroscopic guidance. Injection of radiopaque contrast (Hypaque) delineates the anatomy and often reveals the exact bleeding point. The internal maxillary artery and its branches are occluded using polyvinyl alcohol (Ivalon), dextran microspheres, absorbable gelatin sponge (Gelfoam), or detachable balloons (39,40). Failure to control the epistaxis may be due to inaccessible branches, collateral circulation, or bleeding arising from the ethmoid arteries.

Potential complications of embolization include all the risks of transfemoral catheterization (i.e., hematoma, intimal tears leading to peripheral ischemia, and femoral nerve damage), complications of carotid angiography, and complications of embolization itself, which include severe facial pain, trismus, cranial nerve palsies, seizure, and stroke (41).

Miscellaneous

As has already been described, examination of the nose under general anesthetic with a septoplasty to improve visualization (if indicated) and direct cautery to the offending vessels are excellent alternatives to the above techniques. Selective cautery of the bleeder after lateral displacement of the septum, together with transnasopharyngeal cautery using a suction-cautery, has been used successfully (42). Likewise, endoscopic identification of the bleeder and cautery have been described (18).

A rather easily performed, but somewhat rarely indicated or used technique is the injection of the greater palatine foramen with local anesthetic mixed with 1:100,000 epinephrine. Approximately 3 cc of solution is injected with the needle not being placed any deeper than 28 mm into the canal. Any deeper injection may result in direct injection into the infraorbital fissure. The success of this technique probably results from vessel compression by the volume of fluid in a confined space. Its effect is therefore likely to be purely temporary (43).

Cryotherapy (44) and various lasers also have been used but are probably no more effective than standard cautery.

Hereditary Hemorrhagic Telangiectasia

The management of hereditary hemorrhagic telangiectasia (Osler–Weber–Rendu disease) constitutes a tremendous challenge to the otolaryngologist because of the lifelong refractory nature of the epistaxis. These patients require long-term management and usually develop a keen appreciation of how to prevent and even treat their own epistaxis. In general, they will avoid digital trauma, ensure adequate humidification, and become quite adept at treating the mild epistaxis with self-packing using an absorbable material. They usually will be required to be on long-term iron therapy to combat a chronically low hemoglobin. The use of long-term estrogens, either topical or taken systemically, has proved disappointing (45). Estrogens are believed to promote squamous metaplasia of the nasal mucosa and seal endothelial gaps in the malformed vessels, resulting in the nasal mucosa being less vulnerable to trauma. This therapy has well-known feminizing side effects and contraindications that prevent its use except in severely affected patients.

In most patients, this conservative therapy will suffice. On the other hand, if the bleeding becomes persistent or recurrent, further intervention is required. Several methods of cautery, including the use of the carbon dioxide, Nd-YAG, and contact YAG lasers, have been used with varying success (46,47). Repeated cautery using these techniques is usually necessary.

Frustration with these methods has led to the development of some rather innovative surgical procedures to aid the management of these patients.

Septal Dermatoplasty

The purpose of septal dermatoplasty is to replace the vulnerable affected mucosa of the anterior nose with skin (48). This is performed by removing mucosa of the anterior half of the nasal septum, the floor of the nose, and the lateral wall to the level of the middle turbinate. Bilateral alotomies are performed to expose the affected area. The mucosa is stripped, leaving the perichondrium *in situ*. A split-thickness skin graft is harvested from the upper thigh and carefully sutured and packed into the nose to cover the exposed raw area (Fig. 13). Complications include loss of the graft and failure of the procedure due to bleeding from telangiectasia posterior to the graft or reformation of the telangiectasia in the skin graft itself.

Closure of the Anterior Nares

Frustration with the above techniques has led the senior author to adopt an alternative technique aimed

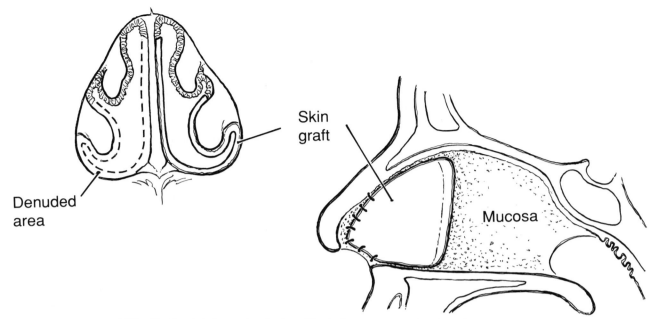

FIG. 13. Septal dermatoplasty: affected mucosa excised and skin grafted.

not at the telangiectasia per se but preventing the drying effects of the inspired air. This is accomplished by closing the anterior nares using a similar technique used in the management of atrophic rhinitis (Young's procedure). A circumferential incision is made in the nasal vestibule at the mucocutaneous junction and then anterior and posterior based flaps are elevated. These are then sutured, creating a double-layered closure (Fig. 14). This procedure is well tolerated by the patient and has proved most successful in a small number of patients. Occasional breakdown of the flaps occurs, particularly inferiorly. This procedure is facilitated by performing an alotomy first.

In conclusion, the ideal management for epistaxis

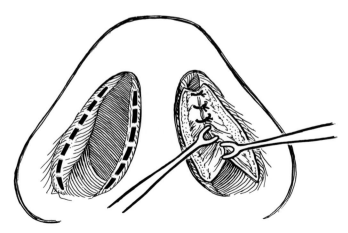

FIG. 14. Closure of the anterior nares using a double-layered flap.

continues to confound and frustrate the otolaryngologist. Never should this condition be taken lightly, as it may result in significant morbidity and occasionally even in mortality.

REFERENCES

1. Petruson B. Epistaxis in childhood. *Rhinology* 1979;17:83–90.
2. Kirchner JA, Yanagisawa E, Crelin ES. Surgical anatomy of the ethmoidal arteries. *Arch Otolaryngol* 1961;74:382–386.
3. Pearson BW, MacKenzie RG, Goodman WS. The anatomic basis of transantral ligation of the maxillary artery in severe epistaxis. *Laryngoscope* 1969;79:969–984.
4. Strumpf DA, Harrop P, Dobbin J, Millman RP. Massive epistaxis from nasal CPAP therapy. *Chest* 1989;95:1141–1142.
5. Kushner FH. Sodium chloride eye drops as a cause of epistaxis. (Letter to the Editor). *Arch Ophthalmol* 1987;105:1634.
6. Buchanan RT, Holtman B. Severe epistaxis in facial fractures. *Plastic Reconstr Surg* 1983;71:768–770.
7. Frable MA, Roman NE, Lenis A. Hemorrhagic complications of facial fractures. *Laryngoscope* 1974;84(11):2051–2055.
8. Moore D, Budde RB, Hunter CR, Mayfield FH. Massive epistaxis from aneurysm of the carotid artery. *Surg Neurol* 1979;11:115–117.
9. Solomons NB, Blumgart R. Severe late-onset epistaxis following Le Fort I osteotomy: angiographic localization and embolization. *J Laryngol Otol* 1988;102:260–263.
10. Myer C, Gluckman JL. Hemangioma of the nasal septum—the "bleeding polyp of the septum." *ENT J* 1983;62(10):58–60.
11. Beran M, Stigendal L, Petruson B. Hemostatic disorders in habitual nose-bleeders. *J Laryngol Otol* 1987;101:1020–1028.
12. Katsonis E, Luke K, Hsu E. Prevalence and significance of mild bleeding disorders in children with recurrent epistaxis. *J Pediatr* 1988;113:73–76.
13. Shaheen OH. Arterial epistaxis. *J Laryngol Otol* 1975;89:17–34.
14. Weiss NS. Relationship of high blood pressure to headache, epistaxis, and selected other symptoms. *N Engl J Med* 1972;287:631–633.
15. Osler W. On a family form of recurring epistaxis associated with

multiple telangiectasias of the skin and mucous membranes. *Bull Johns Hopkins Hosp* 1901;12:333–337.

16. Weber FP. Multiple hereditary developmental angiomata (telangiectasia) of the skin and mucous membranes associated with recurrent hemorrhage: *Lancet* 1967;2:160–162.

17. Hara H. Severe epistaxis. *Arch Otolaryngol* 1962;75:258–269.

18. Wurman LH, Sack JG, Flannery JV, Paulson TO. Selective endoscopic electrocautery for posterior epistaxis. *Laryngoscope* 1988;98:1348–1349.

19. Doyle DE. Anterior epistaxis. A new nasal tampon for fast effective control. *Laryngoscope* 1986;96:279–281.

20. Angell James JE. Nasal reflexes. *Proc R Soc Med* 1969;62:1287–1293.

21. Faribanks DNF. Complications of nasal packing. *Otolaryngol Head Neck Surg* 1986;94:412–415.

22. Thomas SW, Baird IM, Frazier RD. Toxic shock syndrome following submucous resection and rhinoplasty. *JAMA* 1982;244:2402–2403.

23. Hull HF, Mann JM, Sands CJ. Toxic shock syndrome of nasal packing. *Arch Otolaryngol* 1983;109:624–626.

24. Toback J, Fayerman JW. Toxic shock syndrome following septorhinoplasty. *Arch Otolaryngol* 1983;109:627–629.

25. Johnson F. The control of adenoid hemorrhage with a Foley catheter (balloon type). *Arch Otolaryngol* 1956;63:295.

26. Cook TA, Komorn R. Statistical analysis of the alterations of blood gases produced by nasal packing. *Laryngoscope* 1973;85:1802–1809.

27. Cassisi NJ, Biller HF, Ogura JH. Changes in arterial oxygen tension and pulmonary mechanics with the use of posterior packing in epistaxis: a preliminary report. *Laryngoscope* 1971;83:1802–1809.

28. Larson K, Juul A. Arterial blood gases and pneumatic nasal packing in epistaxis. *Laryngoscope* 1982;92:586–588.

29. Jacob JR, Levine LA, Davis H. Posterior packs and the nasopulmonary reflex. *Laryngoscope* 1981;91:279–286.

30. Wang L, Vogel DH. Posterior epistaxis: comparison of treatment. *Otolaryngol Head Neck Surg* 1981;89:1001–1006.

31. Chandler JR, Serrins AJ. Transantral ligation of the internal maxillary artery for epistaxis. *Laryngoscope* 1965;75:1151–1159.

32. McDonald TU, Pearson BW. Follow-up on maxillary artery ligation for epistaxis. *Arch Otolaryngol* 1980;106:635–638.

33. Metson R, Lane R. Internal maxillary artery ligation for epistaxis: an analysis of failures. *Laryngoscope* 1988;98:760–764.

34. Maceri DR, Makielski KH. Intraoral ligation of the maxillary artery for posterior epistaxis. *Laryngoscope* 1984;94:737–741.

35. Kirchner JA. Surgical treatment of nasal hemorrhage. *Surgery* 1961;50:899–904.

36. Ward PH. Routine ligation of the internal maxillary artery is unwarranted. In: Snow JB, ed. *Controversy in otolaryngology.* Philadelphia: Saunders, 1980;320–326.

37. Parnes LS, Heeneman H, Vinuela F. Percutaneous embolization for control of nasal blood circulation. *Laryngoscope* 1987;97:1312–1315.

38. Roberson GH, Reardon EJ. Angiography and embolization of the internal maxillary artery for posterior epistaxis. *Arch Otolaryngol* 1979;105:333–337.

39. Davis KR. Embolization of epistaxis and juvenile nasopharyngeal angiofibromas. *Am J Roentgenol* 1987;148:209–218.

40. Sokoloff J, Wickbom I, McDonald D, Brahme F, Goergen TG, Goldberger LE. Therapeutic percutaneous embolization in intractable epistaxis. *Radiology* 1974;111:285–287.

41. Merland J, Melki J, Chiras J. Place of embolization in severe epistaxis. *Laryngoscope* 1980;90:1696–1704.

42. Anderson RG, Shannon DN, Schaffer SD, Raney LA. A surgical alternative to internal artery ligation for posterior epistaxis. *Otolaryngol Head Neck Surg* 1984;92:427–433.

43. Padrnos RE. A method for control of posterior nasal hemorrhage. *Arch Otolaryngol* 1968;87:181–183.

44. Bluestone CD, Smith HC. Intranasal freezing for severe epistaxis. *Arch Otolaryngol* 1967;85:119–121.

45. Harrison DF. Use of estrogen in treatment of familial hemorrhagic telangiectasia. *Laryngoscope* 1982;92:314–320.

46. Kluger PB, Shapshay SM, Hybels RL, Bohigian RK. Neodymium–YAG laser intranasal photocoagulation in hereditary hemorrhagic telangiectasia: an update report. *Laryngoscope* 1987;97:1397–1401.

47. Mehta A, Livingston D, Levine HL. Fiberoptic bronchoscope and Nd-YAG laser in treatment of severe epistaxis from nasal hereditary hemorrhagic telangiectasia and hemangioma. *Chest* 1987;91:791–792.

48. Saunders WH. Septal dermoplasty—ten years experience. *Trans Am Acad Ophthalmol Otol* 1968;72:153–160.

CHAPTER 39

Minor Intranasal Procedures

Paul J. Donald

The nasal cavity provides the gateway to the sinuses, and any condition that afflicts this cavity can potentially affect the sinuses. There are numerous minor abnormalities and troublesome conditions that involve the nasal cavity that have often simple, but neglected, remedies. A number of miscellaneous conditions have been included in this section because they did not clearly fall into the format of the other chapters.

Congenital and acquired diseases can afflict the nasal cavity, producing symptoms of nasal obstruction, pain, bleeding, discharge, and anosmia. These symptoms, unfortunately, are common presentations of such diverse entities from the common cold to carcinoma, or from a foreign body to Wegener's granulomatosis. A careful history with a conscientious chronicling of symptoms often dismissed by the patients as "my sinus," details concerning trauma and past surgery, supplemented by a meticulous examination before and after shrinkage of the nasal mucosa will usually yield the diagnosis. Introduction of the nasal telescope added a quantum leap to the diagnostic capability of the rhinologist. Computer-assisted tomography (CAT) scanning and magnetic resonance imaging (MRI) are usually unnecessary in these conditions, as an accurate history and thorough clinical examination will usually yield the diagnosis.

MANAGEMENT OF THE DRY CRUSTED NOSE

True ozena, commonplace in the Orient and the Third World, is decidedly rare in the United States and Canada. The characteristic withering of the turbinates, with drying and the production of foul smelling crusts that obstruct the airway, is almost never seen in Western clinical practice. Some drying and crusting in the nose, however, is not uncommon and is especially prevalent in the early weeks following surgical intervention. Moreover, it is almost always seen for pro-

longed periods following major surgical resections such as medial maxillectomy or septectomy. The nasal cavity is not really atrophic; it has a reduced area of functioning mucosa and readily lends itself to drying and subsequent crusting. The humidity produced by the existing mucus blanket is simply insufficient to the task. In addition, the activity of the cilia is reduced as a result of the adverse effects of surgery and medication.

Effective management of nasal drying and crusting is simple and straightforward. In the initial healing phases, it requires the mechanical removal of crusts under direct visualization. If supervening infection has ensued, an appropriate antibiotic should be given systemically. Infections are characterized by a significant foul odor, frank pus, and erythematous mucosa with either edema or a granular appearance. In most instances, the infection is superficial and requires only local measures.

The patient is encouraged to wash out the nose using saline irrigations. Normal saline can be produced at home by dissolving a level teaspoon of salt for each quart of water and boiling for 20 min. The saline can be sealed and stored in the refrigerator for future use. A soft rubber bulb syringe is used and the saline is gently pulsed into the nasal cavity via the anterior nares while the patient leans open mouthed over a sink. The patient should be encouraged to use copious quantities of irrigant until no further crusts are produced, and the nose feels comfortable. These lavages are repeated initially four times daily, and then reduced to twice daily according to the exigencies of the condition.

In addition, the nose is sprayed with a wetting agent on a 1 to 2 hour basis. Saline in a small plastic spray bottle is the most popular since it is convenient to carry, easiest to use, and the most painless to the mucosa. Unfortunately, it is the least effective. The addition of propylene glycol to the saline in a 25% solution

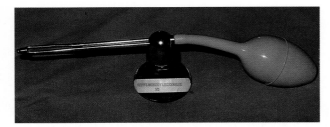

FIG. 1. Atomizer—the most effective means of delivering a nasal spray.

produces a slightly oily, hydrophilic coating to the mucosa that is a much more effective wetting agent. It has the unpleasant side effect of a slight burning sensation in the mucosa. The saline needs to be used more frequently than the propylene glycol solution. The best delivery system is an atomizer (Fig. 1) that produces a generous spray of small diameter droplets. Because of the bulk of the apparatus and the unesthetic appearance of using such a contraption in the nose in public, the demand is slight; therefore the availability is low. An alternative wetting agent that is very effective and less conspicuous since it can be administered in drop form is a solution of 25% glucose in glycerine. This is a rather viscid solution, but it is a very effective moisturizing agent because it is highly hydrophilic. It also carries with it the unfortunate side effect of burning. The use of a room humidifier at night is encouraged. A very effective treatment for enhancing the comfort of the nose with drying and crusting is the application of petroleum jelly with a Q-tip to the nasal vestibule.

In many patients with nasal drying, there is a secondary vestibulitis with inflammation and cracking of the vestibular skin. There is often drying and crusting along the nasal septum anteriorly, and when the crusts are removed digitally, bleeding ensues. The use of an antibacterial ointment such as bacitracin or polysporin will remedy the infection and mollify the septal crusting. Weekly trimming of the vibrissae will reduce bacterial colonization and hasten resolution of the vestibulitis. Once the infection is clear, the substitution of the petroleum jelly for the antibiotic ointment is important to eliminate the possible emergence of topical skin sensitivity to the antibiotic.

SEPTAL PERFORATION

Historically, septal perforation is in a way a curious reflection of the times. In the 19th and early 20th centuries, one of the commonest causes was syphilis. Following the introduction of penicillin, an iatrogenic etiology following septal surgery was the commonest cause. In the past two decades, cocaine abuse has emerged as one of the most frequently seen reasons for septal perforation. Moreover, the badly abused mucosa secondary to cocaine produces the closest North American equivalent to ozena. Currently, perforation as a complication of septal surgery probably remains the commonest cause. Cautery for repeated epistaxis using either electrical, chemical, or laser may cause perforations. This is especially true in patients suffering from Osler–Weber–Rendu disease. Factitious ulceration secondary to nasal picking may occasionally result in perforation, often much to the consternation and even protestations of the patient when made aware of this occurrence. A more complete list of causes is found in Table 1.

Certain precautions must be taken during septal surgery to avoid septal perforations. One of the ways to avoid this complication is to stay in the submucoperiosteal plane. Dissection over sharp septal prominences, especially adjacent to the maxillary crest, even with the most meticulously careful technique often results in perforations. The mucosa here tends to be thinner, more atrophic, and vulnerable to injury. Friable mucosae in patients who are cocaine abusers or who have any chronic inflammatory process are predisposed to perforations. Most of these close spontaneously without difficulty. However, through-and-through perforations are especially prone to become permanent. When such an injury becomes apparent, interposition of a thin piece of straight septal bone between the septal lacerations and closure with direct suturing usually ensure a trouble-free postoperative course. The use of the small dacryocystorhinostomy needle with a 4-0 chromic catgut suture grasped with a Castrovejeo needle holder facilitates closure in the tight confines of the nose.

TABLE 1. *Causes of nasal septal perforations*

1. Injury	3. Inhalant irritants
Nasal septal surgery	Cocaine
Cautery for epistaxis	Chromic acid fumes
Cryosurgery for	Sulfuric acid fumes
turbinates	Lime and cement
Nose picking	dust
Knife wounds,	Tar and pitch
nasotracheal intubation	Salt
Hematoma following	Glass dust
blunt trauma	Sodium carbonate
2. Inflammation and	Calcium nitrate
ischemia	Calcium cyanide
Septal abscess	Arsenicals
Syphilis	Mercurials
Tuberculosis	Phosphorus
Typhoid	4. Neoplasms
Diphtheria	Carcinoma
Wegener's granulomatosis	Leukemia
Lupus erythematosus	
Sarcoidosis	

From ref. 1, with permission.

Many patients with septal perforations are asymptomatic and are discovered only as an incidental finding. This is especially true for those perforations located most posteriorly in the septum and for very large perforations. The smaller ones, and those located in the more anterior portion of the nasal cavity, are more inclined to be symptomatic. These are characterized mainly by bleeding, crusting, and a whistling sensation on nasal breathing. Those involving the most caudal extremity of the nasal septum may cause columellar retraction. If the perforation extends to the nasal dorsum beneath the upper lateral cartilages, this may lead to a saddle deformity of the nose (Fig. 2).

A simple nonsurgical solution to septal perforation is the placement of a septal button (2). These buttons, fashioned from Silastic, fit like a collar stud into the perforation, thus markedly reducing crusting and usually eliminating bleeding. The biggest drawback to this technique is that many patients cannot tolerate them.

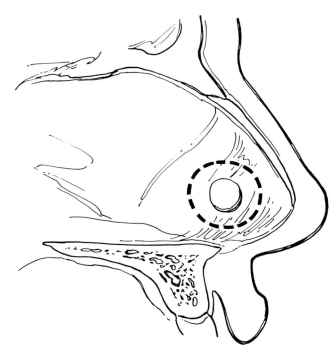

FIG. 3. Septal perforation outlined sufficiently wide so that adequate tissue will be present when the mucoperichondrium is inserted through the hole to close without tension.

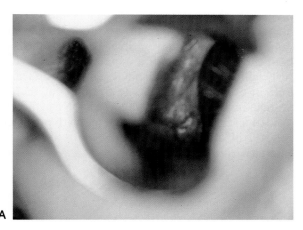

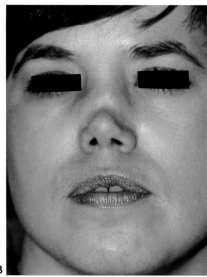

FIG. 2. A: Septal perforation. **B:** Anterior nasal dorsal collapse producing the classic saddle deformity.

This device has had very limited success in my experience.

For perforations approximately 12 mm or less, surgical intervention is indicated, provided of course that the patient is symptomatic. Perforations larger than 15 mm are almost impossible to close. Many procedures have been described to close these holes, and the ones most successful in my hands will be presented. The basic principle invoked is to establish a two-layered mucosal closure while avoiding the overlap of suture lines.

The procedures can be done under local or general anesthesia, with the former being preferred. Local infiltration beneath the mucoperichondrium of both sides of the septum is done. On one side of the perforation, a circumferential incision is outlined such that a cuff of mucoperichondrium when elevated will close the hole on the opposite side without tension (Fig. 3). The cuff of mucoperichondrium is elevated around and through the perforation, bearing in mind the thin nature of the atrophic mucosa that exists at the margins of the perforation. An eventration of the mucosa at this point prejudices a good postoperative result. The Cottle, Freer, and Woodson elevators are very helpful in the dissection, which may be slow and tedious. Once the mucoperichondrium has been elevated and inverted through the perforation to the opposing nasal cavity, it is approximated with a 4-0 or 5-0 chromic catgut suture

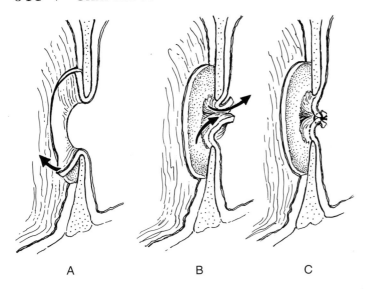

FIG. 4. Cross-sectional diagram showing perforation being closed on the side opposite the elevation. **A:** Incision and beginning elevation of cuff of mucoperiosteum around perforation. **B:** Tissue cuff inverted through perforation. **C:** Raw edges approximated on opposite side.

(Fig. 4). A dacryocystorhinostomy needle driven with a Castrovejeo needle is most effective.

On the side from which the septal perforation cuff was cut, a large bare area now exists. This is closed using a large bipedicled flap of mucoperichondrium raised on the side above the perforation. The flap is pulled down like a window shade to cover the defect. Occasionally, a small flap from the inferior side of the perforation down even to the floor of the nose needs to be advanced slightly to achieve the closure (Fig. 5). Care is taken to avoid exposure of the bare area of the inverted mucosa with this elevation and the suture line

of this side must not overlie the suture line of the opposite side. Grafts of temporalis fascia, pericranium, and cartilage have been described for placement between the flaps, but I do not use them. I prefer to have viable vascularized tissue sitting on live vascularized tissue without the interposition of a nonviable graft.

Very light packing of medicated gauze or Telfa strips is done in order to approximate the flaps of the two sides. Packing is removed at 48 to 72 hr. Nose blowing is avoided and a humidification regime with propylene glycol 25% in saline is instituted.

An alternative method of closure is available if the

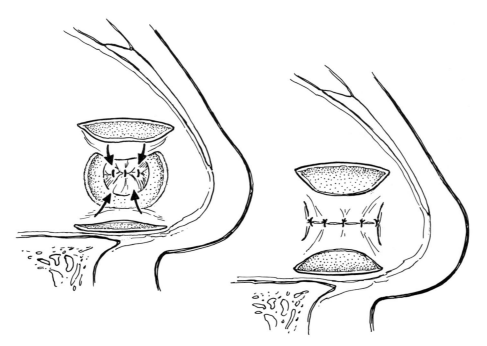

FIG. 5. A bipedicle flap is elevated above the perforation and advanced inferiorly. If approximation of edges is not possible, a smaller similar flap is elevated inferiorly.

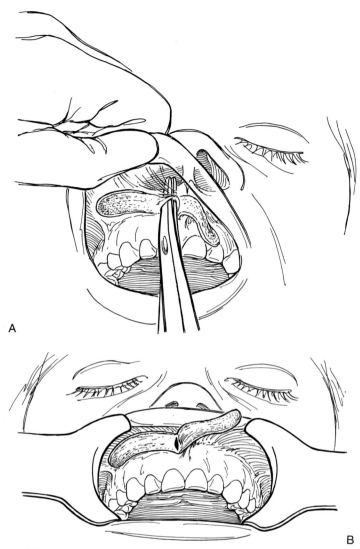

FIG. 6. A generous labial mucosal flap is designed, pedicled on or near the frenulum of the upper lip. In planning, thought must be given to the length necessary to cover the gap, but also to the natural foreshortening that will occur as the flap is rotated around its pedicle as it is placed into the defect. **A:** Scissor dissection into floor of nose. **B:** Gap for passage of flap into nasal cavity.

gap on the side from which the inversion has been taken is too large. It is also useful in those circumstances when a tension-free closure on the side of inversion cannot be achieved without advancement of a single flap or tandem bipedicled flaps (Fig. 5). The mucosa is taken from that of the upper lip and inverted through a gap created in the floor of the nose. This technique will only work when employed in the anterior part of the nose.

A generous flap is outlined on the mucosal surface of the upper lip. The pedicle is at or near the frenulum (Fig. 6). Scissor dissection is carried through the soft tissues adjacent to the premaxilla to perforate through the floor of the nose adjacent to the septum (Fig. 7A).

The flap must be made long enough to not only cover the defect but to accommodate the natural foreshortening that will occur as the flap is rotated 90° around its pedicle. Maintaining a 2:1 ratio of flap length to width is necessary to ensure continuous viability of the flap's distal end. The flap is delivered through the floor of the nose and sutured in place (Fig. 7B). Obviously, the pedicle cannot be sewn at the inferior edges of the defect and a permanent nasal labial fistula results from the pedicle's passage. This does not seem to present a problem.

Gentle packing is done, removed at 48 to 72 hr, and a course of nasal humidification begun. This latter technique has been the most successful in my own practice.

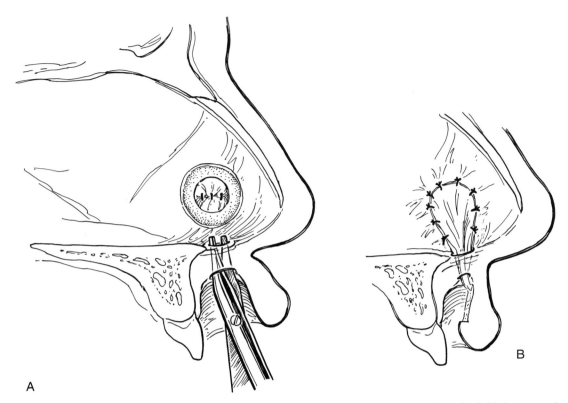

FIG. 7. A large perforation with inversion, which necessitates the construction of a labial mucosal flap tunneled through the floor of the nose to achieve closure on the raw side. **A:** Raw surface presenting scissor elevation to allow passage of flap. **B:** Closure of defect with labial mucosal flap.

FOREIGN BODIES

Possibly the most exotic tales in medicine relating to surgical problems center around the presentations and removal of foreign bodies introduced by accident or design through the various orifices of the body. The nose is no less the subject of such events (Fig. 8). One of the most spectacular foreign body reports is by Malhotra et al. (3), who described a patient involved in a motor vehicle accident. The man was a pedestrian who was struck by a jeep on a country road. He presented some weeks later with symptoms of nasal obstruction. A sinus series revealed a door handle from the jeep lodged in the maxillary sinus and extending into the nasal cavity (Fig. 9).

Usually small articles such as pencil erasers, collar buttons, bits of paper, beads, and small plastic toys are most prevalent. Teeth may present in the nose or maxillary sinus as a foreign body. This is especially true of children with a cleft palate. Organic material such as peas, beans, and seeds are also seen. These foreign bodies are most often seen in small children and are recognized early by a watchful parent. Extraction is then usually not difficult. In some, however,

they go unnoticed and may form the nidus for the formation of a rhinolith.

A rhinolith, or nasal stone, usually arises from the deposition of calcific salts and inspissated mucus around a central nidus. These calcareous deposits are comprised of calcium, magnesium, or sodium salts of phosphate or carbonate.

Foreign bodies can also occur in the paranasal sinuses, but less commonly so. The most spectacular case on record was a patient who had his own toe extracted from his maxillary antrum (4). He had been injured during wartime by a land mine that blew his foot apart and lodged his great toe within his maxillary sinus. Most of the antral foreign bodies are traumatically induced and smaller ones can produce rhinoliths. Sinus rhinoliths seem to be found exclusively in the maxillary sinus (5).

Long-standing foreign bodies and rhinoliths produce symptoms of nasal obstruction and periodic bleeding but are particularly characterized by a foul, fetid rhinorrhea. Those of shorter duration are more inclined to have bleeding. On anterior rhinoscopy, the foreign body is visible as such, but a rhinolith has the appearance of a brownish-green, rough-surfaced entity that

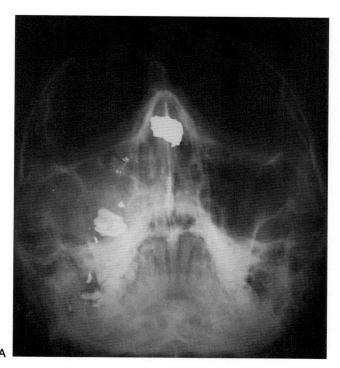

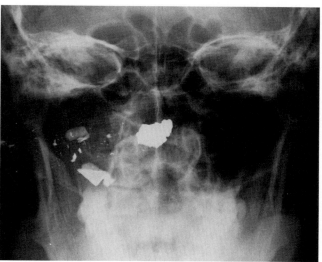

FIG. 8. Multiple gunshot wounds to the face resulting in bullets lodged in the nose, palate, and pterygomaxillary space. **A:** Waters view. **B:** Lateral view.

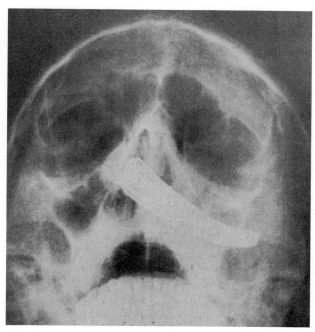

FIG. 9. Jeep door handle in maxillary sinus and nose.

is hard in consistency but has a tendency to crumble. Occasionally, a nasal rhinolith may erode into the maxillary sinuses.

For children in whom the object is not impacted, removal is done after cocaine spray with parental restraint and extraction forceps. However, often in this age group, rhinoliths and impacted foreign bodies require a general anesthetic. In adults, severely impacted rhinoliths also require either a general anesthetic or solid local anesthesia, possibly supplemented by sedation. A lateral rhinotomy may be required to permit

extraction. Bleeding may ensue after extraction, requiring nasal packing.

NASAL ORAL FISTULA

Nasal–labial, nasal–alveolar, and nasal–oral fistulas have manifold etiologies. The commonest cause is cleft palate. Incomplete healing of a cleft palate repair occurs in approximately 0% to 20% of cases (6) and will produce a nasal–oral fistula. The failure rate appears to be related to the severity of the cleft. Musgrove and Bremner (7) reported a 7.7% overall fistula rate in 750 patients. In unilateral incomplete cleft palates, the incidence was only 4.6%, but rose to 12.5% in the bilateral complete deformity.

A nasal–labial fistula is a much more common event if cleft alveolus and cleft lip are present. This is often true in the bilateral deformity (Fig. 10). Congenital syphilis is uncommonly seen in modern times but can produce a nasal–oral fistula (Fig. 11). Severe maxillofacial trauma, especially following gunshot wounds, produce in some instances large fistulas that are exceedingly difficult to close. The same is true of such fistulas resulting from cancer resection, many of which are open to the maxillary sinus as well. A very troublesome fistula that usually communicates with the antrum rather than the nasal cavity is the antral–oral fistula. Antral–alveolar fistulas may be seen after tooth extraction or in cases of complete cleft palate.

Nasal–oral fistulas result in some degree of rhinolalia aperta and nasal regurgitation. Nasal labial fis-

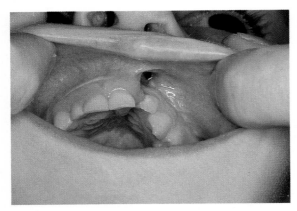

FIG. 10. Nasal–labial fistula in cleft palate patient.

tulas lead to some articulation errors, especially the production of /p/, /b/, or /f/. Antral–oral or antral–alveolar fistulas lead to regurgitation of oral contents as well.

The repair of a nasal–labial fistula requires a combined intranasal and intraoral approach. In the cleft palate patient, this may be accompanied by the placement of a bone graft in the alveolar cleft. Some authorities recommend primary bone grafting to the alveolar defect at about 3 to 4 months after closure of the lip defect and the maxillary arch segments are well aligned. A graft of autogenous rib or cancellous bone chips are placed in the gap and the gingival flaps are sutured overtop these implants (8,9). There is some concern about interfering with growth and development of the maxilla. Great care must be taken in these children to avoid damage to the nasal–vomerine suture area. The more standard approach is to do the alveolar cleft repair at about 8 to 11 years of age (10,11). Iliac crest cancellous bone is packed into the defect and gingival flaps are transposed across the gap (Fig. 12) (11).

Closure of a nasolabial fistula can be done under local or general anesthesia. Local infiltration of the an-

terior septum and the floor of the nose is done as well as in the buccal mucosa and alveolar ridge. A circular incision is created in the labial mucosa extending around the circumference of the fistula. Because the alveolus is involved in part, but the mucosa is somewhat brittle and friable, the circle is eccentric with the widest margin on the labial side (Fig. 12A). The incision is made with a #15 blade, augmented by an angled Beaver blade. The mucosa is elevated toward the fistula and then through the fistula into the nasal cavity. Sufficient freeing up of the edges is done such that a tension-free closure can be accomplished within the nose (Fig. 12B).

The next step is to close the oral side. A rotation advancement flap is created from the labial mucosa from the fistula edge to a considerable distance along the afflicted side anywhere from the second premolar to the second molar tooth (Fig. 13A). At the selected level, the flap is back-cut toward the gingival buccal sulcus. The flap is elevated to this level and now rotated into the defect (Fig. 13B). At the level of the alveolar cleft, closure may be accomplished by raising paired anterior and posterior flaps (Fig. 12A). By incising near to the cleft on one side, for instance, anteriorly on the left side of the alveolus, and dissecting it through the cleft, it can be used to cover the defect remaining posteriorly by the elevation of a similar flap posteriorly on the right. Cancellous bone chips obtained from the hip are packed into the bony gap. The mucosal flaps of gingiva are approximated over the grafts. The upper ends of the flaps are approximated to the rotation advancement flap of labial mucosa swung into the oral side of the nasal–labial fistula (Fig. 13B).

The patient is placed on a liquid diet for 7 to 10 days. A light anterior pack of medicated gauze is placed in the nose and removed 48 to 72 hr later. The patient is admonished to avoid nose blowing and digitalization of the nose. Teeth brushing must carefully avoid the area of the fistula and advice against oral swishing should be done for the first couple of weeks postoperatively.

COLLAPSE OF NASAL VALVE

Once of the most distressing forms of nasal obstruction is stenosis or collapse of the nasal valve. Stenosis of the valve area will be discussed under the heading of synechiae and webs; and this section will address only the problem of valve collapse. The most common cause of this disorder is surgery to the nasal dorsum. During the process of lowering the dorsum, the mucosa of the dome area (Fig. 14) of the nose may be cut across. In some patients there may be a too vigorous resection of the upper lateral cartilage or there may be absorption of cartilage. The loss of support in this area

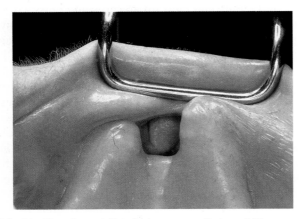

FIG. 11. Nasal–oral fistula in congenital syphilis.

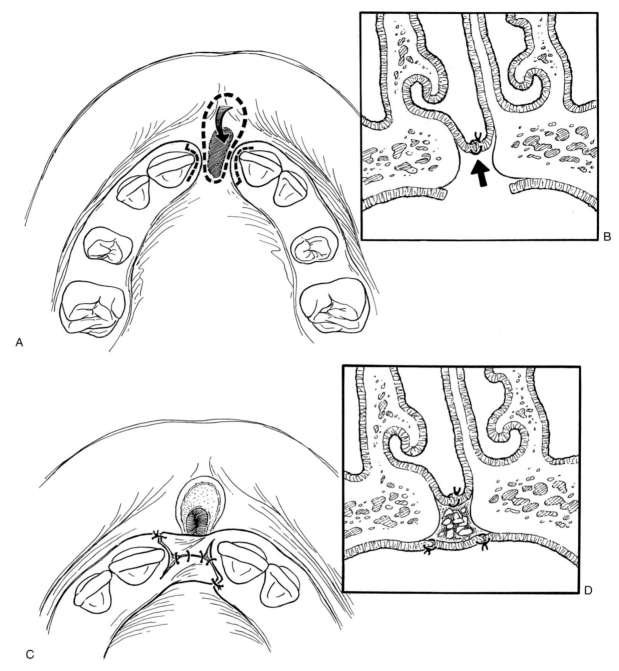

FIG. 12. Closure of nasal–alveolar and labial fistula. **A:** Flaps outlined for closure of both alveolar and labial fistula. **B:** Labial flaps elevated and inserted into the nasal cavity to close nasal side. **C:** Alveolar gingival flaps transposed and alveolar cleft closed leaving raw area in region of nasal–labial fistula. **D:** Alveolar fistula packed with cancellous bone from the iliac crest.

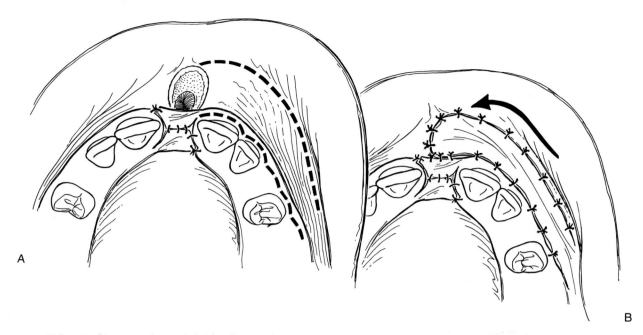

FIG. 13. Closure of nasal–labial fistula. **A:** Labial mucosal flaps on oral side outlined. **B:** Rotation advancement flap of labial and buccal mucosa created to close defect on oral side.

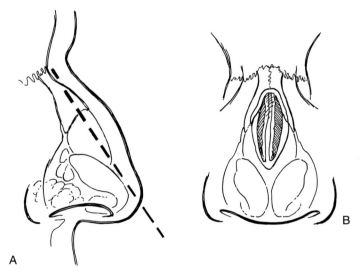

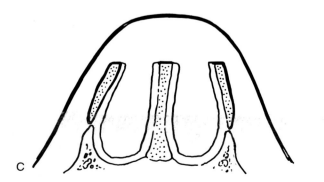

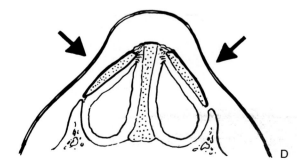

FIG. 14. Mucosal cut in nasal dome as part of hump removal with scar in nasal valve area. **A:** Plane of excision of dorsal hump. **B:** Open roof. **C:** Open nasal cavity and section through valve area. **D:** Subsequent dome scar and collapse of lower lateral cartilages.

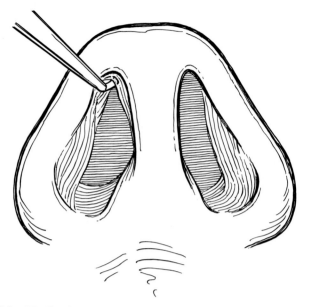

FIG. 15. Buck curet used to establish valve collapse. Dome elevated with curet producing an improved nasal airway.

will cause the lateral wall of the nose to prolapse toward the septum. Even a minor degree of narrowing produces the sensation of nasal obstruction. Another common type of collapse is seen in the elderly as the cartilage loses elasticity and strength and the supportive connective tissues lose their tightness and become relaxed.

The best method of determining whether valve collapse is responsible for the obstruction is the gentle insertion of a Buck curet into the nose and the gentle elevation of the lateral nasal wall during inspiration (Fig. 15). If the obstruction is relieved, then the diagnosis is made. Stucker has devised a test in which a prong of a bayonet forceps is inserted into each nostril. Both lateral walls are elevated simultaneously. Relief of obstruction gives the diagnosis. The valve area can be propped open with grafts. I prefer to carve an outwardly curved graft from irradiated cartilage. A piece with a natural curve is chosen and the graft carved and trimmed. The graft needs to extend from the pyriform crest to the nasal dorsum. The curve in the graft should be directed laterally to the nasal cavity. Too long or too fat a graft will produce an undesirable bulging of the nasal dorsal skin.

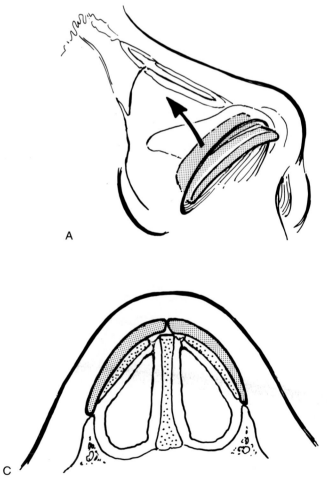

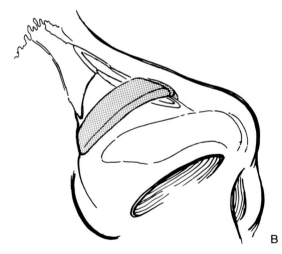

FIG. 16. Carved irradiated cartilage graft propping open a collapsed nasal airway. **A:** Graft inserted into limen vestibuli. **B:** Graft sitting between pyriform rim bone and nasal dorsum opening nasal valve. **C:** Cross-section showing cartilage graft holding valve area open.

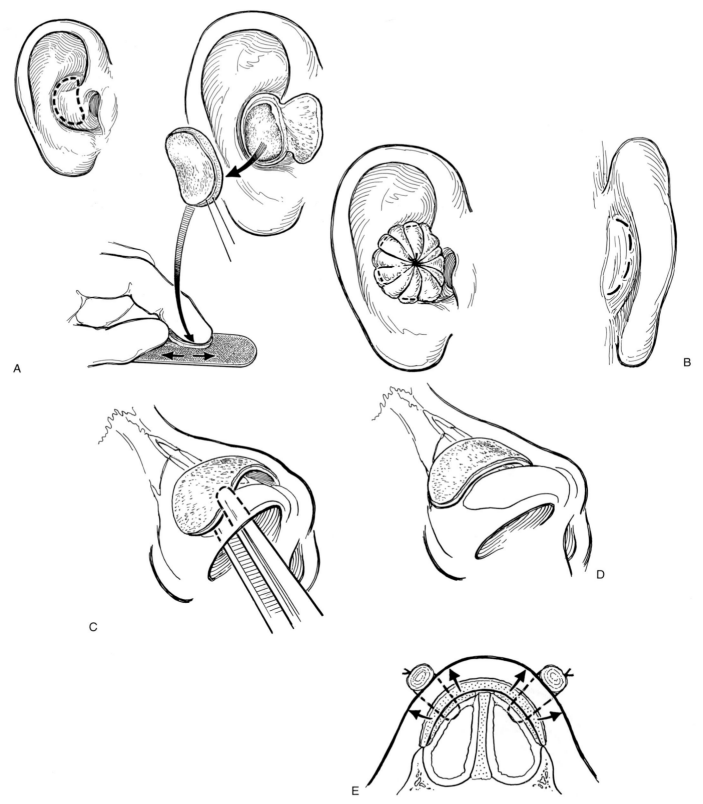

FIG. 17. Conchal graft reconstruction of nasal valve (Stucker). **A:** Conchal perichondral graft harvested. **B:** Tie-over bolster placed at donor site. **C:** Lima bean-shaped cartilage graft trimmed and thinned. **D:** Conchal graft placed into nasal dorsum over upper lateral cartilages through an open rhinoplasty. **E:** Graft secured by through-and-through sutures in nasal dorsum. Intranasal sutures are in the vertical plane of the nose and extranasal sutures are in horizontal plane.

After intranasal anesthesia is secured, an injection of the limen vestibuli is done. An intercartilaginous incision is made and a pocket is created from over the upper lateral cartilage to the edge of the pyriform crest.

The graft is placed in the pocket and trimmed as necessary with the convex side facing laterally (Fig. 16). The curve of the cartilage carries the nasal valve laterally. The limen incision is sutured carefully and the nose is lightly packed with medicated gauze or Telfa strips for 2 days. This procedure produces a slight widening of the nose, but the results in terms of improved breathing are lasting.

Stucker has devised an alternate procedure that is more complex, but very effective. He uses an external rhinoplasty incision and elevates skin over the nasal dorsum. Careful skin elevation is carried down to the pyriform crest. A piece of conchal cartilage is harvested using an anterior periantihelical incision (Fig. 17A). The conchal cartilage is removed and the wound dressed with two tie-over bolsters both front and back of the ear (Fig. 17B). The cartilage is trimmed until a "lima bean-shaped" piece is obtained (Fig. 17C). A disposable emery board is used, along with a #15 blade, to thin the cartilage down and to feather the edges. The graft is placed over the dorsum such that it overlies the upper lateral cartilages (Fig. 17D). The cartilage is secured by placing through-and-through sutures in the nose. The suture is placed in the dome at two sites caudally and rostrally. The needle passes through all layers from mucosa through nasal dorsal skin. The sutures are placed in a vertical direction in the nose, but in a horizontal manner on the nasal skin (Fig. 17E). This is to align the sutures in the lines of minimum tension of the nasal skin and minimize scarring. These sutures are left for 10 to 14 days, thus avoiding the need for packing. Stucker has been able to relieve obstruction in all cases.

SYNECHIAE AND WEBS

One of the most easily remedied causes of nasal obstruction is the surgical amelioration of webs and synechiae. They come about usually as the result of either trauma or surgery. Occasionally, severe necrotizing infection may be the cause as well. In addition to nasal obstruction, the patient may complain of crusting. Prevention during surgery is relatively simple by the placement of Silastic or other barriers between any sites in which juxtaposed abrasions occur. Another way in which synechiae may form is from the organization of a fibrinous clot that forms after ethmoidectomy, especially in the allergic patient. Judicious suctioning on a daily basis or every 2 days will usually eliminate this problem.

On examination, a fleshy connection between the nasal septum and adjacent turbinate indicates a synechia. A web, on the other hand, is seen as a raised area on the floor of the nose or along the nasal dome.

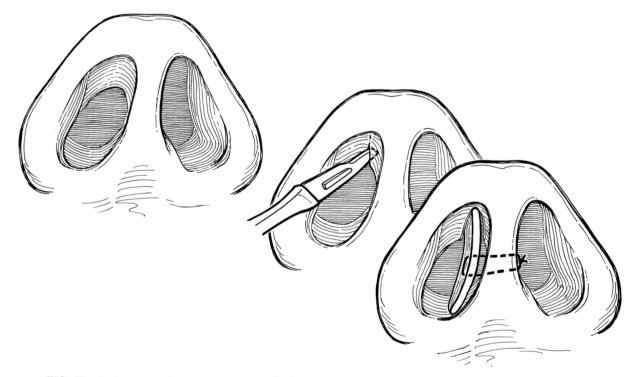

FIG. 18. An intranasal web managed by incision and insertion of Silastic splint fixed to the nasal septum.

The simplest method of handling a synechia is by sharp incision and the placement of an intervening Silastic splint. A web can be handled in a similar fashion (Fig. 18), but recurrence is more common than when Z-plasty is used. When fashioning the Silastic splint, it is important to be sure to leave no sharp edges that may injure the mucosa. A notch is cut to fit over the nasal sill to help anchor the splint. The splint is fixed in place with an absorbable suture. The suture is kept from pulling through the opposing side of the septum by running it through a Silastic button. The splint remains *in situ* from 10 days to 3 weeks.

The most effective way of effacing an intranasal web is by the use of Z-plasty. In the region of the valve, a single Z-plasty will usually solve the problem. The central limb of the Z is placed along the crest of the web. The posterior limb is next cut at one extremity of the central limb and the anterior limb at the other end (Fig. 19). If the web is thick, then any intervening fibrous tissue is excised. The flaps should be kept of sufficient substance so that they will maintain their integrity when transposed and be substantial enough to hold a suture. The anterior flap is transposed first and secured in place posteriorly with 5-0 chromic sutures. The posterior flap is next secured anteriorly. The web will be effaced and the central part of the Z will be transposed to the line of and often directly in the nasal valve (Fig. 19C).

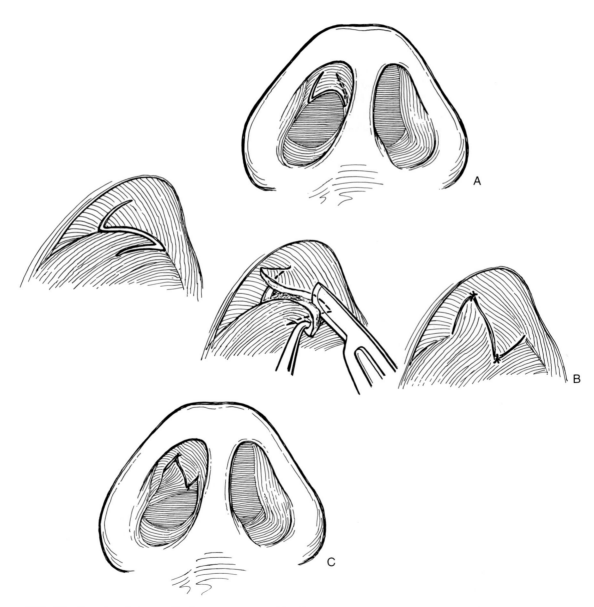

FIG. 19. Nasal web in vault of nose managed by Z-plasty. **A:** Incisions outlined. **B:** Flaps elevated and intervening fibrous tissue excised. **C:** Flaps transposed and web effaced.

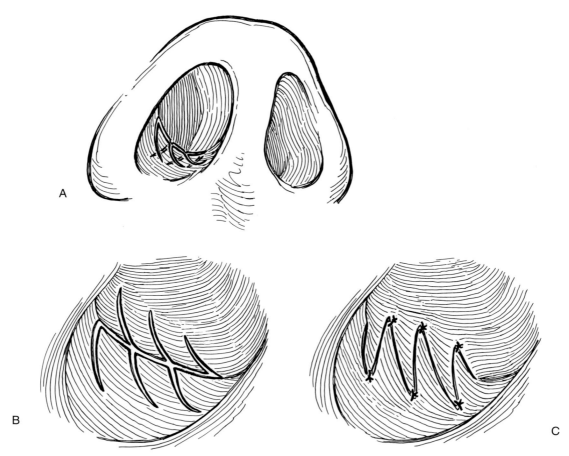

FIG. 20. Nasal web on floor of nose. **A:** Multiple Z-plasties drawn. **B:** Flaps elevated and scar tissue excised. **C:** Flaps transposed and web effaced.

On the floor of the nose, multiple Z-plasties may be used as visualization is easier. The flaps are transposed and fixed in position with multiple 5-0 chromic sutures (Fig. 20). A light medicated gauze dressing may be placed for 24 to 48 hr. Once removed, the wound should be treated with four times daily applications of antibiotic ointment.

REFERENCES

1. Fairbanks DNF, Fairbanks GR. Nasal septal perforations, prevention and management. In: Goldman JL, ed. *The principles and practice of rhinology.* New York: Wiley, 1987.
2. Kern EB, Facer GW, McDonald TJ, et al. Closure of nasal septal perforations with a Silastic button. *Otorhinolaryngol Digest* 1977;39:9–17.
3. Malhotra C, Arora MML, Mehra YN. An unusual foreign body in the nose. *J Laryngol Otol* 1970;84:539.
4. Bradley PF. Foreign bodies in the paranasal sinuses as a complication of facial injuries. *Br J Oral Surg* 1971;8:192.
5. Fairbanks DNF, Barr NL Jr. Foreign bodies in the nose and paranasal sinuses. In: English GM, ed. *Otolaryngology,* Philadelphia: Lippincott, 1990; chap 24.
6. Oneal RM. Oronasal fistulas. In: Gralob WC, Rosenstein SW, Bzoch KR, eds. *Cleft lip & palate: surgical, dental & speech aspects.* Boston: Little Brown, 1971;490.
7. Musgrove RH, Bremner JC. Complications of cleft palate surgery. *Plast Reconstr Surg* 1960;26:180.
8. Kernahan DA, Rosenstein SW. Treatment of complete clefts of the primary and secondary palate at Children's Memorial Hospital, Chicago, Illinois. In: Hotz M, Gnoinski W, Perko M, Nussbaumer H, Haubensak R, eds. *Early treatment of cleft lip & palate.* Lewiston, NY: Hans Huber Publishers, 1986;71–75.
9. Schmid E. Experience gathered and results obtained with primary osteoplasty. In: Hotz M, Gnoinski W, Perko M, Nussbaumer H, Haubensak R, eds. *Early treatment of cleft lip & palate.* Lewiston, NY: Hans Huber Publishers, 1986;80–84.
10. Boyne PJ, Sands NR. Secondary bone grafting of residual alveolar and palatal clefts. *J Oral Surg* 1971;30:87–92.
11. Semb G. A study of facial growth in patients with unilateral cleft lip and palate treated by the Oslo-CHP Team. *Cleft Palate Craniofac J* 1991;28:1–21.

Index

Note: Page numbers followed by *f* indicate figures; those followed by *t* indicate tables.

Maxillary sinusitis
    with oroantral fistula, 601
    pain from, 542
    surgical management of
        antral lavage, 247–249, 247f
        Caldwell-Luc procedure,
            251–254, 252f–254f
        nasoantral window, 249–251,
            249f, 251f
Maxillectomy
    infrastructure, 440, 440f
    medial, 438–439, 439f
    radical, 440–441, 440f
    suprastructure, 439–440, 439f
MCTC (metrizamide computed
        tomography cisternography), of
        CSF leakage, 566–567
Meatus, 34, 35f
Medial canthus tendon, 404–406,
        404f–407f
    treatment of, 413–418, 415f–418f
Medial maxillectomy, 438–439, 439f
Mefoxin (cefoxitin), 62
Melanoma, 434
    MRI of, 94
    pathology of, 79–80, 80f
Memory cells, 109
MEN (multiple endocrine neoplasia),
        527
Meningiomas, 431
Meningitis, 194
Meningoceles, nasal, 610f, 613
Meningoencephaloceles, 613, 613f,
        614f
Meningoencephalocytoceles, 613
Mesenchymal chondrosarcoma, 545
Messerklinger technique, 11
Metabolic food reaction, 134t
Metachronous carcinoma, 68, 68f
Metaplasia, in mucosa, 46–47, 47f
Metastases, 93, 436
    lymphatic, 453–454
Methacrylic acid, for frontal
        osteoplasty, 227–230, 228f, 229f
Methicillin, 62
Metrizamide computed tomography
        cisternography (MCTC), of
        CSF leakage, 566–567
Microadenomas, 525–526, 538
Microapocrine secretion, 47
Microbiology, 57
    of antibiotics, 61–63
    of bacterial sinusitis, 58
    of chronic sinusitis, 58–59
    of mycosis, 59–61, 60f, 61f
    of other infections, 61
    of viruses, 59
Microvilli, 45, 45f, 49
Middle meningeal artery, 451
Middle turbinate flap, for CSF
        rhinorrhea, 568, 572, 573f

Midface degloving incision, 438, 438f
Midfacial defects
    alterations at surgical resection to
        enhance prosthetic prognosis
        for, 512–513, 513f
    prosthetics for, 513–518, 515f–517f
Migraine, 547–548
Mixed cellular rhinitis, 150
Mixed squeeze, 158
Molds, allergic reaction to, 114–115
Moraxella catarrhalis, 58, 59
    sinusitis due to, 163, 168
Mosher, Harris, 3–4
Moxalactam (Moxam), 62
MRI. See Magnetic resonance
        imaging (MRI)
Mucoceles
    CT and MRI of, 89–90, 90f, 184,
        185f
    intracranial, 197–198
    sphenoid, 538
Mucociliary transport, in sinusitis, 162
Mucolytic agent, for sinusitis, 167
Mucopyocele
    from frontal sinus fracture,
        369–372, 370f–372f
    from frontonasal duct fracture, 388,
        388f
Mucor, 59
Mucormycosis
    indolent form of, 281, 281f, 282f
    orbital complications of, 178,
        280–281, 280f
    pathophysiology of, 280–282
    rhinocerebral, 59–60, 60f, 279–280
    treatment of, 281–283, 284t
Mucosa, histology of, 44–48, 45f–47f
Mucosal flaps, for nasofrontal duct
        patency, 214–216, 215f–217f
Mucosal preservation, 12
Mucous blanket, 50, 50t
Mucous flow, 51–54, 51f–54f
Mucous retention cysts, CT of, 88–89
Multiple endocrine neoplasia (MEN),
        527
Muscle contraction headaches, 549
Mycetoma, 274, 274f
Mycobacterium leprae, 57, 61
Mycosis, 59–61, 60f, 61f
Myofascial pain dysfunction
        syndrome, 549

N
Nafcillin, 62
    for orbital complications of
        sinusitis, 187
Nares, closure of anterior, 638–639,
        639f
Nasal capsule, 17
Nasal cycle, 55

Nasal defects, 508
    alterations at surgical resection to
        enhance prosthetic prognosis
        for, 508–511, 509f–512f
    prosthetics for, 513–518, 515f–517f
    surgical reconstruction vs.
        prosthetic restoration for, 508
Nasal-labial fistula, 647–648,
        648f–650f
Nasal olfactory placodes, embryology
        of, 15, 17f
Nasal-oral fistula, 647–648, 648f–650f
Nasal packing, for anterior epistaxis,
        630–631, 631f
Nasal pit, 15, 18f
Nasal provocative testing, 115–116
Nasal sac, 15, 18f
Nasal stone, 646–647
Nasal-vagal reflex, 630
Nasal valve, 55
    collapse of, 648–653, 650f–652f
Nasion, 401, 402f
Nasoantral window, 249–251, 249f,
        251f
Nasoethmoid fractures, 95–96, 96f
Nasofrontal duct, 44
    patency of, 214, 124t
Nasofrontoethmoidal complex,
        fractures of
    anatomy of, 401–407, 402f–408f
    diagnosis of, 409–411, 409f–411f
    etiology and pathophysiology of,
        407–409, 409f
    treatment of, 412–418, 412f–418f
Nasolacrimal duct
    anatomy of, 401, 403f
    embryology of, 19
Nasolacrimal duct drainage system
        (NLDS) cyst, 614
Nasolacrimal duct system obstruction,
        congenital, 614
Nasopalatine artery, 237, 238f
Nasopharyngeal angiofibroma,
        pathology of, 74–75, 74f, 75f
Nasopharyngeal carcinoma, pathology
        of, 70, 70f, 71f
Nasopharyngeal packing, for posterior
        epistaxis, 632–635, 633f, 634f
Nasopulmonary reflex, 633
Natural killer (NK) cells, 102, 103
NCAMs (neuronal cell adhesion
        molecules), 453
Neoplasms. See Tumors
Neuralgias
    facial, 544–546
    glossopharyngeal, 544–545
    postherpetic, 546–547
    secondary, 546–547
    Sluder's, 545–546, 545t
    trigeminal, 544
Neurilemomas, 430